ATLAS OF ALLERGIES

SECOND EDITION

EDITED BY
Philip Fireman, MD
Professor of Pediatrics
Director, Division of Allergy, Immunology & Rheumatology
Children's Hospital of Pittsburgh
Pittsburgh, Pennsylvania

Raymond G. Slavin, MD
Professor of Internal Medicine & Microbiology
Director, Division of Allergy & Immunology
St. Louis University School of Medicine
St. Louis, Missouri

FOREWORDS BY
Elliott Middleton, Jr., MD
John W. Yunginger, MD

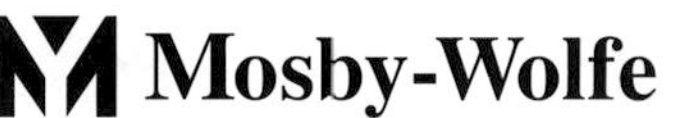

Mosby-Wolfe

London Baltimore Barcelona Bogotá Boston Buenos Aires Caracas Carlsbad, CA Chicago Madrid Mexico City Milan Naples, FL
New York Philadelphia St. Louis Seoul Singapore Sydney Taipei Tokyo Toronto Wiesbaden

Published in 1996 by Mosby-Wolfe, an imprint of Times Mirror International Publishers Limited

Printed by Grafos S.A. Arte sobre papel, Barcelona, Spain.

ISBN 0 7234 21811

For full details of all Times Mirror International Publishers Limited titles, please write to Times Mirror International Publishers Limited, Lynton House, 7–12 Tavistock Square, London WC1H 9LB, England.

A CIP catalogue record for this book is available from the British Library.

Project Managers:	Elaine Graham
	Deborah Russell
	Ellen Sarewitz
Developmental Editor:	Deborah Russell
Designers/Layout Artists:	Chris Read
	Tim Read
Cover Design:	Pete Wilder
Illustration:	Peter Gardiner
Production:	Jane Tozer
Index:	Angela Cottingham
Publisher:	Fiona Foley

Forewords

Atlas of Allergies is a gem of a book filled with useful information compiled by one authority in adult and one in pediatric allergy and immunology. This broad base at once makes the book of value to specialists and primary care physicians alike. Since the publication of the first edition, much new information about these common maladies has been acquired. This is reflected in a greatly expanded chapter on asthma, including new information on occupational asthma. Moveover, there is a very useful extension of information on occupational allergies, including occupational rhinitis and dermatitis. Over several decades the field of allergy and immunology has evolved some experimental diagnostic and therapeutic techniques which have not been validated. These unproven techniques are discussed objectively in the second edition of *Atlas of Allergies*. This book should certainly be in the library of every practicing allergist/immunologist and will be useful also to specialists such as otolaryngologists and dermatologists, in addition to primary care physicians and medical students.

Elliott Middleton, Jr., MD
Professor of Medicine and Pediatrics Emeritus
SUNY at Buffalo, New York

The first edition of this text, edited by a pediatric allergist and an internist allergist who are seasoned professionals, proved popular with a wide range of health professionals, including medical students, primary care physicians, and specialists. As implied by the title, the book contains many illustrative photographs and a multitude of useful tables and figures, but it is not simply a picture book. The accompanying text describes the proper diagnosis and treatment of a wide range of allergic disorders.

The second edition builds and expands the material presented in the first edition. The chapter on asthma is more extensive, and the chapter dealing with occupational asthma now includes sections on occupational rhinitis and occupational dermatitis. A discussion on unproven techniques is now included in the chapter on diagnostic allergy testing. The discussion of regional distribution of allergens now provides information about common European allergens.

As changing patterns of health care delivery evolve in the United States and Europe, there is an increasing need for succinct, accurate, and practical information on asthma and allergic diseases; this text fulfills these needs.

John W. Yunginger, MD
Allergy/Immunology Section
Department of Pediatrics
Mayo Medical Center, Rochester, Minnesota

Contributors

Robert C. Arffa, MD
Associate Professor of Ophthalmology
University of Pittsburgh
School of Medicine
Pittsburgh, Pennsylvania

S. Allan Bock, MD
Department of Pediatrics
National Jewish Center for Immunology and
Respiratory Medicine
Denver, Colorado

Gilbert A. Friday, Jr., MD
Professor of Pediatrics
Children's Hospital of Pittsburgh
Pittsburgh, Pennsylvania

Mary Jelks, MD
Allergy and Immunology Research
Universtiy of South Florida
Tampa, Florida

Leslie C. Grammer, MD
Professor of Medicine
Northwestern University
Chicago, Illinois

Macy I. Levine, MD
Clinical Professor of Medicine
University of Pittsburgh
School of Medicine
Pittsburgh, Pennsylvania

David P. Skoner, MD
Assistant Professor of Pediatrics
Children's Hospital of Pittsburgh
University of Pittsburgh
Pittsburgh, Pennsylvania

Michael D. Tharp, MD
Associate Professor of Dermatology
University of Pittsburgh
School of Medicine
Pittsburgh, Pennsylvania

Lee Wiley, MD
Department of Ophthalmology
St. Vincents Health Center
Eire, Pennsylvania

Contents

Dedication

We dedicate this book to the two who have had the greatest influence on our lives and our careers; the two who shared our achievements and our disappointments, who lifted us when we were down, and tempered our enthusiasm when we were up – our wives and best friends, Marcia Levick-Fireman and Alberta Cohrt-Slavin.

Acknowledgements

The authors appreciate the efforts of their many professional colleagues who wrote or co-wrote chapters or contributed their teaching materials to this Atlas. Without their valuable collaboration, we could not have completed this project.

To our respective secretarial staff, especially Carol Wagner and Marge Smith, we applaud their essential hard work. To all of those at Mosby-Wolfe who participated in organizing and preparing this Atlas, we express our sincere thanks.

In particular, we acknowledge the assistance of the project managers, Elaine Graham, Deborah Russell, and Ellen Sarewitz, and the illustrator, Peter Gardiner, who helped make this *Atlas of Allergies* a reality.

Philip Fireman, MD
Raymond Slavin, MD

Preface

It is gratifying to the Editors that the First Edition of *Atlas of Allergies* was so well received. This indicates to us that there is a need in medical practice for such an Atlas. The positive response of the readers, particularly with regard to the illustrations, photographs, figures, and tables was a compliment to the efforts and talents of our group of contributors. Many colleagues commented that they utilized portions of the Atlas for their own teaching and lectures. Thus, the First Edition of the *Atlas of Allergies* was a most satisfying endeavor for us.

Our field continues to move forward, and the last few years have seen many new developments which we have incorporated into this second edition. The work place occupies an ever more prominent arena for allergic disease. Therefore, the previous chapter on Occupational Asthma has been changed to Occupational Allergies, which now includes occupational rhinitis and dermatitis. Many new insights have been gained into bronchial asthma, along with promising therapeutic approaches, and this chapter has been greatly expanded. Allergy is obviously a world wide concern and we are pleased to add an international character to the *Atlas of Allergies* by significantly revising Chapter Two to include the geographic distribution of inhalant pollen allergens in Europe, Canada, and Mexico as well as the United States. The prevalence of allergic disease has resulted in many new approaches to both diagnosis and management. Some have not been subjected to careful scientific scrutiny and should be avoided. We have now included a discussion of unproven techniques in the chapter on Diagnostic Tests. Most of the other chapters have been significantly revised and updated. This provides an easy-to-read format of the most up-to-date and state of the art information on allergic diseases. We anticipate that this Second Edition will continue to be a readily available resource for those interested in allergic disease.

Philip Fireman, MD
Raymond G. Slavin, MD

CHAPTER 1

Immunology of Allergic Disorders

Philip Fireman

Syndromes that are now identified as allergic diseases have been described for centuries, but the concept of an immunologic basis for allergic disease was not introduced until the twentieth century. During the past 30 years, advances in immunology have changed the clinical practice of allergy. Allergists now understand the mechanisms for many of the diagnostic and therapeutic procedures that had developed empirically, but without well-controlled documentation of efficacy, over the previous 75 years. In addition, these important advances in immunology have influenced the professional organizations in allergy and the residency and fellowship training programs to such an extent that this branch of medicine is now frequently referred to as the specialty of Allergy and Immunology.

TERMINOLOGY

It is important to define the terms common in allergy practice. The manner in which the words *immunology, immunity, allergy, hypersensitivity*, and *atopy* are used has, at times, revealed confusion regarding their meaning. *Immunology* was initially described as the study of antigen–antibody interactions in which the host became resistant to disease, and the term implied a beneficial host-defense induced by the antigen. This type of *immunity* is referred to as specific or *acquired immunity* to a specific antigen. However, there are host-defense mechanisms which are not specific to given antigens or microbes; this type of immunity is referred to as innate or *natural immunity*. While it is appropriate for the study of infectious diseases, the limited definition of immunology above does not describe the body's response to non-infectious environmental factors, such as pollens, drugs, and other potential antigens. In this book, immunology is used to mean the study of antigens, the subsequent development of specific antibodies or sensitized cells, and the reaction between antigen and antibody, whether beneficial or not.

Hypersensitivity indicates a heightened or exaggerated immune response that develops after more than one exposure to a given antigen. Hypersensitivity is usually considered synonymous with *allergy*. An antigen responsible for an allergic reaction is an *allergen*. The term allergy was introduced by Clemens Von Pirquet in 1906, to designate an altered reactivity to a foreign substance after prior experience with the same material, whether this response was helpful or harmful to the host. This concept of allergy, popularized by Gell and Coombs, may have merit in that it permits an organized and systematic approach to the pathogenesis of immunologic diseases. Nevertheless, the term allergy, as commonly used in clinical practice, indicates an adverse reaction, and describes the pathophysiologic responses that result from the interaction of an allergen with antibodies and/or lymphocytes in a patient previously exposed and sensitized to that allergen (**1.1**). This immunologic definition of allergy is accepted by almost all but not every allergist, since non-immune processes can influence the pathogenesis of allergic diseases with recognized immune etiologies.

The terms *atopy* and *atopic* are frequently used in reference to allergic diseases. Derived from the Greek word meaning 'strange', they were introduced by Coca and Cooke in 1923 to describe allergic diseases, such as asthma, allergic rhinitis (hay fever), and atopic dermatitis (infantile eczema), that showed a familial predilection and an implied genetic predisposition. Other allergic diseases, such as contact dermatitis and serum sickness, showed no familial tendency and were referred to as non-atopic. It was also recognized that serum from these allergic individuals contained a factor subsequently described as a skin-sensitizing antibody. This heat-labile serum factor could passively sensitize the skin of a non-sensitive individual and, after intradermal challenge with a specific allergen, the passively sensitized skin showed a positive wheal-and-flare reaction within 20 minutes (**1.2**). This passive transfer test, also known as the Prausnitz–Kustner or PK test, provided documentation of the presence of a specific serum antibody important in the pathogenesis of allergic diseases. More than 90% of these antibodies are now identified as immunoglobulin E (IgE). Many allergists use the term atopic instead of *allergic* to identify those families and patients with predisposition toward asthma, hay fever, or infantile eczema.

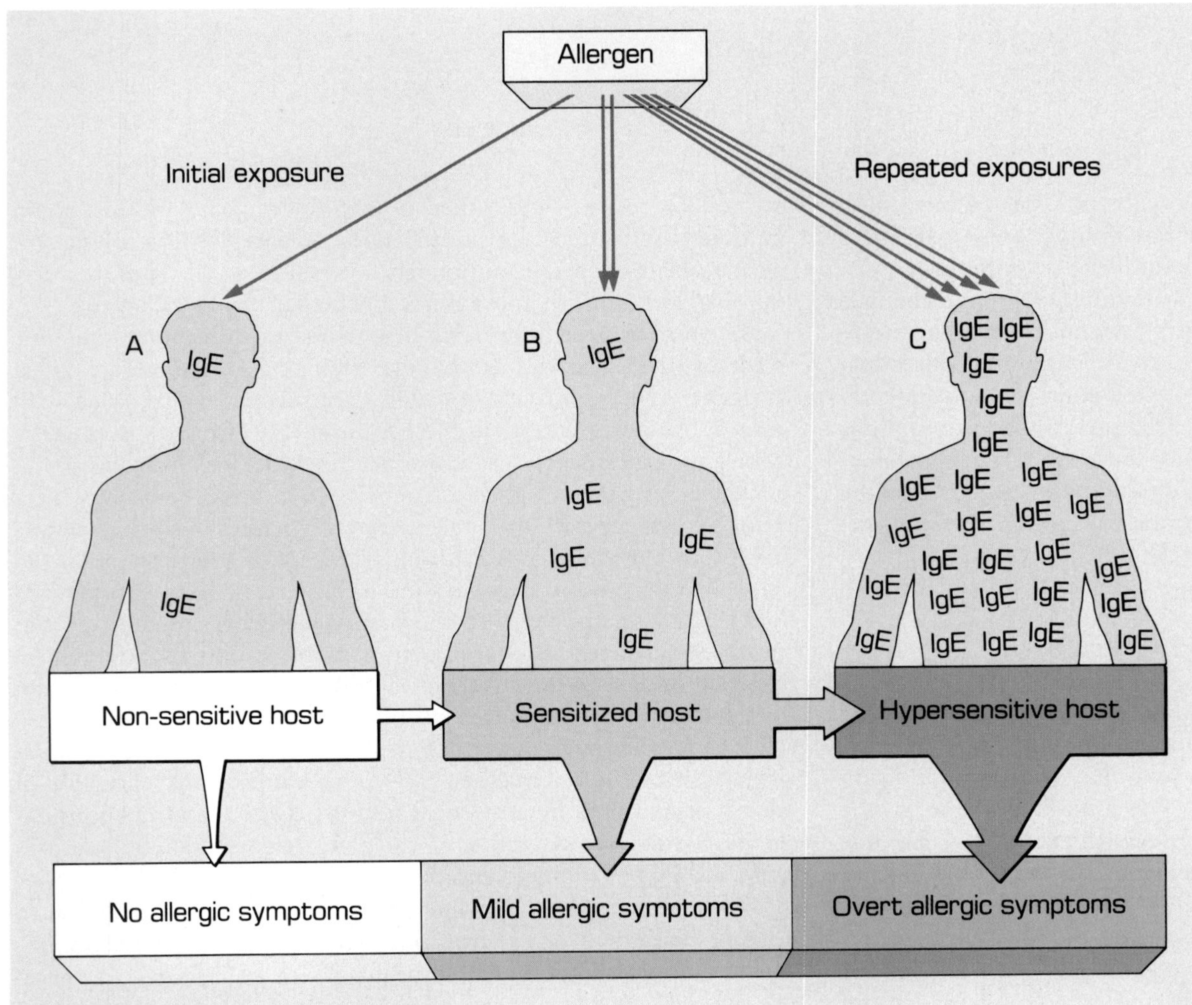

1.1 Hypersensitivity and allergy. (A) Upon initial exposure to an allergen, there are no overt manifestations of allergic disease because the patient is non-sensitized. However, the allergen will initiate an immune response which results in the synthesis of IgE and sensitization of the susceptible (atopic) host. (B) Upon subsequent, repeated exposures, this sensitized individual synthesizes increased amounts of IgE, thus becoming hypersensitive. (C) From this point onward, re-exposure to this specific allergen provokes the overt manifestations of allergic disease.

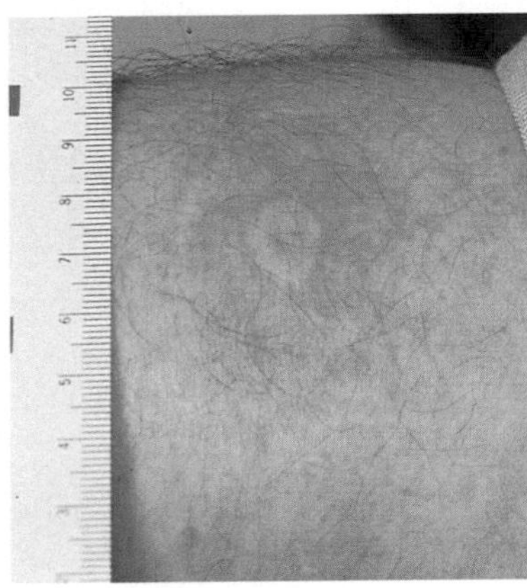

1.2 IgE-mediated wheal-and-flare reaction of passively sensitized skin. This photo was taken 20 minutes after allergen injection into a skin site containing IgE antibodies to the allergen. This Prausnitz–Kustner (PK) test is no longer used in clinical practice, given the risk of passive transfer of viral diseases. The skin reaction is usually accompanied by pruritus. It begins within minutes after allergen is injected, and peaks in 20 minutes. The reaction usually subsides within an hour, unless a late-phase IgE reaction ensues.

CELLS INVOLVED IN ALLERGIC REACTIONS

The immune system of man consists of several lymphoid organs, including lymph nodes, spleen, thymus, and other lymphoid tissues, such as the bone marrow, respiratory tract, and intestinal tract. These lymphoid tissues contain a number of different cells which respond in various ways upon exposure to an allergen. All of the cells of the immune system are derived from pluripotent hematologic stem cells which probably arise in the primordial bone marrow. These cells differentiate via two major pathways into either progenitor lymphoid or progenitor myeloid cells (**1.3**). This cell differentiation is influenced by several cell-derived substances described as cytokines. Some cytokines, which also promote intercellular communication as well as cellular proliferation and growth, are referred to as interleukins, and are discussed later in this chapter. The lymphoid cells are heterogeneous, both morphologically and functionally.

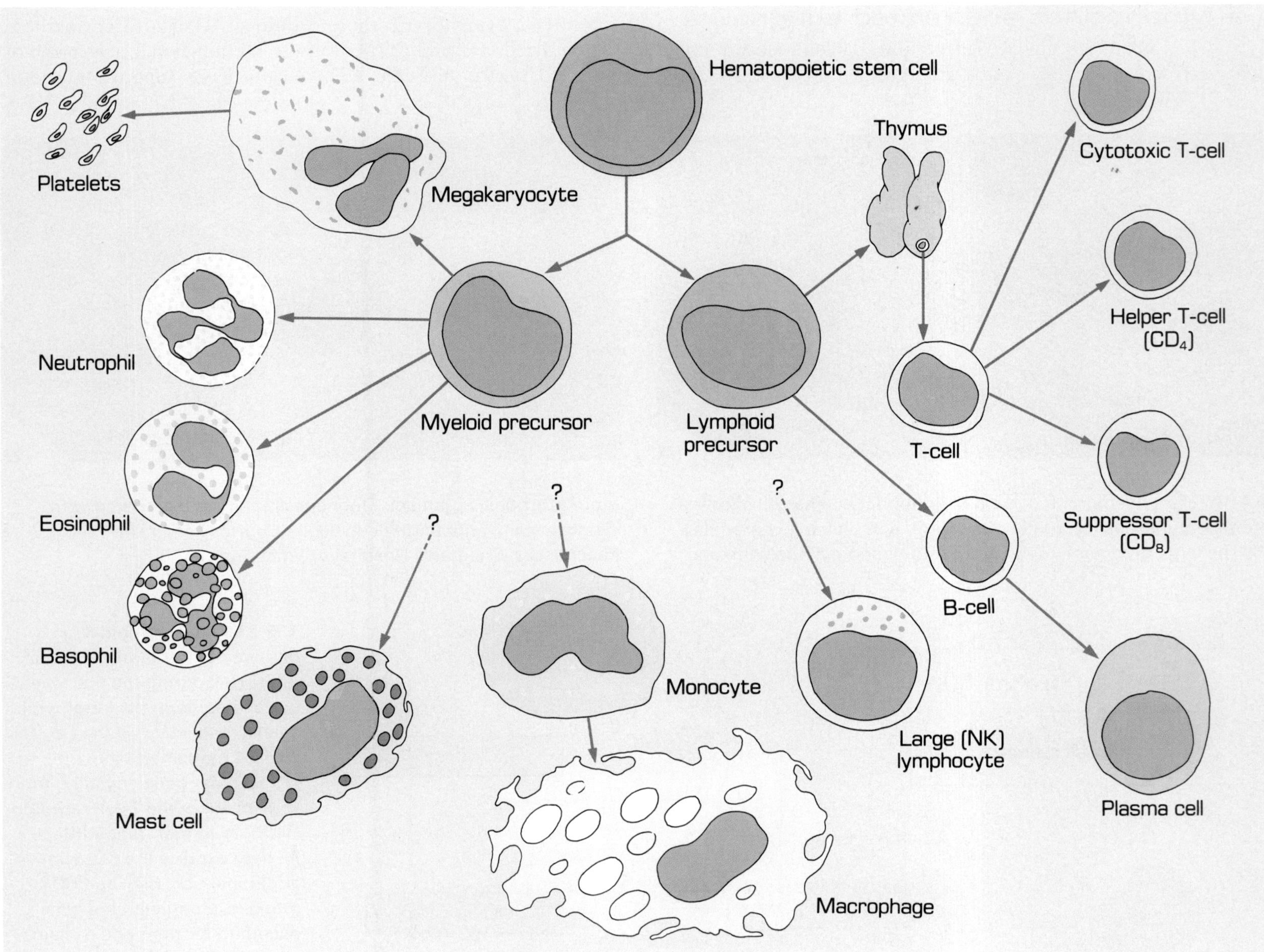

1.3 Ontogeny of the cells participating in the immune allergic response. All of these cells differentiate from pleuripotent hematopoietic stem cells that develop into the two distinct progenitor lineages: one for lymphoid and the other for myeloid cells. From the progenitor lymphoid cells, the T-cells develop under the environmental influences of the thymus. They then differentiate into the various T-cell subpopulations, including T-cytotoxic, T-helper (CD_4), and T-suppressor (CD_8) cells. Other lymphoid progenitor cells develop into B-cells, which further differentiate into Ig-secreting plasma cells. Lymphoid cells also develop into the large, granular lymphocytes, the so-called non-T, non-B (null), or natural killer (NK) cells. The myeloid cells differentiate into the neutrophils, eosinophils, and basophils. (Modified with permission from Roitt *et al.*, 1995.)

LYMPHOCYTES

Using light microscopy and histologic stains, two types of lymphocytes can be distinguished: the agranular, small lymphocytes (**1.4A**), and the large, granular lymphocytes, also called the natural killer (NK) cells (**1.4B**). The small lymphocyte population consists of T-cells which differentiate in the thymus, and B-cells which probably mature in the bone marrow. T-cells make up about 65% of the peripheral blood lymphocytes, whereas B-cells comprise 5–15%. The remainder are non-T, non-B large granular lymphocytes.

T-lymphocytes and related subgroups

T- and B-cells appear similarly in peripheral blood smears under light microscopy, but they can be distinguished on the basis of cell surface proteins which serve as cell markers, and function as receptors for antigens, immunoglobulins, complement, and other, as yet ill-defined factors. These proteins have been employed as antigens, using hybridoma technology to make antibody probes which, together with flow cytometry techniques, have defined the differentiation of T-cell subpopulations.

The developmental pathway of the T-lymphocyte is illustrated in **1.5**. During the first weeks of pregnancy, the embryonic intrathymic T-cells only manifest the cluster of differentiation-2 (CD-2) cell surface marker, as well as the gene which codes for the γ-chain of the T-cell antigen receptor (TCR). With further differentiation, the intrathymic lymphocytes show additional CD and TRC markers. Those T-cells bearing CD_4 constitute the functional helper and/or inducer T-cells, and the CD_8 T-cells have suppressor and/or

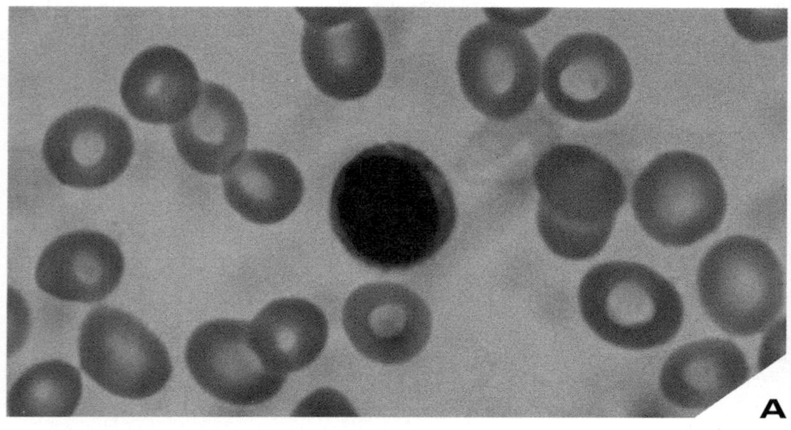

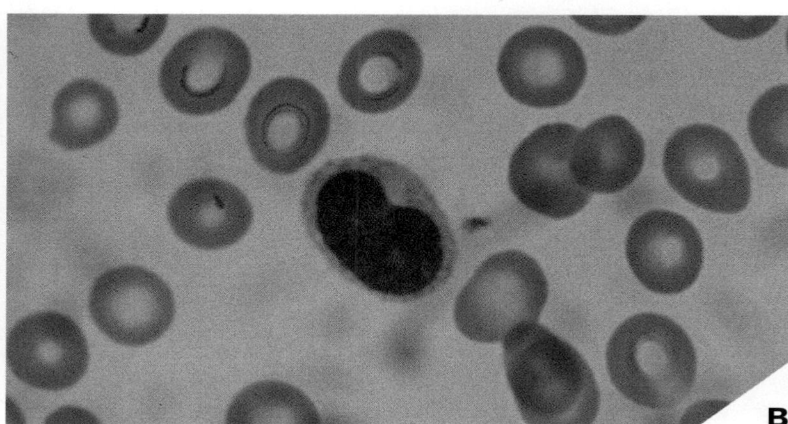

1.4 (A) Light micrograph of a small lymphocyte. The cell shows a prominent nucleus, very little cytoplasm, and only a few granules. (B) The large granular lymphocyte contains more cytoplasm, and more azurophilic granules. Both specimens were prepared with Wright's stain, and magnified ×6000. (Courtesy of Dr Lila Penchansky, Children's Hospital of Pittsburgh.)

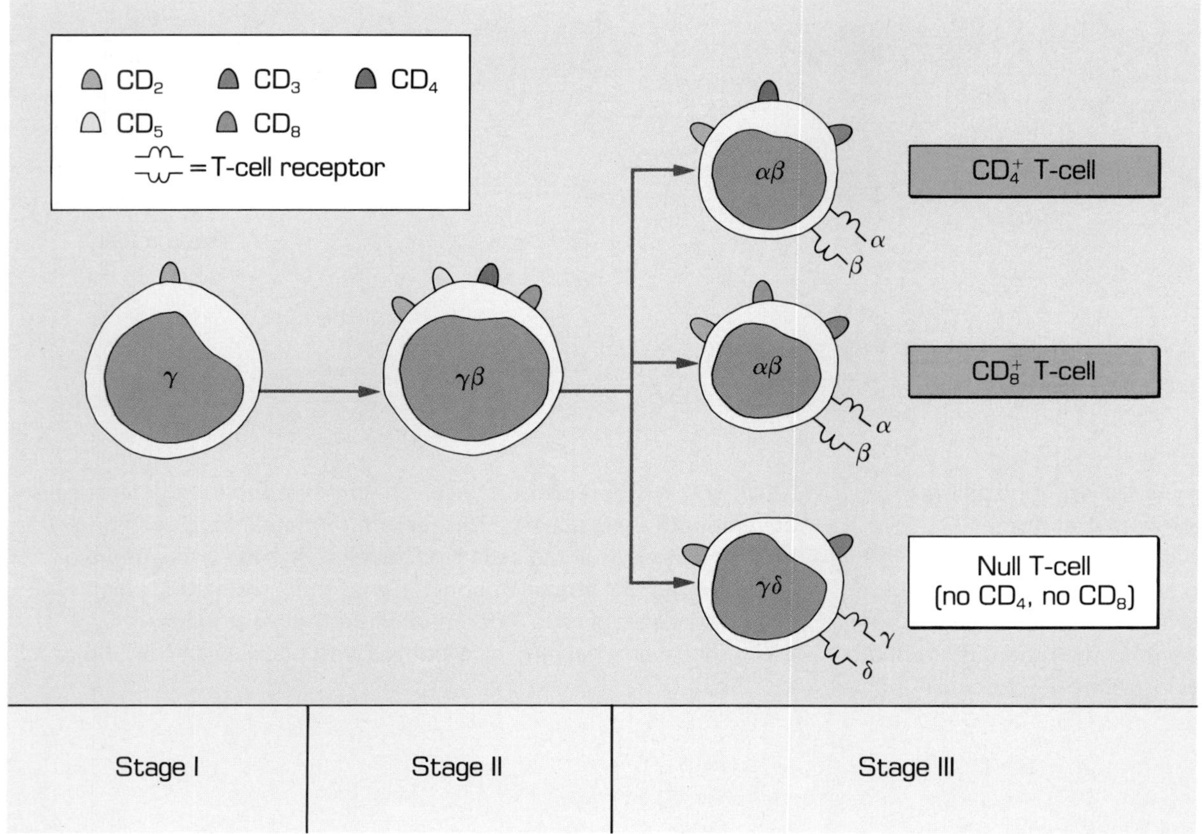

1.5 The developmental pathway of the T-lymphocytes. In Stage I, during the first week of development, the intrathymic T-cells manifest only the CD_2 cell surface marker and the intracellular gene encoding for the γ-chain of the T-cell receptor (TCR). With maturation (Stage II), they express the CD_2 with additional CD_4, CD_5, and CD_8 markers, along with the gene encoding for the γ and β chains of the TCR. At further maturation (Stage III), the T-cells appear in the peripheral blood as well as in the tissues, and they manifest the CD_4 (helper) or CD_8 (suppressor) markers on two non-overlapping subpopulations. These CD_4 and CD_8 cells now express on their surfaces the TCR α and β chains, whereas the non-CD_4, non-CD_8 subpopulations (null cells) have the TCR with the γ and δ chains on their cell surfaces.

immunoregulation functions. The specifics of embryonic and later lymphocyte differentiation are still being defined.

The differentiation of T-cells is also influenced by antigen recognition in association with products of the major histocompatibility complex (MHC). Once an antigen is processed by the antigen-presenting cells (APC), T-cells equipped with the appropriate TCRs for that antigen will recognize and bind to the antigen, which is presented in association with HLA-D (histocompatibility locus antigen-D) molecules (**1.6**). The antigen stimulated T-cells then elaborate a cascade of various cytokines, including interferon-gamma (IFN-γ) (**1.7**). The IFN-γ stimulates the APC to elaborate interleukin-1 (IL-1) which, in turn, interacts with the antigen-activated T-cells, triggering production of IL-2. Under the influence of IL-2, the antigen-activated T-cells begin to divide. Recently, the CD_4 T-helper/inducer cells have been further defined into H_1 and H_2 subsets with unique profiles of cytokine production and effector function.

The TH_1 subset of CD_4 T-cells secretes IL-2 and interferon-gamma (IFN-γ), which are the principal effectors of cell-mediated immunity and expression of delayed-type hypersensitivity. The antibodies (primarily IgG and IgM) stimulated by TH_1 cells are effective at activating complement and opsonization of antigens for phagocytes. On the other hand, TH_2 subsets of CD_4 T-cells produce IL-4, which stimulates IgE antibody, IL-5, which activates and stimulates eosinophils, and IL-13, which together with IL-4 suppresses cell-mediated immunity. Exposure to helminths and allergens induces TH_2 cells, which promote IgE synthesis. Microbes that stimulate production of IL-2 and IFN-γ induce TH_1-dominated responses (*see* **1.7**).

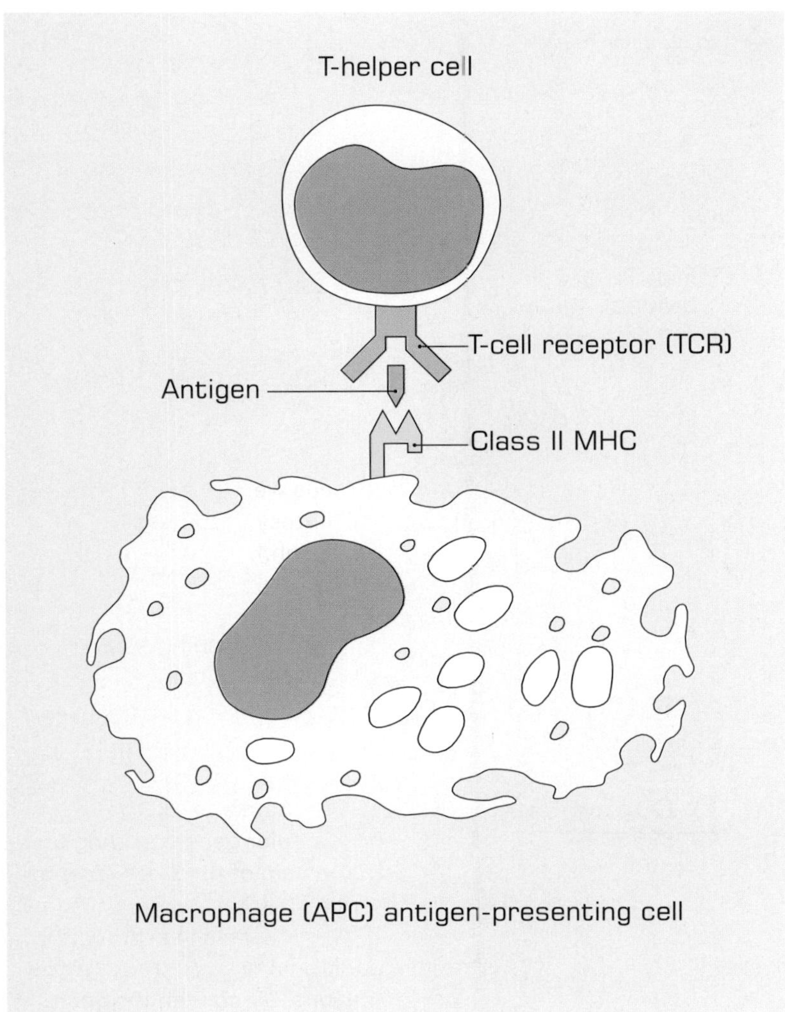

1.6 A likely model for the reaction occurring between the Class II major histocompatibility complex (MHC) surface markers on the antigen-presenting cells (APC), and the specific T-cell antigen receptors (TCR) on the surfaces of the sensitized T-cells. The indentations in the MHC and TCR structures depicted here represent the possible contact and interaction sites for the antigen. It has been shown that the TCR recognizes antigens only if there is a close association with the histocompatibility-D (HLA-D) region.

Cytokines

The effector phases of both natural and acquired specific immunity are in large part mediated by protein hormones called cytokines. In natural immunity these cytokines come largely from mononuclear phagocytes and are sometimes called monokines. In response to antigens, the activated lymphocytes produce cytokines, which can be referred to as lymphokines. In addition, both lymphocytes and macrophages produce another family of cytokines, colony-stimulating factors, which stimulate the growth and differentiation of stem and immature bone-marrow cells or leukocytes. Since cytokines are principally produced by leukocytes with biological activity directed at other leukocytes, they are categorized as interleukins (IL), and many cytokines have been designated numerically as IL-1, IL-2, IL-3, etc. Cytokines initiate their action by binding to specific receptors on the surface of the targeted cells, which may be itself (autocrine action), a nearby or adjacent target (paracrine action), or a distant target stimulated by circulating cytokines (endocrine action). Cytokine functions are complex due to their varying characteristics. Many of the cytokines are produced by several different cell types. They may also have their activity directed at several different cell types, have multiple different effects on the same target, initiate the synthesis of other cytokines, or up- and down-regulate the action of other cytokines. At the present time cytokines may be categorized into four categories of function (**1.8**).

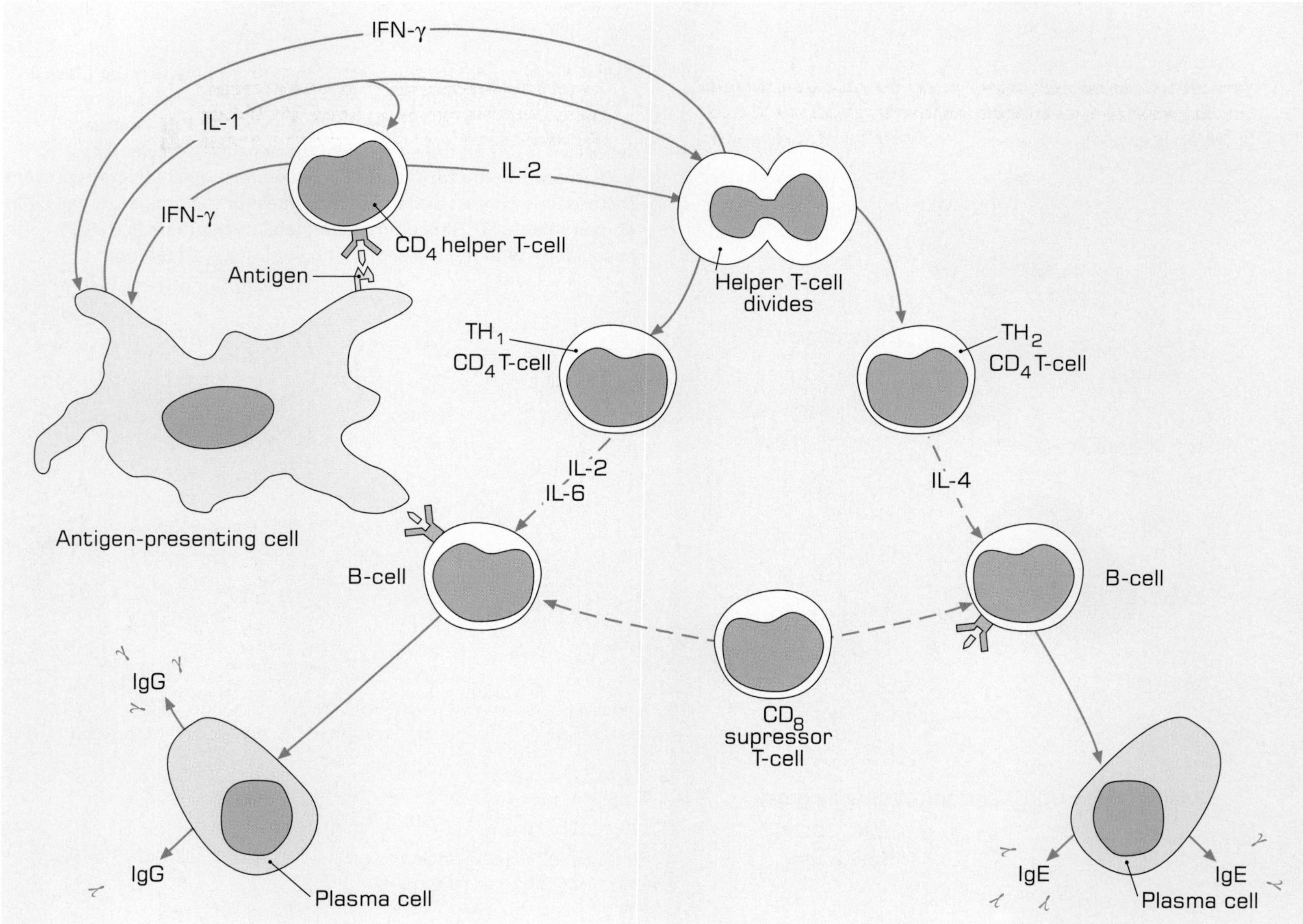

1.7 The current conception of T-lymphocyte, B-lymphocyte, and macrophage interactions in tissues manifesting immune responses to allergens. The important antigen-presenting cells (APC) in the lymphoid tissues are the dendritic macrophages which are capable of both processing antigen and interacting with antigens or T-lymphocytes via the appropriate T-cell receptors (TCR). The binding of the antigen stimulates the T-cell to produce cytokines, including interferon-gamma (IFN-γ), which, in turn, stimulates the APC to initiate synthesis of several additional cytokines, including interleukin (IL)-1. This acts upon the antigen-activated T-cells, stimulating the synthesis and release of IL-2. Under the influence of IL-2, the T-cells proliferate, differentiating into various subpopulations. The CD_4 T-helper cells consist of at least two subpopulations, H_1 and H_2. Once stimulated, the CD_4 T- cells continue to release cytokines. IL-2 promotes proliferation and stimulation of the T-cells, B-cells, natural, and cytotoxic killer cells, TH_2 cells produce IL-4 which acts on B-cells to promote immunoglobulin syntheses, including IgE. IL-5 and IL-6 also stimulate and activate B-cell production of immunoglobulins.

The cytokine mediators of natural immunity are listed in **1.9**. These polypeptides contribute to the inflammation that protects against viruses and bacteria. The cytokine interferon (IFN) consists of IFN-α, for which mononuclear phagocytes are the source, and IFN-β, which comes from fibroblasts. IFN inhibits viral replication, activates NK cells which kill virus, increases MHC molecule expression, and inhibits cell proliferation. Tumor necrosis factor (TNF) is produced mainly from endotoxin (Lipopolysaccharide) stimulated macrophages, but also from stimulated T-cells and activated NK and mast cells. Therefore, TNF also functions as a link between acute inflammation and the specific immune response. IL-1 is produced by not only macrophages, but also many types of epithelial and endothelial cells. Like TNF, IL-1 mediates acute inflammation and can provoke fever and acute-phase reactants. IL-6 is produced by macrophages, vascular endothelium, fibroblasts, and other cells in response to IL-1 and TNF. It participates in the activation of B-cells

CYTOKINES – CATEGORIES OF FUNCTION

1. Mediator of natural immunity
2. Regulator of lymphocyte activation, growth, and differentiation
3. Regulator of immune-mediated inflammation
4. Stimulation of growth and differentiation

1.8 The categories of function of cytokines.

CYTOKINES – MEDIATORS OF NATURAL IMMUNITY

Cytokine	Cell source	Cell target	Primary effects on each target
Interferon (α, β)	Mononuclear phagocyte (α), fibroblast (β)	All cells	Antiviral, antiproliferative increased class I MHC expression
	NK cell		Activation
Tumor necrosis factor	Mononuclear phagocyte, T-cell	Neutrophil	Activation (inflammation)
		Endothelial cell	Activation (inflammation, coagulation)
		Hypothalamus	Fever
		Liver	Acute-phase reactants
		Muscle, fat	Catabolism (cachexia)
		Thymocyte	Costimulator
Interleukin-l	Mononuclear phagocyte, other	Thymocyte	Costimulator
		Endothelial cell	Activation (inflammation, coagulation)
		Hypothalamus	Fever Acute-phase reactants
		Muscle, fat	Catabolism (cachexia)
Interleukin-6	Mononuclear phagocyte, endothelial cell, T-cell	Thymocyte	Costimulator
		Mature B-cell	Growth
		Liver	Acute-phase reactants
Chemokines Interleukin-8 RANTES	Mononuclear phagocyte, endothelial cell, fibroblast, T-cell, platelet	Leukocytes	Leukocyte chemotaxis and activation

Abbreviations: MHC, major histocompatibility complex; NK, natural killer.

1.9 Cytokine mediators of natural immunity.

and, to a lesser degree, T-cells. The chemokines are a newly described family of cytokines that stimulate leukocyte motion (chemokinesis) and directed movement (chemotaxis) and are produced by a variety of cells. Most chemokines, including IL-8, act on neutrophils. Another chemokine, RANTES (produced by activated T-cells) acts on CD_4 T-cells and monocytes.

Cytokines that regulate lymphocyte activation, growth, and differentiation are listed in **1.10**. IL-2 is the major autocrine growth factor for T-lymphocytes. It is also a paracrine activator from CD_4 and CD_8 T-cells, whereby it stimulates the synthesis of other T-cell cytokines. IL-2 also activates B-cells, thereby stimulating antibody synthesis, and stimulates NK cells into lymphokine activated killer (LAK) cells. IL-4 is produced by the TH_2 subset of CD_4 T-cells and stimulates production of IgE by isotype switching. It also inhibits macrophage activation and blocks the effect of IFN-α. IL-4 is also a growth factor for mast cells and stimulates expression of endothelial adhesion molecules, especially VCAM-1. Transforming growth factor B is synthesized by T-cells and macrophages. It typically inhibits immune responses, but may be important in IgA isotype switches.

Cytokines that regulate immune-mediated inflammation are listed in **1.11**. IFN-γ is produced by the CD_4 TH_1 subset, nearly all CD_8 T-cells, and NK cells. It is the means by which T-cells activate macrophages and TH_1 responses, while suppressing TH_2 cells and eosinophil responses. Lymphotoxin (LT) is produced by activated T-cells and activates neutrophils, endothelial cells, and NK cells via the same receptor as TNF. IL-10 is produced primarily by the TH_2 subset of CD_4 T-cells, but also by TH_1 cells, B-cells, and macrophages. Its activities are to inhibit cytokine production by macrophages and macrophage function. IL-5 is produced by the TH_2 subset of CD_4 T-cells and activated mast cells. Its functions are to stimulate the growth and differentiation of eosinophils. IL-12 is produced by many cells, including T-cells, B-cells, NK cells, and macrophages. It stimulates NK cells and differentiates CD_4 cells into its TH_1 subset, as well as stimulating differentiation of CD_4 T-cells into active cytotoxic lymphocytes.

Cytokines which mediate the growth and differentiation of bone-marrow progenitor cells are called colony stimulating factors (CSF). They are listed in **1.12**. Different CSFs act on bone marrow cells at different stages of maturation and are necessary for normal bone marrow function by stimulating hematopoiesis. Interestingly, many of the CSF's genes are located on human chromosomes 5, including IL-3 and granulocyte macrophage (GM) CSF. The genetic loci for IL-4 and IL-5 are also on chromosome 5.

T-cell receptors and surface molecules

The interaction between the T-cell antigen receptors on T-helper (CD_4) cells and the peptide MRC on the APCs is enhanced by several other cell surface molecules. The APC cell membrane contains the ligand called intercellular adhesion molecule-1 (ICAM-1),

CYTOKINES – MEDIATORS OF LYMPHOCYTE ACTIVATION, GROWTH, AND DIFFERENTIATION

Cytokine	Cell source	Cell target	Primary effects on each target
Interleukin-2	T-cells	T-cell	Growth; cytokine production
		NK cell	Growth, activation
		B-cell	Growth, antibody synthesis
Interleukin-4	CD_4 T-cell	B-cell	Isotype switching to IgE
		Mononuclear phagocyte	Inhibit activation
		T-cell	Growth
Transforming growth factor β	T-cells, mononuclear phagocyte, other	T-cell	Inhibit activation and proliferation
		Mononuclear phagocyte	Inhibit activation
		Other cell types	Growth regulation

Abbreviations: NK, natural killer; Ig, immunoglobulin.

1.10 Cytokine mediators of lymphocyte activation, growth, and differentiation.

CYTOKINES – MEDIATORS OF IMMUNE-MEDIATED INFLAMMATION			
Cytokine	**Cell source**	**Cell target**	**Primary effects on each target**
Interferon-gamma (IFNγ)	T-cell, NK cell	Mononuclear phagocyte	Activation
		Endothelial cell	Activation
		NK cell	Activation
		All	Increased class I and class II MHC molecules
Lymphotoxic (LT)	T-cell	Neutrophil	Activation
		Endothelial cell	Activation
		NK cell	Activation
Interleukin-10	T-cell	Mononuclear phagocyte	Inhibition
		B-cell	Activation
Interleukin-5	T-cell	Eosinophil	Activation
		B-cell	Growth and activation
Interleukin-12	Macrophages, other cells	NK cells	Activation
		T-cells	Activation (growth and differentiation)
Migration inhibition factor	T-cell	Mononuclear phagocyte	Conversion from motile to immotile state

Abbreviations: NK, natural killer; MHC, major histocompatibility complex.

1.11 Cytokine mediators of immune-mediated inflammation.

CYTOKINES – STIMULATION OF CELL GROWTH AND DIFFERENTIATION			
Cytokine	**Cell source**	**Cell target**	**Primary effects on each traget**
c-Kit ligand	Bone marrow stromal cell	Pluripotent stem cell	Activation
Interleukin-3	T-cell	Immature progenitor	Growth and differentiation to all cell lines
Granulocyte macrophage CSF (GM-CSF)	T-cell, mononuclear phagocyte, endothelial cell fibroblast	Immature progenitor	Growth and differentiation to all cell lines
		Committed progenitor	Differentiation to granulocytes and mononuclear phagocytes
		Mononuclear phagocyte	Activation
Macrophage CSF	Mononuclear phagocyte endothelial cell fibroblast	Committed progenitor	Differentiation to mononuclear phagocytes
Granulocyte CSF	Mononuclear phagocyte, endothelial cell fibroblast	Committed progenitor	Differentiation to granulocytes
Interleukin-7	Fibroblast, bone marrow stromal cells	Immature progenitor	Growth and differentiation to B-lymphocytes

1.12 Cytokines that stimulate cell growth and differentiation are colony stimulating factors (CSF).

whose receptor on T-cells is the lymphocyte function-associated antigen-1 (LFA-1). ICAM-1 is also present on monocytes, fibroblasts, epithelial cells, and endothelial cells. The LFA-1 receptors are also present on monocytes, granulocytes, and NK cells. The role of these molecules in cellular adhesion appears important, and their role in cell-to-cell interaction is still under investigation (**1.13**).

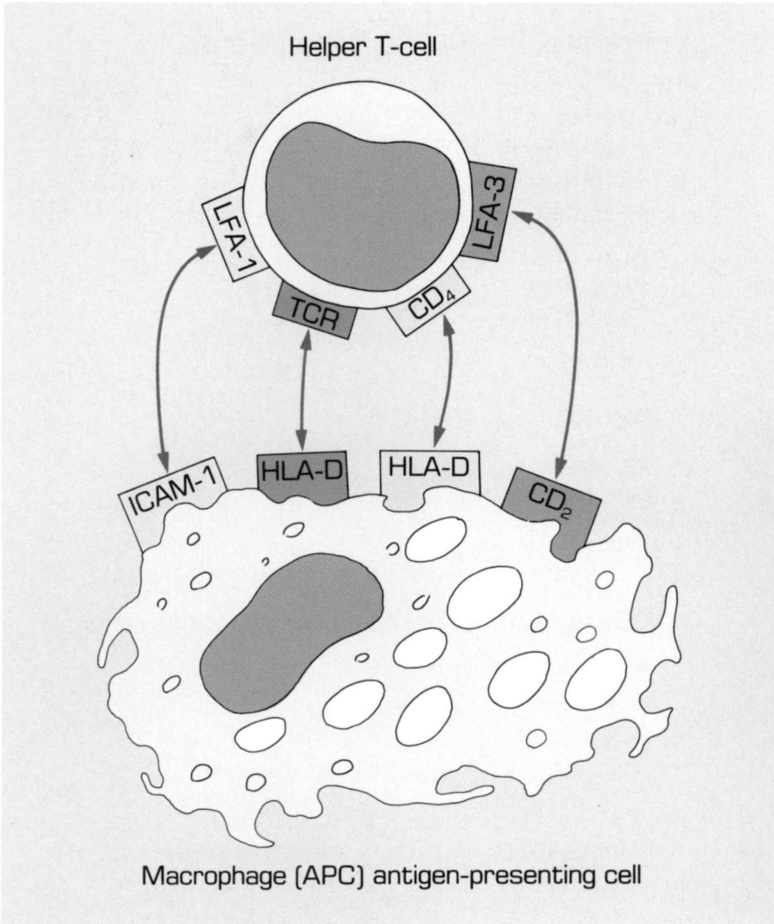

1.13 The surface interactions between an antigen-presenting cell (APC) and a sensitized T-helper cell. The intercellular adhesion molecule-1 (ICAM-1) on the surface of the APC interacts with the lymphocyte function-associated antigen-1 (LFA-1) on the surface of the T-helper cell. The presence of CD_2 on the APC, and its interaction with the LFA-3 molecule on the T-cell, enhances the interaction between the T-cell receptor (TCR), the CD_2 receptor, and the HLA-D protein on the APC.

B-lymphocytes

The B-lymphocytes are defined by the presence of endogenously produced immunoglobulins – antibody molecules associated with the cell surface membranes, that function as specific antigen receptors. These membrane markers can be detected by staining the B-lymphocytes with anti-human immunoglobulins (**1.14**). Most of the peripheral blood B-cells express surface IgM and IgD antibodies, with a few having IgG, IgA, or IgE markers. A number of other markers are also present on B-cells (**1.15**).

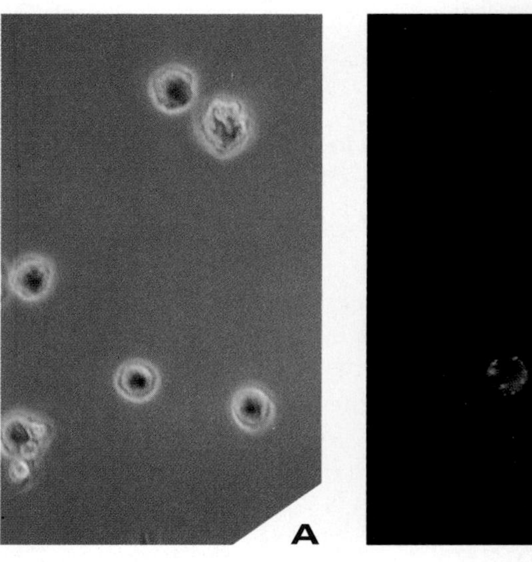

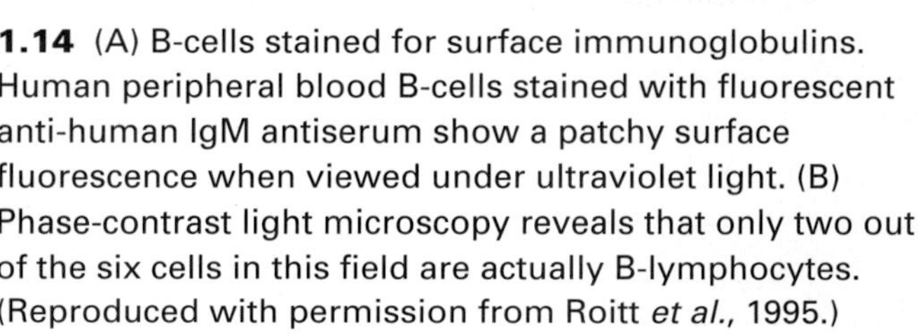

1.14 (A) B-cells stained for surface immunoglobulins. Human peripheral blood B-cells stained with fluorescent anti-human IgM antiserum show a patchy surface fluorescence when viewed under ultraviolet light. (B) Phase-contrast light microscopy reveals that only two out of the six cells in this field are actually B-lymphocytes. (Reproduced with permission from Roitt *et al.*, 1995.)

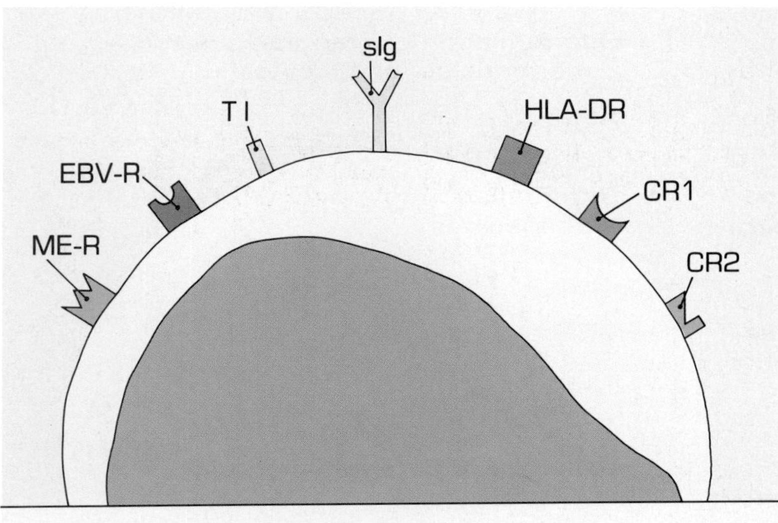

1.15 Cell-membrane markers on human peripheral blood B- lymphocytes. SIg is the receptor for serum immunoglobulins (usually IgM). HLA-DR is the Class II major histocompatibility complex (MHC) receptor. CR_1 and CR_2 are the receptors for complement components C_{3b} and C_{3a}, respectively. T_1 is the marker for T-lymphocytes, and EBV-R is the receptor for the Epstein Barr virus. ME-R is the receptor for mouse erythrocytes, a marker for immature B-cells seen in lymphoproliferation disorders. (Modified with permission from Roitt *et al.*, 1995.)

Like the T-cells, the B-cells also bind to peptide antigens on the surfaces of antigen-presenting cells. However, B-cells do not require the presence of HLA-D. This reaction with antigen activates the B-cells which, under the influence of the T-cell elaborated cytokines, IL-4, IL-5, and IL-6, proliferate and differentiate into tissue plasma cells. The plasma cells contain intracytoplasmic immunoglobulin (**1.16**), and are typically found in the germinal follicles of lymphoid tissue. They synthesize and secrete the immunoglobulins. A single plasma cell appears to be capable of producing only one immunoglobulin isotype.

MONOCYTES

Macrophages and antigen-presenting cells (APC)

The mononuclear phagocyte system constitutes the second major cell population of the immune system. All of these originate in the bone marrow and differentiate into varied morphologic types (**1.17**). In the peripheral blood these cells are called monocytes (**1.18**). In tissues these cells mature and become macrophages, which some pathologists refer to as 'histiocytes'. In response to a

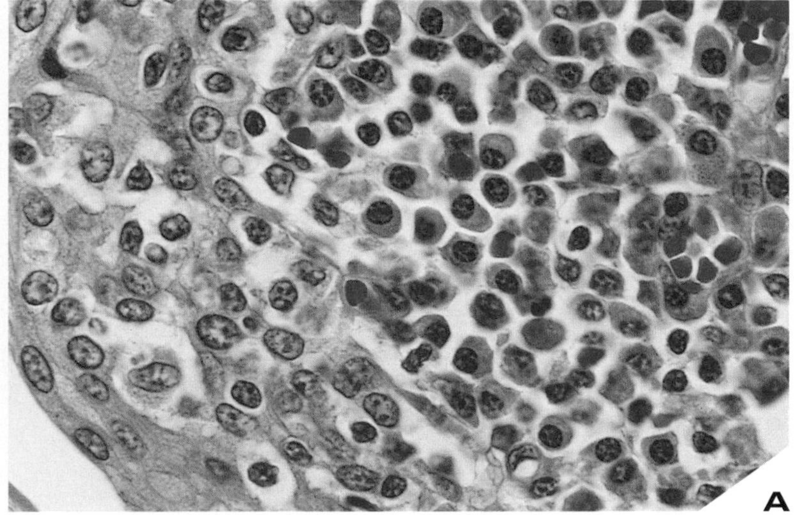

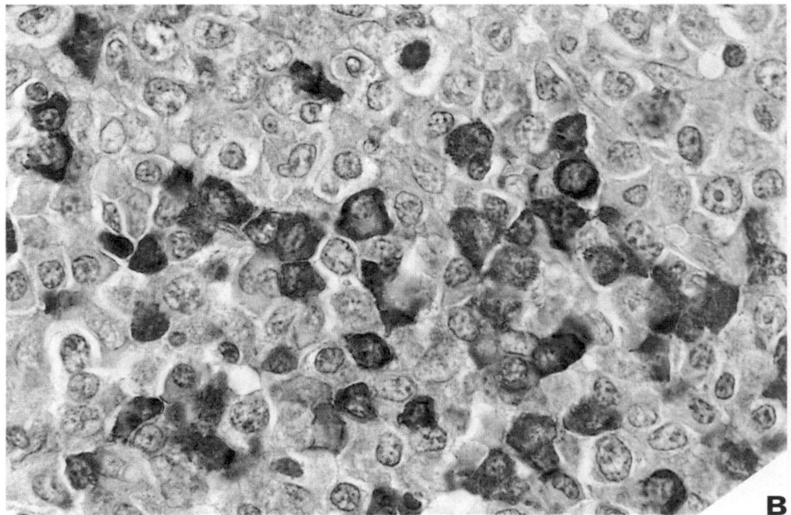

1.16 (A) Photomicrograph showing abundant plasma cells beneath the squamous epithelium of the tonsil. The plasma cells have eccentric oval nucleii with clock-like condensation of the chromatin, and amphophilic (blue) cytoplasm with a paranuclear clearing. The specimen was stained with hematoxylin and eosin, and magnified ×75. (B) Histochemical staining of intracytoplasmic immunoglobulin in plasma cells. Human plasma cells treated with immunoperoxide-conjugated antihuman IgG (heavy chain) show considerable intracytoplasmic staining. The specimen was magnified ×210. (Courtesy of Dr Ronald Jaffe, Children's Hospital of Pittsburgh.)

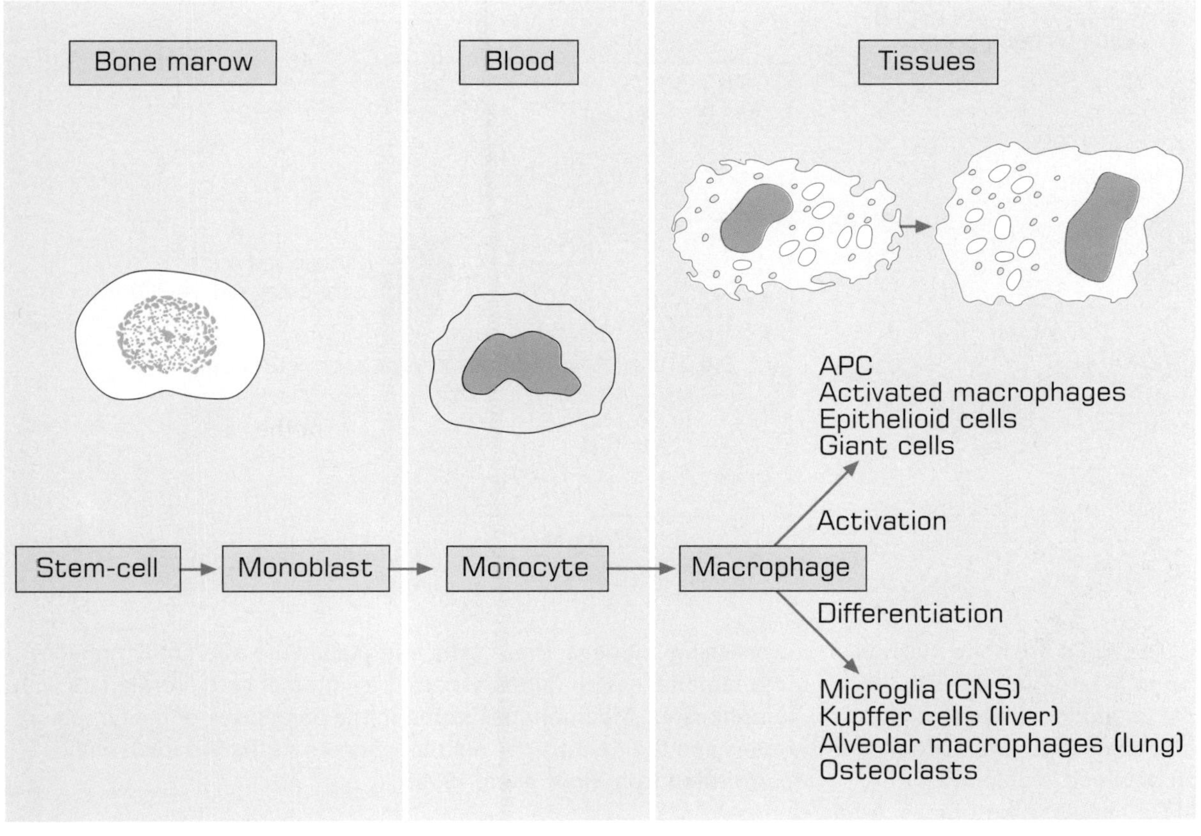

1.17 Maturation of mononuclear phagocytes from stem cells and monoblasts in the bone marrow to monocytes in the peripheral blood to macrophages in tissues. Macrophages are found in all organs and connective tissues. In specific locations these macrophages are differentiated by pathologists as microglia cells in the central nervous system (CNS), 'Kupffer cells' that line the sinusoids of the liver, alveolar macrophages in the pulmonary airways, and osteoclasts in bone tissue. Activation of macrophages promotes both the natural and specific immune reactions. They function as accessory cells with antigen presentation and promote lymphocyte activation. The antigen-presenting cells (APC) when activated may change their histologic appearance into epitheliod and giant cells.

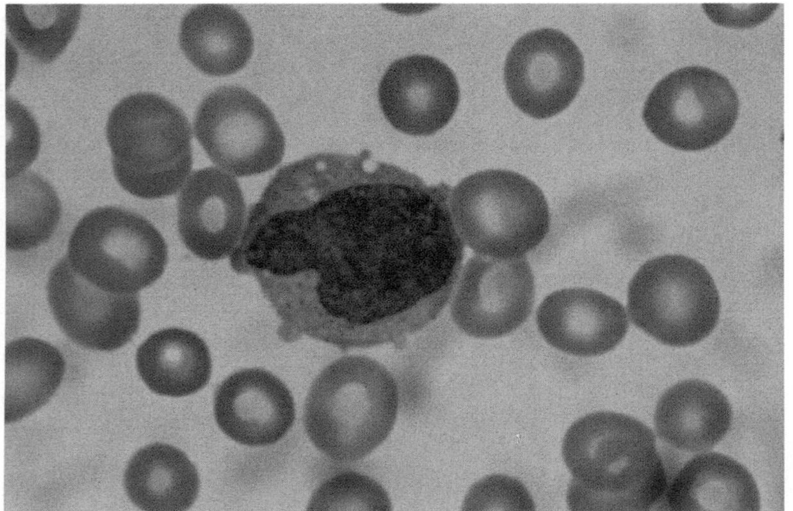

1.18 Morphology of the monocyte. Peripheral blood monocytes have typical horseshoe-shaped nucleii. They are larger than most peripheral blood lymphocytes. This cell can function as a phagocytic macrophage and as an antigen-presenting cell. The specimen was prepared with Wright's stain, and magnified ×4500. (Courtesy of Dr Lila Penchansky, Children's Hospital of Pittsburgh.)

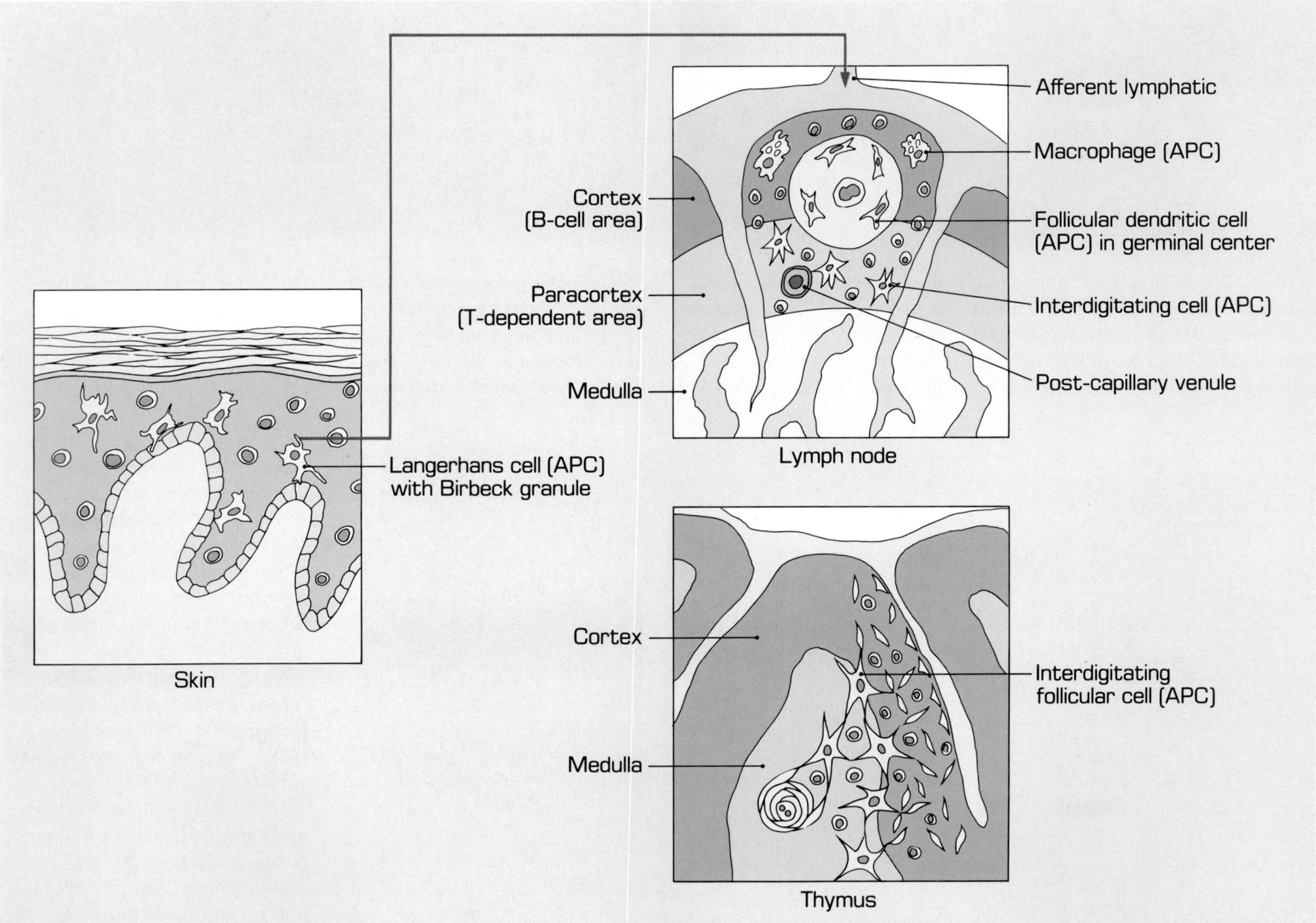

Afferent lymphatic
Macrophage (APC)
Cortex (B-cell area)
Follicular dendritic cell (APC) in germinal center
Paracortex (T-dependent area)
Interdigitating cell (APC)
Medulla
Post-capillary venule
Lymph node
Langerhans cell (APC) with Birbeck granule
Skin
Cortex
Interdigitating follicular cell (APC)
Medulla
Thymus

1.19 Antigen-presenting cells (APCs). The APCs are bone marrow-derived mononuclear macrophages found in large numbers in the skin and lymphoid tissue. In the skin, APCs are identified as Langerhans cells, which are found in the epidermis. Their cytoplasm contains Birbeck granules, the function of which is unknown. HLA-DR determinants are present on the APCs' cellular membranes. After processing antigens, these cells migrate via the afferent lymphatics into regional lymph nodes, where they interact and interdigitate with lymphocytes. Macrophages found in the paracortex of the lymph nodes and the thymus can also function as APCs. (Adapted with permission from Roitt *et al.*, 1995.)

variety of stimuli, these macrophages can assume different forms – pathologists identify macrophages with abundant cytoplasm as epithelial cells and when the inflammation causes the macrophages to fuse, they form multinucleated giant cells. Macrophages play a role in natural as well as specific acquired immunity. In natural immunity, the macrophages function as the principle scavenger cells in tissues, along with the polymorphonuclear leukocytes. They phagocytose microbes and foreign substances, as well as injured or dead red blood cells, leukocytes, or other tissues. In addition these cells secrete enzymes, nitric oxide, and lipid-derived mediators, such as prostaglandins, which control the spread of infection but also contribute to inflammation and injury. The macrophages also produce cytokines (IL-1, TNF, IL-6) and growth factors, which also participate in inflammation.

Mononuclear phagocytes function as both accessory and effector cells in the immune response. As APCs, the macrophages express on their cell surface proteins that promote T-cell activation. These antigen stimulated T-cells secrete cytokines that, in turn, activate the macrophages, which are stimulated to become more efficient effector cells in the processes of phagocytosis than the prior non-stimulated macrophages. Because the macrophages also express surface receptors for antibodies and complement proteins, they can bind and phagocytose antibody-coated particles much more avidly than non-antibody complexed substances. In this manner, the macrophages also participate in the humoral immune response. The ability of macrophages and lymphocytes to stimulate each other presents an important amplification mechanism for immunity (**1.19**).

Dendritic cells

Dendritic cells are accessory cells that are as important in the induction of the immune response as APCs. These cells are of two types, interdigitating dendritic cells and follicular dendritic cells (**1.19**). The interdigitating dendritic cells are thought to originate in the bone marrow and are abundant in the T-cell rich areas of lymph nodes and spleen. In the skin these dendritic cells are called Langerhans cells, which are extremely efficient at presenting antigens to CD_4 T-cells. Follicular dendritic accessory cells are present in the germinal follicles of lymph nodes, spleen, and mucosal-associated lymphoid follicles. These accessory cells probably are important in regulating the magnitude of the immune response.

GRANULOCYTES

The myeloid precursor cells can also differentiate into polymorphonuclear granulocytes under the influence of granulocyte monocyte colony stimulating factor (GM-CSF), which is also produced by stimulated T-cells. These granulocytes represent 60–70% of the peripheral blood leukocytes, and are relatively short lived – about 2 or 3 days. In contrast, monocytes, macrophages, and T-cells may circulate for months or years. On the basis of the histologic staining of their cytoplasmic granules, the granulocytes are characterized as neutrophils, eosinophils, or basophils.

Neutrophils and eosinophils

Neutrophils represent 90% of the granulocytes in the peripheral blood (**1.20B**). Their primary role is phagocytosis and the killing of ingested organisms. These cells have no apparent immunologic specificity, but are very important in acute and chronic inflammation. The eosinophils (**1.20A**) comprise 2–5% of peripheral blood leukocytes in normal healthy individuals. They participate in the inflammatory process, and their numbers are increased in the tissues, secretions, and peripheral blood (>600/mm^3) of many patients with allergic disease. Eosinophil levels are also elevated in parasitic disease. IL-1 enhances the accumulation as well as release of neutrophils from the bone marrow, and IL-6 influences the maturation

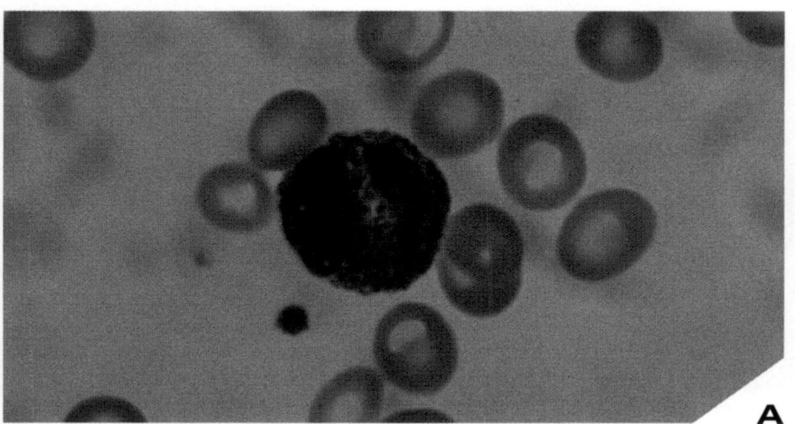

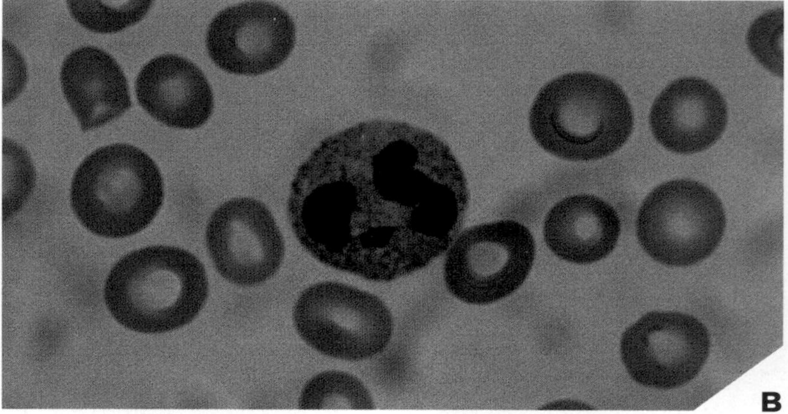

1.20 (A) Morphology of the eosinophil. This photomicrograph of a blood smear shows an eosinophil with its multilobed nucleus and reddish-stained cytoplasmic granules. The specimen was prepared with Wright's stain, and magnified ×4500. (B) Morphology of the neutrophil. This photomicrograph of a peripheral blood smear stained with hematoxylin and eosin shows the polymorphonuclear shape and neutrophilic cytoplasm typical of neutrophils. (Courtesy of Dr Lila Penchansky, Children's Hospital of Pittsburgh.)

of neutrophils. IL-5 promotes the differentiation of eosinophils.

Like neutrophils, eosinophils are also capable of phagocytosis and the killing of ingested organisms, especially parasites, but this is not their only or primary function with regard to allergic diseases. They are attracted to sites of inflammation by chemotactic factors released by T-cells, basophils, and mast cells. Upon degranulation, they release several toxic proteins, identified as major basic proteins (MBP), and eosinophil-derived neurotoxin, as well as histaminase and aryl sulfatase, which inactivate histamine and leukotrienes, respectively. It has been suggested that, besides being active participants in allergic inflammation, the eosinophils may also participate in down-regulation of the allergic response.

Basophils and mast cells

Basophils are derived from progenitor myeloid cells, whereas mast cells develop from a progenitor mononuclear or stem cell. IL-3 and IL-4 promote the development of mast cells from bone-marrow cell suspensions *in vitro*. Mast cells are heterogenous, with one population present in connective tissue and another present in the mucosal tissues of the gastrointestinal tract and the respiratory system. Basophils (**1.21**) make up less than 1% of peripheral blood cells, and are found only occasionally in the tissues. On the other hand, mast cells (**1.22**) are found only in the tissues.

Basophils and mast cells both have receptors for immunoglobulins, especially IgE, and they are essential in the expression of allergic diseases. However, these cells can also participate in non-IgE-mediated inflammation. The granules of basophils and mast cells contain mediators of inflammation, especially histamine. Other mediators, including prostaglandins and leukotrienes, are generated from the phospholipid membranes of these cells during inflammation (**1.23**). These mediators promote the pathophysiologic changes responsible for many of the allergic patient's symptoms.

The cell surface membrane markers on granulocytes are summarized in **1.24**. Platelets are also derived from pleuripotential bone-marrow stem cells, and may participate in a variety of allergic diseases. Their specific role in allergic disease is, however, unclear.

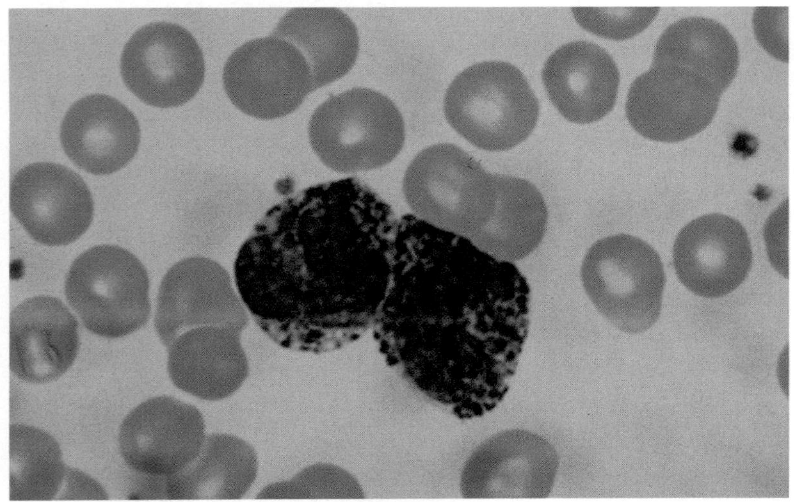

1.21 Morphology of the basophil. This photomicrograph of a peripheral blood smear shows a typical basophil, with its dark violet–blue granules. The specimen was stained with Wright's, and magnified ×4500. (Courtesy of Dr Lila Penchansky, Children's Hospital of Pittsburgh.)

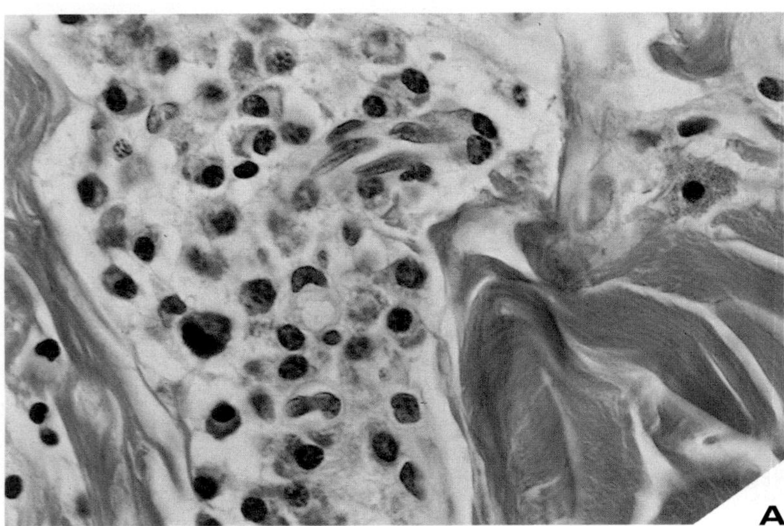

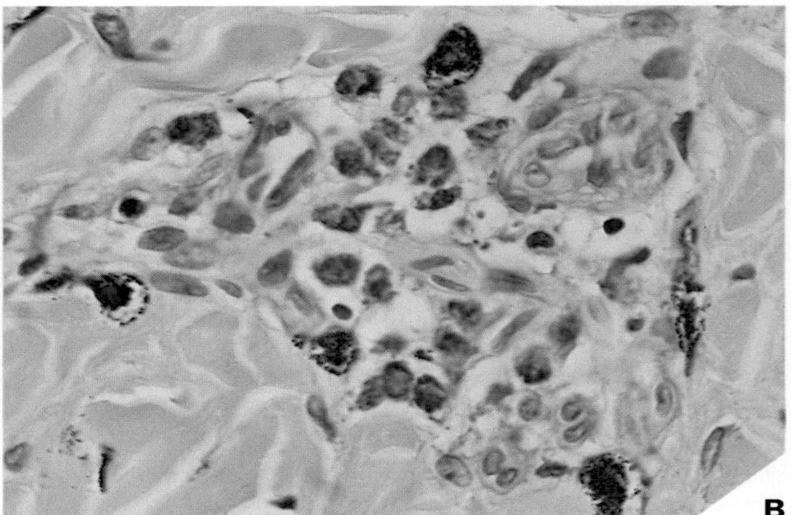

1.22 (A) Histology of the dermis. Inflammatory cells, predominantly plasma cells, surround a small vessel in the dermis. A mast cell is present. Note that the nucleus of the mature mast cell is smaller and rounder than that of the plasma cell, and in the hematoxylin and eosin stain, the cytoplasmic granules of the mast cell are barely visible (magnification ×210). (B) A perivascular dermal space, similar to that shown in (A). Giemsa stain reveals the mast cells by staining the granules intensely metachromatic (purple). There are at least five mast cells in this field, which is magnified ×210. (Courtesy of Dr Ronald Jaffe, Children's Hospital of Pittsburgh.)

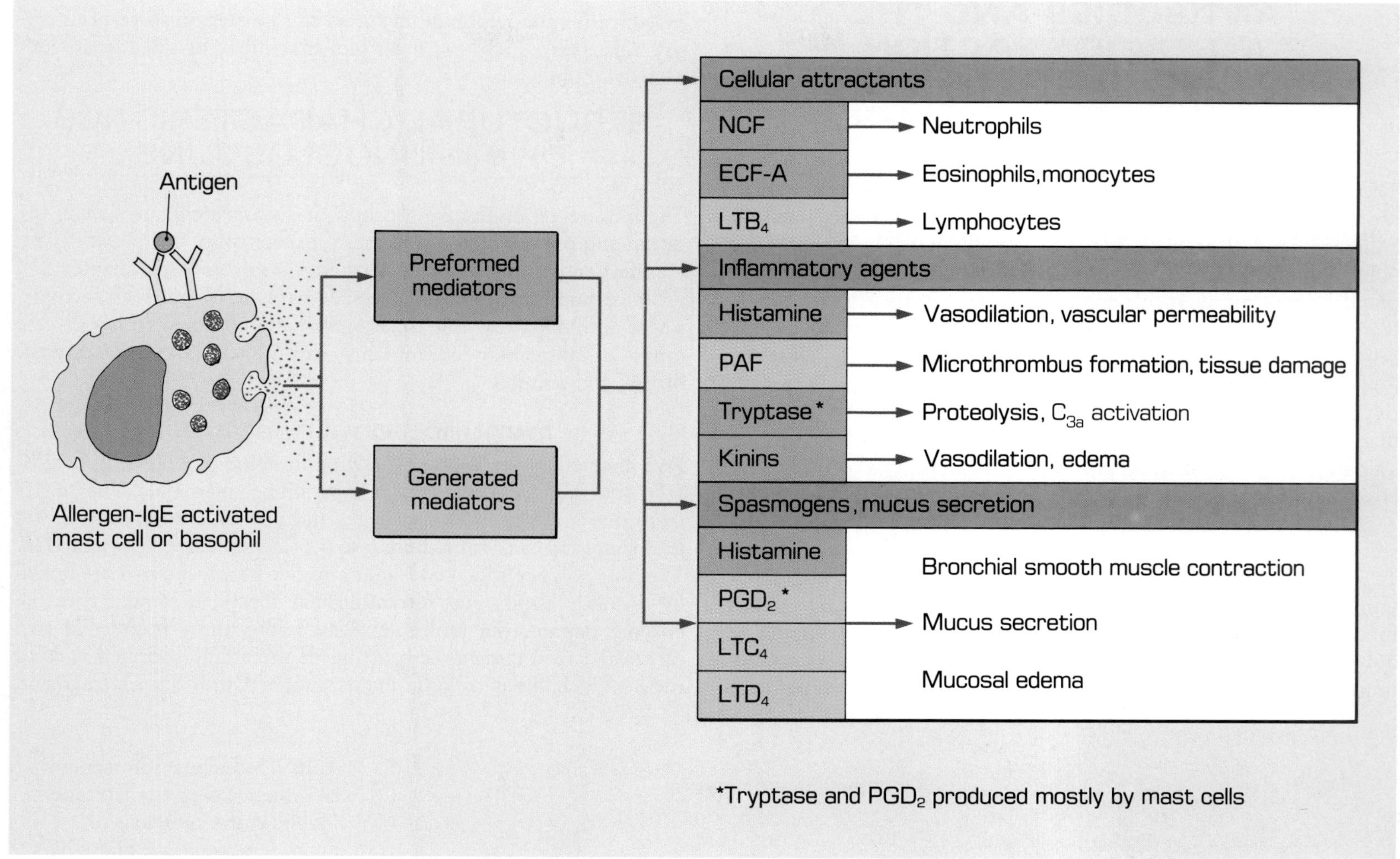

1.23 Pathophysiologic and inflammatory effects of mediators derived from mast cells and basophils. The preformed (granule-associated) mediators, and those generated from the phospholipid cell membranes via the arachidonic acid cascade, have multiple activities. The cellular attractants draw a variety of cells, including neutrophils, eosinophils, monocytes, and lymphocytes, to the site of allergic reaction. These mediators also promote inflammation by direct action on tissues, causing vasodilation, edema, smooth muscle contraction, and mucus secretion (LT, leukotriene; PAF, platelet activating factor; PG, prostaglandin; ECF, eosinophil chemotactic factor). (Adapted with permission from Roitt *et al.*, 1995.)

CELL SURFACE MARKERS AND GRANULOCYTE ENZYME CONTENT

					Enzyme content			
	FceR (IgE)	**FcgR (IgG)**	**$C_{3a}R$, C_{5a} R**	**CR_1, CR_3**	**Peroxide**	**Acid phosphatase**	**Alkaline phosphatase**	**Tryptase**
Basophil	+	+	+	+	+	-	-	-
Mast cell	+	+	+	+	-	+	+	+
Eosinophils	±	+	+	+	+	+	-	-
Neutrophils	–	+	+	+	+	+	+	-

1.24 Cell membrane surface markers on mature human granulocytes. All cells possess Fc receptors for IgG (FcR). Only basophils and mast cells have the high-affinity receptors for IgE. All cells carry receptors for complement components, with C_{3a} and C_{5a} being the most important for chemotaxis, and CR_1 and CR_3 being involved in phagocytosis and adherence. Granulocytes differ qualitatively in their enzyme content; mast cells are characterized by the presence of tryptase.

ANTIBODIES AND THE ALLERGIC REACTION

CELL ACTIVATION AND ANTIBODY SYNTHESIS

The lymphoid system and its cellular components are essential to the synthesis of the antibodies involved in the allergic reaction. (Allergens and their characteristics are discussed in Chapter 2.) After being processed by macrophages and presented to the lymphoid system, an allergen's antigenic determinants activate the T-lymphocytes (**1.25**). These activated helper CD_4 T-lymphocytes, via cell-to-cell interaction and the elaboration of cytokines, assist the bone-marrow-derived B- lymphocytes in initiating antibody synthesis. The T-cell-derived cytokine, IL-4, plays a central role in the regulation of IgE synthesis. The IL-4-dependent IgE synthesis can be amplified by IL-5 and IL-6, whereas IL-1 and IL-2 have little or no effect on IgE synthesis.

The B-lymphocytes mature into plasma cells that synthesize and secrete the specific immunoglobulin antibodies. After sensitization, T- and B-lymphocytes continue to cooperate in the regulation of immunoglobulin synthesis, with the subpopulations of CD_8 T-cells functioning as suppressor cells in the essential role of stopping or down-regulating immunoglobulin synthesis. Without this capacity to reduce antibody production, the patient would end up with excessive immunoglobulin levels, as can be seen in some proliferative diseases, such as multiple myeloma or Waldenstrom's macroglobulinemia.

STRUCTURAL CHARACTERISTICS OF IMMUNOGLOBULINS

The immunoglobulins are a group of glycoproteins present in the serum and tissue fluids. All humans, except those few patients who manifest an immunoglobulin deficiency syndrome (*see* Chapter 17), produce immunoglobulin molecules capable of antibody activity. These antibodies are able to recognize and combine with a diverse range of antigenic determinants from bacteria, viruses, fungi, plants, and animals.

Immunoglobulin isotypes

Five distinct classes (isotypes) of immunoglobulins, IgG, IgA, IgM, IgD, and IgE, are recognized in most higher mammals. They differ from one another in size, charge, and chemical composition. Yet they share the basic four-chain polypeptide structure shown in **1.26**. The four polypeptides – two light and two heavy chains – are linked by disulfide bonds plus intermolecular forces. If treated with the enzyme papain, the molecule cleaves into three fragments: two identical Fab fragments, consisting of the amino terminal ends of the heavy chains with light chains attached, and one Fc fragment,

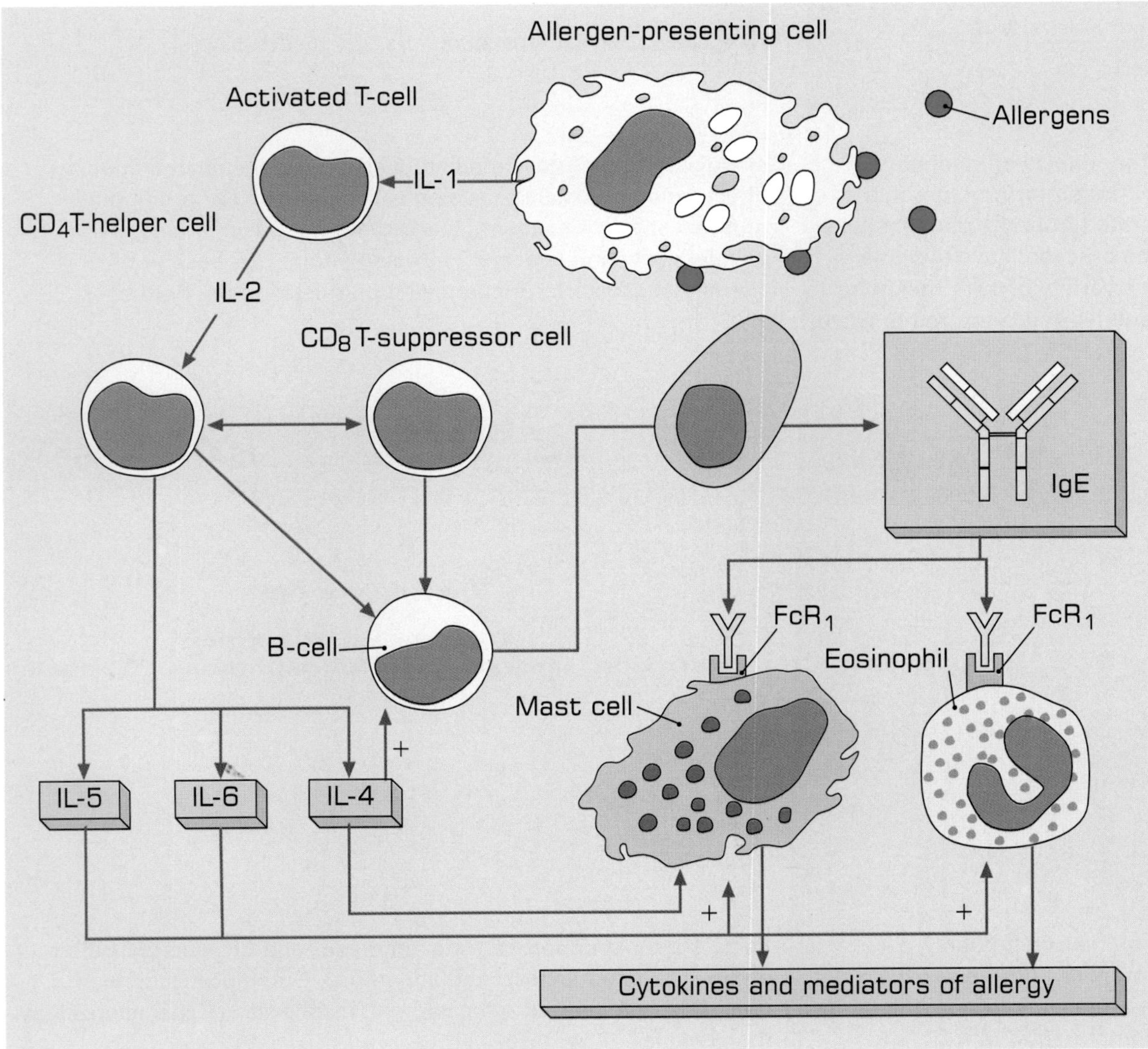

1.25 The cellular interactions by which allergen sensitization results in the synthesis of allergen-specific IgE antibodies. Allergens are processed by the macrophages (APCs), which synthesize IL-1. This substance stimulates and activates the T-cells which begin producing IL-2, thereby stimulating the CD_4 cells to produce other interleukins. IL-4 helps promote IgE synthesis, and these antibodies are then able to sensitize the patient's mast cells or basophils via the high-affinity receptors. T-cells and cytokines not only cooperate in the initiation of IgE antibody synthesis, they also regulate its synthesis through both stimulation and suppression of B-cell function. The plasma cells are ultimately responsible for synthesis of IgE as well as the other immunoglobulins. The eosinophils also have receptors (FcR_1) for IgE. Eosinophils are stimulated by IL-5 and IL-6, as well as by TNF from the mast cells.

consisting of the carboxy terminal ends of the heavy chains. The designation Fab refers to the antigen binding fragments of the immunoglobulin antibody, which are uniquely adapted to combine with one and only one antigenic or closely similar determinant. The variable regions of the heavy (V_H) and light (V_L) chains show marked variation in amino acid sequence and composition in different antibody molecules. These amino acid sequences determine the specificity of the antigen binding sites of the Fab fragment.

The Fc fragment of the molecule contains the site that determines the deposition of antigens that bind the Fab portion of the molecule. The Fc fragment bears the site for interaction with the complement system components, and for binding to various cells including neutrophils, monocytes, and macrophages.

Heavy and light chains

The five immunoglobulin isotypes, IgG, IgA, IgM, IgD, and IgE, differ from one another in the structure of their respective heavy (H) chains, which are designated by the corresponding Greek letters γ, α, μ, δ, and ε, respectively. There are two types of light (L) chains, designated κ and λ. Of IgG molecules, 65% have two κL chains and two γH chains, and 35% have two λL chains and two γH chains. A similar distribution is found for IgA and IgM molecules.

A single plasma cell appears capable of producing only one type of H and one type of L chain. H and L chains are synthesized independently on ribosomes of different sizes. Most probably, one L and one H chain combine to form half of a molecule, and then the two halves combine to form the four-chain immunoglobulin. Formed within the cells, the molecules are then transported through the cell membrane to the interstitial fluids.

The differences among the various immunoglobulins are shown in **1.27**. IgG and IgE are present in the serum as monomeric structures with molecular weights of 150,000 and 180,000, respectively, while IgM is a pentamer with a molecular weight of 900,000. IgA is also present in the serum, and is the predominant immunoglobulin

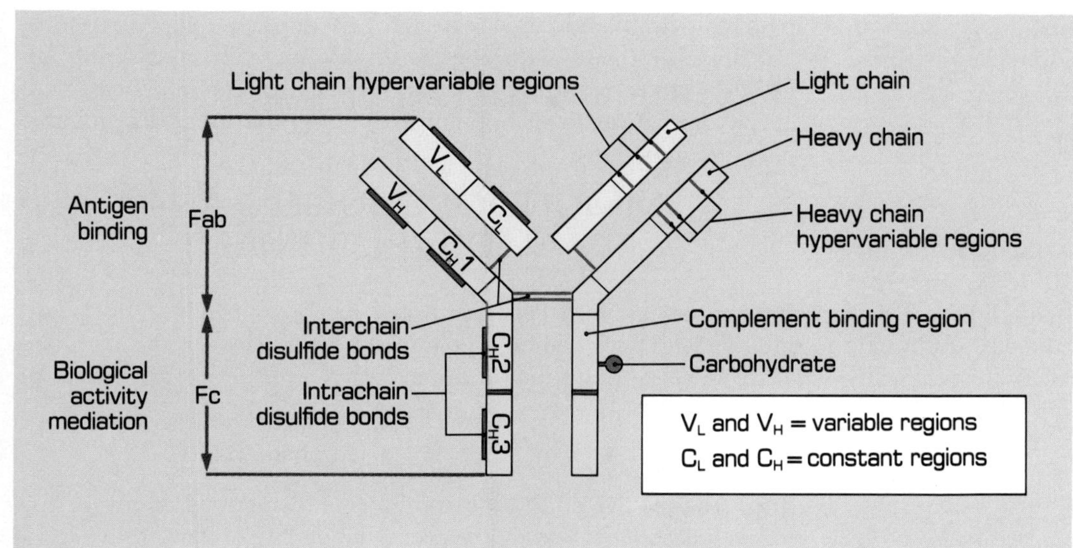

1.26 Structural characteristics of the immunoglobulins. All immunoglobulins manifest a basic chain polypeptide structure with two light (L) chains, and two heavy (H) chains linked by disulfide bonds. Enzymatic treatment with papain produces three peptides: two identical Fab fragments, which contain the L chains and the posterior portions of the H chains, and a single Fc fragment, which contains the carboxyl terminal ends of the H chains.

STRUCTURAL AND METABOLIC PROPERTIES OF IMMUNOGLOBULINS

	IgG_1	IgG_2	IgG_3	IgG_4	IgM	IgA_1	IgA_2	sIgA*	IgE
Heavy chain	γ_1	γ_2	γ_3	γ_4	μ	α_1	α_2	α_1, α_2	ε
Adult mean serum level (mg/ml)	9	3	1	0.5	1.5	3.0	0.5	0.05	5×10^{-5}
Molecular weight	1.5×10^5	1.5×10^5	1.7×10^5	1.5×10^5	1×10^6	1.6×10^5	1.6×10^5	3.8×10^5	1.9×10^5
Placental transfer	+	+	+	+	–	–	–	–	–
Complement fixation	++	+	+++	–	+++	–	–	–	–
In secretions	–	–	–	–	–	–	–	++	+

*secretory IgA

1.27 The structural and metabolic properties of the immunoglobulins.

in the nasal, salivary, bronchial, optic, and intestinal exocrine secretions. The secretory IgA exists as a dimeric form in which two IgA monomers are joined together by another protein synthesized in epithelial cells and called the secretory or transport piece. IgA is normally present in the serum as either a monomer or a polymer. IgE has also been detected in secretions, but secretory IgE, unlike secretory IgA, appears to be physiochemically similar to serum IgE, and does not contain a secretory piece.

IgG comprises four subclasses designated as subtypes 1, 2, 3, and 4 (*see* **1.27**). IgA has two subtypes, and IgM, IgD, and IgE have one subtype. The properties of these different subclasses are determined by differences in the L chains.

Genetic markers have been discovered on the class-specific H chains of the immunoglobulins, permitting classification of individuals according to these differences. For IgG, these markers are called Gm types, and almost 30 have been identified. It has been shown that injection of IgG of one Gm type into an individual producing IgG of a different Gm type results in the formation of antibodies against the injected IgG. Antibodies that developed against a 'foreign' Gm antigenic determinant were found to produce an allergic systemic reaction when the patient was reinjected with the 'foreign' IgG.

IMMUNOGLOBULIN CONCENTRATIONS

IgG accounts for most of the immunoglobulins found in normal human serum (70–80%). There is less IgA (10–15%) and IgM (5–10%), and minute amounts of IgE (<1%) and IgD (<0.1%) (**1.28**). The immunoglobulins have differences in electrophoretic mobility, but these differences are not clinically useful in specifically quantifying the serum levels of each isotype. IgE levels are best measured in serum by sensitive radioimmunoassay or ELISA procedures; the nephelometry or agar precipitation techniques, such as those used for the measurement of IgG, IgA, and IgM, are not sufficiently sensitive.

Normal immunoglobulin levels

The normal adult serum level for IgG is 10 mg/ml; for IgA it is 2.0 mg/ml, for IgM it is 1.5 mg/ml, and for IgE it is 0.0002 mg/ml. The serum concentration of each immunoglobulin is determined by its synthetic and catabolic rate. The normal biologic half-life of IgG is 23 days, which is the longest of the five immunoglobulins. IgE has the shortest half-life (i.e., 2.3 days). IgG, IgA, and IgE are distributed almost equally between the intravascular and extravascular compartments, while IgM and IgD are found primarily in the intravascular compartment.

Abnormal immunoglobulin levels

Statistically higher mean serum IgE concentrations are present in patients with allergic diseases, such as asthma and allergic rhinitis, but not all patients with allergic disease have elevated serum IgE (**1.29**). Marked elevation of serum IgE may be seen in patients with atopic dermatitis, bronchopulmonary aspergillosis, and helminthic parasitic infections.

IMMUNOGLOBULINS AND FETAL DEVELOPMENT

B-lymphocytes with cell membrane receptors for IgM, IgE, IgA, IgG, and IgD are demonstrable in the fetus between the 10th and 12th weeks of gestation, and may reach adult levels by the end of

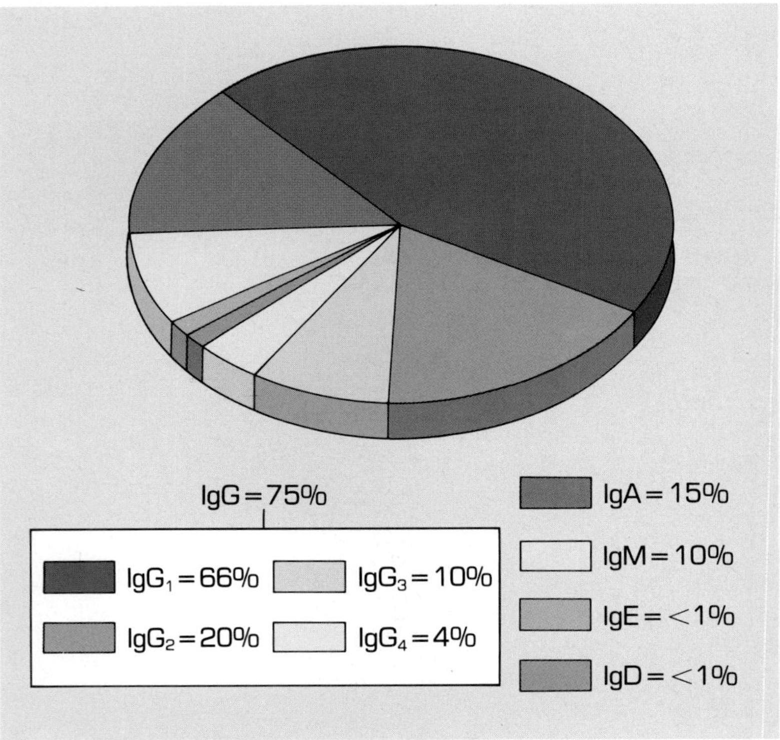

IgG = 75%
IgG$_1$ = 66%
IgG$_3$ = 10%
IgG$_2$ = 20%
IgG$_4$ = 4%
IgA = 15%
IgM = 10%
IgE = <1%
IgD = <1%

1.28 The relative adult concentrations of the various serum immunoglobulins. Serum IgG accounts for 75% of the serum immunoglobulins, whereas IgE accounts for less than 1% of normal adult serum levels. Of the IgG subclasses, subclass 1 comprises 66% of the total IgG concentration.

the second trimester. However, synthesis of the corresponding quantities of serum immunoglobulins does not generally begin until after birth, unless the fetus is infected, or antigens gain access to fetal tissues. In these cases, serum immunoglobulins (usually IgM and IgA) may be synthesized in appreciable amounts prior to birth.

Unlike maternal IgG, maternal IgE, IgM, and IgA do not traverse the placenta. Consequently, the mother who is allergic cannot passively sensitize her fetus; the fetus is, in a sense, protected from the mother's allergic antibodies. Thus, with the exception of IgG, which comes from the mother, the infant is deficient in the other immunoglobulins at birth (*see* **17.9**). As maternal IgG is catabolized, the infant's total serum IgG decreases from birth until 3–6 months of age, when synthesis of the child's own IgG increases. Endogenous IgG, along with IgM, IgA, and IgE, gradually increases during the first year of life, but adult concentrations are not reached until 3–6 years of age. Serum IgE increases above adult levels before and during adolescence, stabilizes during the middle years, and gradually decreases in old age.

FUNCTIONAL ASPECTS OF IMMUNOGLOBULINS

Biologic activity of the isotypes

As mentioned earlier, antibody activity has been demonstrated in all the immunoglobulin isotypes except IgD (**1.30**). There are differences in biologic activity among antibodies developed in the different immunoglobulin isotypes. These differences reside in the variable portion of the heavy chains that are unique for each immunoglobulin. Serum IgG, serum IgM, and secretory IgA are capable of viral neutralization, but serum IgE and IgA are not. Toxin neutralization is carried out by serum IgG, but not serum IgM or IgE. Bactericidal activity against Gram-negative organisms is carried out for the most part by IgM, with minor involvement of IgG. IgG subtype 1 contains most of the IgG antibodies to protein antigens such as tetanus toxin; IgG subtype 2 contains antibodies to the capsular polysaccharide antigens of *Streptococcus pneumoniae* and *Haemophilus influenzae.* IgG subtype 3 antibodies are ill-defined. IgG subtype 4 may also

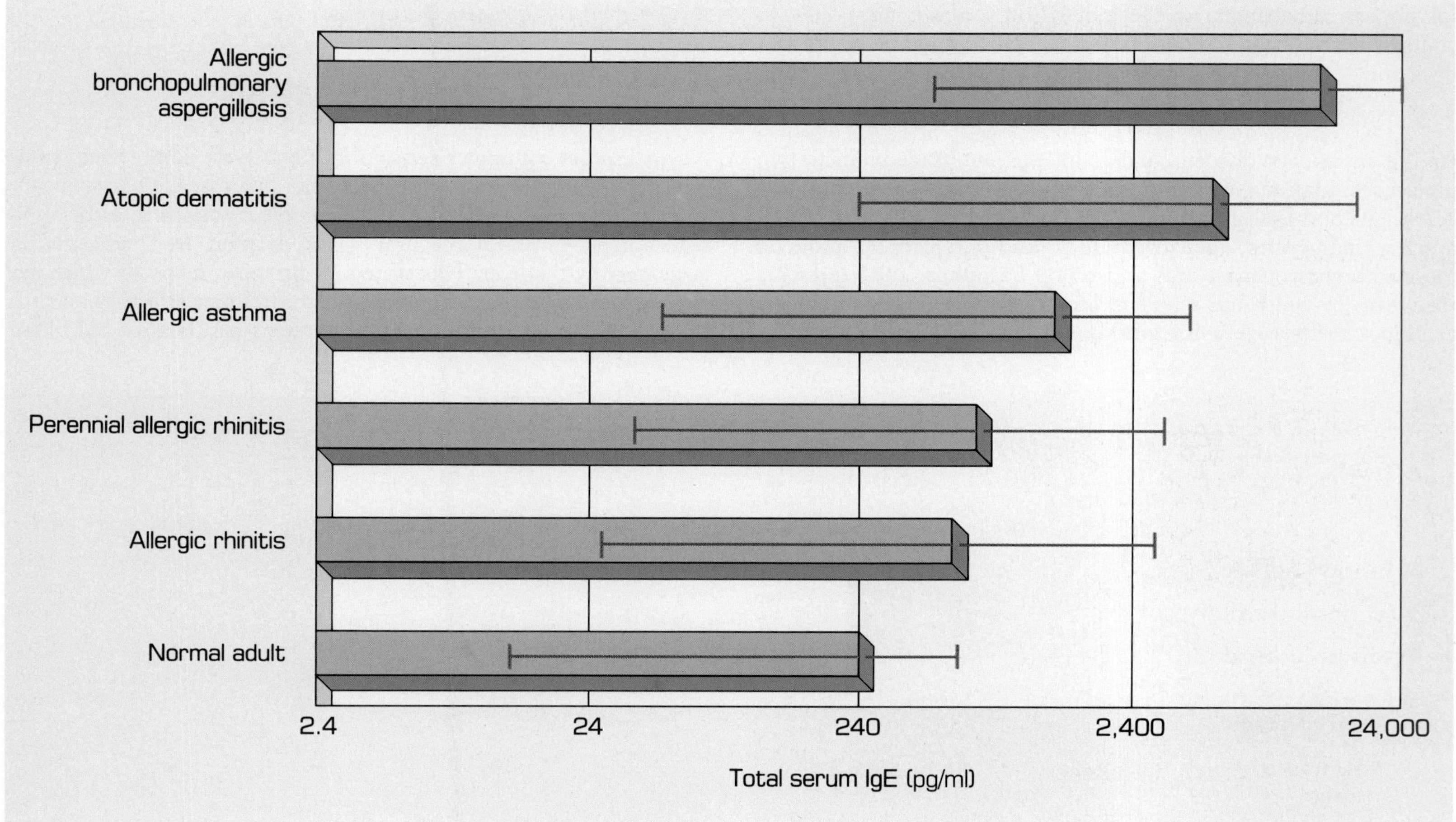

1.29 Serum IgE levels (expressed in pg/ml) are increased in approximately 33% of adult patients with either seasonal or perennial allergic rhinitis, and in about 66% of adult patients with allergic asthma. Though mean serum IgE concentrations of both groups are statistically higher than normal, one-third of patients with allergic asthm and two-thirds of those with allergic rhinitis have normal IgE levels. Approximately 90% of atopic dermatitis patients and 99% of allergic bronchopulmonary aspergillosis patients have elevated serum IgE levels.

may also initiate immediate hypersensitivity reactions, but much less commonly than IgE.

One of the identifying characteristics of the sensitized allergic individual is the presence, in the serum and tissues, of an antibody that is capable of eliciting a wheal-and-flare reaction within 20 minutes of a cutaneous allergen challenge. Initially, the synthesis of skin-sensitizing antibody, primarily but not exclusively IgE, was thought to be a phenomenon limited to individuals with a so-called atopic constitution. However, it is now accepted that production of IgE can be induced in virtually all humans by an appropriate allergen stimulation or immunization. In addition to IgE production, a variety of immune responses occur in allergic patients after natural exposure to, or intentional immunization with, a given allergen. These responses include the development of sensitized T-lymphocytes responsible for cell-mediated immune responses, and the production of a spectrum of antibodies that may be associated with the IgG, IgA, IgM, and IgE immunoglobulins.

Although IgE antibodies have been shown to be synthesized in response to a variety of antigens, including parasites, bacteria, and other infectious agents, they generally have no neutralizing, bactericidal, or opsonizing activities. The antibody activities of secretory IgE appear to be similar to those of IgE in serum or in tissues. In contrast, secretory IgA shows antiviral capacities, while serum IgA does not.

Antigen binding

An IgE antibody is divalent, and an allergen molecule binds to two molecules of IgE via the Fab portion of the antibody molecules (*see* **1.26**). IgG and IgA are also divalent, and IgM may have up to 10 antigen binding sites. The Fc peptide of IgE reacts with receptors on the membranes of mast cells and blood basophils, and represents the means by which IgE is able to bind to tissue sites. Fc fragments can block the passive sensitization of skin by IgE antibodies in the PK test. If the Fc fragment of IgE is treated with mercaptoethanol, which disrupts disulfide bonds, it loses its ability to attach to the mast cell or basophil receptors.

Immunoglobulin–mast cell interactions

Although there is a relatively low concentration of IgE in the serum, IgE has an extremely high affinity for the mast cells and blood basophils. The IgE affinity for basophils was calculated at 10^9 per mole as compared with 10^5 per mole for IgG. This represents a ten thousand-fold difference. IgE has a relatively rapid catabolism as compared with IgG. Although cutaneous sensitization with IgE antibody may persist for weeks, the half-life of IgE in circulation is only 2.3 days, as compared with 3–4 weeks for IgG.

Generally, there are between 10,000 and 30,000 IgE molecules on the surface of a blood basophil, and full saturation may indicate that there are as many as 100,000 IgE receptor sites on that cell. The affinity of IgE for the mast cells or basophils appears to be the same in allergic and non-allergic individuals. Owing to an increased IgE synthesis, the basophil receptors of allergic individuals are likely to be more highly saturated than those in normal subjects. Apparently, normal individuals have more unoccupied IgE receptors on their tissue mast cells or basophils.

COMPLEMENT

Normal serum contains a series of proteins – the complement components – which interact with each other in a cascade-like sequence so as to mediate a variety of immunologic reactions in association with antigen–antibody reaction. These proteins are synthesized in large part by the liver. This system of proteins, many of which are enzymes, non-specifically implements the immune effects of an antibody by opsonization of bacterial antigens and lysis of red blood

STRUCTURAL AND METABOLIC PROPERTIES OF IMMUNOGLOBULINS

	IgG_1	IgG_2	IgG_3	IgG_4	IgM	IgA	sIgA*	IgE
Antibody activity	+	+	+	+	+	+	+	+
Viral neutralization	+	+	+	±	+	–	+	–
Toxin neutralization	+	?	?	?	–	?	?	–
Bactericidal activity (Gram-negative)	–	–	–	–	+	–	–	–
Antibodies to polysaccharide antigen	±	++	–	–	–	–	–	–
Wheal-and-flare reactivity	–	–	–	±	–	–	–	++

*secretory IgA

1.30 Selected antibody activities of the various immunoglobulins.

cells. In addition, several peptides generated during the complement cascade have multiple effects in activating inflammation and cellular phenomena (**1.31**).

Proteins of the complement system form two interrelated enzyme cascades, termed the classical and the alternative pathways, which provide two routes to the cleavage of C_3, which is the central player in the complement system (**1.32**). Each enzyme precursor is activated by the previous complement component or complex, which often has proteinase activity. This converts the enzyme precursor into its catalytically active form. During this limited proteolysis, a peptide fragment is cleaved and a membrane binding site is exposed, resulting in initiation of the next complement sequence. Since each enzyme can amplify several enzyme precursors, the system can amplify this cascade of events.

COMPLEMENT PROTEINS

The classical complement components are numbered C_1 to C_9, but the sequence of their activation does not follow the numerical order (*see* **1.32**). Rather, they interact in the following sequence: C_1, C_4, C_2, C_3, C_5, C_6, C_7, C_8, and C_9. The C_1 complex is composed of C_{1q}, C_{1r}, and C_{1s}. There is one proteinase inhibitor in the classical pathway, which is specific to C_1, a serine proteinase. This C_1 inhibitor is discussed later, in the context of protein deficiency in hereditary angioedema (*see* Chapter 16). The alternative pathway involves several additional serum proteins, factors B, D, H, and properdin. It bypasses activation of C_1, C_4, and C_2.

COMPLEMENT ACTIVATION

IgG and IgM, but not IgA and IgE, have the capacity to activate the classical or complete complement sequence (*see* **1.32**). Since complement activation is important for bacterial phagocytosis or lysis, IgG and IgM play a major role in immunity to infectious diseases. The recognition unit of the complement system is the C_1 complex, and the process begins when the C_{1q} component binds to immunoglobulin. Only certain IgG subclasses (IgG_1 and IgG_2), as well as IgM, can fix C_1. When C_{1q}, C_{1r}, and C_{1s} interact, C_1 esterase

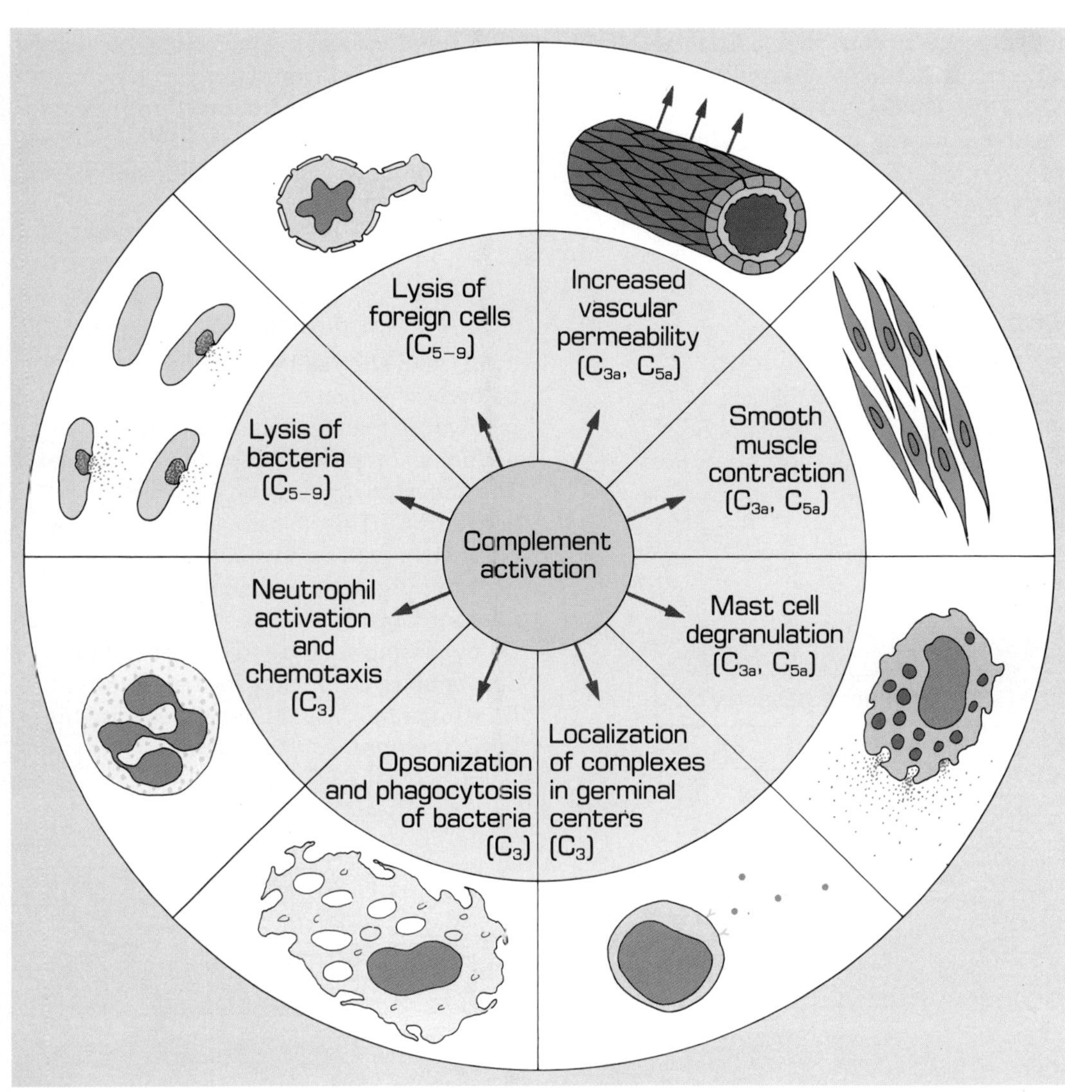

1.31 The multiple effects of complement activation. Complement components participate in various aspects of inflammation. After the complement reaction is initiated, the generation of C_{3a} and C_{5a} increases vascular permeability, causing smooth muscle contraction and mast cell degranulation. C_3 facilitates the action of immune complexes and the opsonization and phagocytosis of bacteria. C_3 and C_5 activate neutrophils, attracting them by chemotaxis to phagocytize the opsonized bacteria. Components C_5–C_9 bind to cell membranes, resulting in lysis of bacteria, red blood cells, or foreign cells. (Adapted with permission from Roitt *et al.*, 1995.)

is generated. The C_{1s} splits the peptide C_{4a}, leaving C_{4b} which reacts with C_{2b}, to form the enzyme $C_{14b,2b}$. This enzyme splits the C_3 anaphylatoxin (C_{3a}) from C_3. The remainder, C_{3b}, acts on C_5 to form C_{5a}. The C_{5b} becomes fixed to a cell membrane, and this is followed by the sequential interaction of C_6, C_7, C_8, and C_9 to form the $C_{5b,6,7,8}$ complex, which disrupts the cell membrane and causes cytolysis.

Biologic effects of C_{3a} and C_{5a} (anaphylatoxins)

The anaphylatoxins, C_{3a} and C_{5a}, can mimic the IgE-mediated reaction. It is important for the allergist to appreciate that complement activation can provoke what appears to be an IgE-mediated syndrome. For example, C_{3a} causes smooth muscle contraction (i.e., bronchospasm), and reacts with mast cells to cause the release of histamine and other mediators. It also enhances vascular permeability, with resultant urticaria or angioedema. C_{5a} is 10–20 times more active than C_{3a}, with wider biologic activity. However, it may be present in lower concentrations. It also causes smooth muscle contraction, mast cell degranulation, and increases vascular permeability. C_{5a} is a major chemotactic factor for neutrophils, and it also initiates the bactericidal activity of these cells. C_{5a} switches on neutrophil production of leukotriene B_4. The alternative pathway can also be initiated in the absence of antibody–antigen interaction. This pathway also results in the activation of C_{3a}, which binds to Factor B. In the presence of properdin, the alternative pathway is potentiated and prolonged.

IMMUNOGENETIC ASPECTS OF ALLERGIC (ATOPIC) REACTIONS

The familial nature of allergic diseases has been recognized for years, and a positive family history of atopic disease has been reported in about 75% of allergic patients. Though the tendency for developing allergic disease is clearly familial, the specific clinical allergic reaction is not directly inherited, since the host response is dependent on the appropriate environmental exposure. If there is no exposure to the allergen, there is no allergic disease, regardless of familial predisposition. Family studies comparing the allergic high-IgE phenotype to the non-allergic low-IgE phenotype suggested a simple, recessive inheritance for high IgE levels. However, studies of IgE levels in monozygotic and dizygotic twins were not conclusive. Although a major portion of the variation in IgE levels is genetic, other factors are likely to be involved.

Investigations of inbred animals suggested that specific antibody synthesis to a well-characterized antigen is controlled, in part, by immune response (Ir) genes linked to the major tissue histocompatibility locus (HLA). Analogous Ir genes linked to HLA have been described in humans. Ragweed hay-fever symptoms and positive skin tests to the purified ragweed antigen E correlated highly with a particular HLA haplotype in successive generations of allergic families. The observed haplotype varied from family to family, suggesting that the Ir genes for this response were linked to (not associated with) HLA. The responses to complex multiple allergens, such as those used in clinical practice, may be dominated by the

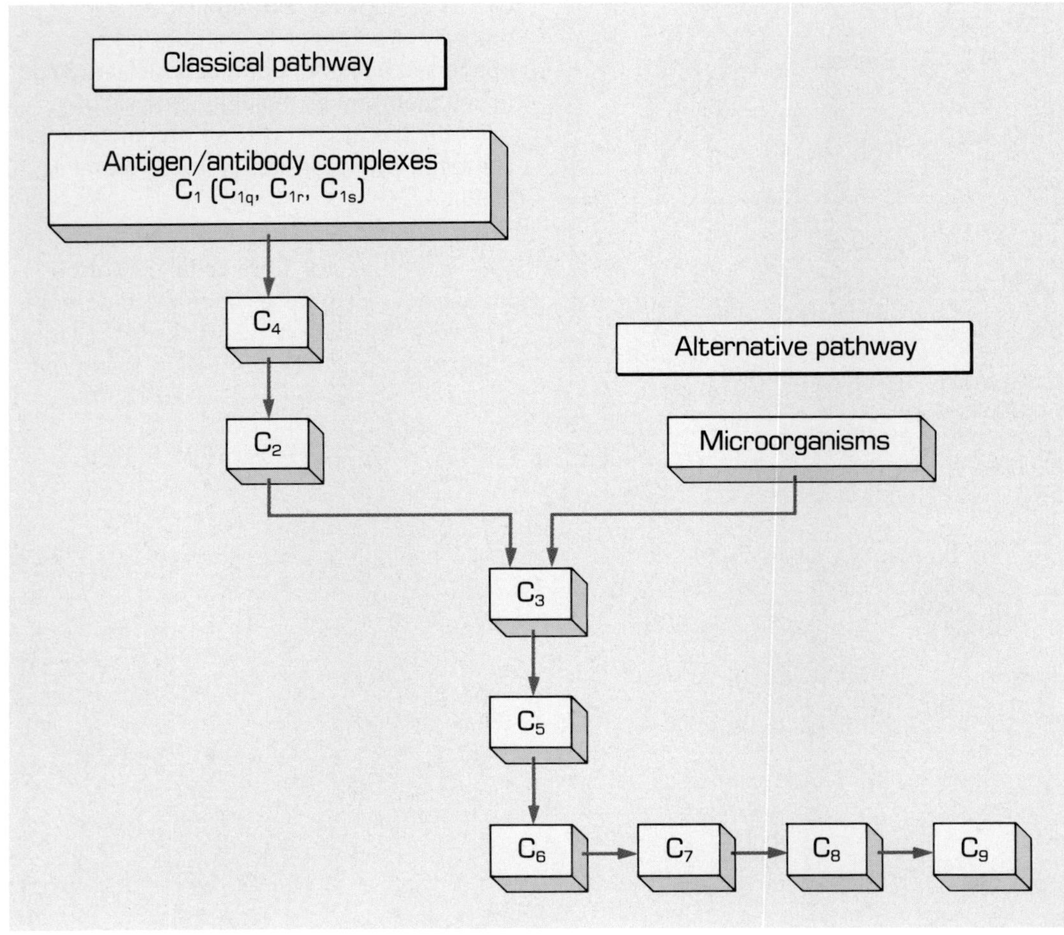

1.32 Activation of the two complement pathways. Activation of the classical pathway is initiated when the antigen-antibody complexes act on the C_1 complex. The activated C_{qrs} acts on C_4, which activates C_2. This, in turn, cleaves C_3. The alternative pathway, usually initiated by non-immune factors, including microorganisms, involves direct cleavage of C_3, bypassing C_1, C_4, and C_2. Thereafter, C_3 activation of C_5 initiates the next sequence – C_5 acting on C_6, C_7, C_8, and C_9, to form the C_5–C_9 membrane attack complex.

general level of IgE production rather than by the presence of specific HLA-linked Ir genes. Recently, a dominant autosomal trait was uncovered in allergic families, through use of restrictive enzymes, and the IgE immune response gene has been linked to chromosome 11. However, these studies have not been confirmed, and other studies suggest the gene is located on chromosome 5. A multi-factorial mode of inheritance has also been proposed, and many investigators feel that several loci may be involved in the expression of allergic disease.

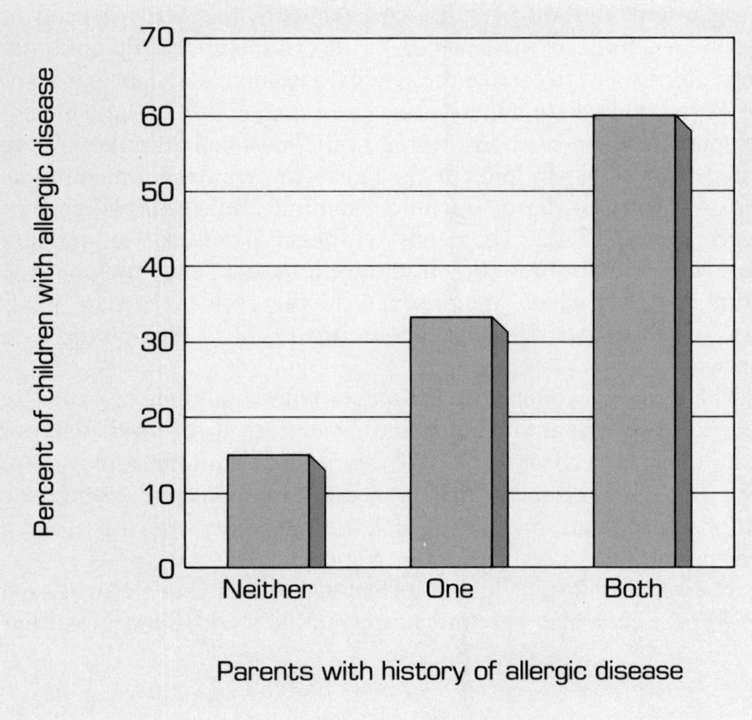

1.33 Risk of allergy in families in which neither, one, or both of the parents have a history of allergic disease. The greater the parental history of allergic disease, the greater the risk of atopy in the offspring.

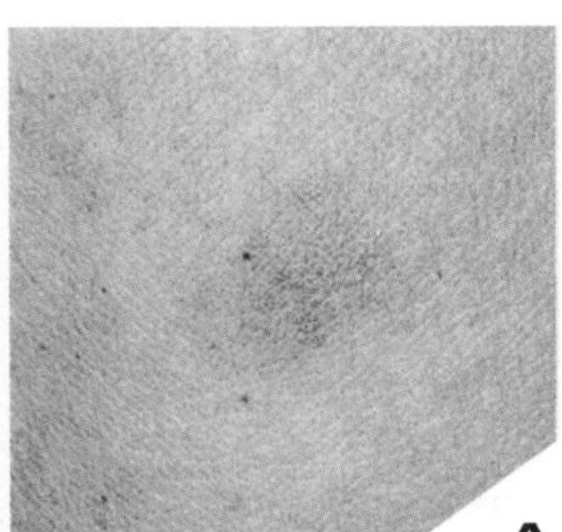

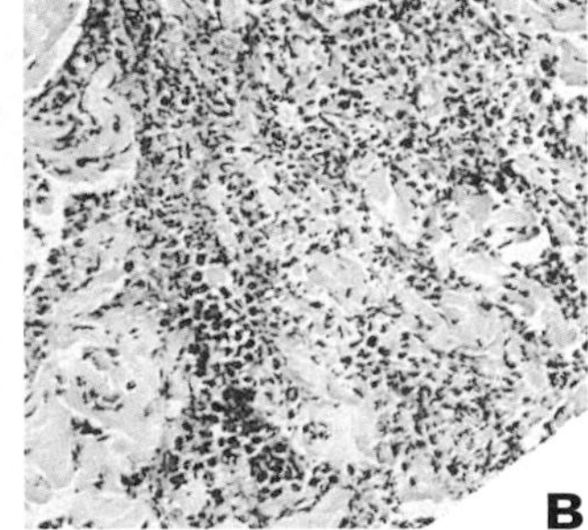

1.34 Clinical and histologic appearance of delayed (tuberculin) type hypersensitivity. (A) The erythema and induration of the skin is maximal 48–72 hours after intradermal injection of antigen. (B) Histologically, the delayed hypersensitivity skin reaction appears as a dense dermal infiltrate of mononuclear cells, including small lymphocytes and macrophages. (Reproduced with permission from Roitt *et al.*, 1995.)

Parents often become concerned with the risk of having allergic children if one or both of them have allergic problems or if they already have an affected child. Retrospective family studies suggest that when both parents are affected, allergic disease is present in about 60% of the offspring, and that when only one parent is affected, about 30% of the children are allergic (**1.33**). When both parents are non-allergic, only 12% of the children are allergic. Since environmental exposure is probably the same for siblings in a given family, the risk of developing allergic disease is probably the same for each pregnancy, unless the family initiates preventive tactics to reduce antigen exposure. Many clinicians suggest breast feeding, during the first year of life, to reduce the possibility of cow's milk allergy. It remains to be proven that avoidance of inhalant allergens during infancy reduces the incidence of respiratory allergy.

CLASSIFICATION OF IMMUNOLOGIC REACTIONS IN ALLERGIC DISEASE

The manifestations and expressions of allergic disease are dependent on many variables, which include the genetic constitution of the sensitized individual, the nature of the allergen involved, the route of allergen administration to the sensitized subject, the biologic properties of the antibodies or sensitized cells, and the local tissue response to the allergen–antibody interaction. If a suspected allergen is applied to or injected into the skin of a previously sensitized allergic subject, several different responses occur. The allergic or hypersensitivity cutaneous reactions can be classified as immediate, early, and late-phase reactions, Arthus (immune complex), and delayed (48 hour) hypersensitivity.

IMMEDIATE HYPERSENSITIVITY

The immediate hypersensitivity reaction usually develops within 20 minutes of challenge with the antigen, and is manifested as a wheal-and-flare skin response (*see 1.2*). Studies have demonstrated that an antibody (usually IgE immunoglobulin), present in either serum or tissues, is responsible for the immediate hypersensitivity response.

Biopsy and microscopic examination of an immediate hypersensitivity reaction at 15–30 minutes reveals little cellular infiltrate – perhaps a few neutrophils and occasional eosinophils, and some local edema (*see 3.2*). It is the immediate hypersensitivity reaction that is the basis for much of the so-called allergy skin testing performed by clinical allergists and immunologists (*see* Chapter 3).

DELAYED OR LATE RESPONSES

Depending on allergen concentration, some allergy patients show a late (2–6 hours) allergic response in addition to the immediate reaction. Biopsy of the late-phase IgE reaction reveals moderate inflammation, an increased number of neutrophils, with many basophils and eosinophils. The cutaneous delayed hypersensitivity reaction peaks 24–48 hours after antigen challenge, and is characterized by local erythema and induration (**1.34**).

The delayed reaction is not dependent on a serum antibody, but rather on a cell-mediated immune reaction involving sensitized T-lymphocytes. Microscopic examination of a cutaneous biopsy of delayed hypersensitivity skin reaction reveals moderate mononuclear cellular infiltrate, consisting primarily of small lymphocytes (**1.30**).

These different cutaneous manifestations are not mutually exclusive, and may be elicited in the same host, depending on the variables listed above.

GELL AND COOMBS CLASSIFICATION SCHEMA

In order to better comprehend the concepts of allergy, including the cutaneous immediate and delayed hypersensitivity reactions, Gell and Coombs proposed a classification of the immunopathologic mechanisms. As shown in **1.35**, Gell and Coombs separated the reactions by which a specific antigen can induce cellular and tissue injury into four groups: Type I (immediate or anaphylactic), Type II (cytotoxic or cytolytic), Type III (antigen–antibody complex or Arthus), and Type IV (delayed or cell-mediated). These four reactions patterns are not mutually exclusive; often more than one of them occurs in the same patient. For example, in a reaction to penicillin, urticaria often develops, representing a Type I response involving IgE. Concurrently, a hemolytic anemia can result from the cytolysis of sensitized red blood cells due to penicillin and complement (Type II). Serum sickness symptoms might result from the formation of a toxic complex composed of penicillin, antibody, and complement (Type III). Further, a contact dermatitis, mediated by sensitized T-lymphocytes reacting to the penicillin (Type IV), may also arise.

Type I reaction

The Type I reaction of Gell and Coombs is referred to as the immediate, anaphylactic, or homocytotropic antibody reaction (*see* Chapter 4). This reaction might also be called the atopic phenomenon, and it is responsible for many of the common allergic diseases. Clinical examples include asthma, hay fever, urticaria, angioedema, and anaphylaxis.

In the Type I reaction, mast cells or peripheral blood basophil leukocytes are passively sensitized by homocytotropic IgE antibodies, which are synthesized by plasma cells on stimulation by appropriate allergens. The binding of IgE to the mast cells involves the Fc portion of the IgE molecule and a receptor on the cell surface. During this initial sensitization phase, there is no overt deleterious host reaction. On subsequent challenge, however, this same allergen combines with its specific IgE antibody at the cell membrane of the sensitized mast cell and/or the blood basophil. This combination of allergen and antibody results in a sequence of energy-dependent enzyme reactions, with alteration of the cell membrane that initiates the synthesis and release of the specific pharmacologic mediators of the Type I immediate hypersensitivity reaction (**1.36**). These mediators may be preformed and stored in the mast cell granules or generated from phospholipids of the mast cell or basophil membrane. The preformed mediators include histamine and eosinophil chemotactic factor (ECF-A). The newly synthesized mediators of anaphylaxis are metabolites of arachidonic acid, and include the prostaglandins, which are products of the cyclo-oxygenase pathway, and the leukotrienes, which are the result of the lipoxygenase pathway.

The Type I reaction usually occurs within minutes of exposure to an appropriate antigen, but may be sustained for hours without additional antigen contact. After the mast cells and basophils have been through a refractory period of several hours, they resynthesize the pharmacologic mediators of hypersensitivity, and once again become capable of responding to a specific allergen.

The specific intracellular biochemical events that occur during the Type I response are not entirely understood on a molecular

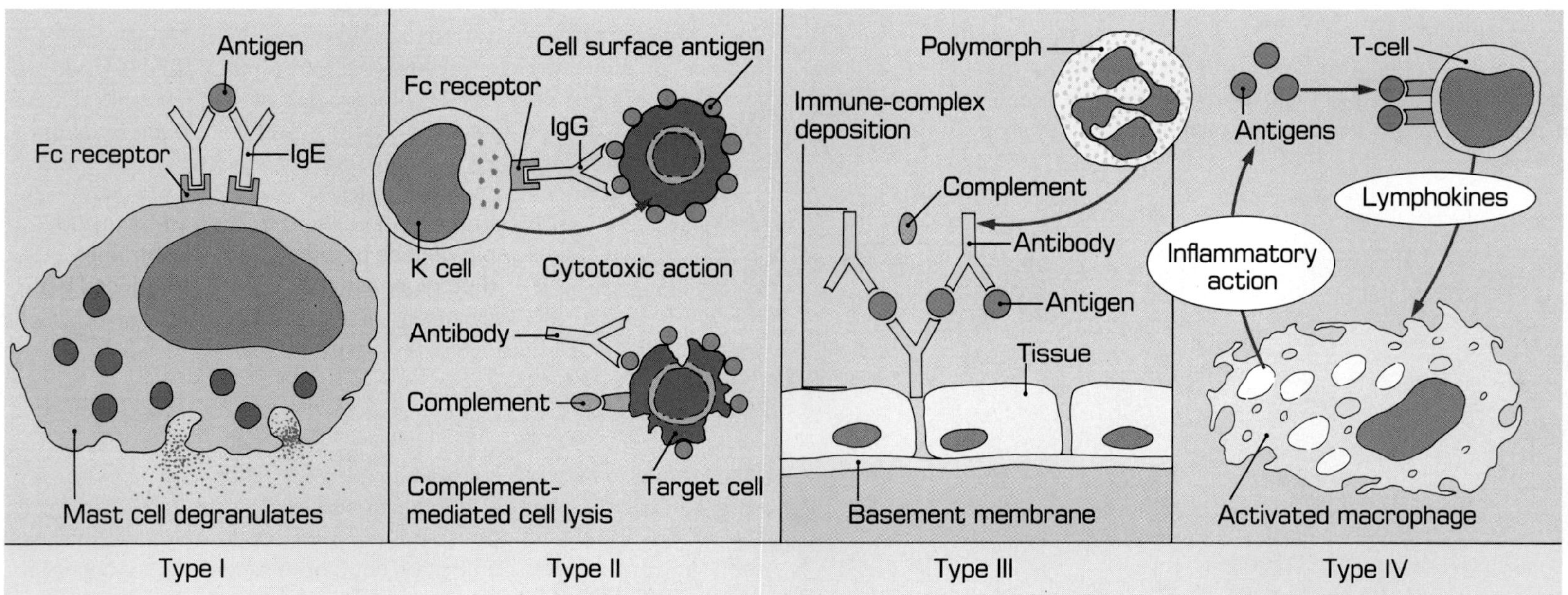

1.35 Summary of the four types of hypersensitivity reactions. Type I: mast cells bind IgE via Fc receptors. On encountering antigen, the IgE becomes cross-linked, inducing degranulation and release of mediators. Type II: antibodies are directed against antigens on an individual's own cells (target cells). This may lead to complement-mediated lysis or cytotoxic action by killer cells. Type III: immune complexes are deposited in the tissues, complement is activated, and polymorphs are attracted to the site of antigen deposition, causing local damage. Type IV: Antigen-sensitized T-cells release lymphokines following a secondary contact with the same antigen. Lymphokines induce inflammatory reactions, activating and attracting macrophages which release mediators.

level, but *in vitro* studies suggest that mediator release is promoted by those processes that decrease intracellular cyclic adenosine monophosphate (AMP). It has been noted that adrenergic agents, especially the more selective β-adrenergic agents, increase intracellular cyclic AMP, and thereby inhibit histamine release. Theophylline, a methylxanthine derivative, is a phosphodiesterase inhibitor. Cyclic AMP is normally catabolized by phosphodiesterase; if phosphodiesterase is inhibited by theophylline, intracellular cyclic AMP is increased, and less histamine may be released. Calcium and magnesium appear to be essential to the release of histamine from sensitized mast cells and basophils *in vitro*.

Interaction of IgE antibodies and an allergen at the mast cell membrane does not appear to be capable of activating the complement sequence by the classical pathway; however, complement activation by the alternative pathway may occur. In most situations, the immunologic effectors of the Type I immediate hypersensitivity allergic reaction have been shown to be IgE antibodies; it should be emphasized, however, that it is the inflammatory mediators (e.g., histamine, prostaglandins, and leukotrienes) that are responsible for the pathophysiologic changes observed in the clinic.

Type II reaction

The Type II reaction described by Gell and Coombs is referred to as the cytotoxic or cytolytic reaction. In this allergic situation, circulating IgG and IgM antibodies react with antigens that may actually be portions of cells, such as erythrocytes and their membranes, or with an unrelated antigen, such as a drug that has become associated with these cells. The fact that the antigen is a cell or a cell-constituent indicates that this reaction may be expressed as a form of autoimmunization or isoimmunization in clinical situations. In most cases, both IgM and IgG are involved in this reaction, as is the complement system. The complement-activated mediators are responsible for an inflammatory reaction. The cell that functions as the antigen or carries the appropriate antigenic determinant is usually destroyed or altered; there may be injury to erythrocytes, leukocytes, and platelets, and other cytotoxic reactions may be involved in this mechanism. Clinical examples of Type II reactions include autoimmune hemolytic anemia, transfusion reactions, hemolytic disease of the newborn, Goodpastures's syndrome, and drug-induced, antibody-dependent hemolytic anemia, leukopenia, and thrombocytopenia. It is the destruction or alteration of a target cell that differentiates this type of immunologic injury.

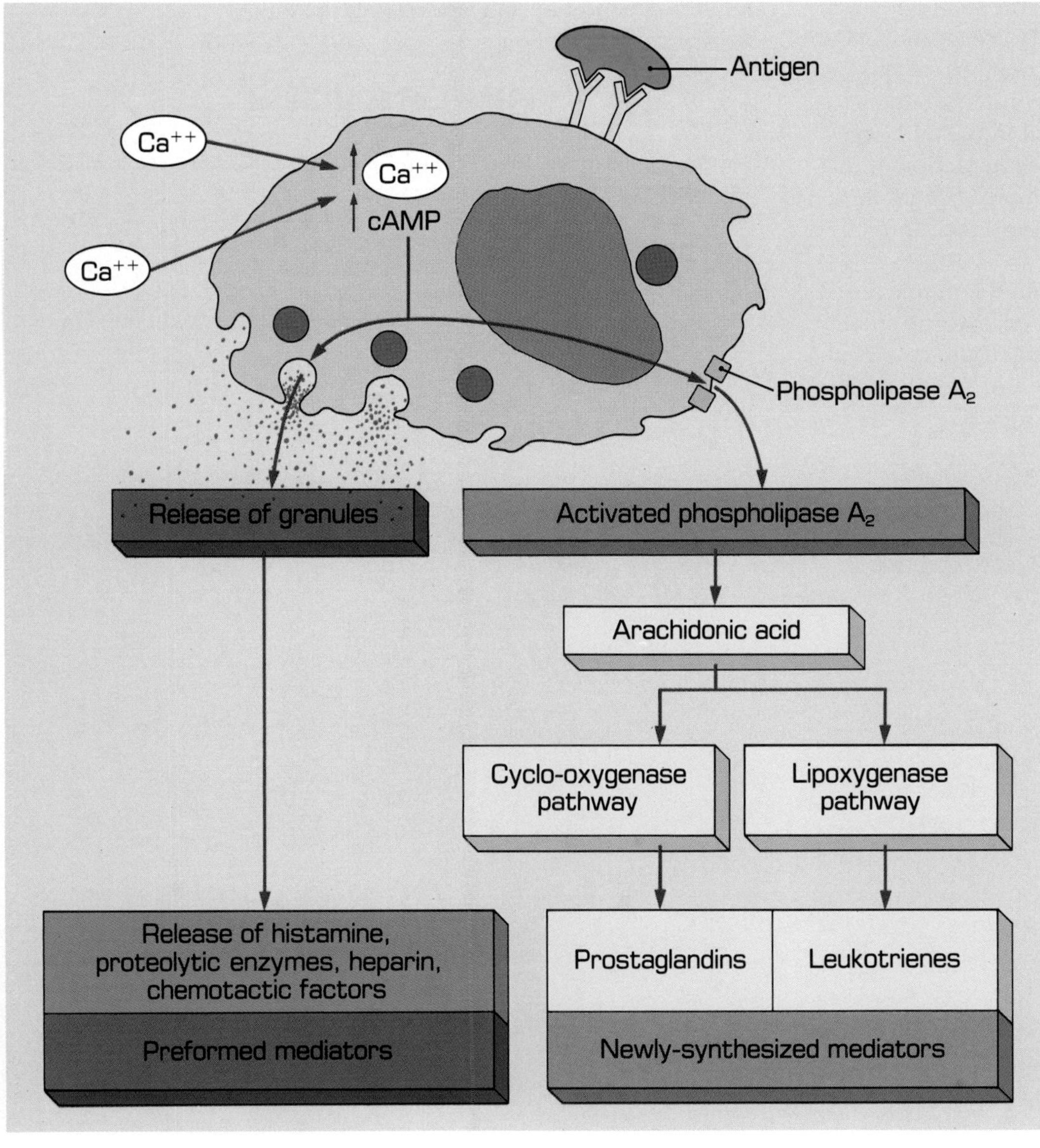

1.36 Mast cell activation. Immunologic triggers (antigen or IgE) perturb the mast cell membrane, causing a calcium ion influx which is essential to degranulation. Microtubule formation and movement of granules to the cell membrane lead to a fusion of the granules with the plasma membrane. In this way, the granule-associated mediators are released into the intercellular space. Plasma membrane activation allows phospholipase A_2 to release arachidonic acid, which is then metabolized by either lipoxygenase or cyclo-oxygenase enzymes, depending on the mast cell type. The end products of these two distinct pathways include prostaglandins and thromboxane (cyclo-oxygenase pathway), and leukotrienes (lipoxygenase pathway). (Reproduced with permission from Roitt *et al.*, 1995.)

Type III reaction

The Type III reaction is referred to as immune-complex injury or tissue damage. In this immunopathologic reaction, serum IgG antibodies interact with an antigen, but not necessarily at a cell surface or membrane. Antigen–antibody complexes are formed, usually in moderate antigen excess, when antigen and antibody concentrations are appropriate. These microprecipitates or complexes aggregate in and near blood vessels. They may induce inflammation in the tissues in which they are deposited, which leads to vascular damage and thrombosis. Frequently, these antigen–antibody complexes are formed in areas of high blood flow, with deposition occurring in such tissues as the kidneys, lungs, and walls of small blood vessels.

The antigen–antibody complexes activate the complement system, and components C_5, C_6, and C_7 attract polymorphonuclear leukocytes to the reaction site. Phagocytosis of the complexes may lyse many of the leukocytes, with the resultant release of the enzymes and other mediators responsible for the observed inflammation and tissue destruction. Clinical examples of this Type III reaction include serum sickness syndrome, acute post-streptococcal glomerulonephritis, and some collagen vascular diseases, especially systemic lupus erythematosus.

Type IV reaction

The Type IV reaction of Gell and Coombs is the cell-mediated immune response or delayed hypersensitivity reaction. The immunopathologic response in the Type IV reaction appears to be dependent on sensitized small T-lymphocytes; serum antibodies to the appropriate antigens have not been implicated in the pathogenesis of this immune reaction. There is no apparent interaction of the antigen with humoral antibodies, either at the cell membranes or in tissues, and it has been proposed that the antigens react directly with the sensitized lymphocytes.

After challenge with an antigen, the cell-mediated immune reaction results in the accumulation of mononuclear cells at the site of tissue injury within 24–48 hours. Activation of macrophages, local proliferation of mononuclear cells, and the release of lymphokines are important in the development of the delayed hypersensitivity, cell-mediated immune reaction. The lymphokines are the mediators of the cell-mediated delayed hypersensitivity reaction; these biologically active molecules include migration inhibitory factors, leukocyte chemotactic factors, lymphocytotoxin, lymphocyte-stimulating factor, and, perhaps, transfer factor. Complement does not appear to be involved in this reaction. Cell-mediated delayed hypersensitivity represents the pathophysiologic basis for contact dermatitis (*see* Chapter 14), as well as for many aspects of organ transplant and skin graft rejection phenomena. In certain pulmonary diseases (e.g., tuberculosis, fungal diseases, and sarcoidosis), the observed tissue damage and inflammation appear to be due to cell-mediated, delayed hypersensitivity responses of the hosts to various antigens.

CONCLUSION

The advances in immunology of the past several decades have enhanced our understanding of allergic diseases. Immunology has provided the clinician with a rational mechanism for many of the accepted diagnostic and therapeutic measures. It is anticipated that immunology will be the basis for a new and better understanding of diagnosis and therapy in the future. Subsequent chapters of this book further define and describe the major allergic diseases and the immunologic mechanisms underlying them.

REFERENCES

Abbas AK, Lichtman AH, Paber JS: *Cellular and Molecular Immunology*, Saunders, Philadelphia, 2nd edn, 1994.

Middleton E, Reed C, Ellis EF (eds): *Allergy: Principles and Practice,* C.V. Mosby, St Louis, 3rd edn, 1988.

Paul W: *Fundamental Immunology*, Raven Press, New York, 3rd edn, 1994.

Roitt IM, Brostoff J, Male DK: *Immunology*, Mosby, London, 4th edn, 1995.

Samter M, Talmage DW, Frank MM, *et al.*: *Immunologic Diseases,* Little, Brown & Co., Boston, 5th edn, 1995.

CHAPTER 2

Allergens

Philip Fireman
Mary Jelks

Allergens are those antigens responsible for clinical allergic diseases. They are usually proteins or glycoproteins capable of inducing synthesis of IgE antibodies, thereby sensitizing the potentially allergic person. Upon re-exposure to the same allergen, the previously sensitized patient manifests the signs and symptoms of allergy, as the allergen reacts with cell-related IgE tissue antibody and the cells generate the mediators of inflammation. It is imperative that the clinician link the circumstances of allergic disease to allergen exposure, as allergens represent important etiologic factors in the pathogenesis of allergy.

As shown in **2.1**, allergens can be classified on the basis of the nature or manner in which the patient is exposed. Those allergens responsible for allergic respiratory diseases, including allergic asthma and allergic rhinitis, are principally inhalants. These aero-allergens are responsible for the majority of all allergic diseases. Foods and other ingestants, including drugs, are also important, especially for allergic gastrointestinal and skin diseases. The contactants are principally responsible for allergic contact dermatitis. In addition to drugs, the injectant group includes the venoms and saliva of insects. This chapter is limited to a discussion of the inhalant allergens, since the other allergens are included and described in the separate chapters on food allergy, drug allergy, contact dermatitis, and anaphylaxis.

The inhalant allergens can be grouped as outlined in **2.2**. Pollens were the earliest known causes of allergic respiratory diseases, being identified as such in the nineteenth century. They remain the most commonly recognized today. The spores of fungi, often referred to as molds by clinicians, are especially important when airborne in those environments in which the humidity supports the growth of these organisms. Animal products, both mammalian and arthropod, have been increasingly recognized during the twentieth century as being causative factors in allergic diseases, as have other organic and inorganic dusts to which sufferers are exposed in the home and workplace.

POLLENS

Pollens are the viable male germinal cells that are essential for the reproduction of most seed plants. The sources of pollens include the trees, grasses, and weeds (**2.3**). Since pollen production is related to the life cycle of a given plant, the pollens usually have a seasonal or cyclic occurrence in the atmosphere. Because of this seasonal variation in atmospheric pollen, the patient who develops pollen allergy manifests a seasonal symptomatology, such as seasonal allergic rhinitis. In some tropical and subtropical regions of the world, however, climatic conditions show little annual variation and pollen prevalence may be perennial with a resultant perennial allergic rhinitis. (For the seasonal pattern of pollen distribution in North America and the seasonal pollen distribution in Europe, *see* **2.11** and **2.12**, respectively.) Algae are relatively uncommon inhalant allergens.

CLASSIFICATION OF ALLERGENS ACCORDING TO ROUTE OF EXPOSURE

Allergens

1. Inhalants
2. Ingestants
3. Contactants
4. Injectants

2.1 Classification of allergens according to the route through which they enter the body.

CLASSIFICATION OF INHALANT ALLERGENS

Inhalant allergens

1. Pollens
2. Fungi (Molds)
3. Animal products:
   — Mammalian
   — Arthropod
4. Dusts
5. Algae

2.2 Classification of inhalant allergens.

MAJOR SOURCES OF ALLERGENIC POLLENS

Sources of pollens

1. Trees
2. Grasses
3. Weeds

2.3 The three main sources of allergenic pollens.

Guidelines for the characterization of those pollens that can become potent allergens were initially postulated by Thommen in 1931 (**2.4**). In general, pollens that are wind-borne (anemophilous) are of greater clinical importance than those carried by insects (entomophilous). Thus, the pollens of attractive, brightly colored flowering plants are infrequently the cause of allergic diseases. These insect-borne pollens tend to be heavy, sticky, and less numerous. For example, the pollens of roses and golden rod are often incorrectly incriminated as important inhalant allergens, since their flowers bloom at the height of the grass pollen and ragweed pollen seasons, respectively. However, florists, landscapers, hobbyists, and others whose occupational or recreational pursuits increase their exposure do become sensitized to the pollens of flowering plants.

The buoyancy, relative size, and density of a pollen can contribute to its dispersion. Ragweed pollen has a long wind-borne range and has been detected many miles offshore. Certain plants are widely distributed and produce large amounts of pollen – a single ragweed plant may release a million pollen grains in one day. Trees, especially conifers such as pine, may release clouds of pollen (**2.5**), but these are generally less allergenic than ragweed. The onset of pollination for ragweed is predictable to within a margin of a few days, a characteristic that is important for clinical diagnosis. The seasonal patterns for the presence of airborne individual pollens is discussed below; clinicians should know the most prevalent pollen allergens in their area, as well as their seasonal patterns. Even though the seasonal appearance of the pollen is predictable, the amount produced in a given season varies, depending upon climatic conditions. Extended dry periods during plant development and growth reduce the eventual pollen production. Also, a rainy day during the pollen season reduces the amount of airborne pollen on that day, whereas a dry, windy day increases the airborne concentration.

In addition to allergen exposure, the allergenicity of the pollen is another important factor. It is not known what accounts for certain pollens being more potent sensitizing allergens than others. As discussed in other chapters, only a subset (10–20%) of the population becomes sensitized and shows allergic symptoms, even though the entire community is exposed to the allergens.

The quantification of pollens has been traditionally accompanied by collecting the pollen grains onto greased microscope slides using the Durham gravity system. It is only during the past two-to-three decades that impact samplers (Rotorod) and suction samplers (Burkard and/or Kramer–Collins) have been used, providing truly quantitative ways of measuring (**2.6**). As described below, the pollen grains have unique microscopic characteristics that are identifiable, making them countable when stained and examined under a microscope. Airborne pollen grains range in size from 5–60 μm. They are principally deposited in the upper airway and, because of their relative size, cannot reach the bronchi. Recently, immunochemical techniques have been developed which can identify the soluble allergen constituents of ragweed pollen. Using aerodynamic air samplers, ragweed allergenic particulates smaller than the intact ragweed pollen have been identified not only during the ragweed pollen seasons, but before and after as well. Such observations indicate that these smaller ragweed allergen particles, which cannot be identified microscopically, could penetrate not only the upper respiratory tract but also the bronchi and bronchioles. These types of studies have become very important in finding other amorphous airborne allergens which cannot be identified using microscopy.

WEEDS

Weeds are commonly defined as those annual plants that grow wildly and have little decorative or agricultural value. The pollens of weeds are common causes of seasonal allergic rhinitis. The distributions of the pollens of various weeds in North America and Europe are shown in **2.11** and **2.12**, respectively. The most notorious in the North America is ragweed, which is not a problem in the rest of

FACTORS CONTRIBUTING TO POLLEN ALLERGENICITY	
1. Wind-borne (anemophilous)	3. Produced in large quantity
2. Buoyant (of small particle size)	4. Potent antigen

2.4 Factors that contribute to the allergenicity of pollens. This schema was initially presented by Thommen in 1931.

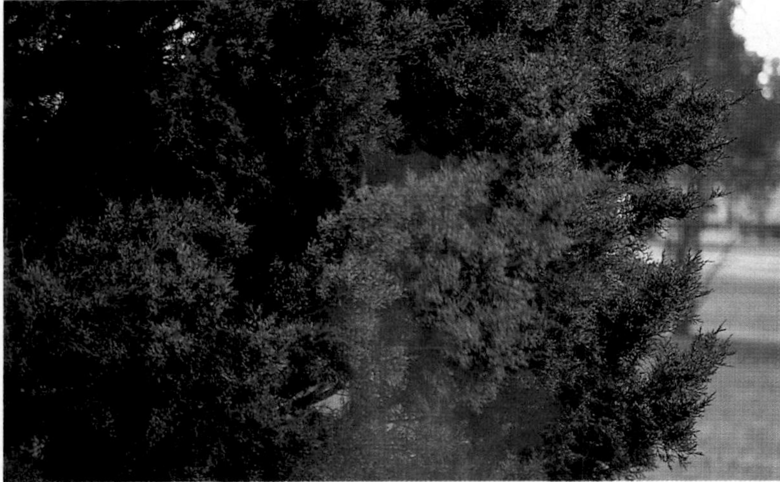

2.5 Cloud of pollen released from a juniper tree.

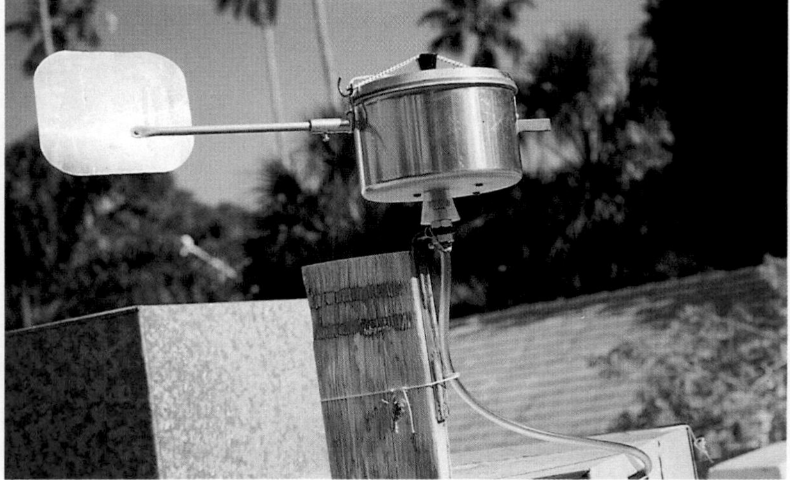

2.6 Kramer–Collins suction air sampler for the quantitative collection of pollens.

the world. It is most prevalent in the midwestern and northeastern areas of North America, where it is widespread (**2.11**). The most prevalant ragweeds are Short and Giant Ragweed – the latter can reach a stately 12 feet (3.7 m) in height (**2.7**) and the former, shown in **2.8**, is now found across all of North America. Its pollen is released in temperate areas as the days become shorter, with peak pollen counts in the northeastern and midwestern areas of the United States from mid-August to mid-September. In the southern and southwestern states, ragweed pollen (**2.9**) can be airborne throughout the spring, summer, and fall.

Botanically, ragweed is a member of the same composite family as many flowering plants, including chrysanthemums, marigolds, asters, some daisies, and sunflowers. These others, however, are only bothersome to those such as florists or gardeners who handle them regularly. Pyrethrum is an insecticide made from the flower heads of certain chrysanthemums, and inhalation of this compound can provoke symptoms in ragweed-allergic patients. The major allergens of ragweed have been isolated and characterized as Amb a I (antigen E) and Amb a II (antigen K). Commercial extracts of ragweed pollen used in clinical allergy testing and immunotherapy are now required by the US Food and Drug Administration (FDA) to be standardized to Amb a I content.

Depending on geographic locale, other weeds can be important allergens as well. English Plantain (**2.10**) can provoke significant allergic rhinitis, which can be confused with grass pollen allergy because English Plantain pollinates in May, June, and July – the same season during which grasses pollinate in the US and Canadian Northeast and Midwest. Sagebush (**2.14**) is found in the Southwestern United States and northern Mexico and is related to ragweed with which it sometimes cross-reacts. Prevelant also in this region are the pollens of Russian thistle and Burning Bush (**2.13**). Other cross-reactive allergenic weeds include Lamb's Quarter and Pigweed (**2.15**) whose pollens are microscopically similar and therefore grouped together by the family name, Chenopod–Amaranth, a combination of two families that have pollens that look alike and cross-react strongly.

Except for ragweed, the most common weeds in Europe (*see* **2.12**) are similar to those found in North America. These include nettle, plantain, dock, sage, mugwort, and Chenopod–Amaranth. Depending on the climate and the local geography, the pollination of weeds frequently coincides with that of grasses in both Europe and North America.

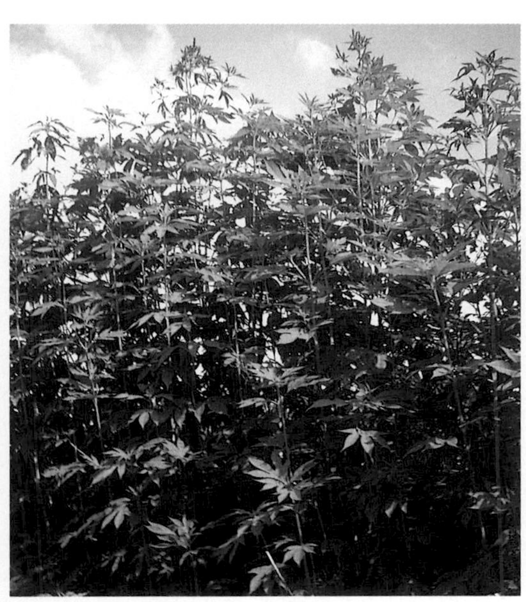

2.7 Giant Ragweed (*Ambrosia trifida*). One of the two common forms of ragweed in North America, this plant can reach heights of up to 12 feet (3.7 m).

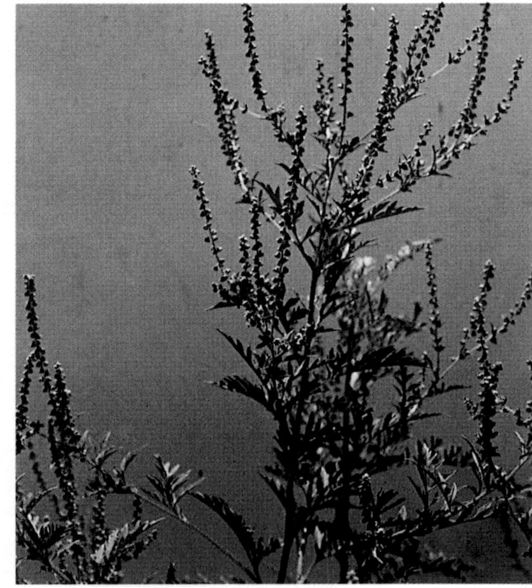

2.8 Short Ragweed (*Ambrosia artemisiifolia*). More widespread than Giant Ragweed, this plant is now found in much of North America, proliferating in more temperate climates. The pollen may be airborne throughout the year in some regions; peak counts generally occur during August and September.

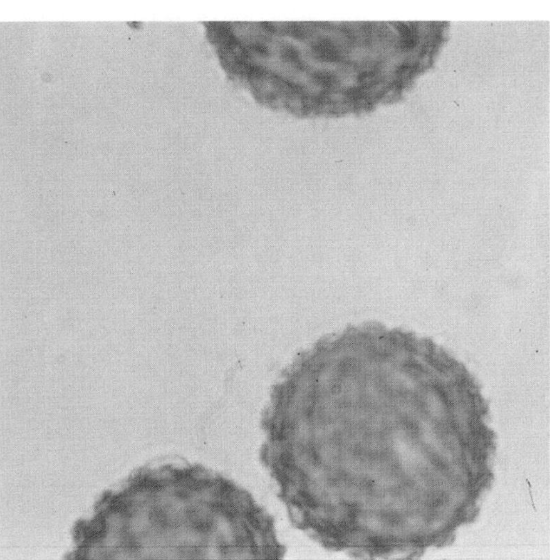

2.9 Ragweed pollen grains. Oil emersion photomicrograph, ×450. (Courtesy of Greer Laboratories.)

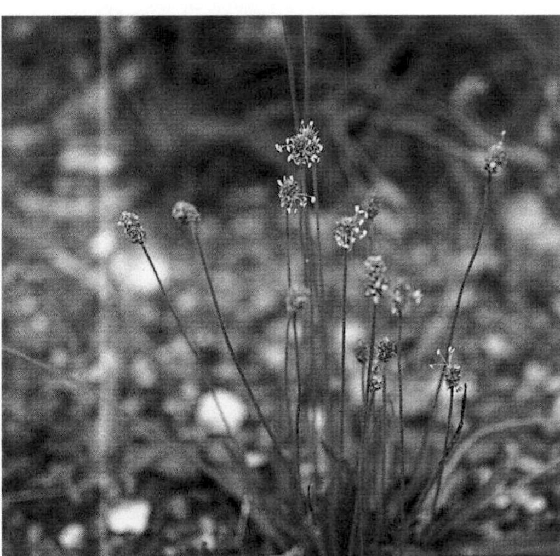

2.10 English Plantain. This plant pollinates during the same season as the grasses. It can trigger allergic rhinitis in some individuals, which may be confused with an allergic response to grass pollens.

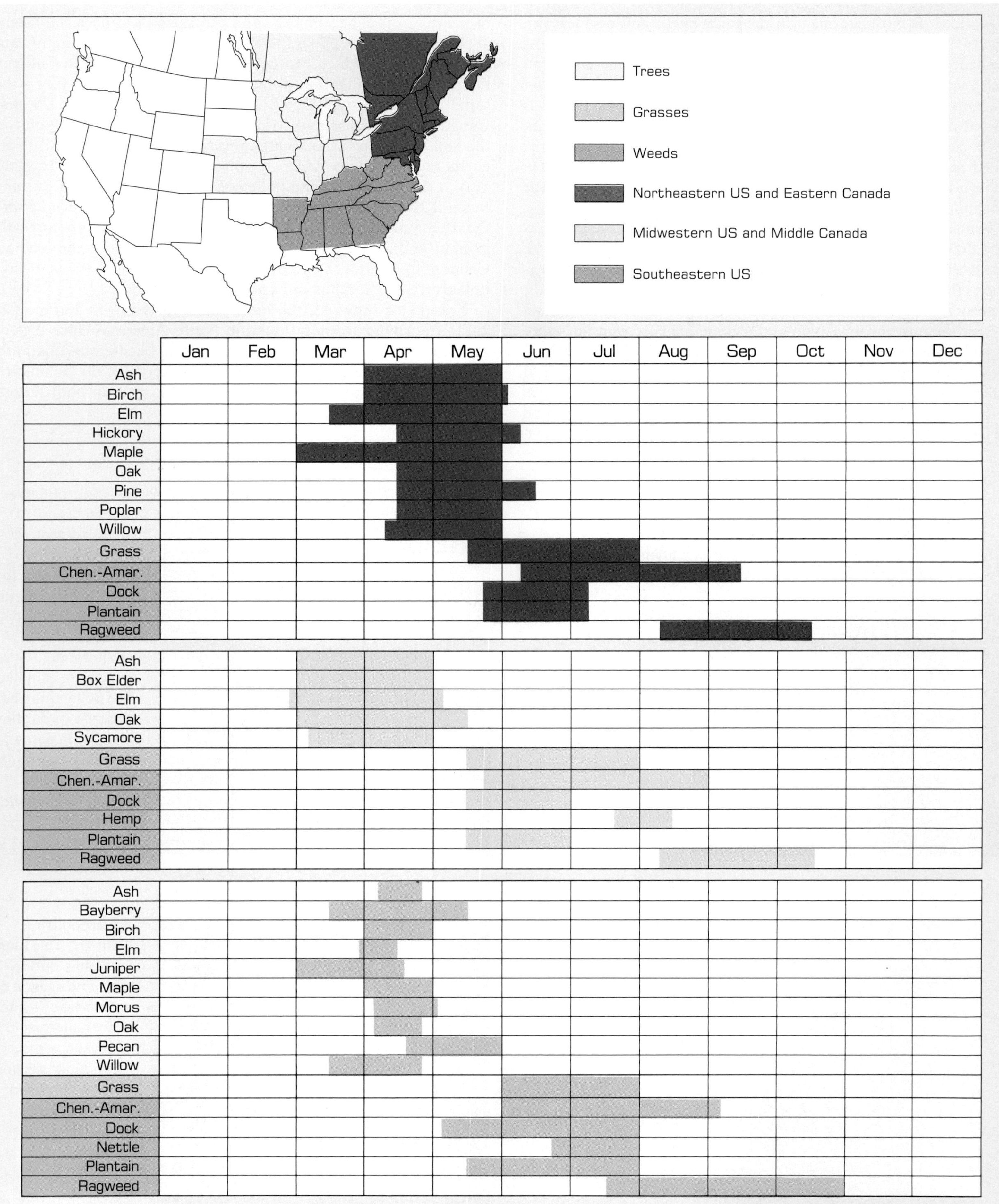

2.11 Geographic distribution of common allergenic pollens in the various regions of North America over the course of 1 year.

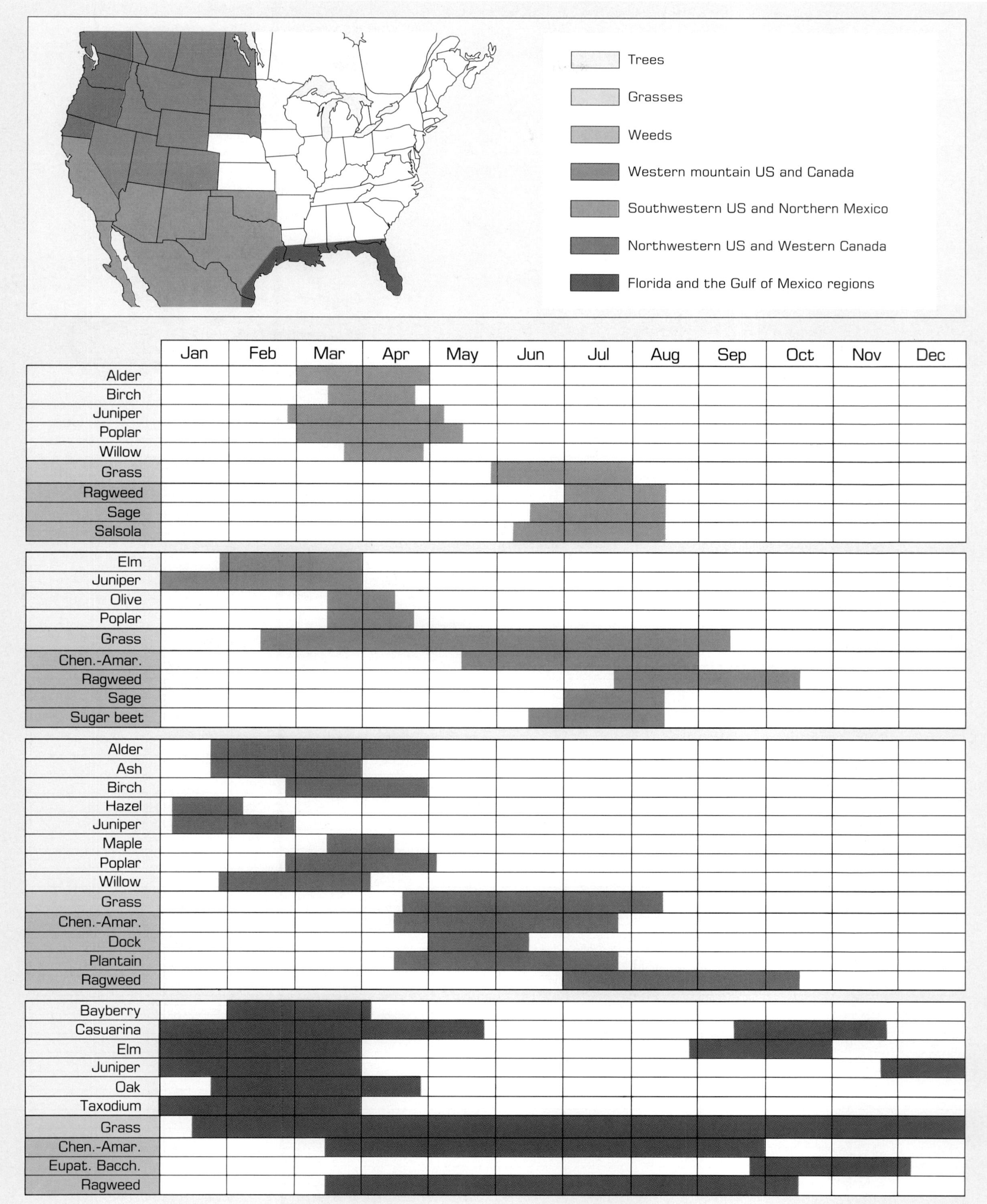

2.11 cont'd Geographic distribution of common allergenic pollens in the various regions of North America over the course of 1 year.

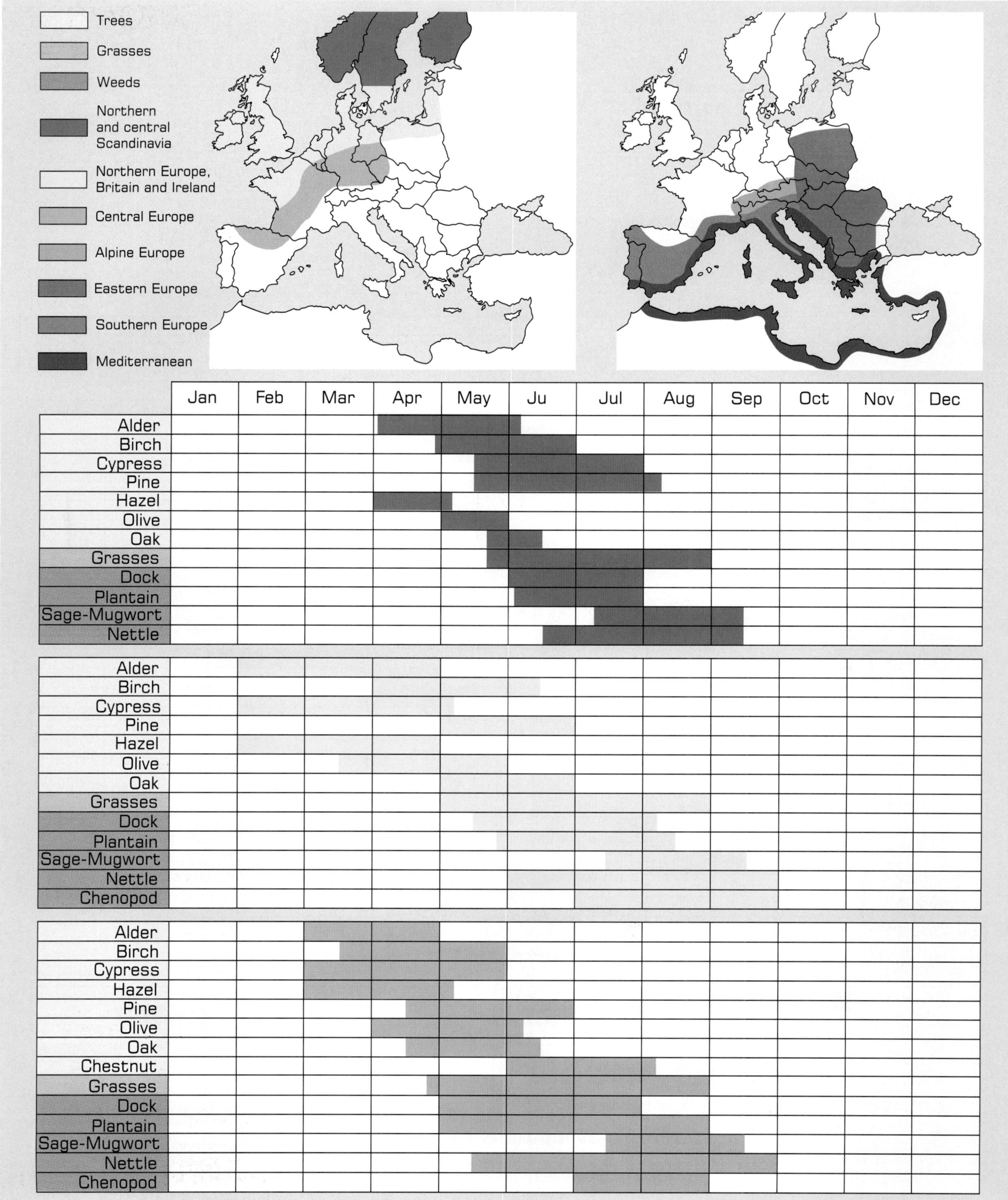

2.12 Seasonal pollen distribution in Europe.

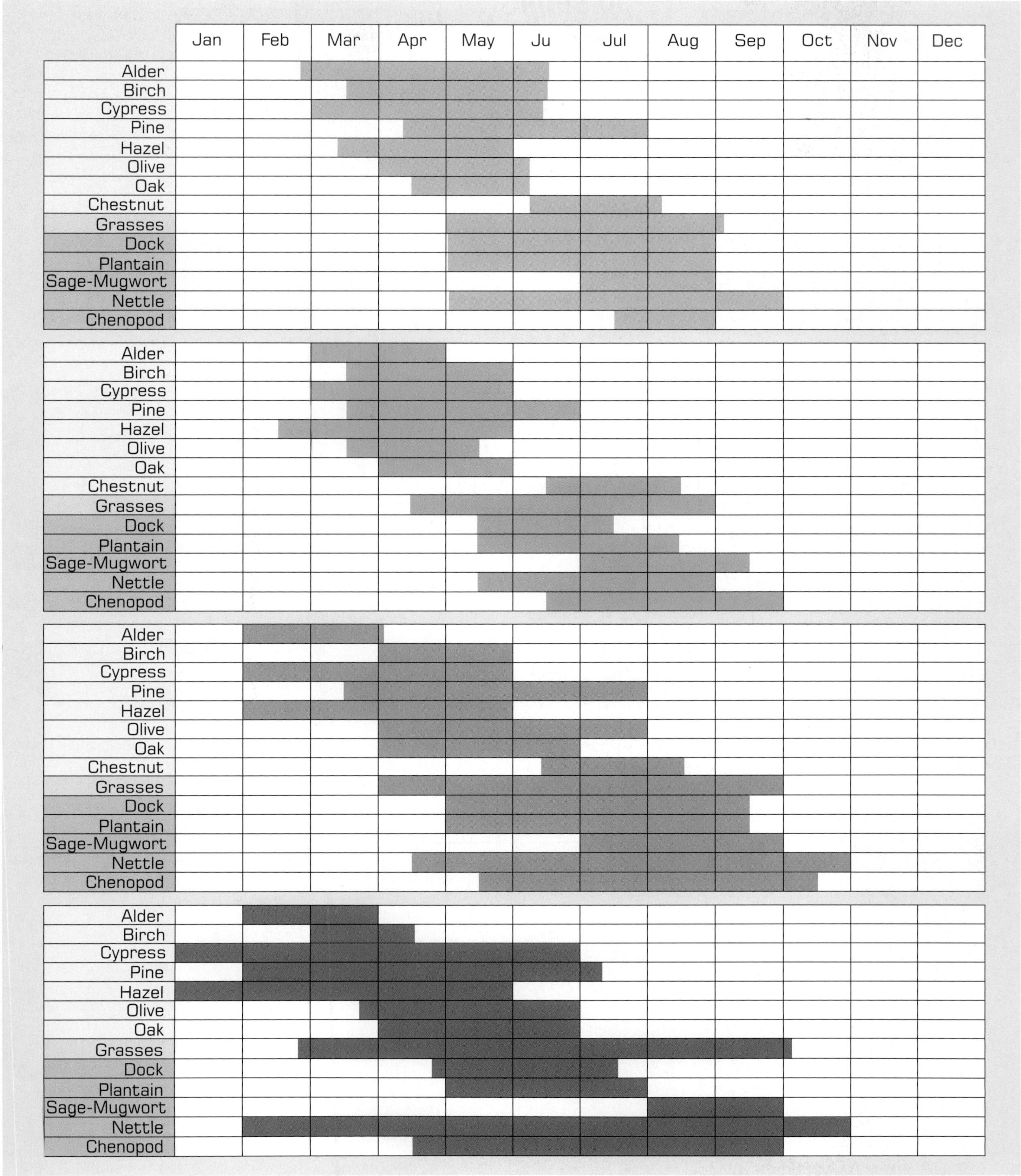

	Jan	Feb	Mar	Apr	May	Ju	Jul	Aug	Sep	Oct	Nov	Dec
Alder												
Birch												
Cypress												
Pine												
Hazel												
Olive												
Oak												
Chestnut												
Grasses												
Dock												
Plantain												
Sage-Mugwort												
Nettle												
Chenopod												

	Jan	Feb	Mar	Apr	May	Ju	Jul	Aug	Sep	Oct	Nov	Dec
Alder												
Birch												
Cypress												
Pine												
Hazel												
Olive												
Oak												
Chestnut												
Grasses												
Dock												
Plantain												
Sage-Mugwort												
Nettle												
Chenopod												

	Jan	Feb	Mar	Apr	May	Ju	Jul	Aug	Sep	Oct	Nov	Dec
Alder												
Birch												
Cypress												
Pine												
Hazel												
Olive												
Oak												
Chestnut												
Grasses												
Dock												
Plantain												
Sage-Mugwort												
Nettle												
Chenopod												

	Jan	Feb	Mar	Apr	May	Ju	Jul	Aug	Sep	Oct	Nov	Dec
Alder												
Birch												
Cypress												
Pine												
Hazel												
Olive												
Oak												
Grasses												
Dock												
Plantain												
Sage-Mugwort												
Nettle												
Chenopod												

2.12 cont'd Seasonal pollen distribution in Europe.

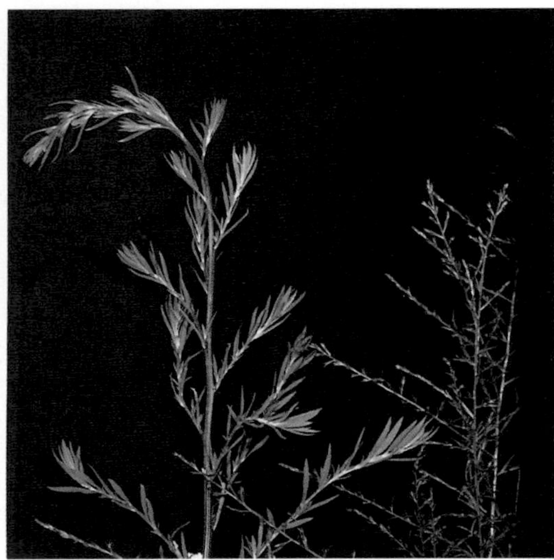

2.13 Burning Bush, also known as Mexican Fireweed (left, foreground), and Russian thistle. These are common, often cross-reactive allergenic plants in the prairie and western North America.

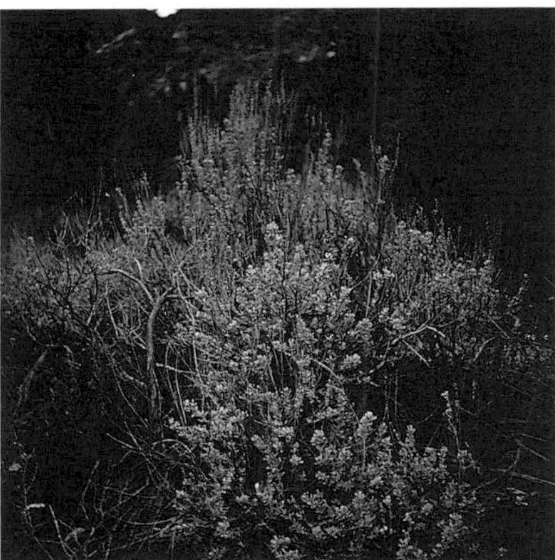

2.14 Sage-brush. This is another of the common allergenic plants in the western regions of North America. (Courtesy of Greer Laboratories.)

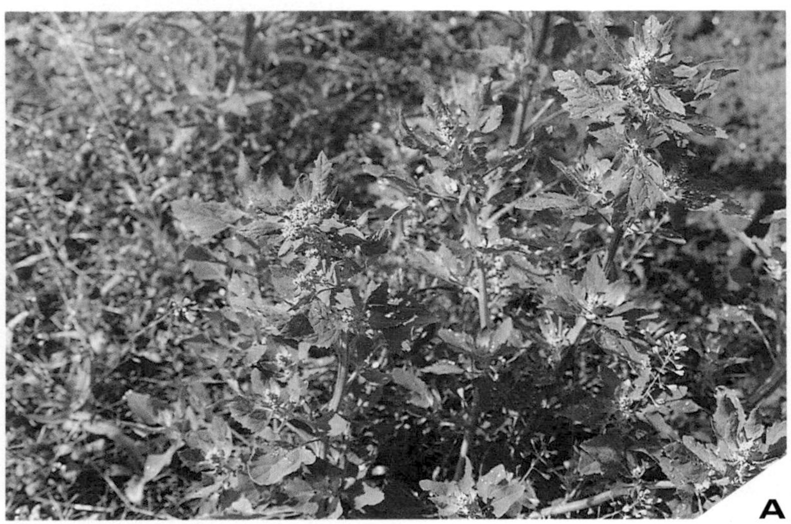

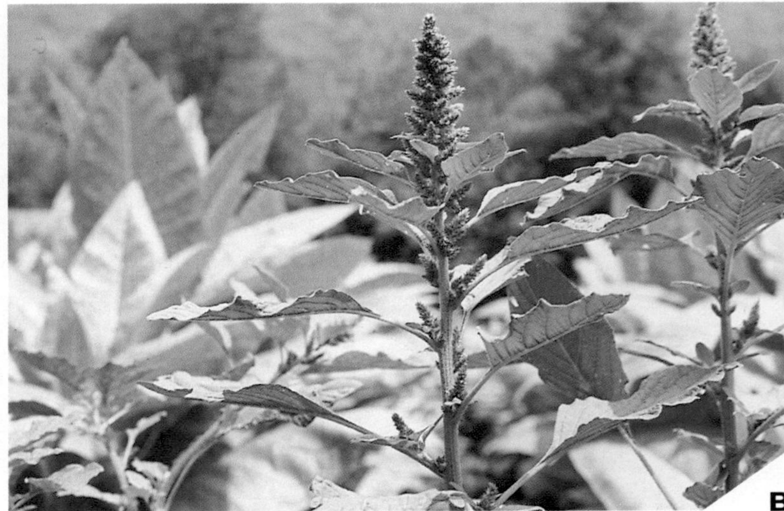

2.15 (A) Lamb's Quarter (*Chenopodium album*) and (B) Pigweed (*Amaranthus retroflexus*). The microscopic similarity between the pollen grains of these two plants has led to their classification under a combined family name of Chenopod–Amaranth.

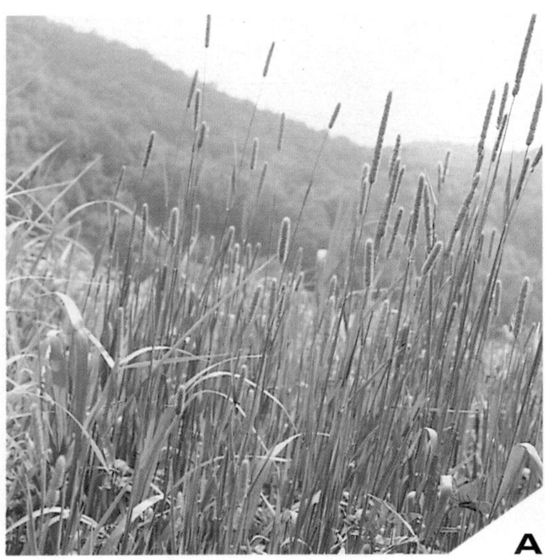

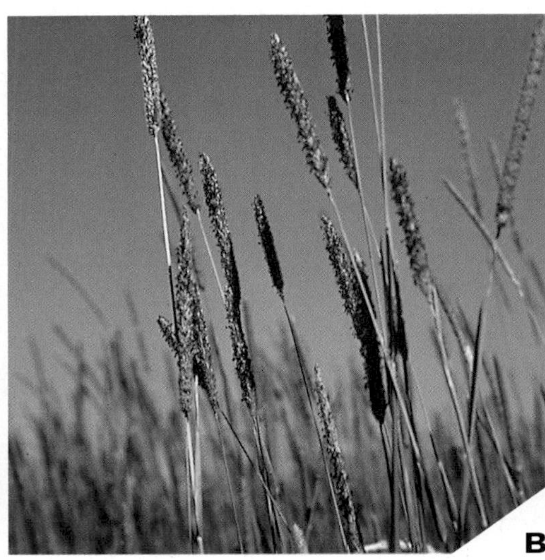

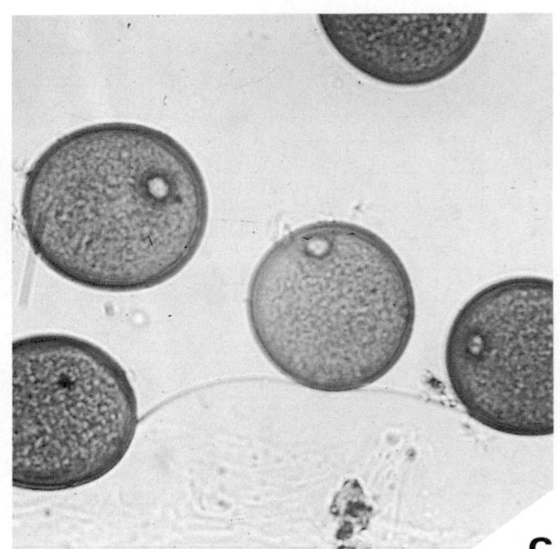

2.16 (A) Timothy grass as it appears in the field. (B) Closer view showing detail of the Timothy grass plant, which is widely cultivated as hay. (Courtesy of Hollister–Stier Laboratories.) (C) Timothy grass pollen. Oil emersion photomicrograph, ×450. (Courtesy of Greer Laboratories.)

GRASSES

In Europe, grasses are the most important causes of pollen allergy. Allergic rhinitis was described initially in England, in 1889 by Blackley, as *hay fever* because of the association of nasal symptoms with the harvesting of the forage grass, Timothy, which is used to make hay (**2.16**). Most of the grasses are cultivated either agriculturally or ornamentally and are prevalent where people live. The considerable production of pollen by these widespread plants contributes to the frequency of symptoms associated with grasses. The pollens of the different grasses vary in size from 20–40 μm, and they all have a single germinal pore which makes them difficult to distinguish microscopically (**2.16C**).

Only about a dozen of the more than 5000 species of grass are important allergens, since many of the grasses do not produce abundant pollen. As shown in **2.11** and **2.12**, the bulk of the airborne grass pollen in the northern United States, Canada, and Europe is present in the late spring and early summer, from May to July. The important early grasses include Sweet, Vernal, and Orchard (**2.17**), which are followed by Timothy, Bluegrass, Fescue, Redtop, and Perennial Ryegrass (**2.18A–2.18C**). All of these grasses show considerable allergen cross-reactivity, but they are allergenically distinct from the

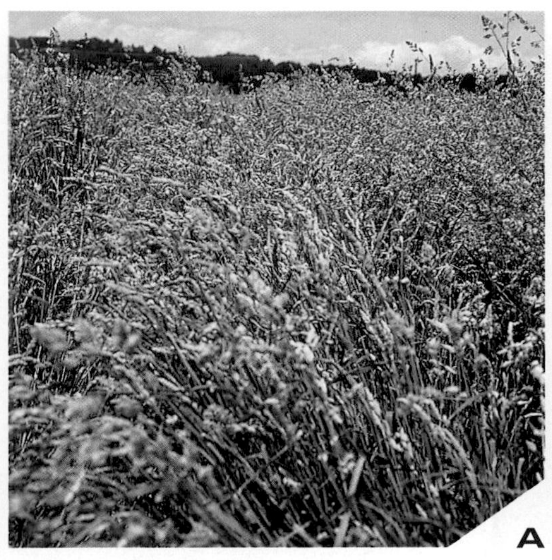

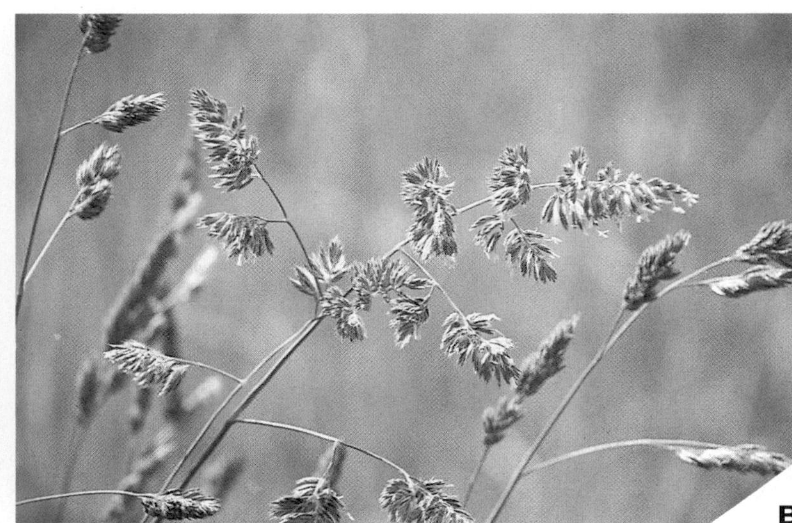

2.17 Orchard grass (A) in the field and (B) close-up. The allergenic pollen of this grass reaches peak levels in the early summer. (Courtesy Hollister–Stier Laboratories.)

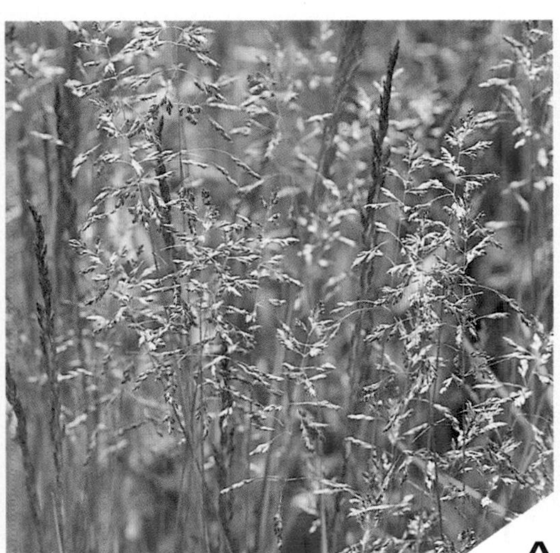

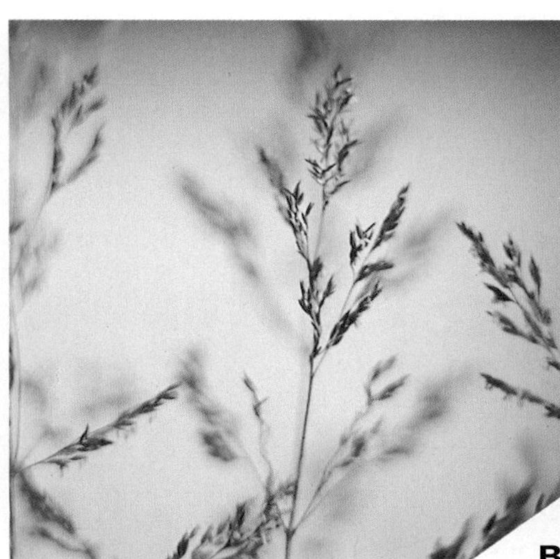

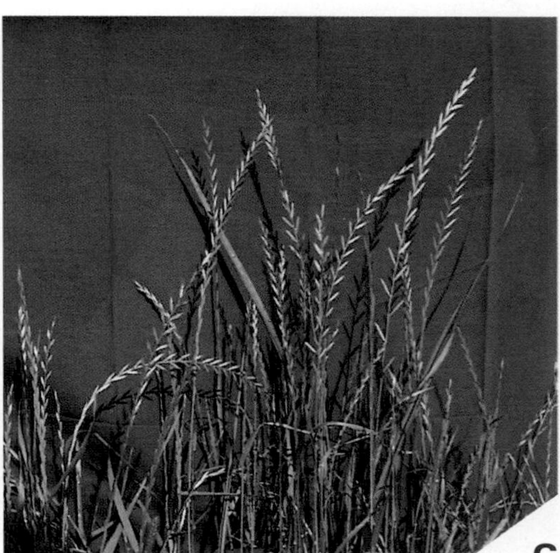

2.18 (A) Bluegrass, (B) Redtop grass, and (C) Perennial Ryegrass. Though allergenically distinct, these three grasses show considerable cross-reactivity. (A and B courtesy of Greer Laboratories.)

southern grasses. In the southern United States, Bermuda grass is found nearly all year round, and Johnson and Salt grasses also have long seasons (**2.19A–2.19C**). In southern Europe and the Mediterranean areas, grasses may pollinate from February to October.

TREES

Tree pollens are prevalent world-wide, but because of a shorter pollen season in most countries, they do not produce as much allergic disease as do the grasses and weeds. The fruit-bearing trees, such as apple, pear, peach, etc., are insect-pollinated and their pollens are not relevant in most clinical allergy. Still, trees should not be ignored. In much of North America and Europe, the pollen seasons for trees precede those of the weeds and grasses, making any unseasonal symptoms easy to relate to the tree pollens. There is some cross-reactivity among the tree pollens, as among the grass pollens.

In the Mediterranean and southern Europe areas, cypress and hazel tree pollens can appear as early as January, whereas in the northeastern forests of North America and Europe, the earliest tree pollens appear in March and April, with the release of pollen from the birch, elm, maple, ash, alder, and hazel trees (**2.20A–2.20D**). Birch is a major allergen in Scandinavian countries. Oak trees (**2.21A–2.21C**) shed more pollen than many other plants, and are present in all of Europe

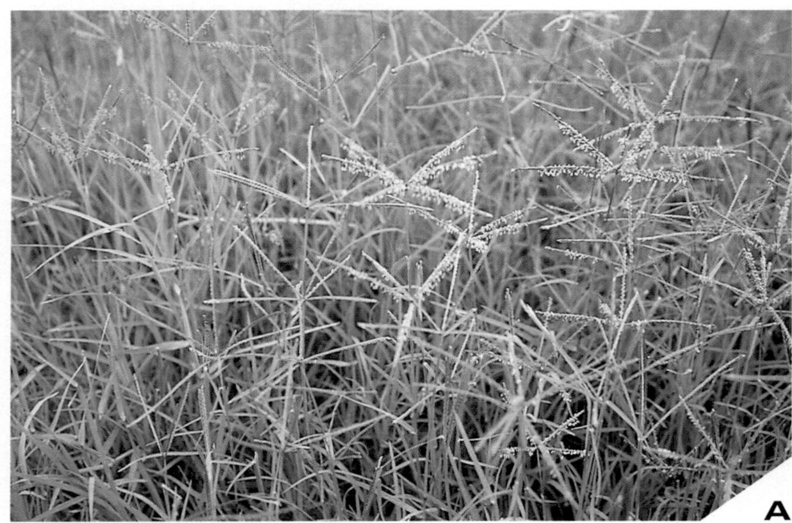
A

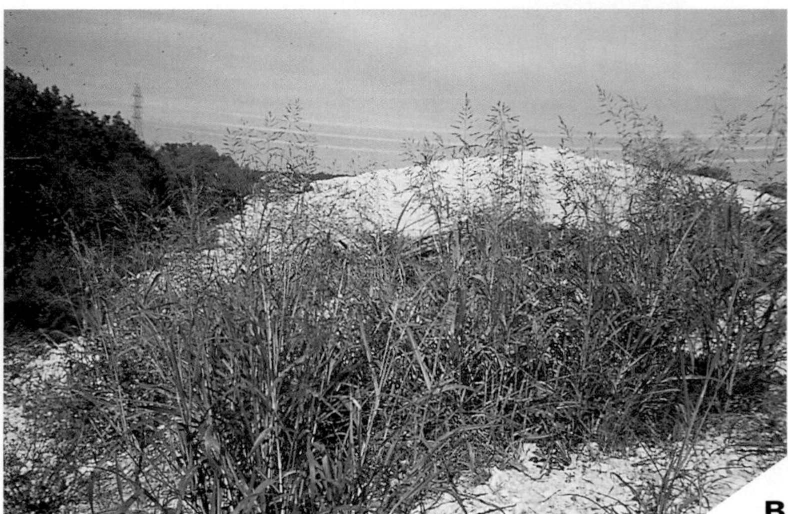
B

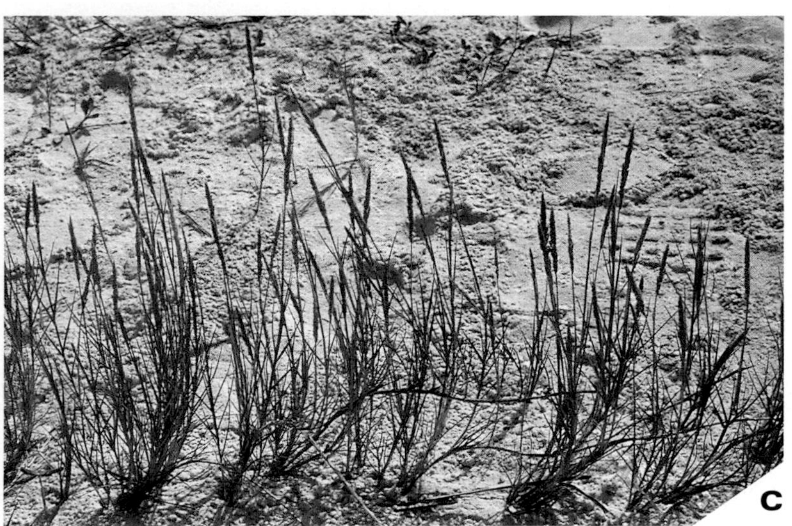
C

2.19 (A) Bermuda, (B) Johnson, and (C) Salt grasses. These three plants have long seasons in the southern regions of North America. (A and B courtesy of Hollister–Stier Laboratories.)

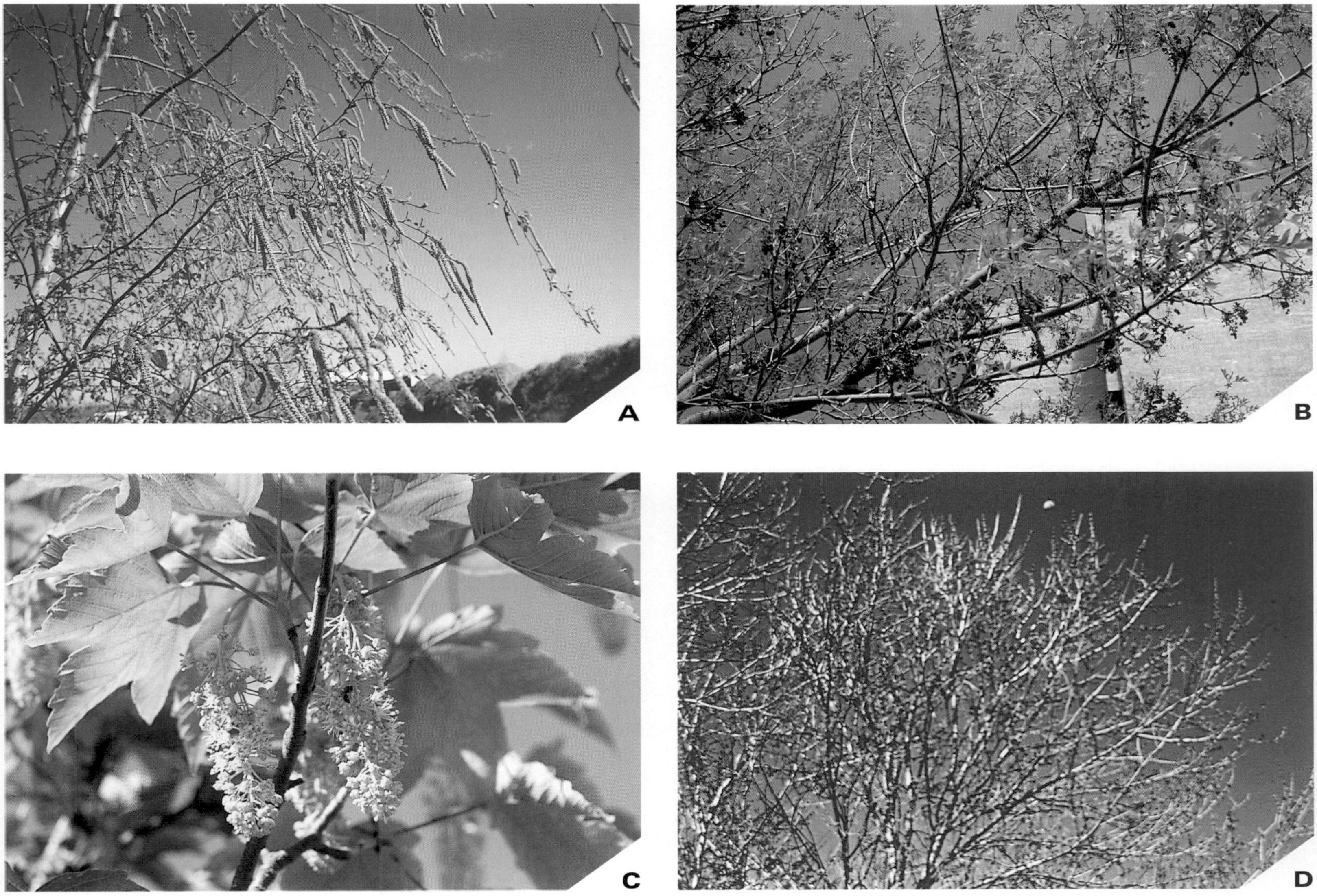

2.20 (A) Birch, (B) Ash, (C) Maple, and (D) Red Maple trees in spring bloom. Pollens from these trees begin to reach peak levels in the very early spring. (Courtesy of Hollister–Stier Laboratories.)

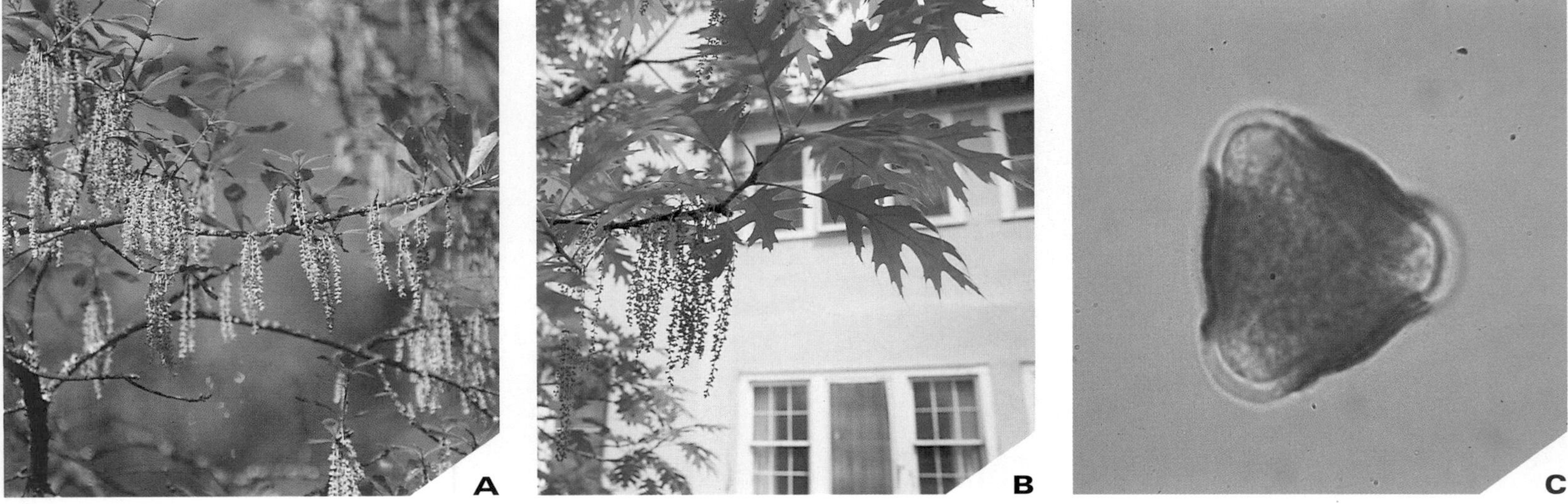

2.21 (A) Water Oak and (B) Black Oak as they appear in the spring. (C) Oil emersion photomicrograph of Oak pollen, ×450. (Courtesy of Greer Laboratories.)

and North America except Alaska and Hawaii. In the northern areas, airborne oak pollens are present in April and May, whereas in the southern areas these and others can appear as early as February. In general, the conifer (pine) trees produce large amounts of pollen, but cause modest allergies, with the exception of the Mountain Cedar (**2.22**) in Texas and the Japanese Cedar in California and Japan.

FUNGI (MOLDS)

Fungi are saprophytic organisms that are present throughout the world. Most fungi, even mushrooms, produce airborne spores that can become important inhalant allergens. As allergens, fungi can be detected both out- and indoors, and may show seasonal or perennial presence. It is helpful in clinical practice to group the mold spores as field (seasonal) or storage (perennial), even though this classification may not always be precise (**2.23**). Like the pollens, some of the molds can be collected and identified microscopically by outdoor air samplers, and they tend to show seasonal patterns in temperate climates. Their numbers increase in the air during the warm months, decrease when hard frost prevents growth, and they are absent when the ground is snow covered. In those areas of the world without a winter season, outdoor mold spores can be perennial aero-allergens. Alternaria and Cladosporium (Hormodendrum) (**2.24A–2.24C**) are the most numerous in late summer and early fall. These molds are saprophytic fungi and grow on decaying leaves and dead plants. They are often increased atmospherically in the daytime. Some, such as Drechslera (Helminthosporium), grow abundantly on grasses, cereal crops and in the soil and are more numerous in subtropical climates.

The storage molds, such as Aspergillus and Penicillium (**2.25A** and **2.25B**), can grow in areas with a lower humidity, by 15% or more. These are the organisms most typically found in sheds, barns,

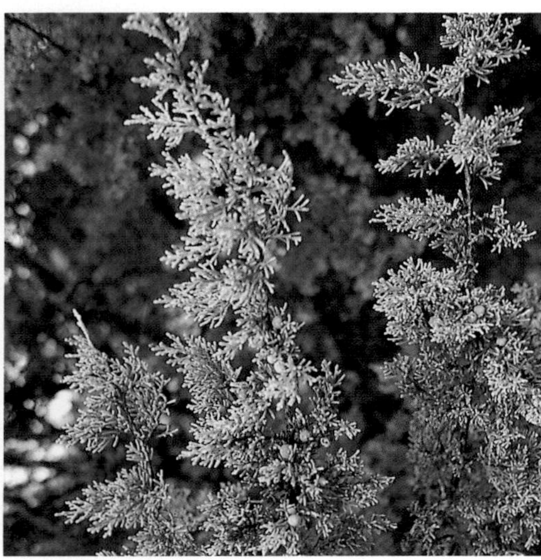
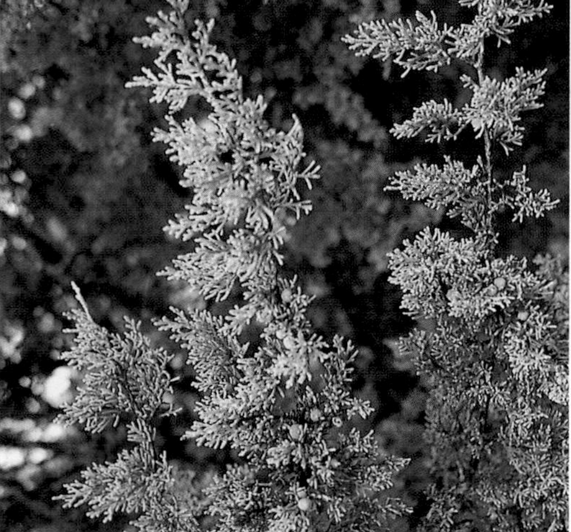

2.22 Mountain Cedar. This is one of the conifers that causes allergic responses in sensitive people. (Courtesy of Hollister–Stier Laboratories.)

CLASSIFICATION OF COMMON ALLERGENIC FUNGAL (MOLD) SPORES

Field (seasonal)	Storage (perennial)
— Alternaria	— Aspergillus
— Cladosporium (Hormodendrum)	— Penicillium
— Helminthosporium, Drechslera	— Epicoccum
— Epicoccum	

2.23 Classification of common allergenic fungal (mold) spores.

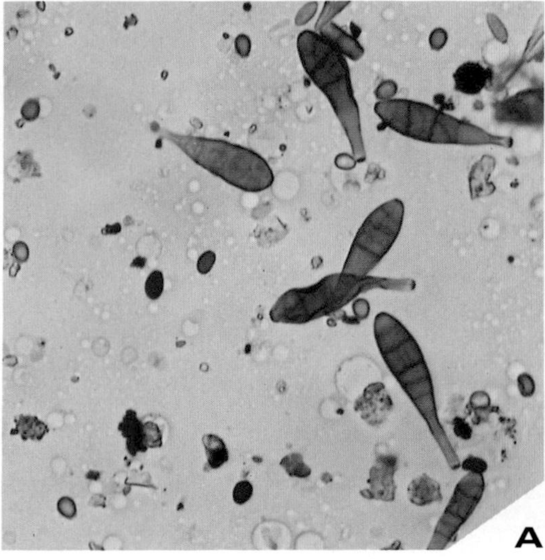

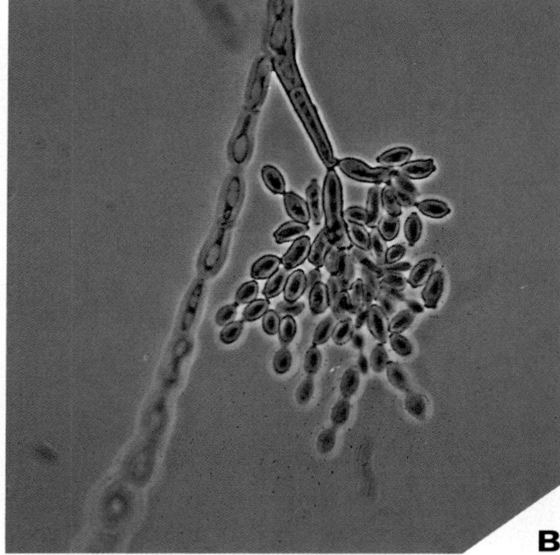

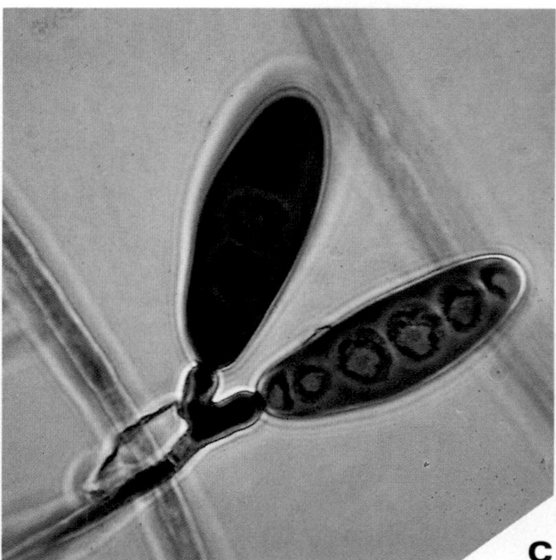

2.24 Photomicrograph of spores of (A) Alternaria (courtesy of Dr William Solomon), (B) Cladosporium, and (C) Drechslera (Helminthosporium). (B and C courtesy of Greer Laboratories.)

and homes, especially in basements and crawl spaces. Aspergillus is also commonly found in rotted or stored grains or vegetables. Penicillium is the green 'mildew' seen typically on items stored in damp basements. Epicoccum can be found both in storage areas and in a seasonal aero-allergen. Molds can also often be found in damp bathrooms and greenhouses. Vaporizers, humidifiers, and air conditioners which have water storage units can become contaminated with fungi, then becoming a source of aerosolized mold spores. The potential of fungal allergy should not be ignored since recent studies have indicated that about 25% of asthmatics in large cities, such as London and Cleveland, Ohio, had positive immediate skin tests to Aspergillus.

The detection of storage molds in an indoor environment can be accomplished by placing uncovered plates of growth media, such as Sabouraud's, in the suspected room or area for 10 minutes. After incubating the plates, the growing fungal colonies are identified and enumerated. Aerodynamic air sampling can be used to inoculate culture plates, and immunochemical detection of fungal allergens has been employed recently to detect mold allergens in office buildings with mold-contaminated air conditioning or ventilation systems.

ANIMAL PRODUCTS

Airborne animal allergens are important causes of clinical allergy. It has been known for years that exposure to domestic animals, either as household pets or as livestock, can provoke respiratory allergy (**2.26**). Symptoms of allergy have occurred not only in owners of dogs and cats, but also in veterinarians, farmers, and laboratory workers exposed to horses, cattle, sheep, and rodents, including rabbits, rats, mice, and guinea pigs. The hair or fur of these animals was initially incriminated as allergenic, but in truth it is neither buoyant nor of a suitable size to become an inhalant allergen. It has subsequently been shown that the desquamated epithelium, also known as dander, that is attached to the hair becomes aerosolized and is a potent allergen (**2.27**). Epithelial desquamation is a constant process in mammals and is a continual source of aerosolized, highly allergenic proteins.

It is common for animal allergic individuals to develop urticaria at sites where they have been licked by a cat or dog, or scratched by its claws or teeth. Among the house pets, cats seem to cause the more prominent symptoms. Recent studies have shown that the

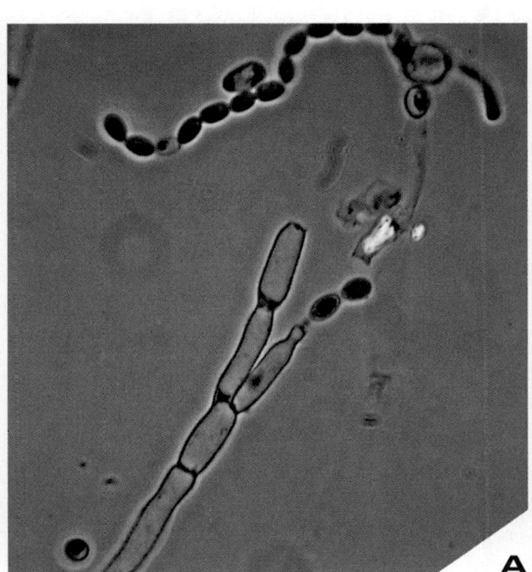

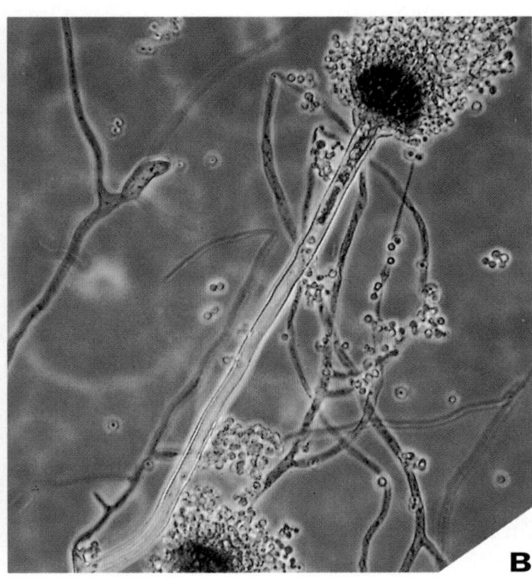

2.25 Photomicrographs of (A) Penicillium spores and (B) Aspergillus flavus spores. Both of these common storage molds can grow in low-moisture conditions. They tend to be found in sheds, barns, and basements. (Courtesy of Greer Laboratories.)

ANIMAL SOURCES OF INHALANT ALLERGENS

Mammalian
Cat, dog, horse, cattle, sheep,
Rabbit, guinea pig, rat, mouse

Birds

Arthropods
House dust mite, cockroach

2.26 Classification of animals known to produce inhalant allergens.

ANIMAL INHALANT ALLERGENS

Epidermal	Excretions
— Dander (desquamated epithelium)	— Saliva
— Cuticle (body)	— Urine
	— Feces

2.27 Common inhalant allergens from animal sources.

most important cat allergen is found in both saliva and sebaceous glands of the skin. A cat deposits saliva on its fur during grooming, and large amounts of this allergen can be aerosolized or recovered when the animal is brushed or washed. It has also been suggested that cat urine can become aerosolized from litter pans and act as an allergen. Dog allergens have been shown on fur, in dander, saliva, and serum proteins. It has been suggested that some breeds of dogs are less allergenic than others, but this may be more quantitative than qualitative, and related to frequency of grooming.

Rodent inhalant allergens cause illness in about 20% of exposed laboratory animal workers. It is the urinary proteins of mice, rats, and guinea pigs, as well as their dander, that can be allergenic. Remarkable levels of mouse aero-allergens have been found in older New York City tenements as compared to newer suburban middle- and upper-class homes. Feathers of pet birds, as well as of chickens, ducks, and geese, have been found to be a significant source of inhalant allergens, especially when used as down in pillows, bedding, and garments. It is unclear whether it is the pulverized feather or another associated protein that becomes the aerosolized allergen.

Human sperm is a known contactant to other humans in certain cases, and the possibility that human dander is also allergenic to other humans has been proposed but not substantiated.

For years, house dust has been recognized as a potent aero-allergen, but only recently has its principal allergenic component been shown to be a mite (**2.28**). House dust or mattress mites (*Dermatophygoides*), as well as other mite species, are found world-wide, with *Dermatophygoides pteronyssius* being more common in Europe and *Dermatophygoides farinae* more so in the United States. There is, however, considerable overlap. These arthropods cannot be seen without magnification, but they can be identified microscopically with lower power lenses. They feed on human or animal dander, molds, and other high-protein debris found in human environmental dusts. The highest concentrations of mites have been found in mattresses, pillows, rugs, upholstered furniture, and vacuum sweepings. For optimal propagation, mites require temperatures of 25–30°C, and humidity greater than 50%. In temperate climates, they attain their maximum numbers in early fall, but the animals can survive lower temperatures and humidity as well. They are rarely found in arid climates or at high altitudes.

The major mite allergen has been found in the spherical mite fecal particles. The shape and 25 μm size make these particles comparable to many pollens. Moderate amounts of mite allergen are found in the body cuticle. In the United States and England, 10% of the population and 80–90% of allergic asthmatics have positive immediate skin tests to dust mite allergen. Reduction in mite exposure by reducing its environmental concentration leads to lower levels of specific IgE antibody and fewer allergic symptoms. About 10% of house dust allergic patients in the United States do not react to skin testing with dust mites; they are reactive to another allergenic constituent in the environmental house dust.

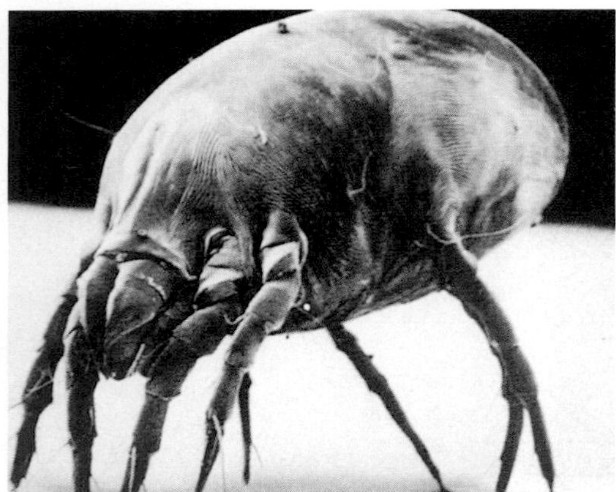

2.28 House dust mite (*Dermatophygoides farinae*). This, and other species of mites, comprise the principal allergenic component of common house dust.

The cockroach can also introduce an important aero-allergen into the household dusts of certain environments. Studies comparing air samples in crowded New York tenements versus suburban middle-class homes showed comparable concentrations of house dust mite allergen, but remarkably higher levels of cockroach allergen in the older urban apartments. Like the dust mite, the major cockroach allergens are related to the gastrointestinal tract or the feces. More studies are needed. Another arthropod, the mayfly, can be an outdoor inhalant allergen during the summer months along the Great Lakes. The major allergen of the mayfly is thought to be in its body.

ENVIRONMENTAL DUST

A variety of inhalant airborne allergens have been defined for various occupations – these are described in detail in Chapter 6. They include organic dusts, such as baker's flour, grain mill dust, enzymes used in laundry detergents, trimellitic anhydride, plicatic acid from wood dust, and toluene di-isocyanate, as well as the salts of nickel, chrome, and platinum. Kapok, a plant fiber from the Kapok tree, is very resilient and has been used in pillows and upholstered furniture. It is impervious to water, making it a useful material for boat cushions and life jackets. When pulverized and airborne, kapok is a potent allergen. It is being replaced by various synthetic polymers in pillows and cushions.

Occasionally, foods become aerosolized allergens during cooking. If inhaled by a sensitive person, certain food allergens may provoke severe respiratory allergy. However, most food-allergic individuals manifest their reactions, which can include respiratory symptoms, after ingestion of the specific food (*see* Chapter 13).

Some clinicians feel that respiratory complaints related to our environment have increased in the past several decades. Such terms as 'Sick Building Syndrome' and 'Twentieth Century Syndrome' have been coined to describe patients whose symptoms might be related to exposure to inhaled substances from closed environments with inadequate ventilation. Some of these complaints may be related to specific inhalant allergies. However, in evaluating such patients, the clinician must be careful not to label chemical or physical irritants as allergens, even if these inhalants provoke symptoms of asthma and rhinitis. Such non-allergic irritants, which can exacerbate respiratory disease, include sulfur dioxide, cigarette smoke, cold air, auto exhaust fumes, hair sprays, perfumed aerosols, and solvent vapors. These substances may directly provoke the activation of mediators of inflammation, such as histamine, which then cause respiratory symptoms without any mediation by an antibody and allergen reaction. To be identified and incriminated as an allergen, these inhalants must induce an IgE-mediated immune response as well as provoke respiratory symptoms.

REFERENCES

Adolphson CR, Gleich GJ, Yunginger JW: Standardization of allergens, in Rose NR, Friedman H, Foley JL (eds): *Manual of Clinical Laboratory Immunology*, American Society for Microbiology, Washington DC, 3rd edn, 1986.

Baer H, Anderson MC, Turkletaub PC: Allergenic extracts, in Middleton E, Jr, Reed CE, Ellis EF (eds): *Allergy: Principles and Practice*, C.V. Mosby, St. Louis, 3rd edn, 1988.

D'Amato G, Spieksma, FTM, Bonni, S: *Allergenic Pollen and Pollenosis in Europe*, Blackwell, Oxford, 1991.

Farnham JE, Vaida GA: A new look at New England tree pollen. *NE Soc Allergy Proc*, 3:320–326, 1982.

Gutman AA: Allergens and other factors important in atopic disease, in Patterson R (ed.): *Allergy Diseases*, J.B. Lippincott, Philadelphia, 3rd edn, p. 123, 1985.

Jelks M: *Allergy Plants that Cause Wheezing and Sneezing*, Worldwide, 1986.

Lewis WH, Vinay P, Zenger V: *Airborne and Allergenic Pollens of North America*, Johns Hopkins Univ. Pr., Baltimore, 1983.

Marsh DG, Goodfriend L, Krig TP *et al*:: Allergen nomenclature. *Bull WHO*, **64**:767, 1986.

Solomon W, Mathews KP: Aerobiology and inhalant allergens, in Middleton E, Jr, Reed CE and Ellis EF (eds): *Allergy: Principles and Practice*, C.V. Mosby, St. Louis, 3rd edn, 1988.

Yunginger JW: Allergens: Recent advances, in *Pediatric Clinics of North America*, 35:981, WB Saunders, Philadelphia, 1988.

CHAPTER 3

Diagnostic Tests in Allergy

Raymond G. Slavin

The diagnosis of allergic diseases should always begin with the procurement of a careful patient history and an appropriate physical examination. When an allergic disorder is suggested on these clinical grounds, there are a variety of procedures that can be used to confirm the diagnosis. Diagnostic tests can also be helpful in ruling out allergic disorders and clarifying the specific responsible antigens or allergens.

SKIN TESTS

Skin testing is the tool used most widely to diagnose clinical allergies. The basic procedure involves delivering an aqueous solution of antigen beneath the stratum corneum and barrier zone of the epidermis. As the antigen combines with IgE antibody fixed to mast cells, mediator substances, particularly histamine, are released from the mast cells. The mediators cause local vasodilation and increased capillary permeability. Wheal-and-flare reactions appear within 15–20 minutes (**3.1** and **3.2A–3.2C**). A typical scoring system is listed in **3.3**. The immediate wheal-and-flare reactions are often followed by late-phase reactions. There is evidence that if high enough concentrations of antigens are presented, 100% of immediate reactions will go on to late phases. These late-phase reactions in the skin are also manifested in the nasal mucosa and bronchi (*see* **3.21**).

There are two types of skin tests – the epicutaneous, also referred to as scratch, puncture, and prick technique (**3.4**), and the intracutaneous or intradermal test.

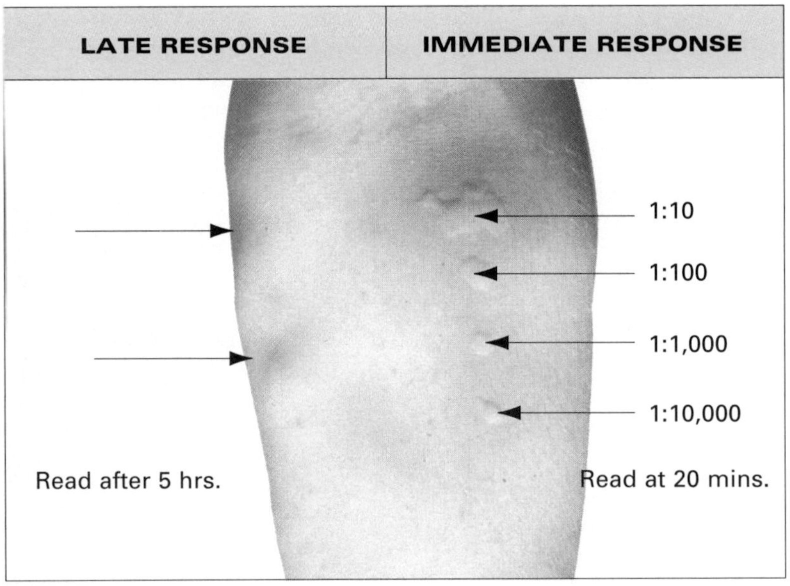

3.1 Skin prick tests with grass-pollen allergen in a patient with typical summer hay fever. Skin tests were performed 5 hours (left) and 20 minutes (right) before the photograph was taken. The tests on the right show a typical end-point titration of a Type I immediate wheal-and-flare reaction. The late-phase skin reaction (left) can be clearly seen at 5 hours, especially where a large immediate response has preceded it. Figures for allergen dilution are given. (Reproduced with permission from Roitt *et al.*, 1995.)

EPICUTANEOUS SKIN TESTS

The epicutaneous method has many advantages. It is easy and safe to perform and causes little discomfort. It is inexpensive and test solutions are stable because they are suspended in 50% glycerine solutions. Positive epicutaneous tests correlate well with clinical symptoms (3.5). One possible disadvantage to this method is that it can result in false-negative reactions due to a lack of sensitivity (3.6).

INTRACUTANEOUS SKIN TESTS

Intracutaneous skin tests are more reproducible than epicutaneous tests and are 100–1000 times more sensitive. Thus, they are associated with fewer false-negative reactions. The drawbacks to intradermal tests are that they are time-consuming and tedious to perform, and are often associated with discomfort and an increased risk of systemic reactions. Even more important, they are more likely to produce false-positive results because of their

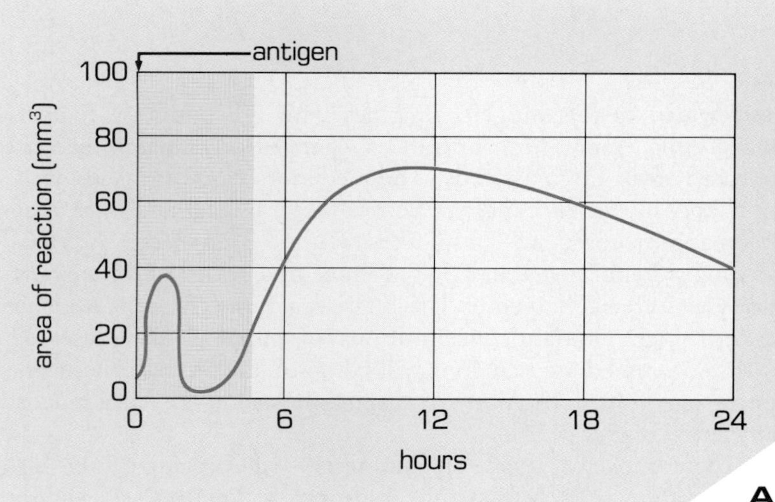

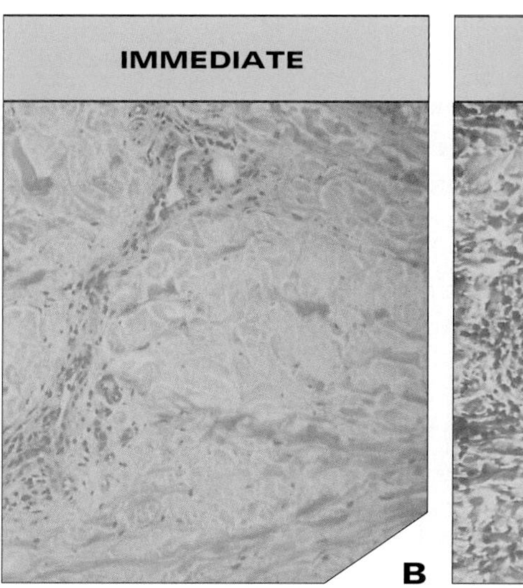

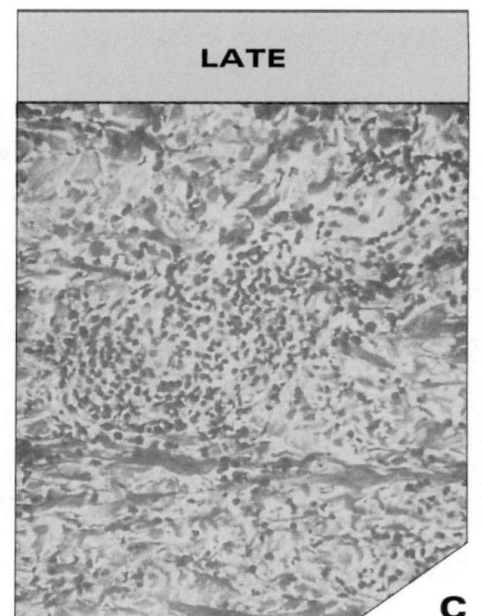

3.2 Immediate and late-phase skin reactions. Using the intradermal method of skin testing, an immediate wheal-and-flare reaction is often followed by a late-phase reaction. (A) This late phase may last for 24 hours, and the reaction is larger and generally more edematous than the immediate response. (B) The immediate type of reaction (here exemplified by a biopsy of chronic urticaria) has a sparse cellular infiltrate around the dermal vessels, consisting primarily of neutrophils. (C) The late reaction has a dense infiltrate with many basophils. The late-phase reaction can be seen following challenge of the skin, nasal mucosa, and bronchi, and may be particularly important in the development of chronic asthma. (Reproduced with permission from Roitt *et al.*, 1993.)

COMMONLY USED SCORING SYSTEM FOR GRADING THE RESPONSE TO HYPERSENSITIVITY SKIN TESTING

Grade	Wheal	Erythema
0(–)	< 3 mm	0–5 mm
1+	3–5 mm	0–10 mm
2+	5–10 mm	5–10 mm
3+	10–15 mm	> 10 mm
4+	> 15 mm or with pseudopods	> 20 mm

3.3 Commonly used scoring system for grading the response to hypersensitivity skin testing. (Adapted with permission from Zitelli, 1987.)

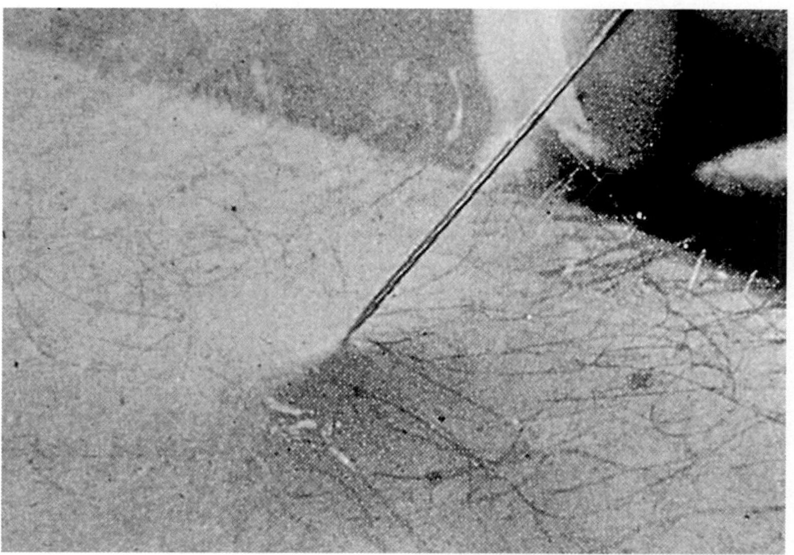

3.4 A needle used to lift and break the skin in the epicutaneous skin-test technique.

increased sensitivity. Mildly positive, intradermal reactions are not considered clinically relevant.

A disposable multi-test applicator has recently gained popularity because of its convenience and the reproducibility of results that it offers (**3.7**); eight epicutaneous tests can be applied at one time (**3.8**). Results compare favorably with those that are obtained by intracutaneous tests.

TEST RESULTS

The value of skin tests, like that of any diagnostic procedure, depends on the knowledge of their interpreter. To be informative, the tests must be related to the clinical context of the patient's history and physical examination. The selection of antigens and the administration of tests requires experience and knowledge. The

ADVANTAGES OF EPICUTANEOUS VERSUS INTRACUTANEOUS SKIN TESTS

Epicutaneous	Intracutaneous
Easy to perform	More reproducible
Safe	More sensitive
Little discomfort	
Inexpensive	
Stable test solutions	
Correlates well with symptoms	

3.5 The advantages of the epicutaneous versus the intracutaneous skin tests.

DISADVANTAGES OF EPICUTANEOUS VERSUS INTRACUTANEOUS SKIN TESTS

Epicutaneous	Intracutaneous
Less sensitive	More time-consuming
	More difficult to perform
	More discomfort
	Increased risk of systemic reaction
	More false-positive results

3.6 The disadvantages of the epicutaneous versus the intracutaneous skin tests.

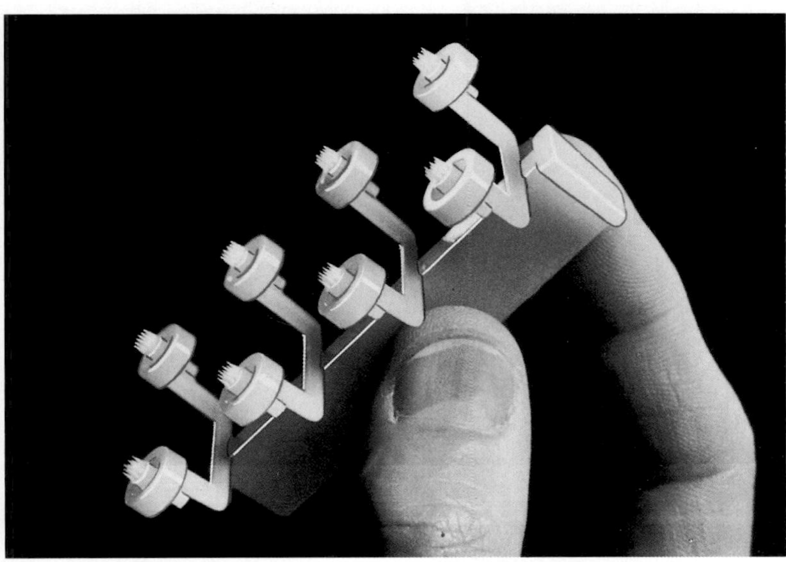

3.7 The multi-test applicator. (Courtesy of Lincoln Diagnostics, Inc., Decatur, IL.)

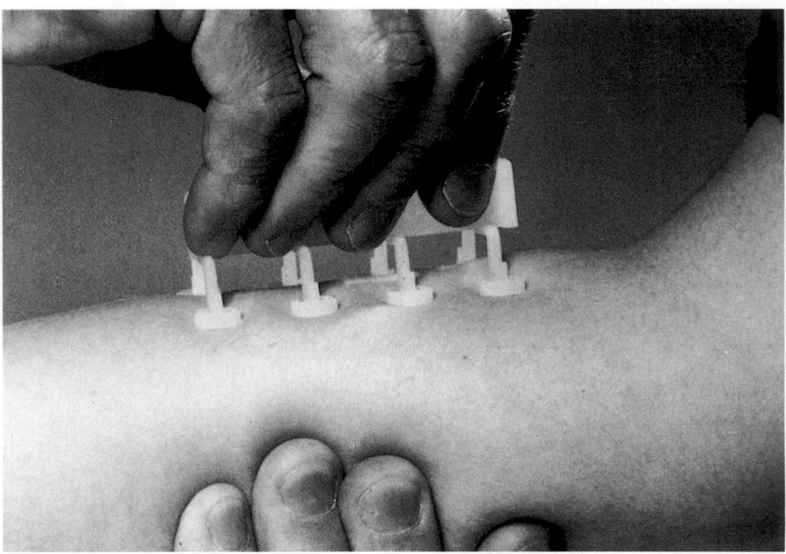

3.8 A multi-test applicator delivers eight antigens at once, simplifying epicutaneous testing. (Courtesy of Lincoln Diagnostics Inc., Decatur, IL.)

physician must be aware of the many reasons for false-positive and false-negative reactions in order to properly interpret test results.

False-negative results

Several circumstances may account for negative skin-test results in a patient who truly has an IgE-mediated allergic disease (**3.9**).

The antigen in solution – a protein – if improperly stored may lose potency with time or exposure to heat, thereby causing a false-negative result. Antigen solutions must be refrigerated and replaced at appropriate intervals.

A false-negative result may also occur due to the improper administration of a test. Too superficial a scratch or prick of the skin or too deep an intracutaneous injection will prevent the allergen solution to reach the skin area in which mast cells are located.

As well, the patient's age must be considered when a skin-test result is negative. In general, the skin of infants and elderly persons is less reactive than that of other age groups. In the same individual the skin on the forearm is less reactive than the skin on the back and responsiveness is lower in the early morning than later in the day. If the patient is chilled and skin temperature lowered, the skin-test response will be lessened.

The refractory period of a test may account for a false-negative result too. Soon after a systemic reaction to an allergen, such as insect venom, penicillin, or food, the patient enters a refractory period during which a skin-test reaction to that substance may be negative. The reason is that specific IgE is consumed by the severe allergic reaction, so a 3–4 week period is needed for the allergic antibody to build back up to its prereaction levels. Therefore, if a patient has a systemic reaction to an allergen, it is best to wait a full 4 weeks before performing skin tests.

Finally, a number of drugs, particularly antihistamines, may inhibit skin reactivity and, therefore, should be discontinued at least 48 hours before skin testing. Astemizole, one of the newer second-generation non-sedative antihistamines, has been shown to inhibit immediate skin-test reactivity for as long as 3 weeks. Whenever a skin test is performed, histamine should be included as a positive control. If the histamine skin-test is negative, further testing should be deferred. A more complete list of drugs that can inhibit immediate skin reactivity is provided in **3.10**. The attribution of inhibiting properties to medications that do not, in fact, inhibit immediate skin-test reactivity is a common error made by physicians. Corticosteroids, theophylline, cromolyn, beta agonists, and decongestants are not presently known to be inhibitory.

REASONS FOR FALSE-NEGATIVE SKIN-TEST RESULTS

1. Improper storage of antigens
2. Improper administration
3. Inherent host factors
   — Age
   — Skin area
   — Time of day
   — Skin temperature
4. Refractory period
5. Inhibiting drugs

3.9 Five reasons for false-negative test results.

DRUGS THAT MAY INHIBIT IMMEDIATE SKIN-TEST REACTIVITY

1. All H1 blocking antihistamines
   — Variable: hydroxyzine, high
   cyproheptadine, low
2. Ranitidine
3. Amitriptyline
4. Desipramine
5. Nortriptyline
6. Imipramine
7. Protriptyline
8. Trimipramine
9. Triavil

3.10 Drugs that may inhibit immediate skin-test reactivity.

False-positive results

When a skin test is positive in the face of a negative clinical picture, several explanations may be offered (**3.11**).

Many factors contribute to the production of non-specifically irritating skin-test solutions. Deviation from a physiologic pH or from the correct osmolarity may cause a false-positive skin-test result. Extracts may contain low molecular weight irritants and it is necessary to dialyze these materials before utilizing them as skin-testing agents. Glycerine, commonly used as a preservative in allergy extracts, causes non-specific irritation at a concentration of 6% if injected intradermally. Injecting too large a volume of extract intradermally may also cause false-positive reactions. The optimal injection volume is 0.02 ml.

Materials that are urticariogenic may cause a wheal and erythema skin-test response in all subjects on a non-IgE-mediated basis. Examples are morphine and codeine. Some food extracts, particularly those from cheese, have a high histamine content and may cause false-positive reactions.

Dermographism may also be responsible for a false-positive test result. It is present in 5–20% of the population, depending on the degree of pressure applied. Skin testing should also include a negative saline control to insure that the patient is not dermographic. A positive response to saline obviously makes other positive skin-test reactions suspect. Premedication with a small amount of antihistamine may serve to ablate the non-specific response while preserving the true IgE-mediated reaction.

As well, positive skin-test reactivity may persist in an individual whose clinical sensitivity has disappeared either spontaneously or through the use of immunotherapy. On the other hand, false-positive results are often harbingers of future sensitivity. The onset of clinical symptoms of allergic rhinitis is generally preceded by a positive pollen prick test. The development of hay fever in college seniors who, as freshmen, had no clinical manifestations of allergies is more than ten times higher in students with initial positive pollen scratch tests than in students with no positive pollen scratch tests (Hagy, 1971). Thus, the risk of developing an allergic condition is considerably greater for individuals with positive skin-test results (**3.12**).

Perhaps the most important reason for the false-positive skin-test reaction is the physician's failure to realize that a positive skin test is not necessarily an indicator of clinical sensitivity. In any group of tested persons there are a certain number of positive responses that are better termed clinically insignificant than false positive. Several studies have pointed out the high incidence of immediate skin-test reactivity in a normal adult population (**3.13**).

REASONS FOR FALSE-POSITIVE SKIN-TEST RESULTS

1. Improper preparation and administration of allergen solution
2. Non-specific histamine release
3. Dermographism
4. Remnant of past sensitivity
5. Harbinger of future sensitivity
6. Disparity with clinical sensitivity

3.11 Six reasons for false-positive skin-test results.

PREDICTIVE VALUE OF IMMEDIATE SKIN TESTS

Epicutaneous skin tests	Incidence of allergic rhinitis 3 years later
Negative	1.7%
Positive	18.2% (p value 0.01)

3.12 Predictive value of immediate skin tests.

ENZYME-LINKED IMMUNOSORBENT ASSAY

TOTAL SERUM IgE DETERMINATION

The discovery of IgE as the antibody responsible for allergic reactions in humans has led to the development of sophisticated techniques for IgE measurement. The two most commonly employed methods for the measurement of IgE are radioimmunoassay (RIA) and enzyme-linked immunosassay (EIA). EIA has largely supplanted RIA because it is non-isotopic, the reagents have long shelf lives, and there are no waste disposal problems (**3.14A** and **3.14B**). This is a competition type of assay.

IgE levels are often elevated in cases of allergic disease, but these levels cannot be considered pathognomonic signs of allergy. IgE levels vary widely, both in allergic and non-allergic individuals. A normal IgE level does not exclude allergy (**3.15**), while definitely elevated levels may be seen in non-atopic people.

ALLERGEN-SPECIFIC IgE

Determination

The radioallergosorbent test (RAST) measures the amount of IgE that is directed to a specific allergen (**3.16**). In this technique, an allergen is bound to a cellulose disc. The patient's serum is added, and any IgE in the serum that is specific for that allergen adheres to the disc. Radiolabeled antibody to IgE is then added. Thus, the IgE in the serum acts as an antibody to the allergen that is fixed to the disc, and as an antigen to the anti-IgE antibody. The amount of radioactivity measured on the disc, therefore, is directly related to the amount of specific IgE antibody present in the serum.

RAST VERSUS SKIN TESTS

Disagreement exists as to the precise role of RAST in everyday allergy practice. There is no question that RAST is more expensive to administer than are skin tests, but proponents of RAST maintain

FREQUENCY OF POSITIVE SKIN TESTS IN ASYMPTOMATIC PATIENTS

Study	Method	Allergen	Allergen
1	ID	Housedust – concentrate	50%
2	ID	Housedust – 1:100	4%
3	ID	Various	9%
4	EC	Various	4%
	ID	Grass	6%
	EC	Various	12%

ID = intradermal
EC = epicutaneous

3.13 The frequency of positive skin tests in asymptomatic patients. (Adapted from Bousquet, 1988.)

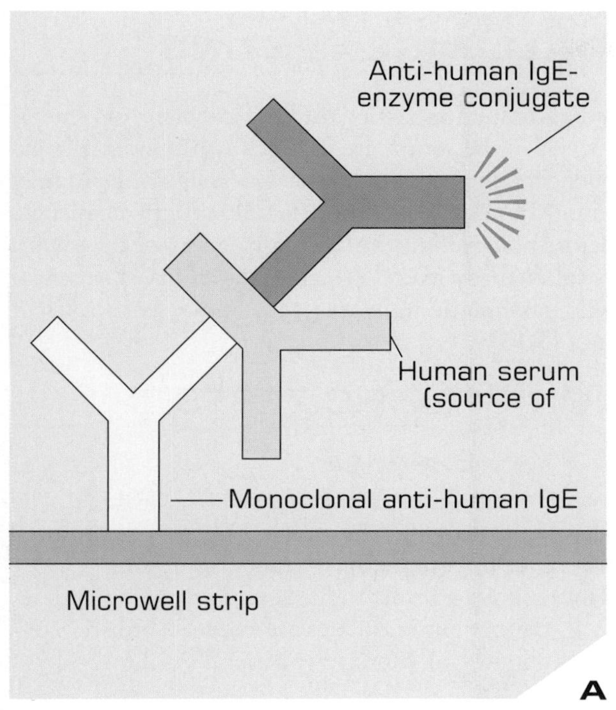

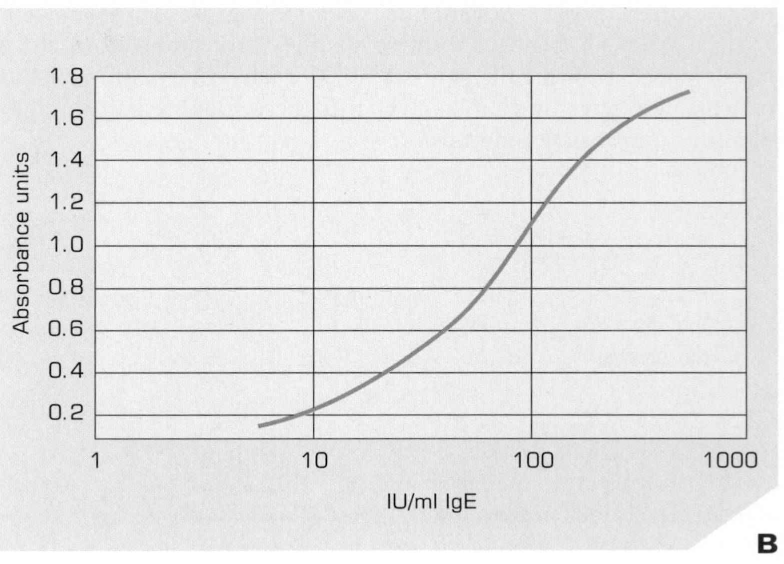

3.14 (A) The enzyme-linked immunoassay (EIA). In this assay, microwell strips are coated with monoclonal anti-human IgE antibody. Test serum is added and IgE is captured. After washing to remove unbound proteins anti-human IgE peroxidase conjugate (or another suitable enzyme) is added to the well. The bound enzyme-linked antibody is quantitated by adding a substrate solution that changes color when hydrolyzed by the enzyme. Therefore, the higher the level of IgE, the more enzyme-linked anti-IgE is bound and the more intense the color that develops, which can be analyzed in a spectrophotometer. (B) The typical normal IgE standard curve.

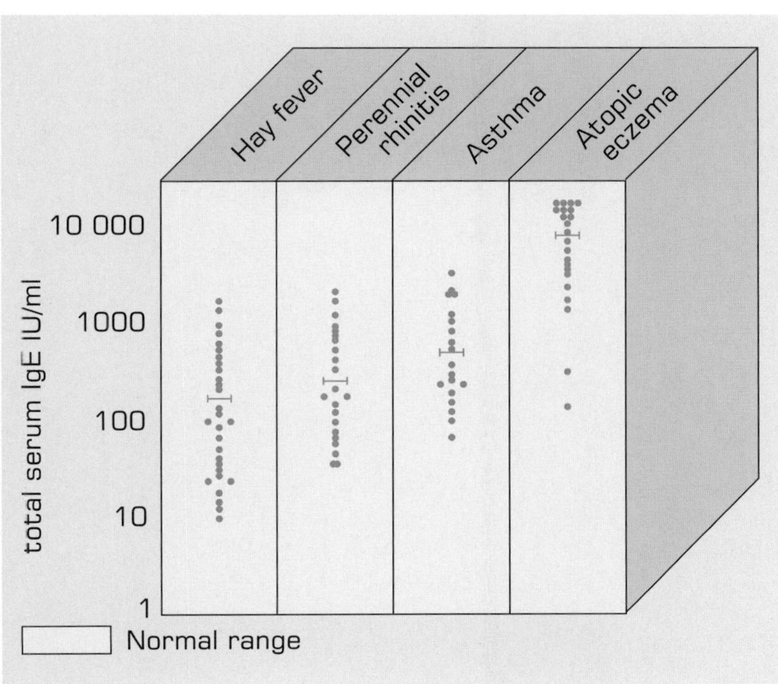

3.15 IgE levels in allergic patients. Each point in this chart represents the serum IgE level of a patient. IgE levels vary over a wide range, but the levels in atopic patients are generally elevated above the levels in normal subjects of the same age. For many atopic individuals with less severe diseases, the serum IgE levels fall within the normal range. IgE titers are usually expressed in international units per ml, by reference to standard sera, where 1 IU = 2.4 ng. The normal range of IgE in non-atopic subjects is shaded yellow. (Adapted with permission from Roitt *et al.*, 1993.)

that it offers several advantages over skin tests. These include greater safety, better quantitative results, protection from drug interference, greater allergen stability, preferability in problem patients, and fewer injections. **3.17** lists these supposed advantages with the appropriate rebuttals.

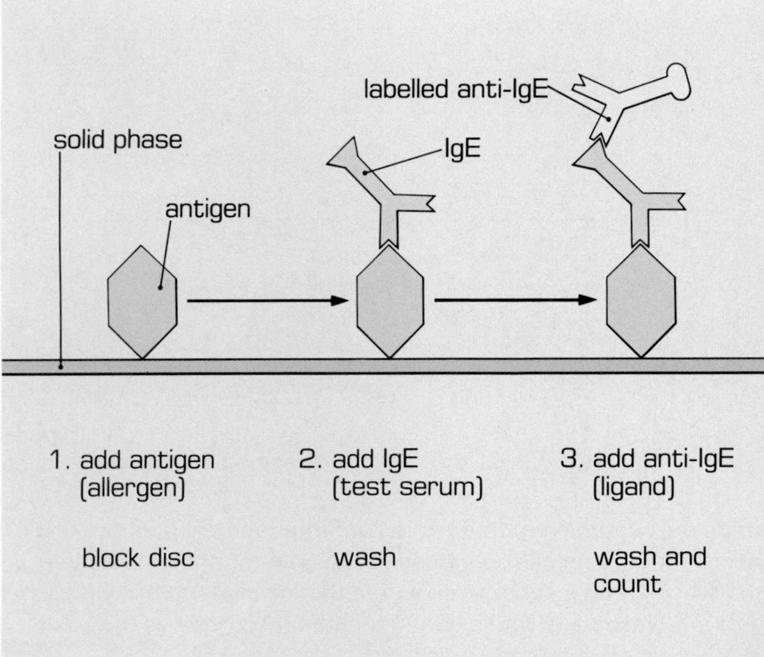

3.16 The radioallergosorbent test (RAST). This test measures antigen-specific IgE in a radioimmunoassay where the ligand is a labeled anti-IgE antibody. The antigen (allergen) is covalently bound to a cellulose disc. Having much more antigen available on the disc permits the high sensitivity necessary to bind the small quantities of IgE present in the test serum. (Adapted with permission from Roitt *et al.*, 1995.)

PROVOCATIVE CHALLENGE TESTING

The skin test and radioimmunoassay for measurement of general and specific IgE levels in the serum are indirect assays of an allergic state. Direct challenge, either by inhaling or ingesting antigens, may be of greater diagnostic use. In addition to the antigen challenge, the general hyper-responsive state of the airway associated with asthma may be evaluated by exercise or by inhalation of chemical substances to which asthmatic individuals are more sensitive than are non-asthmatics (**3.18**).

NON-SPECIFIC TESTS

Exercise

Physical exercise is a major precipitant of bronchial asthma. The diagnosis of asthma can probably be made after 6–8 minutes of exercise and pre- and post-pulmonary function testing (**3.19**). Initially, the patient exhibits a bronchodilation effect, along with an increase in FEV_1. In the patient with exercise-induced bronchoconstriction (EIB), 6–8 minutes of exercise is generally followed by a 20% or greater fall in FEV_1.

Bronchial challenges

Asthma is characterized by enhanced bronchial hyperreactivity. This hyperreactivity can be manifested clinically by the asthmatic's adverse response to cold air, cigarette smoke, fumes, weather changes, and other stimuli that have little or no effect on a non-asthmatic patient. In the doctor's office setting, hyperreactivity can be demonstrated by the patient's responses to a bronchial challenge such as the inhalation of methacholine or histamine (**3.20**). A greater than 20% fall in FEV_1 after the inhalation of a methacholine solution at a concentration of less than 25 mg/ml is indicative of a positive response.

RAST VERSUS SKIN TESTS

RAST advantages	Rebuttals
Greater safety	There is virtually no risk to a carefully performed and administered epicutaneous skin test.
Quantitative results	Though it provides quantitative results, RAST is fraught with technical problems. Studies have shown tremendous variability in results from one laboratory to another.
Not influenced by drugs	Stopping antihistamines 48 hours before skin testing obviates any interference by medications in that technique.
Greater allergen stability	Epicutaneous extracts stored in glycerine are as stable as RAST allergens.
Preferable for children	There is actually less physical and emotional trauma to small children in epicutaneous skin testing.
Preferable for patients with dermographism	Dermographism can be overcome with the use of appropriate antihistamines and lesser downward pressure when epicutaneous skin-testing is performed.
Preferable for patients with widespread dermatitis	It is rare to find a skin condition so severe that a small patch of normal skin cannot be found for skin tests.
Fewer immunotherapy injections	RAST proponents claim that a modification of the RAST makes it possible to place patients in different clinical classes so that immunotherapy can start at higher concentrations, thereby decreasing the total number of injections. A recent, well-controlled study showed that in 98% of allergic patients, the starting dose was the same as the one 'conventional' allergists used.

3.17 The suggested advantages of RAST, with rebuttals.

PROVOCATIVE CHALLENGE TESTS

Non-specific

Exercise

Assessment of airway reactivity
— Histamine
— Methacholine
— Cold air

Specific (antigen)

Bronchial

Nasal

Oral

Injection
— Local anesthetics
— Stinging insects

3.18 Provocative challenge testing.

SPECIFIC TESTS

Bronchial challenges

Specific airway reactivity can be assessed by measuring the patient's bronchial response to the inhalation of certain allergen solutions. There is evidence that skin-test results generally correlate well with bronchial-provocation test results. Therefore, bronchial-challenge testing with specific allergens is generally not necessary in everyday practice. There may be special instances, however, such as in occupational asthma (*see* Chapter 6), or in investigative work, when specific bronchial-challenge testing is indicated. Several bronchial responses have been documented after the inhalation of antigen solutions. **3.21** illustrates the immediate, dual, and late-phase responses that are seen. The 'classic' asthmatic response to inhaled allergens had been thought to be immediate, occurring in all cases within minutes, but it is now estimated that approximately 50% of

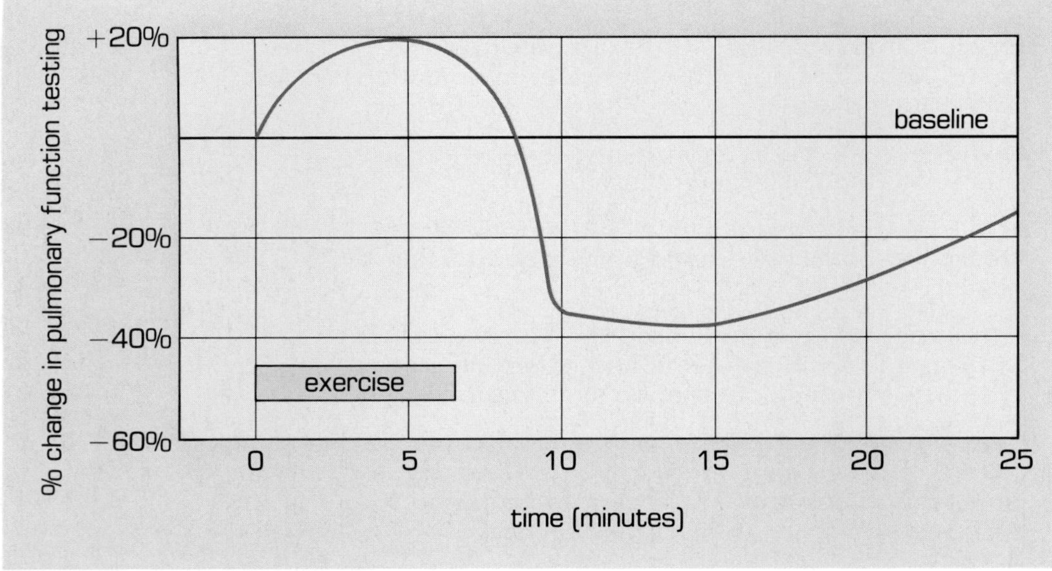

3.19 A classical response in exercise-induced asthma.

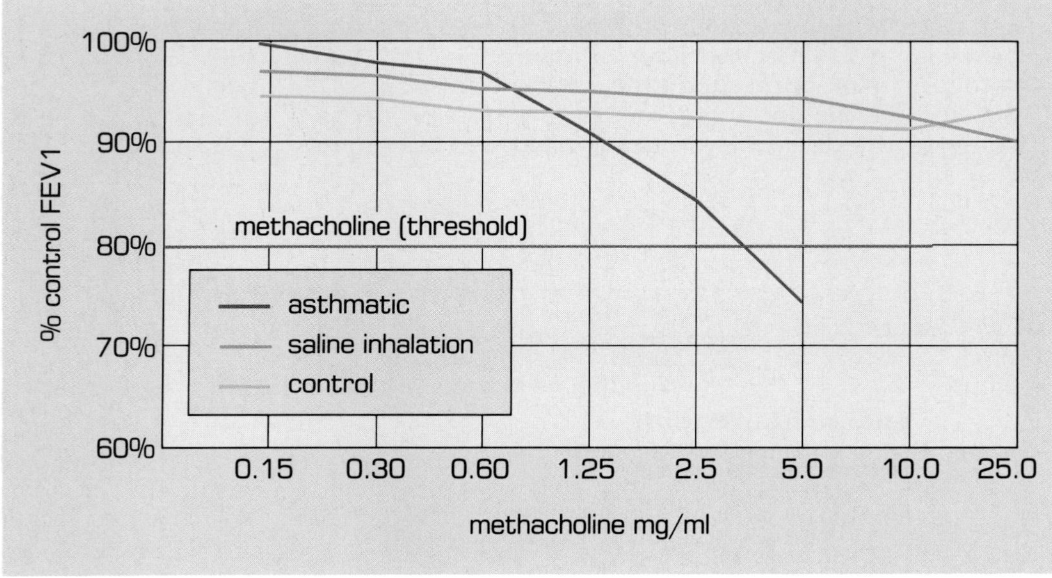

3.20 The effect of methacholine inhalation on an asthmatic patient. The asthmatic subject shows a greater than 20% fall in FEV_1 after inhalation of methacholine 5 mg/ml. Saline inhalation results in no change in FEV_1. A control patient inhales methacholine through a concentration of 25 mg/ml and shows no change in FEV_1.

allergic asthmatics demonstrate a dual immediate and late-phase response. An isolated late-phase bronchial response is seen largely in instances of occupational asthma. Pretreatment with different medications may alter the bronchial responses to antigen inhalation. As seen in Chapter 8, beta agonists block the late reaction, but have no effect on the immediate response; and pretreatment with cromolyn inhibits both bronchial responses.

Nasal challenges

Inhaled antigen solutions can also be used to challenge the nasal mucosa, to diagnose allergic rhinitis. The response can be gauged by the measurement of nasal airway resistance through anterior or posterior rhinomanometry, or by changes in the cellular or mediator content of the nasal mucus. The nasal-challenge technique is useful in studying the pathophysiology of the nose, the action of drugs, and instances of occupational rhinitis (*see* Chapter 6).

Oral challenges

In instances when a suspected allergen is ingested, an oral challenge can be performed. The challenge can be open, in which case both the physician and the patient know the content of the substance ingested, single-blind, with only the doctor knowing the content, or double-blind, with neither the patient nor the physician knowing the content of the challenge. The food or drug can be administered either whole or in a lyophilized preparation contained in an opaque capsule.

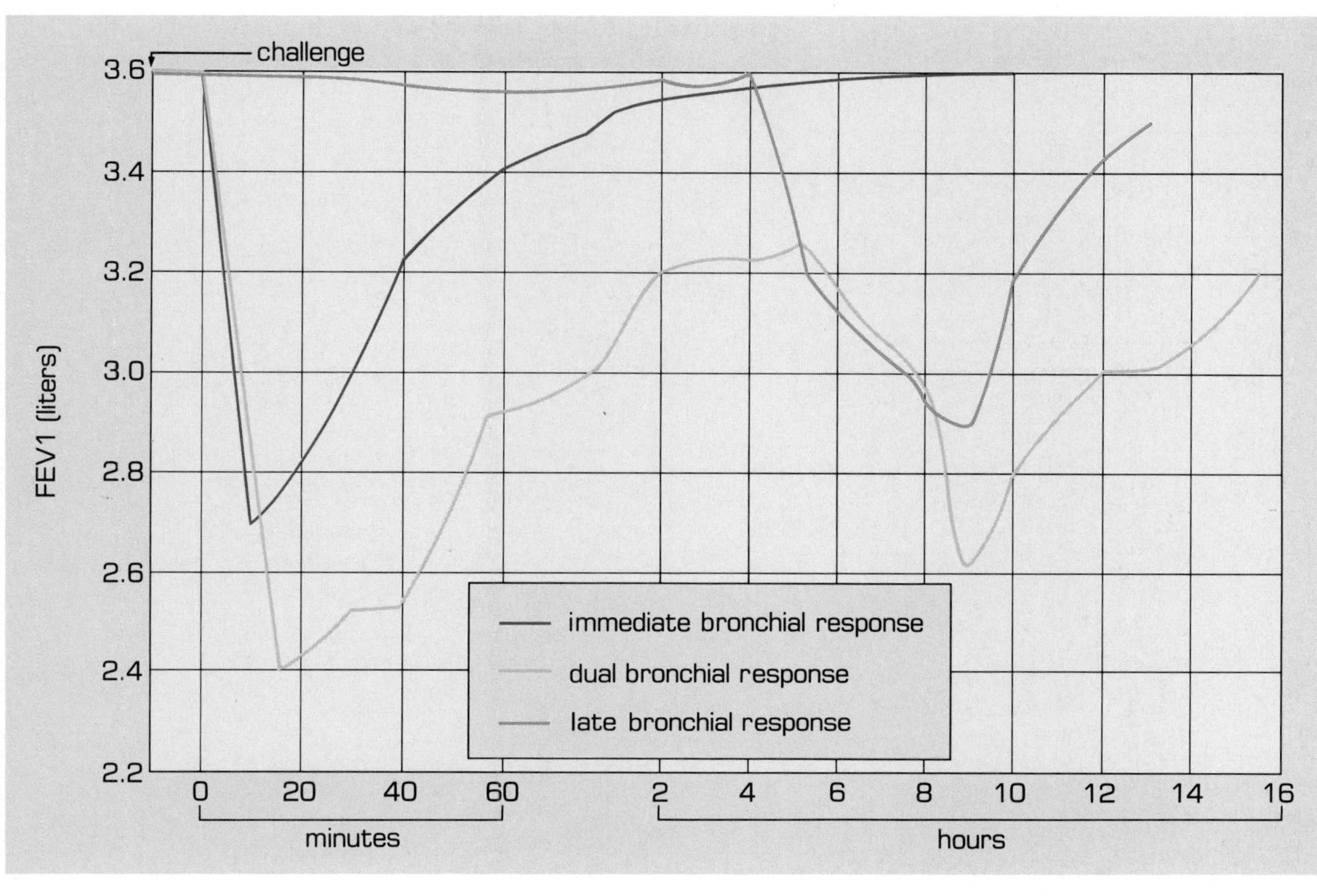

3.21 The different patterns of bronchial response after a bronchial challenge.

Oral challenges serve several purposes. First, double-blind, placebo-controlled food challenges have proven useful in discerning IgE-mediated food sensitivities (*see* Chapter 13). Second, oral challenges can also help diagnose sensitivity to ingested substances, such as aspirin or sulfites, in which the sensitivity is not on an IgE basis (**3.22**). In such instances, skin testing or RAST would be of no use.

Injections

When an antigen causing an IgE-mediated allergic response is delivered by the injectant route, ordinary skin testing or RAST serve as adequate diagnostic procedures. Examples of injectant route allergies are naturally occurring phenomena, such as insect stings, or the iatrogenic administration of penicillin subcutaneously or intramuscularly.

As with oral challenges, some substances that are injected may cause reactions that are not IgE-mediated. Local anesthetics are examples of agents for which skin testing or RAST are of little use in detecting sensitivity. In these instances, a graduated type of challenge up to the full therapeutic dose may be utilized (**3.23**).

A naturally occurring injection, in the form of a Hymenoptera family insect sting, has been carried out at some medical centers. This has been performed in order to determine whether a preceding course of immunotherapy, with venom of that particular insect, had been successful. At present, this is an experimental technique that should only be performed under the most carefully controlled conditions.

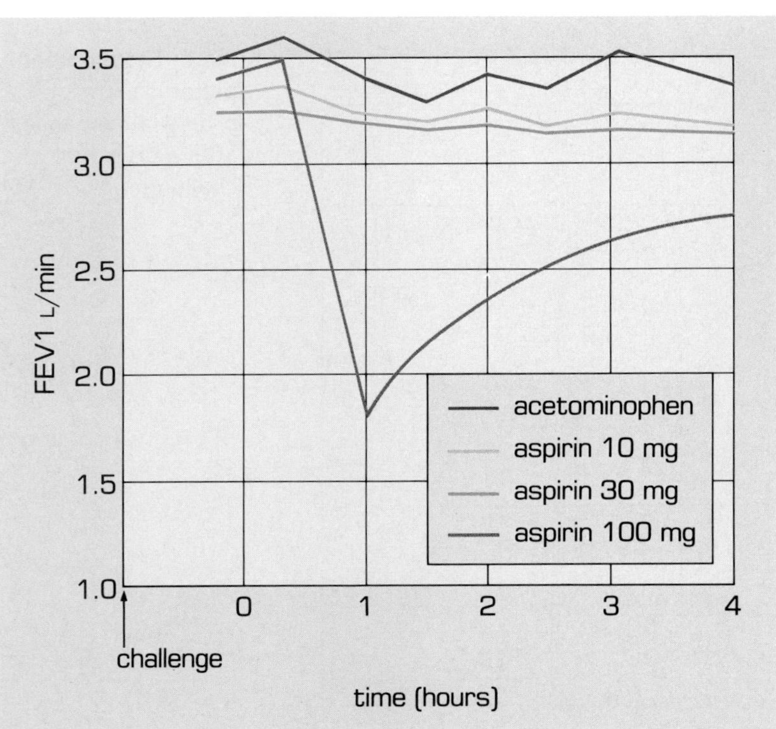

3.22 An aspirin challenge in an aspirin-sensitive asthmatic. A graduated increase in aspirin dosage results in a significant fall in FEV_1 1 hour after ingesting 100 mg. An acetaminophen challenge is negative.

SUGGESTED SCHEDULE FOR LOCAL ANESTHETIC CHALLENGE	
Technique	**Dose**
Puncture	Full strength
Intradermal	0.02 ml diluted 1:100
Intradermal	0.02 ml full strength
Subcutaneous	0.10 ml full strength
Subcutaneous	0.50 ml full strength

3.23 The suggested schedule for a local anesthetic challenge.

UNPROVEN DIAGNOSTIC TECHNIQUES AND THEORIES

In this chapter we have thus far discussed diagnostic techniques that have scientific validity and have been subjected to careful evaluation. A group of practitioners, who often refer to their medical practice as 'clinical ecology', offer allergic patients alternative ways to diagnose allergies; these have no scientific basis and have not been subjected to careful controlled scrutiny. **3.24** lists several diagnostic techniques and theories that are unproven and, indeed, in some instances have been shown to be invalid.

The cytotoxic test is based on the unproven theory that food allergy alters the morphology of leukocytes. Several blind studies have shown the test to be totally invalid. In the provocation–neutralization technique, increasing doses of a substance are administered subcutaneously or sublingually until the patient experiences a 'sensation'. Further concentrations are then given until the patient reports the absence of symptoms. A double-blind placebo control study demonstrated no difference between the test substance and the placebo. Applied kinesiology is based on a claim that allergy impairs the strength of skeletal muscle. There is no scientific basis for this, and no clinical studies of efficacy. Laboratory tests can, indeed, detect both IgG antibodies and immune complexes to food, but there is simply no proof that they are responsible for disease.

Multiple chemical sensitivity embodies the concept that a whole host of symptoms may be caused by exposure to ordinary quantities of synthetic chemicals in our environment. The syndrome is characterized by subjective symptoms only; there are no physical findings and no pathology. There is no scientific evidence that such an entity exists, but the number of patients claiming such sensitivity continues to rise.

Candida hypersensitivity is the concept that the normal presence of *Candida albicans* in the body can cause multisystem, poly-symptomatic subjective illness. Patients are advised to follow a strict diet and take anti-fungal drugs. A well-controlled study demonstrated that anti-fungal agents had no more effect than placebo, and such therapy is inappropriate.

FUTURE DEVELOPMENTS

In this chapter we have reviewed diagnostic tests in allergy and attempted to put the various techniques presently in use into their proper clinical contexts. There is hope that investigative work being performed currently will result in more accurate diagnoses of allergic diseases in the future. In particular, new immunochemical procedures for purifying antigens hold great promise. With better defined and characterized antigens that can be used for both *in vitro* and *in vivo* testing, diagnostic capabilities will be markedly enhanced. Specific organ challenges, especially for the nose and the lungs, are becoming more standardized, as is the double-blind placebo-controlled challenge so essential for the diagnosis of food allergies.

REFERENCES

Bousquet J: *In vivo* methods for study of allergy: skin tests, techniques and interpretation, in Middleton E, Jr, Reed CE, Ellis EF, Adkinson NF, Jr, Yuninger JW (eds): *Allergy: Principles and Practice*, C.V. Mosby, St Louis, Chapter 19, 1988.

Hagy GW, Settipane GA: Prognosis of positive allergy skin tests in an asymptomatic population. *J Allergy Clin Immunol*, **48**:200, 1971.

Homburger HA, Katzmann JA: Methods in laboratory immunology, in Middleton E, Jr, Reed CE, Ellis EF, Adkinson NF, Jr, Yuninger JW (eds): *Allergy: Principles and Practice*, C.V. Mosby, St Louis, Chapter 21, 1988.

Naclerio RM, Norman PS, Fish JE: *In vivo* methods for study of allergy: mucosal tests, techniques and interpretation, in Middleton E, Jr, Reed CE, Ellis EF, Adkinson NF, Jr, Yuninger JW (eds): *Allergy: Principles and Practice*, C.V. Mosby, St Louis, Chapter 20, 1988.

Ownby DR: Clinical significance of IgE, in Middleton E, Jr, Reed CE, Ellis EF, Adkinson NF, Jr, Yuninger JW (eds): *Allergy: Principles and Practice*, C.V. Mosby, St Louis, Chapter 41, 1988.

Roitt IM, Brostoff J, Male DK: *Immunology*, Mosby, London, 4th edn, Chapters 22 & 28, 1995.

Roitt IM, Brostoff J, Male DK: *Immunology*, Mosby, London, 3rd edn, Chapters 19 & 25, 1993.

Skoner DP, Stillwagon PK, Friedman R, Fireman P: Pediatric allergy and immunology, in Zitelli BJ, Davis HW (eds): *Atlas of Pediatric Physical Diagnosis*, Gower Medical Publishing, London, Chapter 4, 1987.

Slavin RG: Choosing the best tests for allergy diagnosis. *Diagnosis*, **10**:45, 1988.

Terr AI: Controversial and unproven methods in allergy diagnosis and treatment, in Patterson R, Grammer LC, Greenberger PA, Zeiss CR (eds): *Allergic Diseases: Diagnosis and Management*, JP Lippincott, Philadelphia, Chapter 26, 1993.

UNPROVEN DIAGNOSTIC TECHNIQUES AND THEORIES

Unproven diagnostic techniques	Unproven theories
Cytotoxic tests	Multiple chemical sensitivity
Provocation–neutralization	Candida hypersensitivity syndrome
Applied kinesiology	
IgG or immune complexes to foods	

3.24 Some unproven diagnostic techniques and theories.

CHAPTER 4

Anaphylaxis

Gilbert A. Friday, Jr.
Philip Fireman

The term anaphylaxis has been used to define the allergic adverse reaction characterized by systemic clinical manifestations that occur in an individual who had been primarily sensitized to a foreign substance upon subsequent re-exposure by any route, whether inhalation, oral, or injection, of the same material. A potentially life-threatening clinical syndrome, it was initially defined in 1902 by Portier and Richet as a fatal reaction to injection of a previously tolerated foreign protein during prophylaxis antisera treatment. Yet, approximately 4500 years earlier, the Egyptians described fatal reactions to Hymenoptera insect stings, which probably represented anaphylaxis.

Over the years, anaphylaxis has gradually come to mean the acute life-threatening syndrome which results from the rapid release of large amounts of chemical mediators of inflammation from mast cells and basophils in response to a specific allergen in a previously sensitized host. The allergens responsible for reactions can be protein, hapten–protein conjugates, lipoprotein, or polysaccharide.

The clinical features of anaphylaxis are produced typically by immunologic mechanisms, but non-immunologic mediated reactions also occur. Immune-provoked anaphylaxis may be mediated by IgE antibody or immune antigen–antibody complexes. Perhaps the most common causes of anaphylaxis today are adverse drug reactions, especially to penicillin. Non-immune anaphylaxis occurs in relation to direct mast-cell degranulating agents, such as opiates, radiocontrast media, and non-steroidal anti-inflammatory agents. Idiopathic anaphylaxis may also occur.

The terms 'anaphylactic' and 'anaphylactoid' refer to similar if not the same syndrome, but have been utilized in the past by some clinicians as meaning IgE-mediated or non-IgE-mediated systemic reactions. Detailed clinical examples of immune and non-immune types of anaphylaxis provoked by drug reactions, insect stings, and exercise are presented later in this chapter.

EPIDEMIOLOGY

Data on the overall prevalence of anaphylaxis are unavailable. The incidence of anaphylactic reactions probably depends upon the degree and frequency of exposure the individual has to a given antigen. Anaphylactic reactions have been described at approximately 2.5 per one thousand (0.25%) for allergen injections administered in aero-allergen immunotherapy of respiratory allergic disease. Fatal anaphylaxis due to penicillin allergy has been reported at a rate of 0.002% for parenteral injections and is much less frequent for oral penicillin therapy. Hymenoptera insect sting anaphylaxis probably accounts for 25–50 deaths per year. The rate of fatal anaphylaxis of any cause is estimated at 0.4 cases per million individuals per year, but may be as high as 2 cases per million per year.

ETIOLOGY

IMMUNE MECHANISM

IgE-mediated reactions

A wide variety of agents are potentially responsible for IgE-mediated anaphylaxis and a partial list of the most common is provided in **4.1**. Antibiotics, such as the penicillins and cephalosporins, cause anaphylactic reactions through a hapten-protein initiated IgE-antibody-mediated mechanism. Proteins, including insulin, chymotrypsin, and venoms, as well as therapeutic agents, such as allergen extracts and various other vaccines, can also be responsible. Foods are a significant source of IgE-mediated anaphylaxis, reactions most commonly occurring with such foods as eggs, shellfish, and nuts (*see* Chapter 13).

Non-IgE-mediated mechanisms

Anaphylaxis may occur during the administration of blood and blood products through a non-IgE immune complex (probably IgG) mechanism. These reactions are provoked by the development of antibodies to the red blood cell antigen or plasma protein, such as immunoglobulin, presumed to be mediated by activation of complement and generation of active C_{5a} anaphylatoxin. Cryoprecipitation and immunoglobulin aggregates can also induce anaphylaxis via fixation of complement. However, administration of blood products containing IgA to selective IgA-deficient patients may induce the development of IgE antibodies to IgA, which could mediate an anaphylaxic reaction.

NON-IMMUNE MECHANISMS

4.2 lists agents that cause anaphylaxis via non-immune mechanisms. Direct mast-cell degranulating agents, such as opiates, curare muscle relaxants, plasma expander polysaccharides (dextran), antibiotics, and iodinated radiocontrast media have been noted to release histamine from basophils and mast cells. Aspirin is also known to cause anaphylaxis through uncertain mechanisms. Aspirin-sensitive patients may also show intolerance to other non-steroidal anti-inflammatory agents, including ibuprofen, indomethacin, and tolmetin. The role of tartrazine and other dyes in producing anaphylaxis is a matter of controversy.

EXAMPLES OF AGENTS CAUSING ANAPHYLAXIS VIA IMMUNE MECHANISMS

IgE mediated

1. **Antimicrobial agents (haptens)**
   Penicillin; cephalosporin; tetracycline; aminoglycoside; streptomycin; amphotericin-B; nitrofurantoin; sulfamethoxazole
2. **Hormones**
   Insulin; TSH; corticotropin; progesterone; ACTH
3. **Enzymes**
   Streptokinase, penicillinase, chymotrypsin, trypsin
4. **Antiserum**
   Tetanus, diphtheria, antitoxins, antithymocyte, antilymphocyte globulin
5. **Venoms (and saliva)**
   Hymenoptera (bees, vespids and wasp, fire ant); Chrysops (deerfly); Triatoma (kissing bug)
6. **Vaccines**
   Tetanus; egg containing vaccines (influenza, mumps); allergen extracts
7. **Foods**
   Milk, egg, wheat, fish and shellfish, legumes (peanuts), nuts (tree)
8. **Miscellaneous**
   Latex, seminal fluid

Complement-mediated

1. **Transfusion reaction associated with IgA deficiency**

4.1 Examples of agents causing anaphylaxis via immune mechanisms.

EXAMPLES OF NON-IMMUNE MECHANISMS OR CONDITIONS CAUSING ANAPHYLAXIS

1. **Direct histamine-releasing agents**
   Succinylcholine; ciproflaxin; vancomycin; pentamidine; radiocontrast media
2. **Arachidonate-mediated**
   Aspirin and non-steroidal anti-inflammatory drugs
3. **Physical**
   Exercise-induced; cold urticaria
4. **Idiopathic**

4.2 Examples of non-immune mechanisms or conditions causing anaphylaxis.

IDIOPATHIC ANAPHYLAXIS

A number of patients are also recognized as having idiopathic anaphylaxis, during which symptoms occur in the absence of any identifiable inciting agent. It is thought that this type of reaction may represent the most severe form of a spectrum of immediate-type reactions due to abnormal and inappropriate mast cell or basophil activation. Exercise-induced anaphylaxis may be included in this category. These individuals have been described as developing anaphylaxis more readily after eating certain foods, such as celery, just prior to exercise. Patients with systemic mastocytosis can also manifest reactions resembling anaphylaxis due to release of histamine and other mediators from the abundant and excessive mast cells.

CLINICAL MANIFESTATIONS OF ANAPHYLAXIS

1. **Cutaneous**
   Pruritus, erythema, urticaria, angiodema
2. **Respiratory**
   Sneezing, rhinorrhea, hoarseness, dysphonia, lump in throat, edema of upper airway (tongue, uvula, vocal cords), tachypnea, bronchospasm (wheezing, decreased breath sounds), apnea, asphyxia
3. **Cardiovascular**
   Tachycardia, dysrhythmia, vascular collapse, arrest (myocardial infarction)
4. **Gastrointestinal**
   Nausea, vomiting, cramps, pain, watery stools (bloody)
5. **Genital**
   Uterine cramps
6. **Neuropsychiatric**
   Seizures, feelings of 'impending doom'

4.3 Clinical manifestations of anaphylaxis.

CLINICAL PRESENTATION

Systemic anaphylaxis frequently involves multiple organ systems of the body, including the skin, respiratory, gastrointestinal, genital, cardiac, and neural systems. These clinical manifestations are outlined in **4.3**. The most important and life-threatening features are those involving the cardiovascular and respiratory tract. Individuals vary greatly in their manifestations of anaphylaxis, especially in the manner of onset and course. It may develop rapidly, reaching peak severity within 5–30 minutes. Late-phase reactions may occur 6–12 hours later and may last 5–30 hours, despite treatment. The typical patient develops generalized itching followed by cutaneous flushing, urticaria, a fullness in the throat, a feeling of 'anxiety', then tightness in the chest, faintness, and, finally, loss of consciousness.

Austen (1974) described the clinical and postmortem findings in six cases of fatal human anaphylaxis, calling attention to the fact that the interval between parenteral administration of an allergen and death ranged from a brief 16 minutes up to 2 hours. The dominant clinical event was laryngeal edema in four of the six patients. One case, however, differed from the rest in that chest pain and shock resulted in death within a few minutes.

CUTANEOUS AND RESPIRATORY SYMPTOMS

Skin manifestations, including pruritus, angioedema, and urticaria (*see* **4.4A**) can predominate. Acute swelling, as seen following a bee sting in **4.4B** may be followed by upper airway swelling and respiratory failure. Involvement of the eyes, nose, and mouth with tearing, redness of the eyes, runny nose, stuffiness, and sneezing may be accompanied by or seen in concert with upper respiratory signs and symptoms of hoarseness or a sensation of narrowing in the throat with stridor, edema of the uvula, and eventually, in some instances, with complete laryngeal obstruction. Lower respiratory symptoms may involve hyperventilation, wheezing associated with bronchospasm and asthma, decreased air exchange, use of accessory muscles, and finally apnea with respiratory arrest.

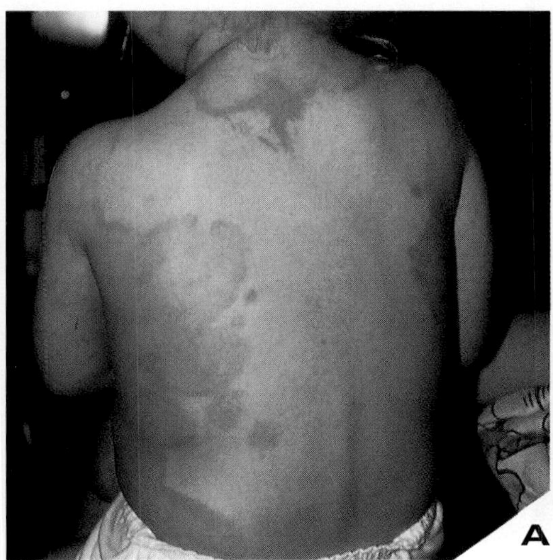

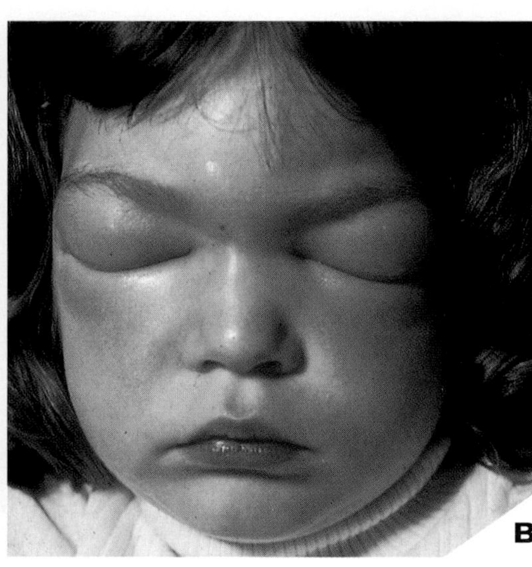

4.4 (A) Acute urticaria associated with anaphylaxis. (B) Facial swelling (angioedema), following a hymenoptera sting, associated with systemic anaphylaxis.

CARDIOVASCULAR AND NEUROLOGIC SYMPTOMS

Cardiovascular signs are very frequent in anaphylaxis and may vary from marked tachycardia to bradycardia or dysrhythmias. **4.5** lists electrocardiographic changes in 186 patients with cardiovascular collapse due to clinical anaphylaxis. Hypotension may eventually lead to cardiac arrest. Myocardial infarction has been reported to complicate anaphylaxis. Neurologic symptoms may be secondary to hypoxia, and include dizziness, weakness, seizures, and even the sensation of 'impending doom'.

PATHOGENESIS

IGE MEDIATION

IgE mediation has been considered responsible for anaphylaxis caused by antibiotics, foreign proteins, foods, drugs, preservatives, and venoms. Anaphylaxis mediated by IgE may occur in both atopic and non-atopic patients, indicating that a prior history of allergic rhinitis, atopic dermatitis, and asthma does not necessarily define an IgE-mediated mechanism as being operative in a particular anaphylactic situation. In fact, anaphylaxis is rarely a consequence of the natural exposure of an atopic individual to an allergen. IgE antibodies on the surface of mast cells mediate anaphylaxis by binding to complete antigens or to antigenic determinants formed by the covalent attachment of haptens (incomplete antigens) to large molecules such as albumin (**4.6**). This interaction leads to the release of mast cell mediators listed in **4.7** and **4.8**.

MEDIATOR RELEASE

The mast-cell mediator identified most commonly in anaphylaxis is histamine, and tissues rich in mast cells are the primary target tissues in anaphylaxis. **4.9** relates histamine plasma levels with some symptoms and manifestation of anaphylaxis. Tryptase, a neutral protease selectively concentrated in the secretory granules of human mast cells, but not basophils, may serve as a marker of mast-cell activation in anaphylaxis.

Anaphylaxis can also follow the release of mediators following massive complement activation, which generates anaphylatoxins C_{3a} and C_{5a} (see **4.6**). These anaphylatoxins bind to mast-cell receptors, alter the cell membrane, and initiate mast -cell degranulation. The mechanisms by which acetylsalicylic acid, other structurally unrelated non-steroidal anti-inflammatory agents, azodyes, and certain preservatives provoke mediator release are not well understood. Non-steroidal anti-inflammatory agents are known to

ELECTROCARDIOGRAPHIC (ECG) CHANGES IN 186 PATIENTS WITH CARDIOVASCULAR COLLAPSE DUE TO CLINICAL ANAPHYLAXIS

ECG Changes	Number of Patients
Supraventricular tachycardia	153
Supraventricular tachycardia with ST elevation	8
Supraventricular tachycardia with ventricular fibrillation	4
Supraventricular tachycardia following transient sinus bradycardia	6
Sinus bradycardia in presence of beta blockers	4
Bradycardia and asystole	2
Rapid atrial fibrillation	4
Other	5

4.5 Electrocardiographic changes in 186 patients with cardiovascular collapse due to clinical anaphylaxis. (Reproduced with permission from Fisher, 1987.)

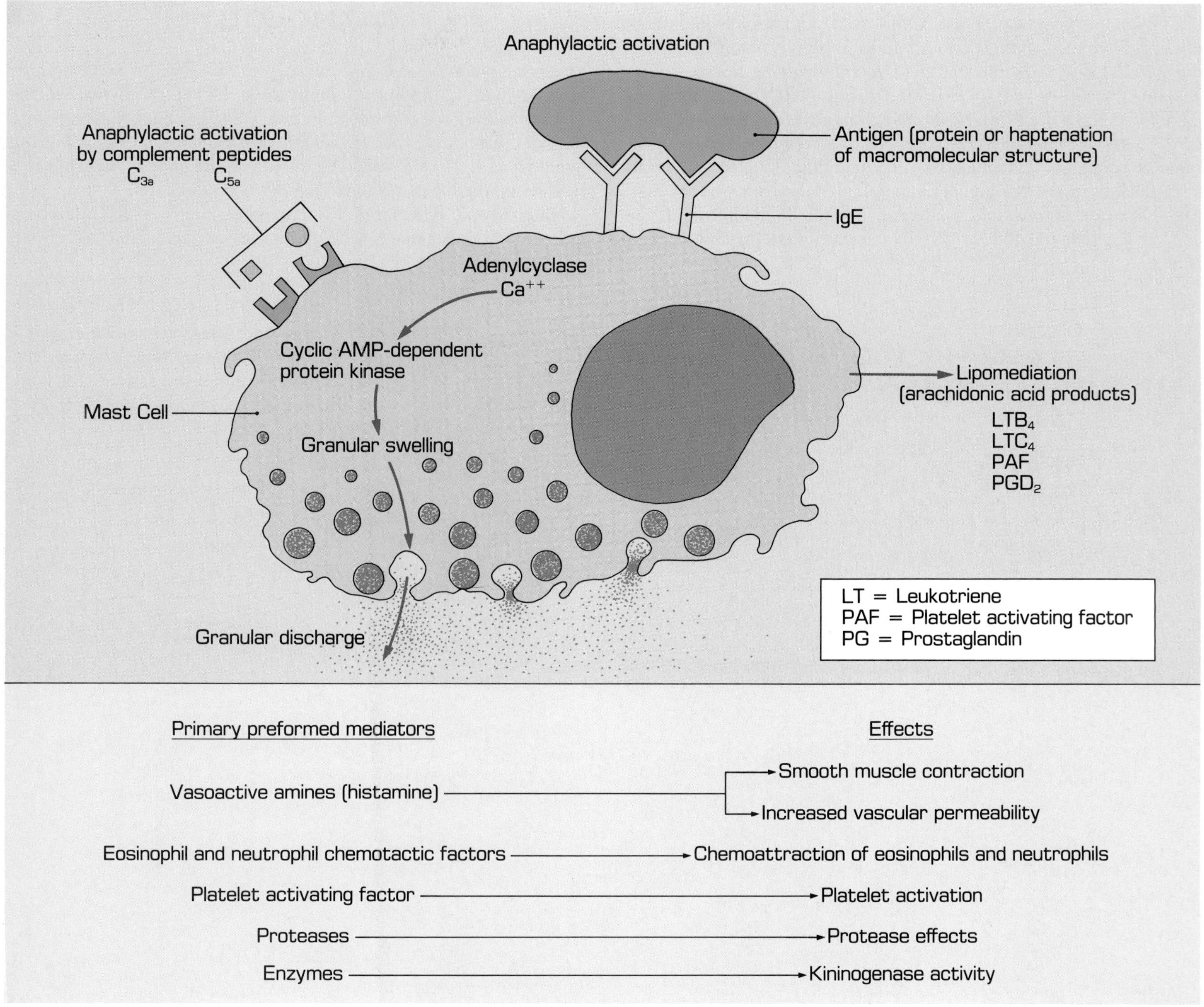

4.6 Activation of the mast cell.

CLASSES OF PREFORMED HUMAN MAST-CELL MEDIATORS

1. Biogenic amines (histamine)
2. Neutral proteases (tryptase, chymase, carboxypeptidase)
3. Acid hydrolases (arylsulfatase)
4. Oxidative enzymes (superoxide, peroxidase)
5. Chemotactic factors (eosinophil, neutrophil)
6. Proteoglycans (heparin)

4.7 Classes of preformed human mast-cell mediators.

MEMBRANE DERIVED HUMAN MAST-CELL MEDIATORS

1. Prostaglandin D_2
2. Leukotrienes B_4, C_4, E_4
3. Platelet activating factor

4.8 Membrane derived human mast-cell mediators.

inhibit cyclo-oxygenase. Their ability to induce anaphylaxis may possibly be related to their potency in inhibiting prostaglandin synthesis by shifting arachidonic acid metabolism to lipoxygenase-dependent pathways (**4.10**) or by activating platelets. Disorders of hemostasis have been observed during anaphylaxis, possibly related to release of heparin from mast cells or alteration of platelets or other components of hemostasis and coagulant. The role of specific mediators in the pathogenesis of anaphylaxis remains speculative. One can assume that a diverse number of mediators act in concert together to produce the clinical pathologic findings.

PATHOLOGY

The principle anatomic and microscopic findings in fatal anaphylaxis include pulmonary emphysema (**4.11**), laryngeal edema (**4.12**), visceral congestion, pulmonary edema, intra-alveolar hemorrhage, urticaria, and angioedema. These findings result from hypoxia and hypovolemia. Autopsy findings may be complicated by therapeutic measures (iatrogenic procedures).

Microscopic evidence (**4.13**) that suggests myocardial infarction, pulmonary hemorrhage, edema, increased bronchial secretions,

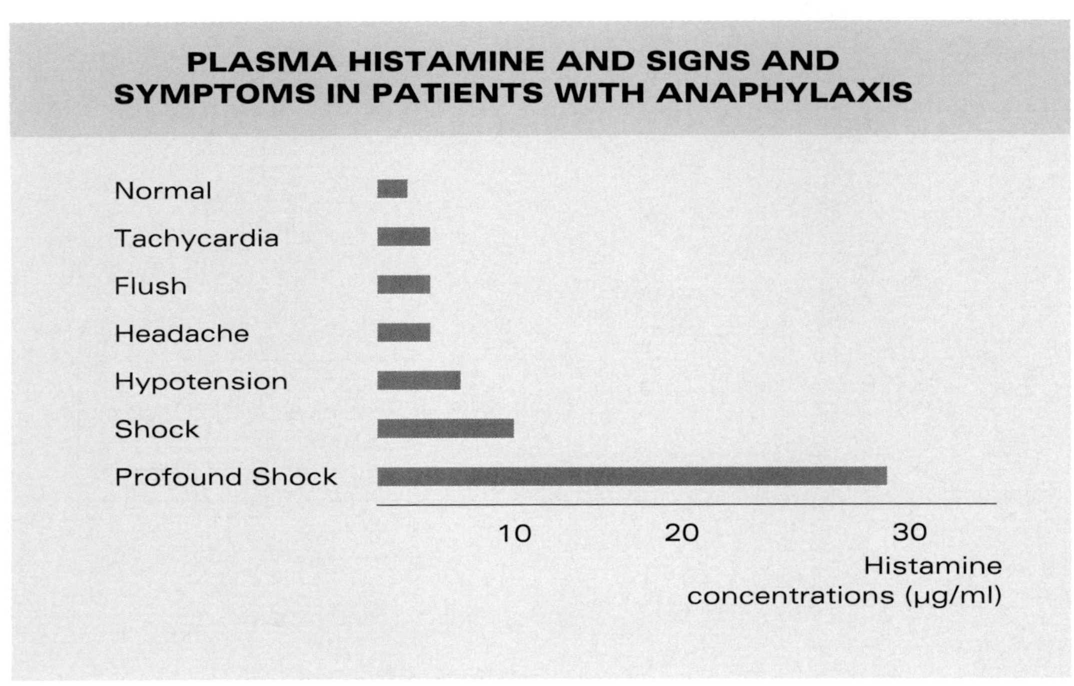

4.9 Symptoms and signs associated with plasma histamine levels in normal subjects and patients experiencing anaphylaxis with varying degrees of severity. (Modified with permission from Fisher, 1987.)

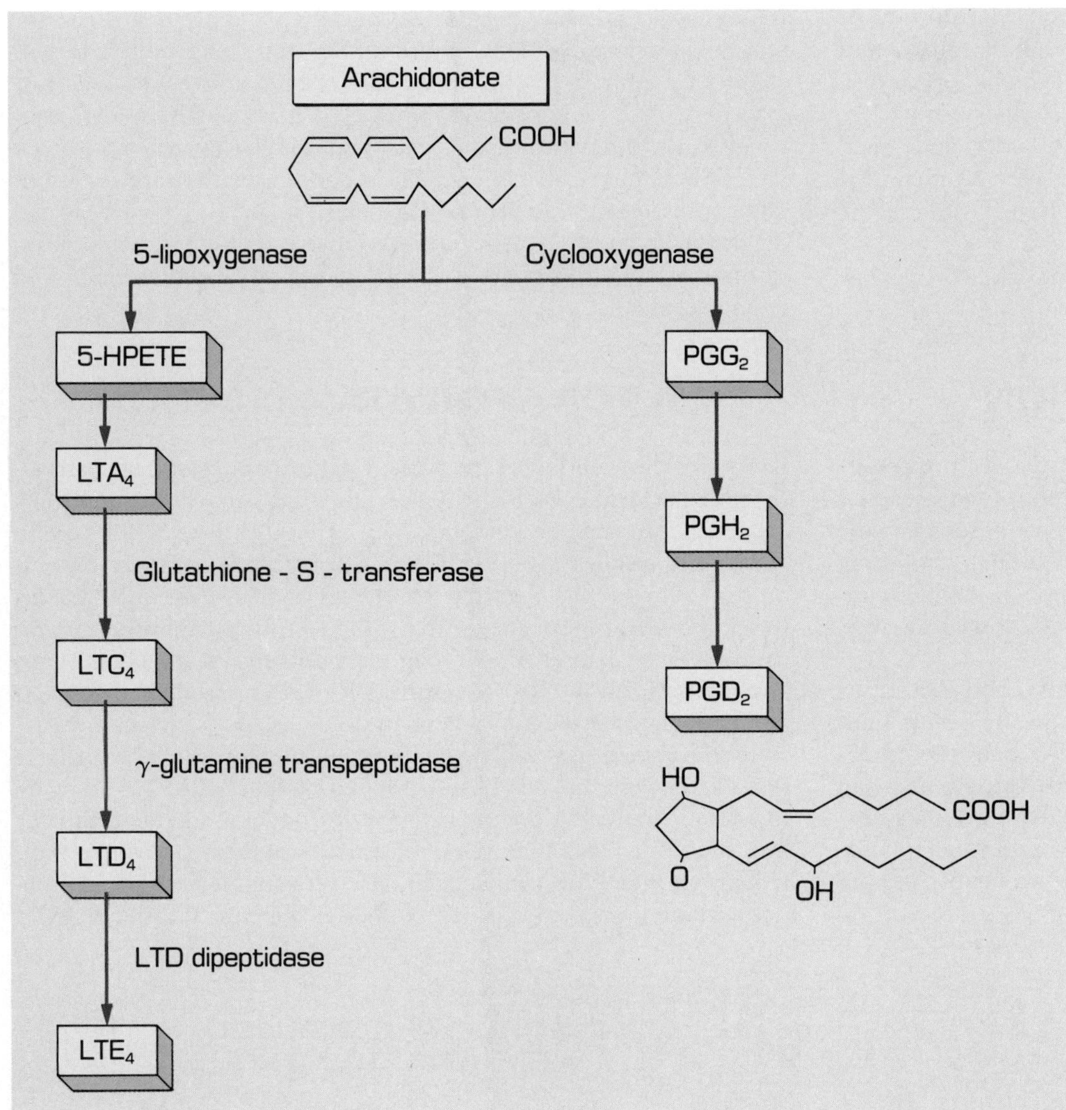

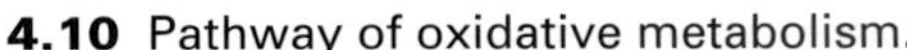

4.10 Pathway of oxidative metabolism.

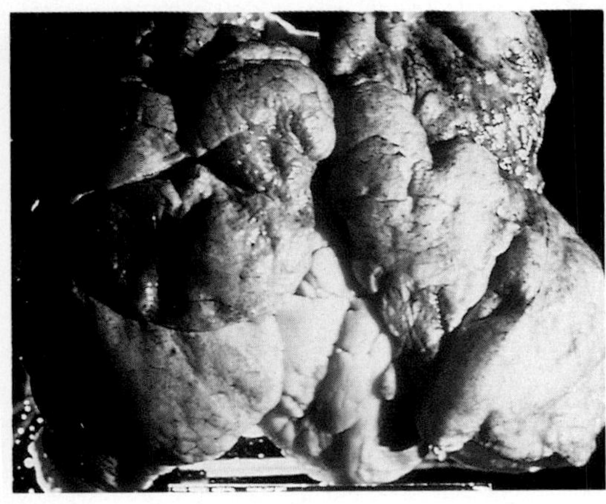

4.11 Pulmonary emphysema.

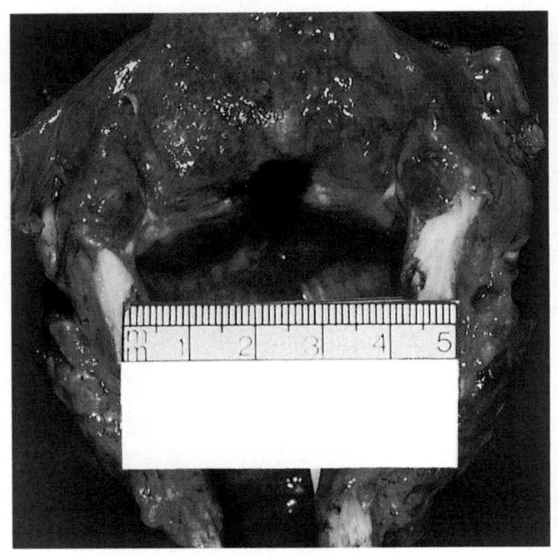

4.12 Laryngeal edema.

peribronchial vascular congestion, and eosinophilic infiltration of the bronchial walls can be found. There is accumulation of thin non-inflammatory fluid in the lamina propria of the hypopharynx, epiglottis, and larynx in up to two-thirds of fatal cases. Other less specific findings associated with systemic anaphylaxis include liver, spleen, and other abdominal visceral congestion, with an increased number of eosinophils in the red pulp of the spleen. Hemorrhagic gastritis may also be seen.

DIAGNOSIS

PHYSICAL EVALUATION

The diagnosis of systemic anaphylaxis has been based on recognition of the clinical features. It is generally, but not always readily, apparent; it must be differentiated from neurogenic vasovagal collapse, which is quite common and presents with similar symptoms (*see* below). The cardinal features of anaphylaxis include acute hypotension, upper airway obstruction, and lower airway (bronchial) obstruction (*see* **4.3**).

The patient with vasovagal collapse (a neuropsychological reaction) can be confused with anaphylaxis. This typically occurs during stressful circumstances, such as during a venepuncture or injection. The patient appears pale, complains of nausea, sweats, has bradycardia, and generally maintains a normal blood pressure. There is no itching, tachycardia, urticaria, or angioedema and, although hyperventilation may intervene, no bronchospasm is noted. Tachycardia is more typical of anaphylaxis.

If laryngeal edema is present during anaphylaxis, hoarseness or aphonia develops. Globus hystericus, the disturbing subjective sensation of a lump in the throat seen in hysteria conversion-behavior disorders, may be considered. However, it is usually milder, nonprogressive, and without any signs of anatomic changes in the pharynx or hypopharynx. Other medical conditions that are occasionally confused with anaphylaxis are listed in **4.14**. This differential diagnosis includes cardiac dysrhythmias, pulmonary embolism, seizures, strokes, hyperventilation, hereditary angioedema, and hypoglycemia.

LABORATORY EVALUATION

Laboratory evaluation of the patient with anaphylactic hypersensitivity is performed to identify the potential causative antigens or agents. It can best be performed by *in vivo* skin tests for certain agents and *in vitro* tests for others. IgE antibody to insect venoms or penicillin can be detected by the more sensitive epicutaneous (prick modification of the scratch) skin test, using appropriate precautions (*see* Chapter 3). Although less sensitive, it may be safer to initially perform *in vitro* serum tests for IgE antibodies to suspected anaphylaxis-provoking allergens, such as foods, which are less well-characterized. Such tests, including radioallergosorbent (RAST), enzyme linked (ELISA), or fluorescence (FAST), eliminate the risk of inducing anaphylaxis by introducing allergen onto or into the skin. Histamine release from leukocytes of sensitive individuals upon *in vitro* challenge are not yet suitable for clinical practice and are limited to research studies at this time. Passive transfer

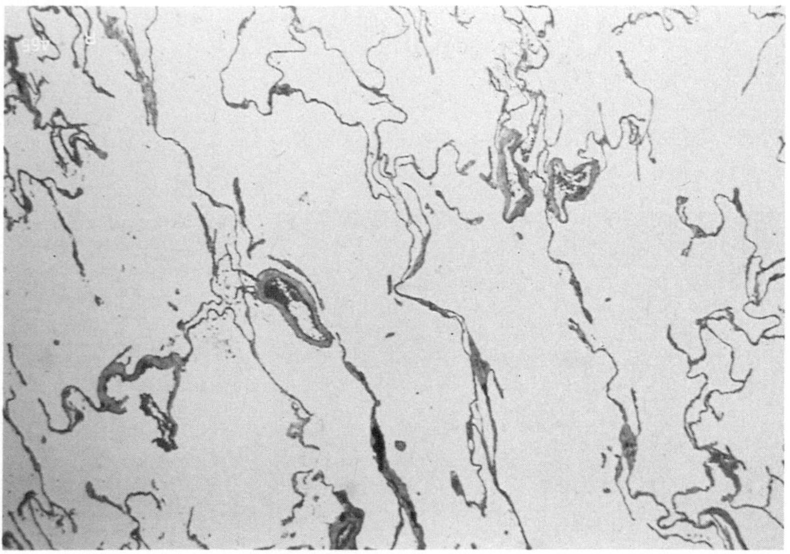

4.13 Microscopic changes: lung.

DISORDERS CONFUSED WITH ANAPHYLAXIS

1. **Cardiac conditions**
   Dysrhythmias, myocardial infarction, arrest
2. **Endocrine problems**
   Carcinoid tumor, pheochromocytoma, hypoglycemia
3. **Pulmonary embolus**
   Pneumothorax, hyperventilation, severe asthma, tracheal foreign body (food, etc.)
4. **Neurologic**
   Head injury, epilepsy, cerebrovascular accident
5. **Other**
   Hereditary angioedema, drug/alcohol reactions, factitious stridor, cold urticaria

4.14 Clinical disorders confused with anaphylaxis.

studies involving normal subjects, as done in the past as Praunitz–Kustner tests, are no longer recommended because of the risk of passive transfer of hepatitis, HIV, or other potentially virus-contaminated sera into the normal recipients. Complement consumption *in vitro* has not been utilized to define anaphylactic mechanisms, although its absence *in vivo* has been noted in exercise-induced anaphylaxis. Histamine levels have been measured and correlated with symptoms of anaphylaxis, but are not yet practical in the clinical management of anaphylaxis. However, serum tryptase levels can be used as an indicator of anaphylaxis.

Oral provocative challenge studies with various foods, chemicals, and drugs can be performed, but may be hazardous if previous experience has been life-threatening. However, sensitivity to aspirin (and other non-steroidal anti-inflammatory agents), tartrazine (yellow dye No 5), and benzoates may be confirmed by carefully graded oral challenge with close monitoring, observation, and measurement of pulmonary function and blood pressure.

TREATMENT AND PREVENTION

The treatment of anaphylaxis can be life-saving. Prompt recognition is essential, since death may occur within minutes. Therapy, as outlined in **4.15**, must be initiated even if there is doubt about the diagnosis, such as in the instance of vasovagal neurogenic reactions following parenteral administration of a vaccine or allergen extract.

TREATMENT OF ANAPHYLAXIS

1. Assess rapidly.
2. Place in recumbent position and elevate lower extremities.
3. Discontinue inciting agent or allergen.
4. Inject epinephrine 1:1000, 0.01 ml/kg (max 0.3–0.5 ml) subcutaneously q 20 min x 3.
5. Establish airway; may require racemic epinephrine by nebulizer or endotracheal tube.
6. Provide supplemental oxygen if needed.
7. Give diphenhydramine 1.25 mg/kg (max 50 mg) IV over 3–5 min.
8. Give cimetidine 5 mg/kg (max 300 mg) or ranitidine 1 mg/kg (max 50 mg) IV over 3–5 min.
9. Establish IV to maintain blood pressure with IV fluids (saline or volume expanders), pressors (dopamine hydrochloride 2–10 μg/kg/min or norepinephrine bitartrate 2–4 μg/min).
10. Give aminophylline 5 mg/kg IV over 20 min then 0.5–1.0 mg/kg/hr for severe bronchospasm.
11. Provide hydrocortisone 5 mg/kg (max 100 mg) IV q 6 hours.

4.15 Treatment of anaphylaxis.

Anoxia is life-threatening and an adequate airway with supplements of oxygen when available is essential. Equipment helpful in this emergency situation is shown in **4.16A** and **4.16B**.

MEDICAL TREATMENT

The initial treatment of anaphylaxis with epinephrine is crucial in:
- Supporting blood pressure.
- Decreasing bronchospasm, which helps maintain an effective airway.
- Decreasing laryngeal edema, especially when given as a racemic epinephrine aerosol.
- Slowing the absorption of injected agents if promptly used to infiltrate the site of injection.

A tourniquet can also be applied above the injection site because this can reduce and compress venous return at the site of an injection and decrease systemic absorption of antigen. It should be released for one of every three minutes.

It is essential to move the patient as soon as possible to an emergency room or intensive-care hospital facility that can manage major complications, such as cardiac arrhythmias, cardiorespiratory arrest, seizures, myocardial infarction, hypovolemia, and obstruction of the airway. Antihistamines (H_1 and H_2 receptor blockers) are suggested and may decrease the potential for cardiac arrhythmias and peripheral vasodilation, as well as possibly urticaria/angioedema and gastrointestinal symptoms. Corticosteroids, although requiring several hours to exert beneficial effects, are indicated and may prevent late-phase reactions.

If a patient who is on therapy with a beta-adrenergic blocking agent, such as propranolol for hypertension, vascular headaches, mitral valve prolapse, or cardiac arrhythmias, develops anaphylaxis, the management may be compromised by the propranolol. Treatment may require massive infusing of fluid to support circulation compromised by the decreased peripheral resistance. In addition, judicious administration of epinephrine, for alpha-adrenergic activity, and isoproterenol to attempt to overcome the beta blockade may be indicated. Therefore, beta-adrenergic blocking drugs should be used judiciously in patients at risk for anaphylaxis.

PREVENTION

The avoidance of potential and future anaphylaxis is of great importance. Steps should be taken to limit exposure to agents known to precipitate and aggravate anaphylaxis (**4.17**). In general, agents given by the oral route, instead of parenterally, provoke anaphylaxis much less frequently. This is especially true for penicillin

EQUIPMENT TO MAINTAIN AIRWAY IN CASE OF ANAPHYLAXIS

Disposable pharyngeal airways (#1, 2, 3, 4, 5)

Self-inflating bag-mask-valve unit - three mask sizes

Endotracheal tubes:

— Uncuffed (ages 2–10 years); sizes 3.0–5.0 mm

— Cuffed (ages 10–adult); sizes 7.0–9.0 mm

Laryngoscope: Medium handle - #2, 3, 4 blades

A

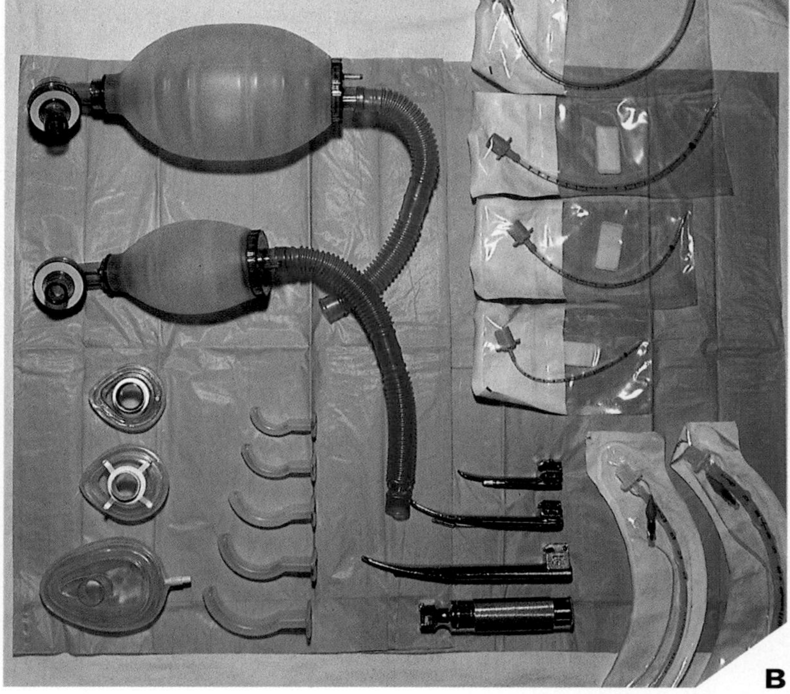

B

4.16 (A and B) Equipment to maintain airway in case of anaphylaxis.

and other anti-microbials, due to the decreased rate of absorption when given orally. If the parenteral route is chosen, the patient should be observed for 20–30 minutes after the injections.

If a drug known to have caused anaphylaxis in the past is urgently needed to treat a life-threatening disease, desensitization can be performed to minimize the severity of the expected reaction. This procedure is described later. Patients should carry on their person medical information regarding known anaphylactic sensitivity and wear a bracelet. Administration of pretreatment corticosteroids and antihistamines (H_1, H_2) to prevent anaphylaxis in selected situations, such as known sensitivity to radiocontrast media, is recommended. Alternative medication, especially antibiotics, should be utilized. It is also now possible to substitute a non-ionic radiocontrast agent to lessen the possibility of anaphylactic reactions to radiocontrast media in susceptible patients.

Avoid using beta-adrenergic blocking agents in patients with a previous history of anaphylaxis. Caution and judgment must be exercised when skin testing allergic patients who are being treated with beta-blockers for any of a variety of illnesses, such as hypertension, migraine, and glaucoma. Immunotherapy for patients taking the beta-blocker drugs should be avoided until alternative drug regimens for the beta-blocker can be instituted.

SELECTED EXAMPLES OF ANAPHYLAXIS

IMMUNOLOGICALLY MEDIATED ANAPHYLAXIS

Stinging Hymenoptera Insect Anaphylaxis

Generalized systemic reactions to stinging hymenopteras have been recognized as potentially life-threatening phenomena related to the IgE antibodies to the various components of venom from the honeybee, yellow jacket, white-faced hornet, yellow hornet, and wasp (**4.18–4.20**). Most fatal reactions to insect venom occur in adults, as noted in **4.21**. The diagnosis of IgE hypersensitivity is best determined by skin testing. For the purposes of immunotherapy, it is important to define the specific insect venom responsible for the reaction. Even more important is deciding whether or not the individual should be tested based on the history of anaphylaxis. Local reactions without systemic anaphylaxis do not warrant allergy testing.

4.22 gives medical indications for the selection of patients for venom skin testing and immunotherapy. Children aged 16 years or

PREVENTION OF ANAPHYLAXIS

1. Avoid exposure to agents known to cause anaphylaxis
2. Use oral rather than parenteral medication
3. Have patients carry information on person concerning anaphylactic sensitivity
4. Avoid beta-adrenergic blocking agents in anaphylaxis-prone patients
5. Pretreat with steroids and antihistamines if patient requires procedure (radiocontrast media) or must have medications

4.17 Prevention of anaphylaxis.

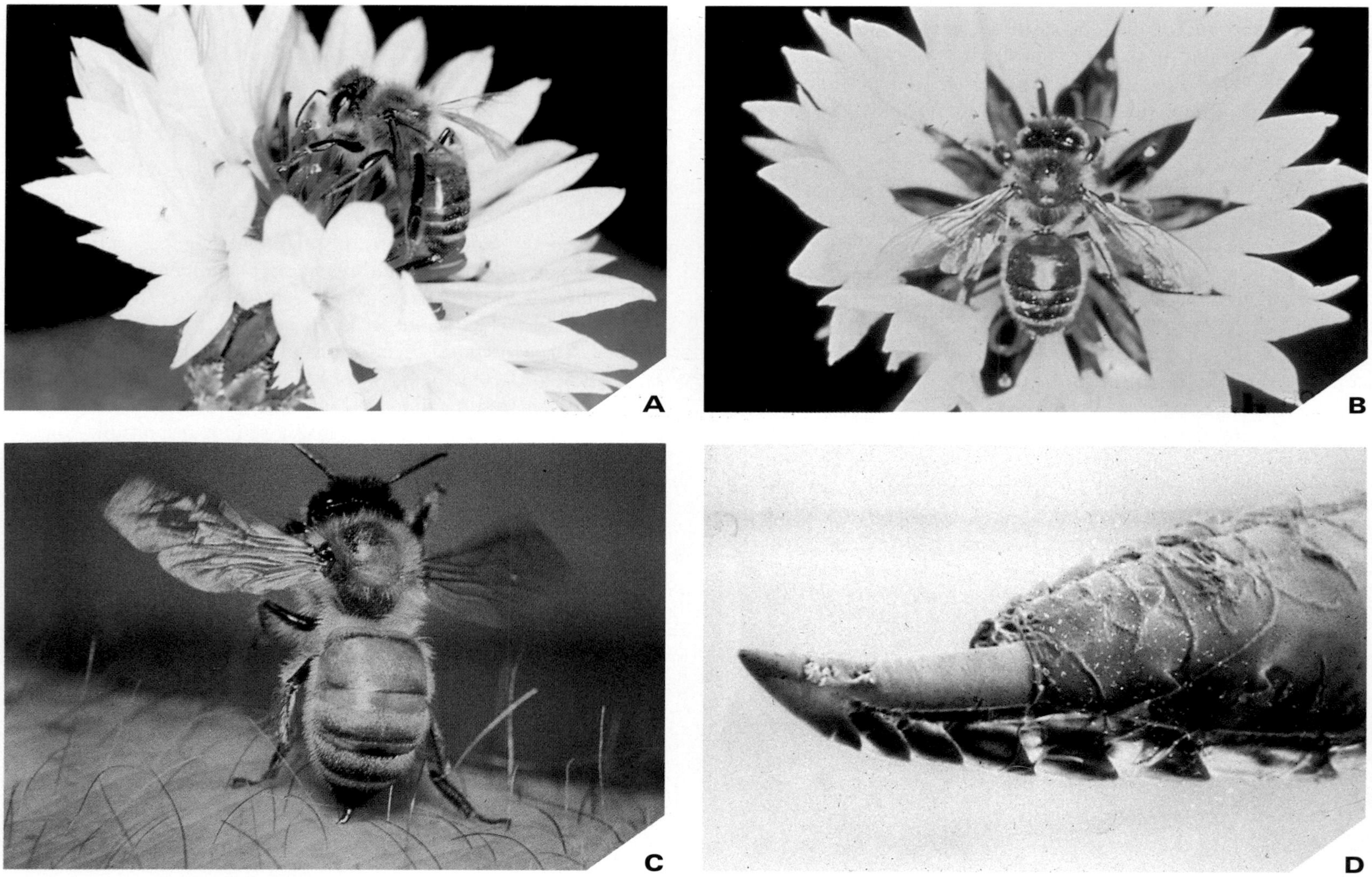

4.18 Hymenoptera (honey bee): (A) Lateral. (B) Dorsal view. (C) Stinging with barbed stinger. (D) Stinger left in skin after sting.

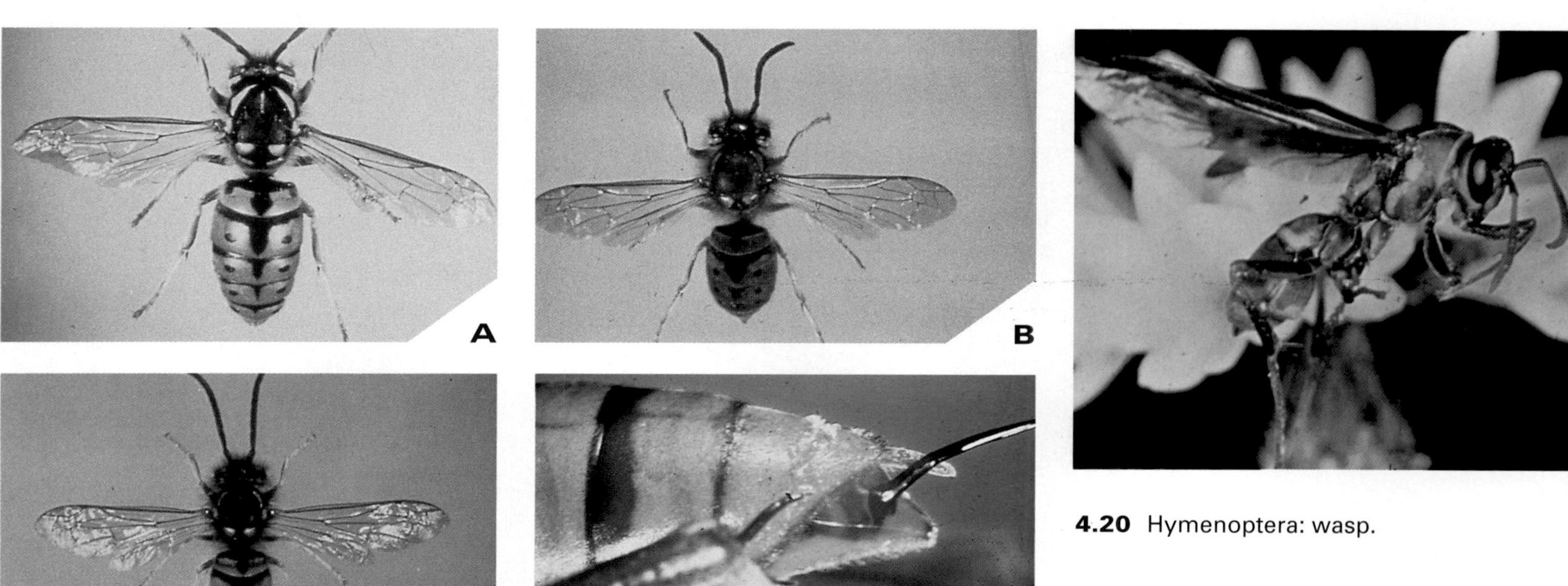

4.19 Hymenoptera (honey bee): (A) Yellow jacket. (B) Yellow hornet. (C) White faced hornet. (D) Yellow jacket with retractible stinger.

4.20 Hymenoptera: wasp.

younger who have experienced only cutaneous manifestations with their allergic reactions, that is, generalized urticaria and angioedema without respiratory or cardiovascular signs or symptoms, do not warrant routine venom immunotherapy.

If the decision is made to provide venom immunotherapy, a schedule should be followed such as illustrated in **4.23A** and **4.23B**.

INSECT STING DEATHS IN THE UNITED STATES

Age (yr)	1979	1980	1981	1982	1983	1983	TOTAL
0–9	1	0	0	0	2	2	3
10–19	1	0	1	0	3	3	3
20–29	1	1	2	3	9	9	9
30–39	4	1	7	4	8	8	24
40–49	10	7	6	16	9	9	48
50–59	7	13	12	13	9	9	54
60–69	13	13	6	10	10	10	52
over 70	1	3	5	8	8	8	25
Total	38	38	39	54	49	49	218
M:F	3:17	25:13	35:4	45:9	43:6	43:6	179:39

Source: National Center for Health Statistics.
M:F = male:female

4.21 Insect sting deaths in the United States. (Reproduced with permission from Graft, 1987.)

SELECTION OF PATIENTS FOR VENOM SKIN-TESTING AND IMMUNOTHERAPY

Classification of sting reaction by history	Venom skin test	Venom immunotherapy
Local	+/–	No
Large local	+/–	No
Systemic:		
(life threatening)	+	Yes
(non-life threatening)		
Adult	+	Yes
Children (<16 years)	+	No
Toxic	+/–	No
Delayed (>24 hours)	+/–	No

4.22 Selection of patients for venom immunotherapy.

DOSAGE REGIME FOR VENOM IMMUNOTHERAPY

Week no.	Vial concentration (ug/ml)	Volume (ml/cm^3)
1	1	0.05
2	1	0.10
3	1	0.20
4	1	0.40
5	10	0.05
6	10	0.10
7	10	0.20
8	10	0.40
9	100	0.05
10	100	0.10
11	100	0.20
12	100	0.40
13	100	0.60
14	100	0.80
15	100	1 cm^3
16	100	1 cm^3
17	no injection	
18	100	1 cm^3
19	no injection	
20	no injection	
21	100	1 cm^3
Begin maintenance q 4 weeks		
25	100	1 cm^3
Continue maintenance q 4 weeks till the end of the first year (52 weeks), then q 6 weeks (if anti-venom IgG level is >3 μg/ml)	100	1 cm^3

A

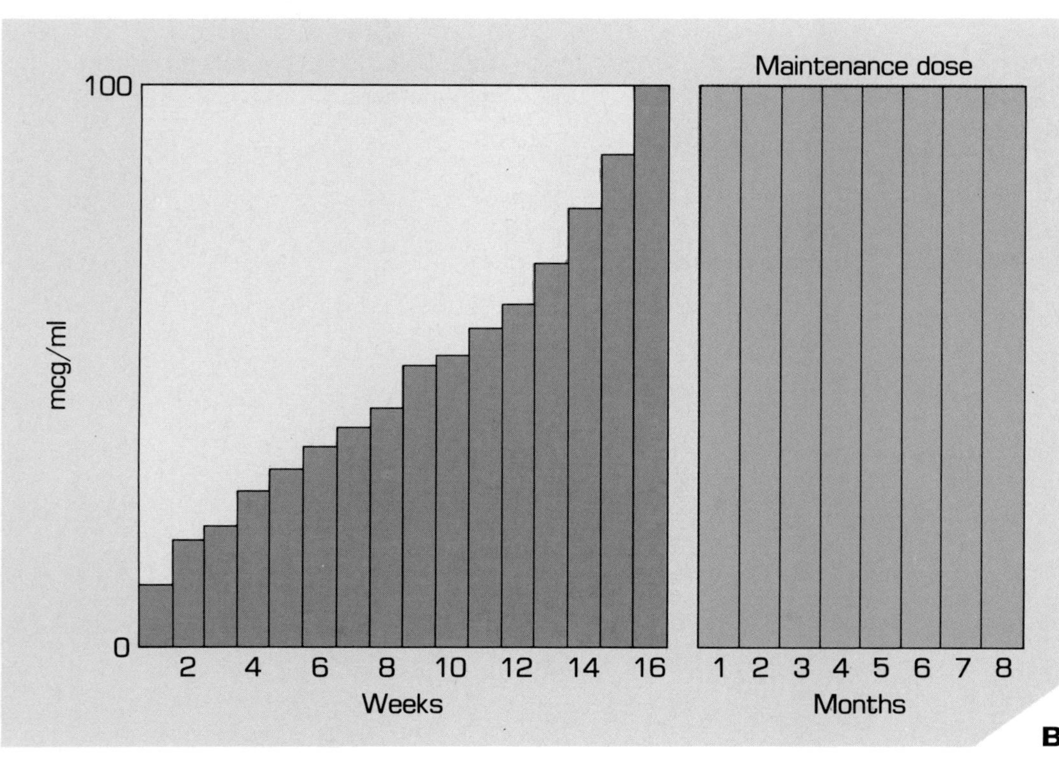

4.23 (A) Dosage regime for venom immunotherapy. (B) Treatment schedule.

Virtually 100% of patients can be protected after increasing the dose of venom to 100 µg, which is approximately equivalent to the amount of venom in two stings. The interval of immunotherapy injections after reaching the maintenance dose is between 4–6 weeks. The duration of the immunotherapy should be at least 5 years. Some clinicians suggest longer periods of therapy, perhaps even for a lifetime, but this is not definitely established at this time. There are no tests to help the clinician decide when to discontinue venom immunotherapy. Protection is probably related to the loss of allergic reactivity of the skin to venom, but this has not been defined for clinical practice. Immunotherapy with whole body extract is contraindicated for bee, wasp, hornet, and yellow jacket insects, but has been shown to be effective for fire ant allergic reactions.

Immune-mediated penicillin anaphylaxis

Drug hapten-protein hypersensitivity can be best illustrated by penicillin allergy. Penicillin anaphylaxis has been estimated to account for 200–500 deaths per year in the United States, or 97% of drug anaphylaxis deaths.

The history of a pruritic macular or urticarial type eruption while taking penicillin is suggestive of allergy. However, the rash may be associated with the infection for which the penicillin is prescribed, and not due to penicillin allergy. A history of life-threatening anaphylaxis with penicillin in a patient who requires penicillin treatment is a serious consideration. The antigenic determinant for most penicillin allergy is the penicilloyl metabolic by-product of penicillin metabolism. Skin testing with benzylpenicilloylpolylysine, the penicilloyl synthetic polypeptide conjugate (Pre-Pen®), an aqueous penicillin G minor determinant mixture, and freshly prepared aqueous penicillin are used to document specific IgE-mediated allergy (**4.24**). If no reaction to skin testing with these reagents occurs, then penicillin can be cautiously administered. If skin tests are positive, then desensitization of a proven allergic individual may be performed orally, subcutaneously, intramuscularly, or intra-

PROTOTYPE OF CHART FOR USE IN CLINICAL SKIN-TESTING FOR PENICILLIN ALLERGY

Puncture	Size of wheel and flare	Puncture	Size of wheel and flare
Pre-pen® (benzylpenicilloyl-polylysine) Aq. Pen-G —100 u —1000 u —10,000 u		Pre-pen® (benzylpenicilloyl-polylysine) Aq. Pen-G —100 u —1000 u —10,000 u	
Aq. Pen-G MD (minor determinant) —100 u —1000 u —10,000 u		Aq. Pen-G MD (minor determinant) —100 u —1000 u —10,000 u	
Diluent control		Diluent control	
Histamine control —1:1000		Histamine control —1:1000	

4.24 Penicillin allergy skin testing.

venously (4.25). During these procedures, personal physician observation and availability of medications and equipment for treatment of anaphylaxis are mandatory (4.15 and 4.16).

Sensitivities to other hapten-protein antigens, including local anesthetic agents, cephalosporin, and insulin, can be similarly evaluated and tested. No skin-testing procedures are available for macrolides, sulfas, or tetracyclines. Provocative challenges with antibiotics, especially parenteral preparations, may be dangerous and should be avoided or performed under constant medical supervision. Failure to react to the skin tests for penicillin allergy guarantees safety from significant anaphylaxis in 98% of patients, but does not rule out late-phase allergic reactions.

NON-IMMUNE-MEDIATED ANAPHYLAXIS

Radiocontrast media

An example of non-immune-mediated anaphylaxis is that seen with ionic iodinated contrast media (sodium meglumine salts of ionic acids). The reported incidence of severe reactions is 1 in 1000 uses of the contrast media, and of deaths is 1 in 1200 to 1 in 75,000 contrast studies. This reaction can be primarily cutaneous, manifesting as pruritus or urticaria, or it can be systemic, with upper airway edema and smooth muscle contraction. Dyspnea due to bronchospasm or shock due to capillary dilation and increased permeability may occur.

PENICILLIN DENSENSITIZATION PROTOCOL

Dose[a]	Units	Route[b]
1	100	PO
2	200	PO
3	400	PO
4	800	PO
5	1,600	PO
6	3,200	PO
7	6,400	PO
8	12,800	PO
9	25,000	PO
10	50,000	PO
11	100,000	PO
12	200,000	PO
13	400,000	PO
14	200,000	SC
15	400,000	SC
16	800,000	SC
17	1,000,000	IM
18	1,000,000	IV

[a]Interval between doses = 15 minutes.
[b]PO = oral; SC = subcutaneous; IM = intramuscular; IV = intravenous.

4.25 Penicillin desensitization protocol.

MEDICATION PROTOCOLS FOR PREVENTION OF RADIOCONTRAST MEDIA ANAPHYLAXIS

1. **Corticosteroids**
   Prednisone 50 mg, PO, 3 or 4 doses, q 6 hours, 18–24 hours.
   Methylprednisolone 100 mg IV, q 6 hours, 18–24 hours.
   Hydrocortisone 200 mg IV, immediately before radiocontrast procedure.
2. **H_1 receptor-blocking antihistamine**
   Diphenhydramine 1.25 mg/kg (max 50 mg) PO or IV.
   Chlorpheniramine 0.08 mg/kg (max 4 mg) PO or IV.
   Hydroxyzine 0.5 mg/kg (26 mg max), PO, q 6 hours, 18–24 hours or immediately before procedure.
3. **H_2 receptor-blocking antihistamine**
   Cimetidine 5 mg/kg (max 300 mg).
   Ranitidine 1 mg/kg (max 50 mg), PO or IV, q 6 hours, 18–24 hours or immediately before procedure.
4. **Beta-adrenergic agents**
   Epinephrine 0.5 mg/kg (max 25 mg), PO, 1 hour before procedure, unless contraindicated by angina, hypertension, or arrhythmias.

4.26 Medication protocols for prevention of radiocontrast media anaphylaxis.

No diagnostic laboratory tests are available. The history of a primary anaphylactic reaction is the important criteria for prophylactic treatment. This can be in the form of pretreating with H_1 and H_2 receptor-blocking antihistamines (diphenhydramine and cimetadine), corticosteroids (prednisone or methylprednisolone), and less commonly beta-adrenergic agents (ephedrine). The use of H_1 and H_2 receptor-blocking antihistamines may reduce the potential for cardiac arrhythmias and peripheral vasodilation. Corticosteroids can prevent potential late-phase reactions. **4.26** outlines protocols for the prevention of this potential anaphylactic reaction.

The recent introduction of non-ionic, low-osmolar contrast media (iohexaol, iopamidol, and sodium meglumine ioxaglate) has greatly reduced the risk of serious anaphylactic reactions to iodinated contrast media. The substitution of these agents for the ionic iodinated, relatively osmolar media must still be preceded by prophylactic medications as noted above.

Exercise-induced anaphylaxis

Another example of non-immune-mediated anaphylaxis occurs in a few individuals with a tendency to develop anaphylaxis during exercise. Signs and symptoms begin with generalized itching followed by flushing, urticaria, angioedema, collapse, choking with respiratory distress, abdominal cramps, and headache. In rare instances, exercise is preceded by the ingestion of specific foods such as celery, fish, shellfish, or any food within 2–4 or even up to 12 hours preceding exercise. Stopping exercise at the first sign of impending anaphylaxis, such as itching, is advisable. Once the reaction is underway, the usual treatment for anaphylaxis is indicated. Prophylactic antihistamine treatment has not been preventive, but antihistamines can be helpful in ameliorating the cutaneous manifestations.

REFERENCES

Austen KF: Systemic anaphylaxis in the human being. *N Engl J Med*; **291**:661, 1974.

Bochner BS, Lichtenstein LM: Anaphylaxis. *N Engl J Med*, 1991:

Fisher M: Anaphylaxis. *Disease-a-Month*, **33**(8):433, 1987.

Graft DF: Venom immunotherapy for stinging insect allergy. *Clin Rev Allergy*, **5**:149, 1987.

Greenberger PA, Patterson R: The prevention of immediate generalized reaction to radiocontrast media in high-risk patients. *J Allergy Clin Immunol*, **87**:867, 1991.

James LP, Austen KF: Fatal systemic anaphylaxis in man. *N Engl J Med*, **270**:597, 1964.

Lieberman P: The use of antihistamines in the prevention and treatment of anaphylaxis and anaphylactoid reactions. *J Allergy Clin Immunol*, **86**:684, 1990.

Marquardt DL, Wasserman SI: Anaphylaxis, in Middleton E, Reed CE, Ellis, EF, Adkinson NF, Yunginger JW, Busse WW (eds): *Allergy: Principles and Practice*, C.V. Mosby, St Louis, Chapter 60, 1993.

Schwartz LB, Metcalfe DD, Miller JS, *et. al.*: Tryptase levels as an indicator of mast cell activation in systemic anaphylaxis and mastocytosis. *N Engl J Med*, **316**:1622, 1987.

Sheffer AL, Austen KF: Exercised-induced anaphylaxis. *J Allergy Clin Immunol*, **73**:699, 1984.

Sheffer AL, Horan RF: Anaphylaxis, in Holgate ST, Church MK (eds): *Allergy*, Gower, London, pp 27.1–27.10, 1993.

Sullivan TJ, Yecies LD, Shatz, GS, Parker, CW, Wedner HJ: Desensitization of patients allergic to penicillin using orally administered B-lactam antibiotics. *J Allergy Clin Immunol*, **69**:275, 1982

Wiggins CA, Dykewicz MS, Patterson R: Idiopathic anaphylaxis: A review. *Ann Allergy*, **62**:1, 1989

CHAPTER 5

Asthma

David P. Skoner

Asthma, a lower airways disease characterized by enhanced responsiveness to various stimuli and manifested by airways obstruction which changes spontaneously or therapeutically, is a common illness in both the pediatric and adult populations. The most widely accepted definition of asthma includes the following characteristics:

- Lower airway obstruction which is partially or fully reversible, either spontaneously or with bronchodilator or anti-inflammatory treatments.
- The presence of airway inflammation.
- Increased lower airway responsiveness to several stimuli, such as cold air or exercise in the natural environment and inhaled methacholine or histamine in a laboratory environment.

The prevalence, morbidity, and mortality of asthma have been increasing since 1970. To lessen its enormous present and future socio-economic impact on our society, asthma must be recognized early and treated appropriately. This chapter reviews our current understanding of the etiology, natural history, symptomatology, identification, and treatment of asthma.

EPIDEMIOLOGY

Approximately 12 million people in the United States have asthma. Care for asthma generally takes place in outpatient settings. Costs for asthma-related care total about 3.6 billion dollars annually. Indeed, asthma accounted for 6.5 million outpatient visits among 640 million total estimated ambulatory care visits in one survey. Prevalence rates for asthma increased by approximately 29% in the period 1980–1987 (**5.1**). Prevalence appears to have increased in all age groups, but the group less than 20 years' old has been the most heavily affected.

There has also been a rise in both the morbidity and mortality associated with asthma during the past 15 years. Asthma accounts for approximately 459,000 hospitalizations per year in the United States. Between 1980 and 1987 an increase of 6% was observed in the hospital discharge rate for asthma. Moreover, approximately three-fold increases in hospital discharge rates were noted between 1970 and 1987. Groups disproportionately represented in these

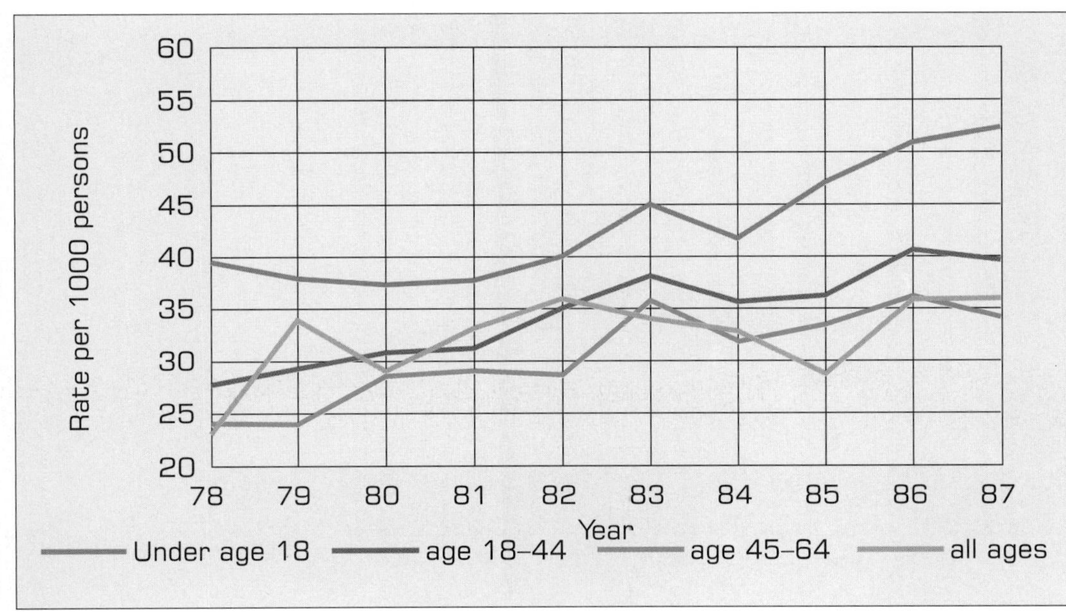

5.1 Asthma prevalence by age groups. (National Health Interview Survey, National Center for Health Statistics.)

statistics included African Americans, who were more than twice as likely as Caucasians to be hospitalized. Our experience at the Children's Hospital of Pittsburgh is shown in **5.2A**. The number of asthma hospitalizations and admissions to the intensive care unit peak during the fall months (**5.2B**) possibly due to infectious agents, environmental allergens, or temperature and humidity changes.

Like morbidity, mortality is also increasing. The death rate due to asthma increased 31% from 1980 to 1987. Indeed, approximately 4360 patients died of asthma in 1987, versus 2891 in 1980. More recent figures from 1991 indicate that there were over 5000 deaths from asthma in the United States (**5.3**). Groups most heavily affected include African Americans and children.

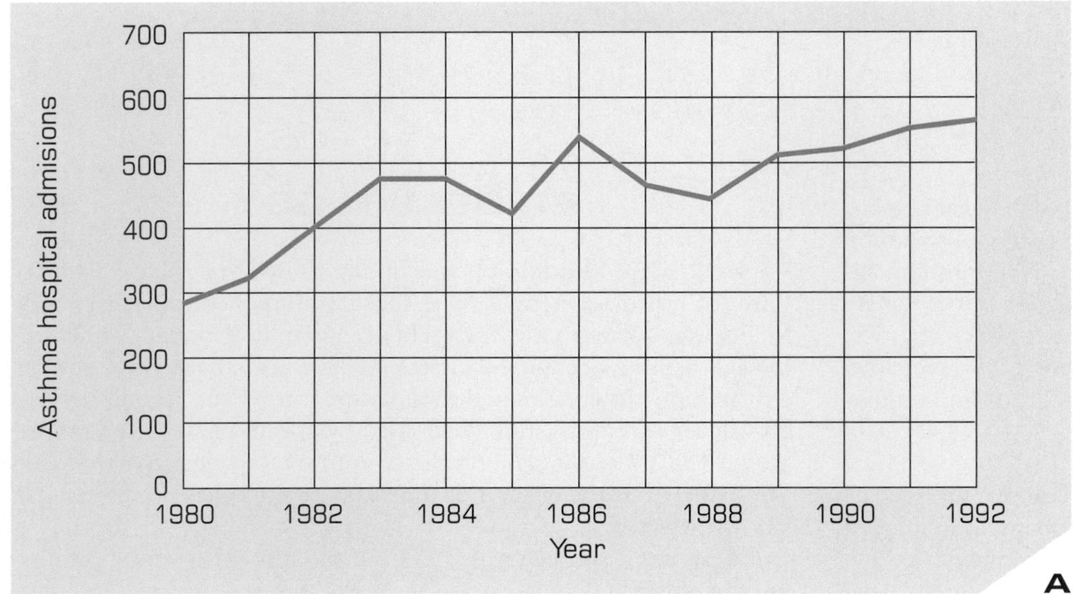

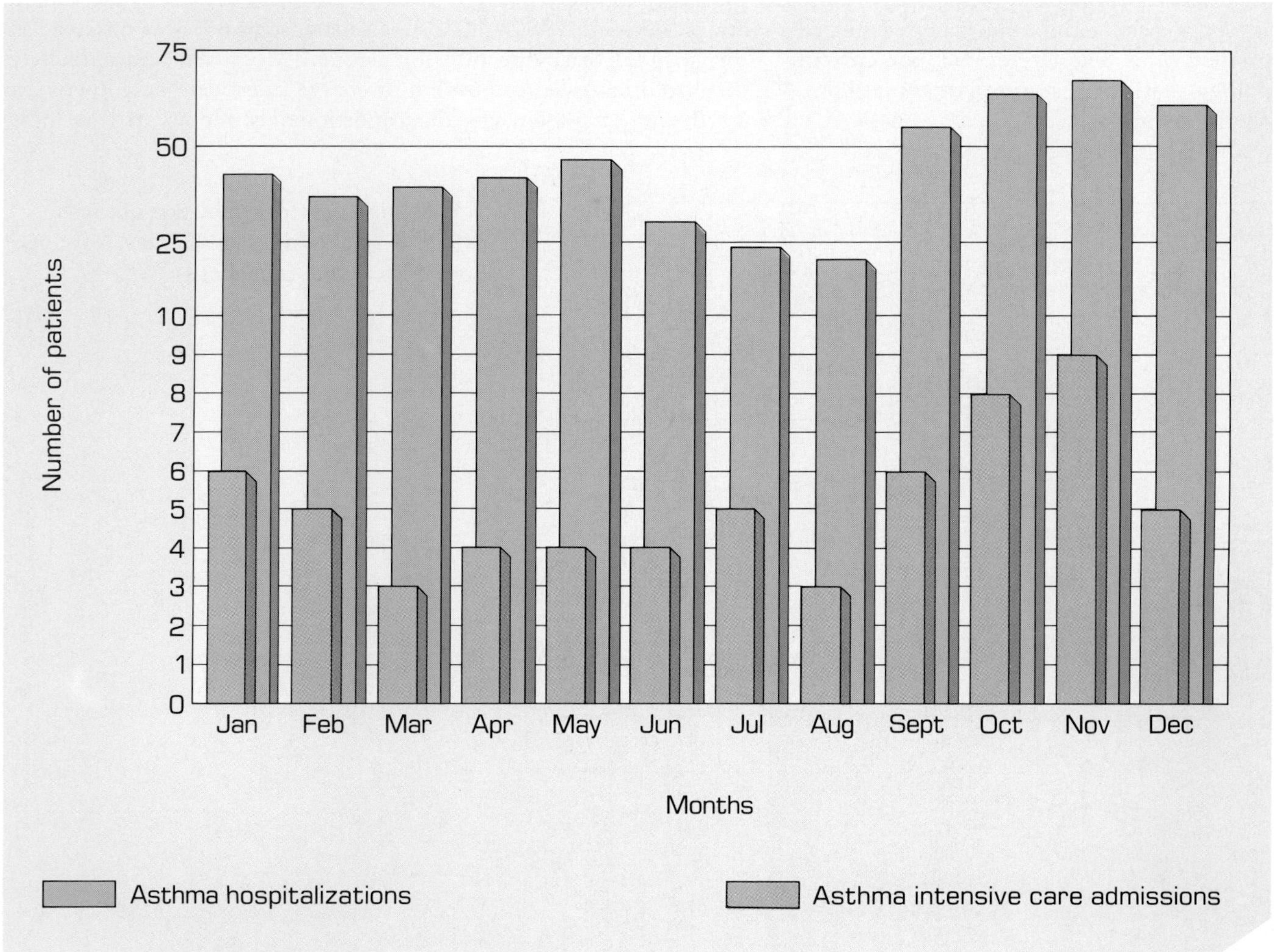

5.2 (A) Hospitalizations for asthma to the Children's Hospital of Pittsburgh. (B) Number of asthma admissions to the Children's Hospital of Pittsburgh (1982–1985) and number of asthma intensive care unit admissions to the Children's Hospital of Los Angeles (1969–1977) by month of year. (B: Adapted with permission from Skoner D. *et al*, *Pediatric Clinics of North America*, **35**(5):1153, 1988, and Richards W. *et al*, *Clin Pediatr*, **18**(6):346, 1979.)

The reason(s) for the rises in prevalence, morbidity, and mortality associated with asthma remain elusive. Possible explanations for this include the lack of access to appropriate medical care and poverty, as often exists in inner cities. In order to counteract these trends, it is essential that patients with documented asthma receive regular medical care and appropriate evaluations, and that physicians and patients engage in comprehensive, frequently reviewed treatment plans. Moreover, the under-diagnosis of asthma is a major problem, since 10–15% of school children have undiagnosed asthma. Therefore, physicians must be cognizant of the likelihood that recurrent episodes of cough and wheezing are frequently due to asthma.

The peak incidence of onset is before the age of 5 years. Available evidence indicates that 5–10% of children in the United States show signs and symptoms compatible with asthma at some time during childhood. Several anatomic and physiologic factors, including a relatively increased peripheral airway resistance and an unstable rib cage with a mechanically disadvantaged diaphragm, may predispose infants and young children to the development of more severe airway obstruction. This may account for the early onset of asthma. In childhood, males are affected 30% more often than females and tend to have more severe disease. Beyond puberty, the sex distribution is equal. Asthmatics with respiratory allergy and eczema usually have a more severe course than those who wheeze only with upper respiratory infections.

CLINICAL PRESENTATION AND DIAGNOSIS

Asthma can present in a number of different ways, ranging from a history of association with upper respiratory infection, allergen exposure, isolated chronic cough or exercise-induced wheezing to repeated episodes of wheezing, shortness of breath, and tachypnea of various levels of severity. The diagnosis of asthma requires the documentation of episodic airway obstruction and the reversibility of that obstruction. Clinically diagnosed asthma most likely represents a heterogeneous group of disorders with many possible underlying causes. This heterogeneity is probably responsible for the variability in presentation observed among different patients with asthma, as well as in the same individual at different times.

In patients less than 6 years of age whose airway obstruction has not been confirmed in the office or emergency-care setting, the diagnosis of asthma is based primarily on historical details about the mode of presentation and response to therapy. The presence of recurrent cough and/or wheezing and the triggering of these symptoms at night-time, or by exercise or cold air exposures, are particularly helpful clues in establishing the diagnosis of asthma.

During asthma exacerbations, patients may have the presence of a lower airway obstruction and the improvement with inhaled bronchodilator confirmed clinically by a physician. In other patients older than 6 years of age, pulmonary function testing may have been

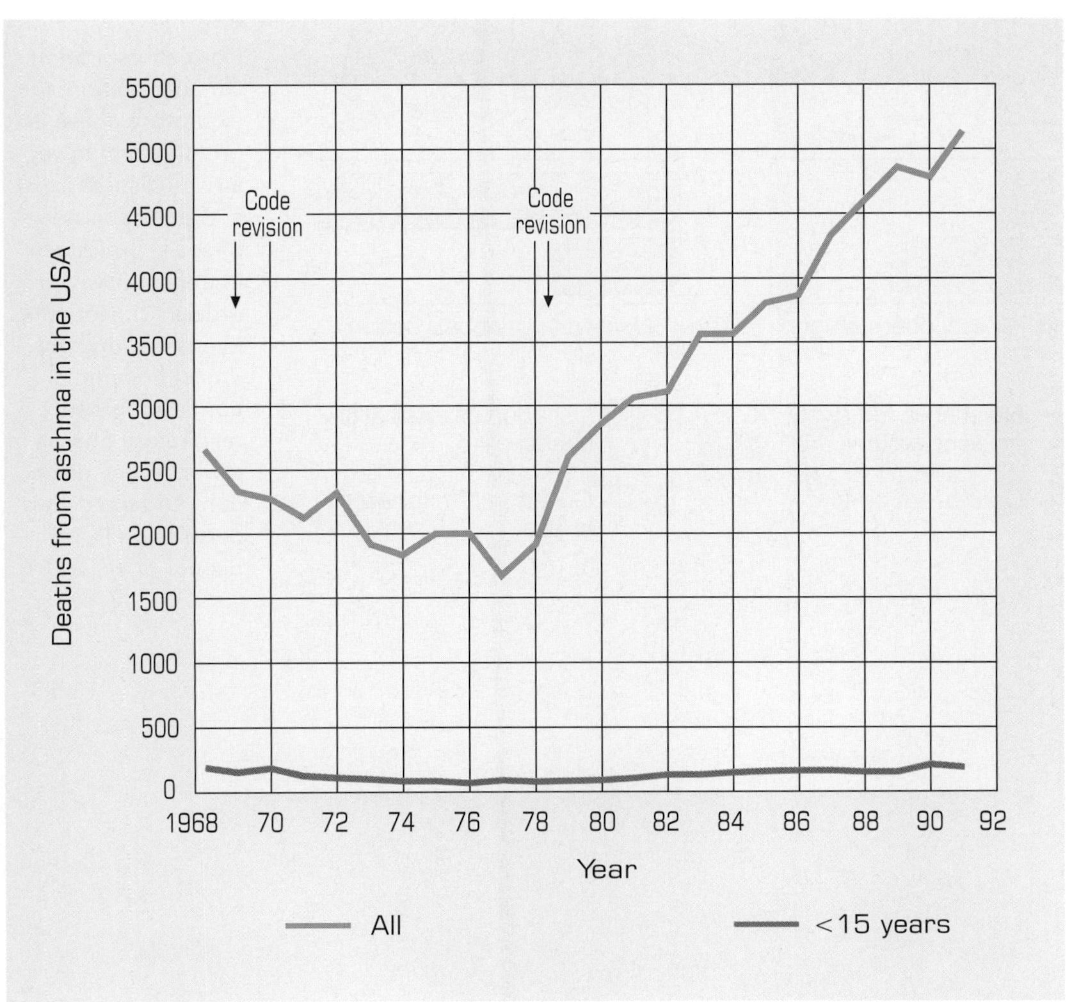

5.3 Asthma mortality by year. (Adapted with permission from Sly, 1994.)

used to confirm the presence of obstruction and the reversibility with inhaled beta$_2$ agonist. Other patients may present with cough as the sole manifestation of asthma. These patients typically have normal pulmonary function tests, with some improvement with the bronchodilator, and manifest airway hyperreactivity to provocative stimuli, such as methacholine, exercise, or cold air (*see* Chapter 3).

During the history and physical examination, particular attention should be focused on the growth pattern, especially in children. Also, the presence of upper respiratory findings compatible with allergic rhinitis (pale, boggy nasal turbinates, suborbital venous congestion – 'shiners' – nasal crease, Denie's lines), and skin manifestations of atopic dermatitis should be noted. The examination should focus on the appearance of a hyper-expanded chest, presence of cyanosis, degree of respiratory distress, use of accessory muscles, wheezing, decreased inspiratory:expiratory ratio, rhonchi, and other findings on auscultation which might indicate pneumonia or atelectasis. The cardiac examination should be geared toward the identification of congenital heart disease in young children and congestive heart failure in adults.

Acute asthma symptoms usually consist of progressively increasing shortness of breath (dyspnea), cough and difficulty breathing, with or without rhinorrhea, low-grade fever, and other manifestations of an upper respiratory infection. On auscultation, expiratory wheezing or a prolonged expiratory phase may be the only manifestations of mild asthma. However, as the obstructive process progresses, the expiratory phase becomes longer (**5.4**) and the musical high-pitched rhonchi louder.

Without appropriate treatment and reversal, signs of hyperinflation (air trapping) develop, with depressed diaphragms, decreased excursions of the chest wall with respiration, and hyperresonance to percussion. Subjectively, the patient experiences chest tightness and anxiety, and works harder to breath. Accessory muscle use (visible contractions of the scalene and/or sternocleidomastoid muscles) and retractions (visible depressions in the chest wall during inspiration) develop with or without a marked degree of wheezing on auscultation. The patient usually assumes an upright posture to maximize air exchange. As respiratory muscles tire, the patient becomes lethargic and cyanotic, even with supplemental oxygen.

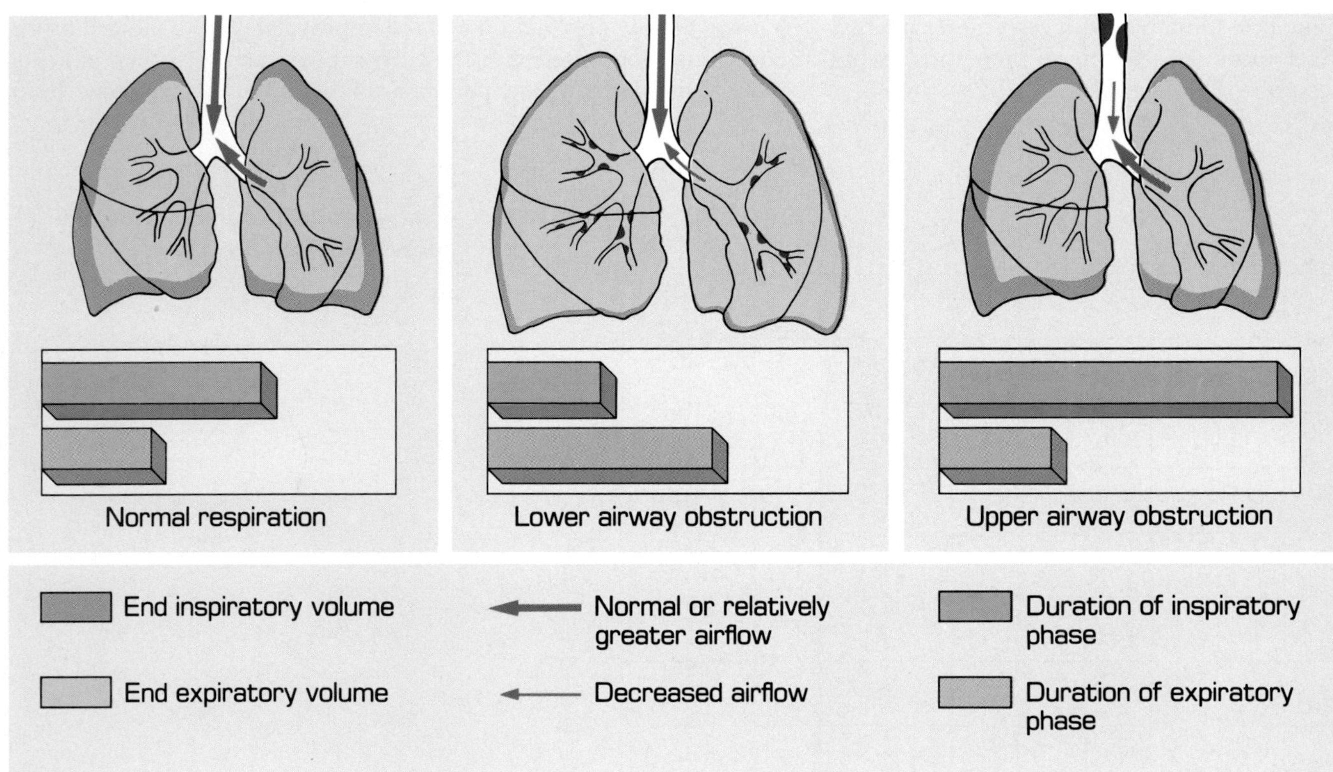

5.4 Characteristic changes in lung volumes and duration of respiratory phases in upper and lower airway obstructive disorders. (A) Normal respiration. On auscultation, the expiratory phase is prolonged in lower airway disorders (B), and the inspiratory phase is prolonged in upper airway disorders (C). Note the increased lung volumes (hyperinflation) during both respiratory phases in lower airway disorders. (Adapted with permission from Skoner *et al.*, 1987.)

Maximum effort to breathe produces feeble air exchange, manifested by decreased intensity and duration or lack of inspiratory breath sounds as air exchange decreases. Consequently, a patient with severe obstruction and impending respiratory failure may not have audible wheezing because too little air is being ventilated to create the sound. With extreme fatigue, respiratory muscles fail, retractions decrease, and respiratory failure is imminent unless appropriate therapy is promptly initiated.

Following the initial examination, serial assessment of the degree of respiratory distress, using a standardized clinical scoring system (5.5), facilitates determination of response to therapy and insures early detection of impending respiratory failure or other complications. Any change in sensorium requires a prompt evaluation for impending respiratory failure.

Between episodes of acute asthma, the physical findings vary with the chronicity of the disease process. In mild asthmatics, the

ESTIMATION OF SEVERITY OF ACUTE EXACERBATIONS OF ASTHMA IN CHILDREN

Sign/Symptom	Mild	Moderate	Severe
PEFR*	70–90% predicted or personal best	50–70% predicted or personal best	< 50% predicted or personal best
Respiratory rate, resting or sleeping (*see* Fig. 7)	Normal to 30% increase above the mean	30–50% increase above the mean	Increase over 50% above the mean
Alertness	Normal	Normal	May be decreased
Dyspnea**	Absent or mild; speaks in complete sentences	Moderate; speaks in phrases or partial sentences; infant's words cry softer and shorter, infant has difficulty suckling and feeding	Severe; speaks only in single words or short phrases; infant's cry softer and shorter, infant stops suckling and feeding
Pulsus paradoxicus***	<10 mm Hg	10–20 mm Hg	20–40 mm Hg
Accessory muscle use	No intercostal to mild retractions.	Moderate intercostal retraction with tracheosternal retractions; use of sternocleidomastoid muscles; chest hyperinflation	Severe intercostal retractions, tracheosternal retractions with nasal flaring during inspiration; chest hyperinflation
Color	Good	Pale	Possibly cyanotic
Auscultation	End expiratory wheeze only	Wheeze during entire expiration and inspiration	Breath sounds becoming inaudible
Oxygen saturation	> 95%	90–95%	< 90%
PCO_2	< 35	< 40	> 40

Note: Within each category, the presence of several parameters, but not necessarily all, indicate the general classification of the exacerbation.
* For children 5 years of age or older.
** Parents' or physicians' impression of degree of child's breathlessness.
*** Pulsus paradoxus does not correlate with phase of respiration in small children.

5.5 Factors used to grade severity of acute asthma exacerbations in children.

examination is usually entirely normal, but wheezing may be elicited in children by gentle manual chest-wall compression, which restricts chest expansion and increases the work of breathing. In contrast, severe asthmatics with a long history of airway obstruction which has not received appropriate therapy, may have signs of chronic lung disease. These include a paucity of subcutaneous fatty tissue and a barrel-chest configuration (**5.6A**). Adults with chronic asthma may produce copious amounts of sputum. Râles, wheezing, rhonchi, and decreased intensity and duration of the inspiratory phase of respiration are commonly found on auscultation. Chest radiography may show areas of atelectasis (**5.6B**).

Asthma should be considered as part of the differential diagnosis in any patient with recurrent or chronic lower respiratory symptoms or signs of lower airways obstruction (**5.7**). Even though a high index of suspicion must be maintained, excessive or erroneous diagnoses may result if they are made hastily, without the appropriate supportive evidence. Patients or their parents must be instructed that physician assessment is essential during suspected episodes of asthma, so that wheezing or other signs of lower airway obstruction and reversibility, if present, can be documented.

Asthma is the most common cause of recurrent episodes of cough and wheezing in both adults and children. Asthma is frequently under-diagnosed, especially in young children who wheeze only during respiratory infections and who are labeled as having bronchitis, bronchiolitis, or pneumonia. Nonetheless, the differential diagnosis of asthma includes a number of other disorders, depending on the age group under consideration. These disorders must be considered, especially in patients experiencing their first episode of asthma.

Any patient with acute asthma who develops symptoms of pleuritic chest pain, severe dyspnea, cyanosis, and tachypnea, as well as physical findings of unilaterally decreased or absent breath sounds, should be evaluated radiographically for pneumothorax (**5.8A**). With tension pneumothorax, the trachea, mediastinum, and cardiac landmarks may be shifted to the opposite side (**5.8B**). Pneumomediastinum and subcutaneous emphysema, usually involving the neck and supraclavicular areas, are more common than pneumothorax. When mild they may be asymptomatic and detected incidentally by radiography (**5.8C**). With more extensive air dissection, the patient may complain of neck and chest pain, and the subcutaneous emphysema (**5.8A**) may be visibly evident as a soft-tissue swelling of the neck and chest which is crepitant (has a crunching sound) on palpation.

Cardiovascular manifestations can also be detected during acute asthma. Heart rate and blood pressure are frequently elevated. Pulsus paradoxus, an exaggerated decrease in systolic blood pressure during inspiration, can serve as an indicator of severity and a guide to therapy. Pulsus paradoxus and the patient's exaggerated use of accessory muscles both correlate highly with the degree of airway obstruction.

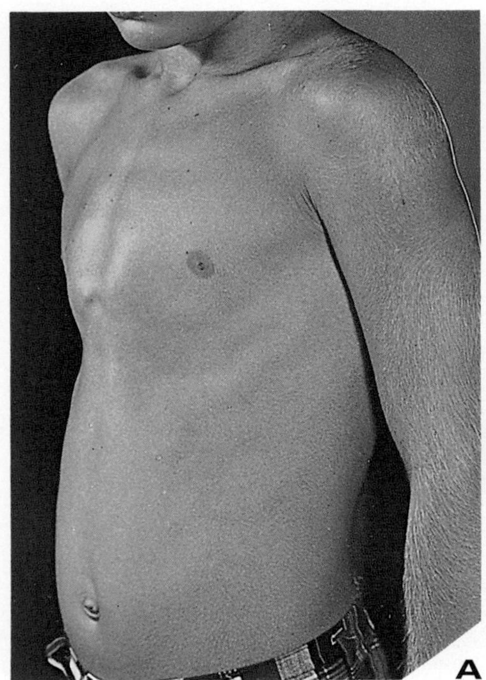

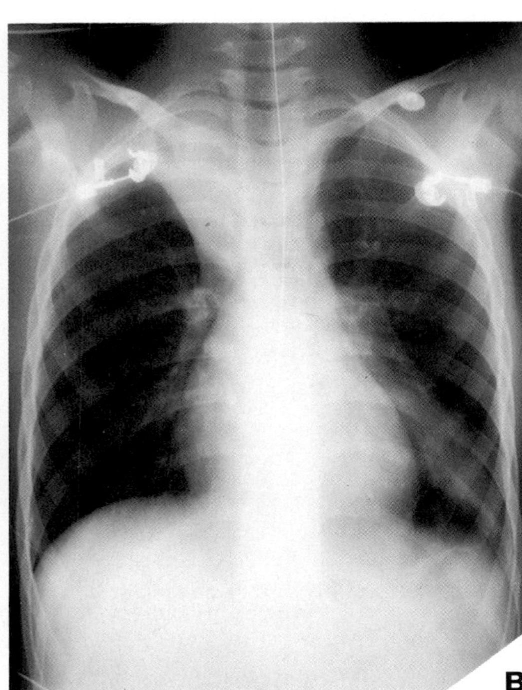

5.6 (A) The barrel-chest configuration of chronic asthma. Physical findings include an increased anteroposterior diameter of the chest and decreased respiratory excursion of the chest wall. (Courtesy of Dr Meyer B. Marks and with permission from Skoner *et al.*, 1987.) (B) Chest radiograph showing right upper lobe and left lower lobe atelectasis in a patient with acute asthma. (Courtesy of Dr Beverly Newman, Children's Hospital of Pittsburgh.)

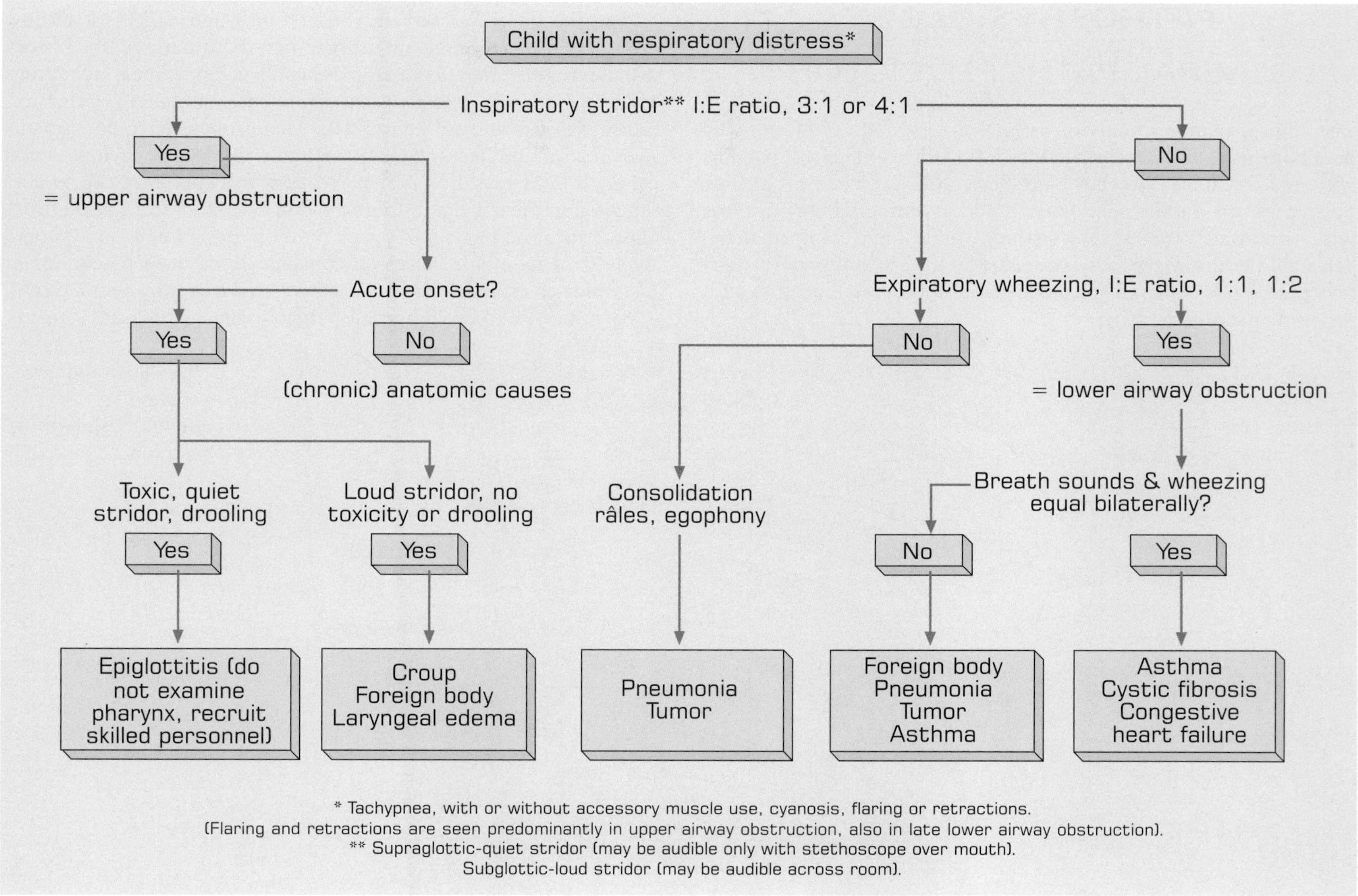

Child with respiratory distress*

Inspiratory stridor** I:E ratio, 3:1 or 4:1

Yes

= upper airway obstruction

Acute onset?

Yes

No

(chronic) anatomic causes

Toxic, quiet stridor, drooling

Yes

Epiglottitis (do not examine pharynx, recruit skilled personnel)

Loud stridor, no toxicity or drooling

Yes

Croup
Foreign body
Laryngeal edema

No

Expiratory wheezing, I:E ratio, 1:1, 1:2

No

Consolidation râles, egophony

Pneumonia
Tumor

Yes

= lower airway obstruction

Breath sounds & wheezing equal bilaterally?

No

Foreign body
Pneumonia
Tumor
Asthma

Yes

Asthma
Cystic fibrosis
Congestive heart failure

* Tachypnea, with or without accessory muscle use, cyanosis, flaring or retractions.
(Flaring and retractions are seen predominantly in upper airway obstruction, also in late lower airway obstruction).
** Supraglottic-quiet stridor (may be audible only with stethoscope over mouth).
Subglottic-loud stridor (may be audible across room).

5.7 Algorithm of differentiating features of upper and lower airway obstructive disorders in children. (Adapted with permission from Skoner *et al.*, 1987.)

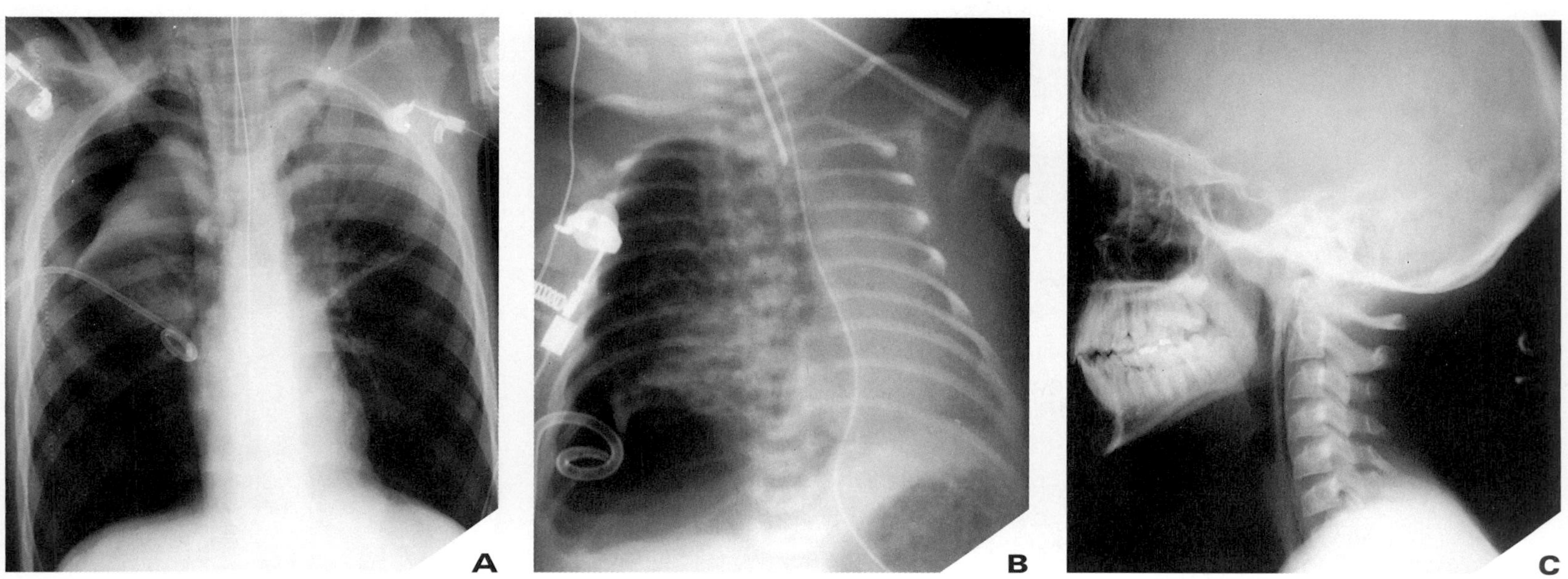

5.8. (A) Chest radiograph showing right-sided pneumothorax in intubated patient with acute asthma and respiratory failure. Also note the marked hyperinflation of the lungs, which can result in cardiac compression (narrow cardiac shadow) and compromise of cardiac venous return, and the extensive right-sided subcutaneous emphysema. (Courtesy of Dr Beverly Newman, Children's Hospital of Pittsburgh.) (B) Chest radiograph showing right-sided tension pneumothorax. Note shifting of mediastinum to the left. (C) Lateral neck radiograph showing spontaneous pneumomediastinum in a child with asthma. Note the dissection of air in soft tissues just anterior to the vertebrae. Clinical manifestations include dysphagia. (Courtesy of Dr Beverly Newman, Children's Hospital of Pittsburgh.)

PATHOPHYSIOLOGY

GENERAL PATHOPHYSIOLOGY

The clinical manifestations of asthma are related to the periodic development of airway obstruction (5.9). When evaluated, patients with mild asthma may have no detectable evidence of airflow obstruction on routine pulmonary function testing. However, those with moderate and severe asthma may have abnormalities detectable both on physical examination and in pulmonary function testing (office-based spirometry and home-based peak expiratory flow measurements).

Despite the variability in the presence and degree of airflow obstruction during sequential office-based evaluations, the history usually reveals that asthma patients develop clinical symptoms after exposure to allergens, environmental irritants, viral infections, exercise, and cold air (5.10). This propensity to develop airway obstruction in response to normally innocuous environmental agents is known as airway hyperreactivity. Its presence can be documented in the clinical pulmonary function laboratory using bronchoprovocation testing, in which pulmonary function is monitored while patients inhale increased concentrations of methacholine or histamine to establish the provocative concentration that causes a 20% fall in FEV_1. Virtually all patients with asthma have airway

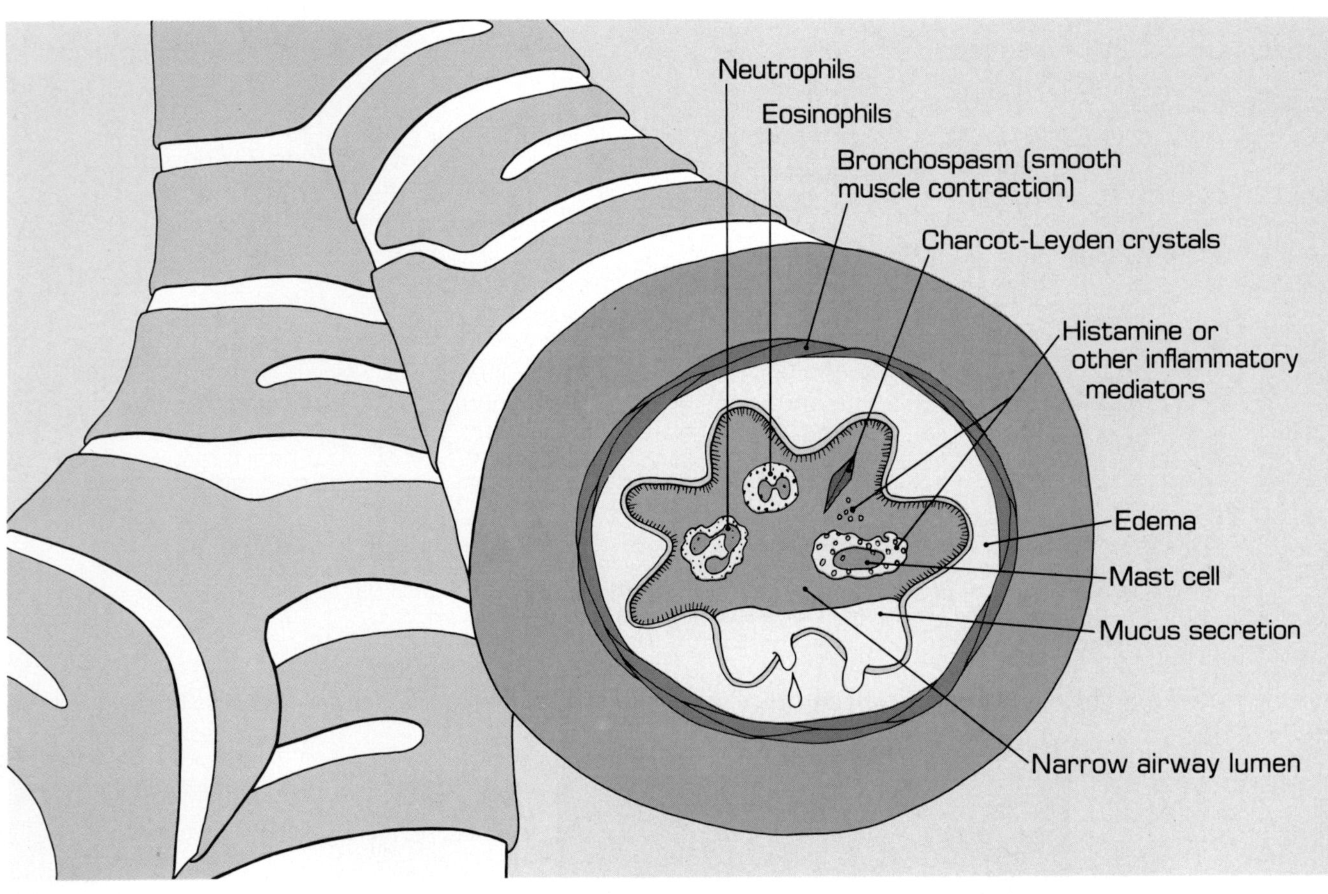

5.9 Illustration of airway pathophysiology in asthma.

ASTHMA TRIGGERS	
1. Infections	— Viral — Bacterial sinusitis
2. Allergens	— Pollens — Animal products — Molds — Dusts
3. Airway factors	— Cold air — Hyperventilation (crying, laughing) — Exercise
4. Irritants	— Noxious gases, odors — Cigarette smoke
5. Pharmacologic	— Aspirin
6. Psychosocial	— Emotions

5.10 Asthma triggers.

hyperreactivity, although patients with other disorders can be affected to a lesser extent (**5.11**).

Other stimuli which can be used to measure the degree of airway hyperreactivity include non-pharmacologic agents such as hyperventilation with cold, dry air and with exercise. Indeed, the clinical severity of asthma, and thus medication requirements, parallel the degree of airway hyperreactivity. As such, airway hyperreactivity is fundamentally important in the pathogenesis of asthma. Severe airway hyperreactivity results in a considerable degree of bronchial liability in asthmatics, such that decreases in airway flow rates can develop precipitously and unexpectedly.

One of the signs of airway hyperreactivity in patients with asthma is an exaggerated fluctuation in morning and evening peak expiratory flow rates (**5.12**). The normal diurnal variability in airflow in non-asthmatics is approximately 10% or less, but the variability may increase dramatically in patients with high degrees of airway hyperreactivity and severe asthma.

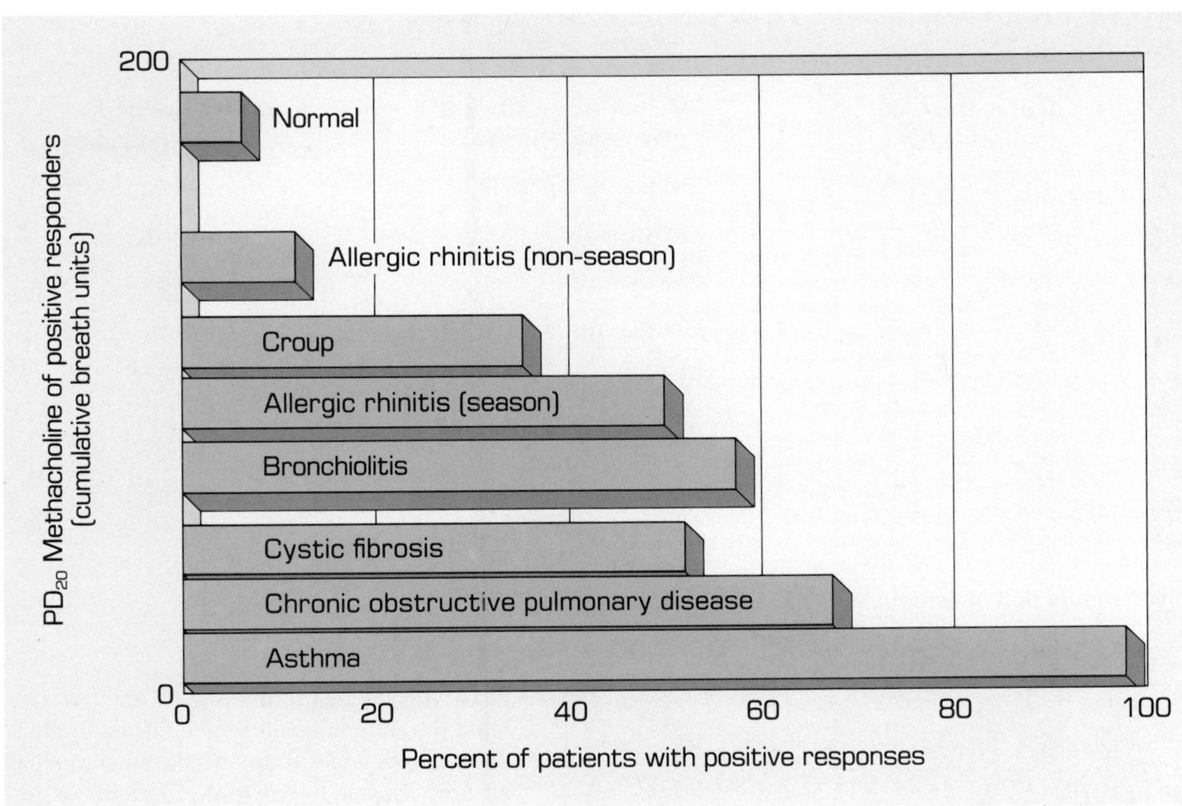

5.11 Relative average levels of airway responsiveness and percentage affected in groups of patients with various respiratory diseases compared to normal. A low PD_{20} (provocative dose of methacholine causing a 20% fall in FEV_1) denotes a high degree of airway hyperreactivity. (Developed from data previously published by Gurwitz, 1981; Taylor, 1985; and Madonini, 1987.)

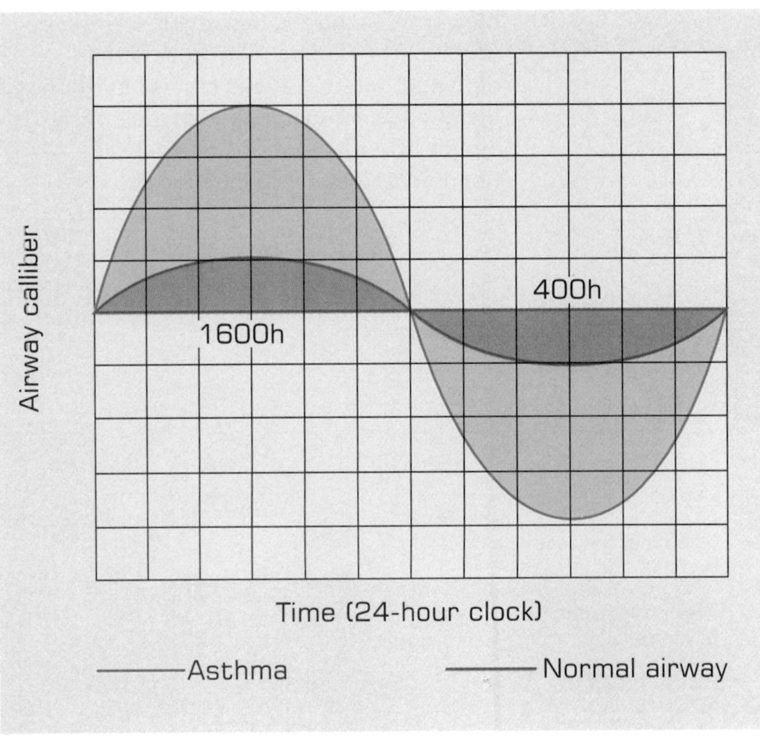

5.12 Illustration of the diurnal variability of airway caliber in asthma patients and normal individuals.

Postulated mechanisms for the development of airway hyperreactivity include airway inflammation, abnormalities in bronchial epithelial integrity, changes in intrinsic bronchial smooth muscle function, changes in autonomic neural control of airways, and the degree of baseline airflow obstruction.

The proposed neurogenic mechanisms include an imbalance of the autonomic nervous system (**5.13**). According to this hypothesis, bronchoconstriction results from a variety of stimuli that lower the threshold of afferent, rapidly adapting vagal irritant receptors. This cholinergic imbalance promotes smooth muscle constriction, which results from efferent vagal parasympathetic output.

One of the primary mechanisms responsible for the development of airway hyperreactivity is believed to be airway inflammation, which has now been documented directly using mucosal biopsies (**5.14**). In asthma, mucous glands and airway smooth muscle become hypertrophied. Moreover, the lower airways are infiltrated

AUTONOMIC NERVOUS SYSTEM FUNCTION IN ASTHMA

Parameter	Beta adrenergic (albuterol)	Alpha adrenergic (phenylephrine)	Cholinergic (pilocarpine)
Cyclic monophosphates	Increase cAMP[a]	Decrease cAMP	Increase cGMP[b]
Smooth muscle	Dilate	Constrict	Constrict
Degranulation (mediators)	Inhibit	Stimulate	Stimulate
Mucus gland	–	Stimulate	Stimulate
Response status	Decreased	Enhanced	Enhanced

[a]cAMP = Cyclic adenosine monophosphate.
[b]cGMP = Cyclic guanosine monophosphate.

5.13 Features of autonomic nervous system function in asthma.

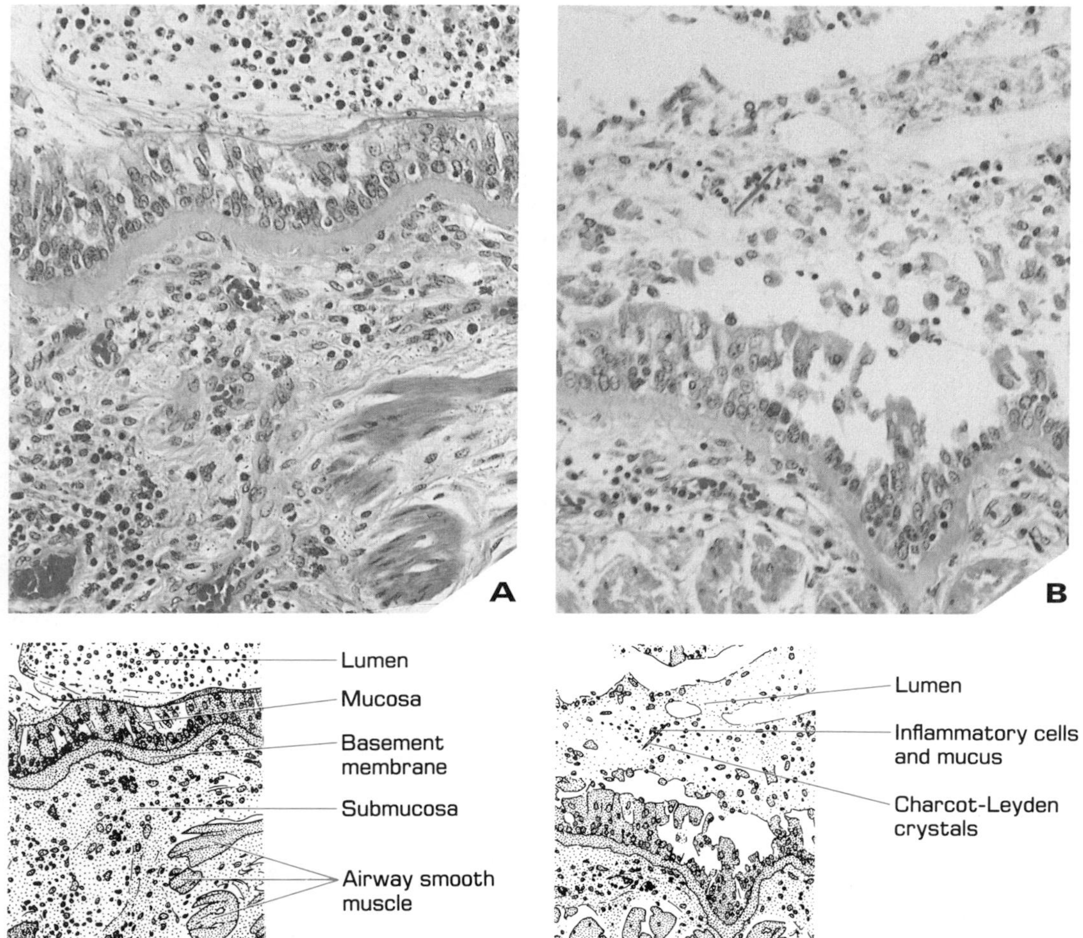

5.14 Airway histopathology in asthma. (A) Note the diffuse eosinophil infiltrate in the submucosa and lumen, intraluminal mucus, smooth muscle hypertrophy, and the appearance of a thickened basement membrane, which may represent collagen deposited along the basement membrane. (B) Note the red-staining, eosinophil-derived Charcot–Leyden crystal, surrounded by mucus and eosinophils in the airway lumen. (Courtesy of Dr Ronald Jaffe, Children's Hospital of Pittsburgh.)

by inflammatory cells, have epithelial disruption, and show signs of mucosal edema. The airway lumen can be occluded by inflammatory debris. The number of participatory cells is likely to be large, and their levels of interactions complex. Indeed, this interaction probably involves inflammatory cells, their mediators (including cytokines), and the cells and tissues which reside in the airways.

Inflammatory mediators probably play a major role in the pathogenesis of asthma. The potential effects of various inflammatory mediators on the airways in asthma are summarized in **5.15**. Many of the more recently described mediators are derivatives of membrane phospholipid-bound arachidonic acid (**5.16**). Some of the cells which release these potent mediators, including basophils and mast cells, may have an inherent enhanced degree of mediator releasability in asthma, thus providing a possible explanation for the observed elevations of plasma mediator levels during laboratory-provoked and naturally acquired acute asthma.

Several types of cells have emerged as important in the development of airway inflammation in asthma (**5.17**). Eosinophils, whose tissue migration and activation may be directed by the secretory products of pulmonary mast cells, macrophages, and epithelial cells, have been linked to alterations in epithelial integrity, abnormalities in autonomic neural control of airway tone, and increased airway smooth muscle responsiveness. Another cell with a likely role in these events is the T-lymphocyte. Indeed, this cell, once activated by antigen, may orchestrate the development and maintenance of airway inflammation through the secretion of pro-inflammatory, soluble cytokines, which have the ability to influence the activation state of a variety of inflammatory cells in both autocrine and paracrine fashions.

Genetics and environment both participate in the pathogenesis of asthma, but their precise roles lack definition. Family history very often reveals affected siblings, parents, or first-degree relatives. This inherited predisposition to asthma is autosomal and epidemiologic surveys suggest a recessive expression. No asthma gene has yet been identified, but recent advances in molecular biology promise to better define the genetic basis for asthma. Certain environmental factors may be prerequisite for its clinical presentation. For example, a propensity to develop airway hyperreactivity may be inherited, but appropriate exposure to certain allergens, respiratory viruses, chemicals, or psychosocial stimuli are associated as triggers for its clinical expression as asthma (see **5.10**).

In addition to a likely genetic predisposition, several environmental factors may contribute to the development of airway inflammation, airway hyperreactivity, and clinical asthma. Allergens are one such factor. Approximately 80% of childhood asthmatics have concomitant inhalant respiratory allergy ('extrinsic asthma') to pollens, molds, dust mite, or animal allergens, while a lower but significant percentage of adult asthmatics are affected by inhalant allergy. Additionally, acute asthma can be triggered by allergen inhalation in the laboratory or in the patient's natural environment. Laboratory experiments have demonstrated that inhalation of a relevant allergen by an allergic asthmatic patient results in the

AIRWAY PATHOLOGY IN ASTHMA – IMPLICATED MEDIATORS AND DRUG EFFECTS

Mediators[a,b]					Drug inhibition/reversal[b]			
PG	**LT**	**LT**	**PAF**	**Pathologic event**	**Beta agonist**	**Methyl-xanthine**	**Cromolyn sodium**	**Cortico-steroids**
+	+	+	+	Smooth muscle constriction	+	+	-	-
+	+	+	+	Mucosal edema	+	+	-	+
+	+	+	+	Mucus secretion	+/-	+/-	-	+
+/-	+[c]	+/-	+	Cell infiltration (chemoattraction)	-	-	+[d]	+

[a] PG = Prostaglandins, LT = Leukotrienes, HIST = Histamine, PAF = Platelet activating factor.
[b] + Positive, – Negative, +/– Variable or unknown.
[c] LTB_4 only.
[d] Via the inhibition of chemotactic mediator release.

5.15 Airway pathology in asthma – implicated mediators and drug effects.

development of an acute decrease in FEV_1 and the onset of asthma symptoms within 30 minutes of exposure (**5.18A**). Such a trigger may cause bronchial mast cells, macrophages, and epithelial cells to release inflammatory mediators, which then trigger the bronchospasm.

Over the ensuing hours, airway function returns to baseline in most patients. If followed, approximately 50% of these patients then experience a second decline in FEV_1 approximately 4–8 hours after exposure, termed a late-phase allergic reaction. Importantly, the degree of bronchial hyperreactivity to non-specific stimuli is

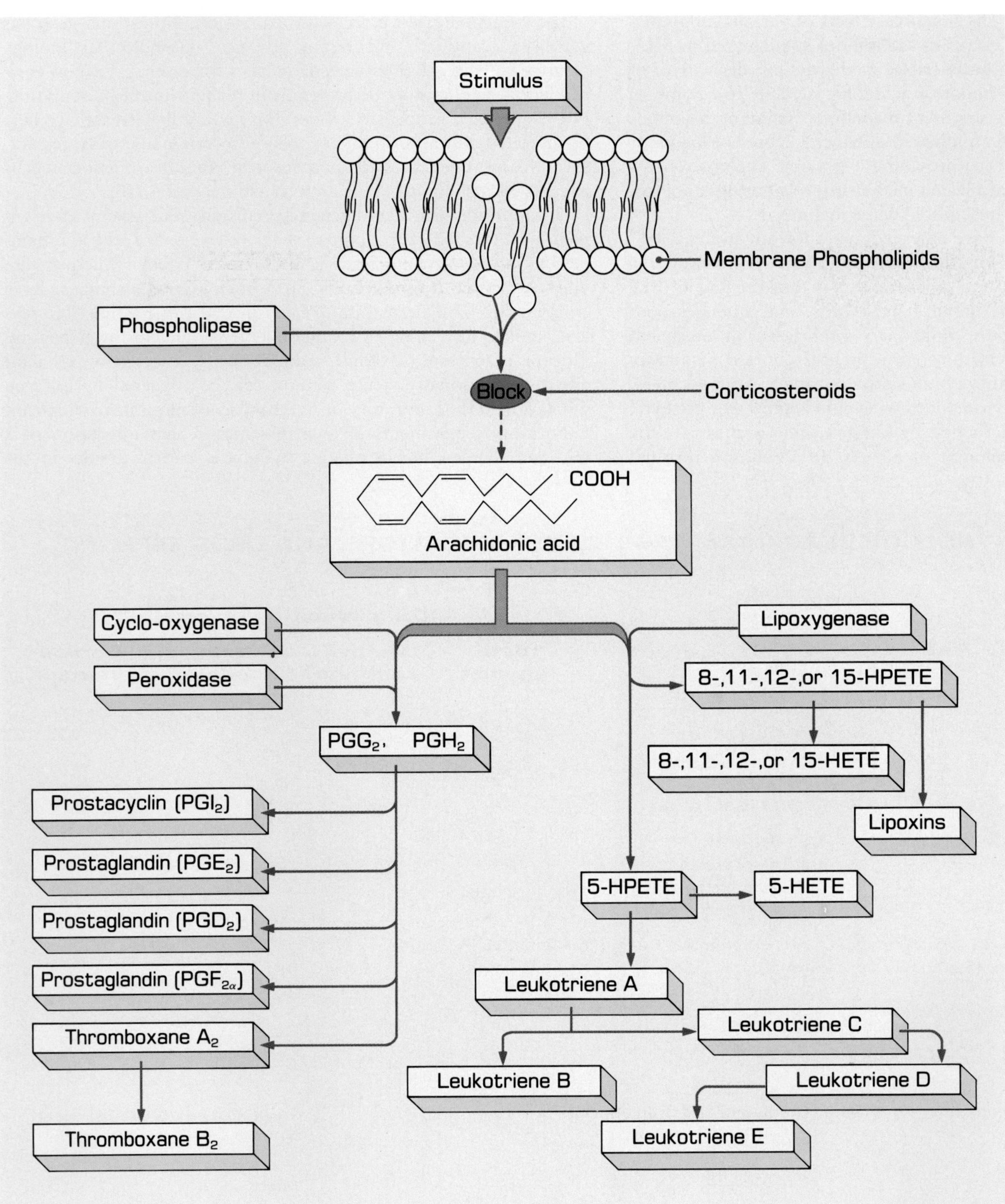

5.16 Inflammatory mediators generated by the cyclo-oxygenase and lipoxygenase pathways of arachidonic acid metabolism.

increased in patients experiencing late-phase allergic reactions (**5.18B**). This is believed to be related to the intense airway inflammation that develops in these patients, manifested by increased numbers of eosinophils in the airways, along with neutrophils, macrophages, basophils, and lymphocytes. The migration of eosinophils and neutrophils into the airways and their activation may be directed by inflammatory mediators released earlier during the immediate allergic reaction. Indeed, patients who experience sequential late-phase bronchial reactions could thus experience progressively heightened levels of airway hyperreactivity, as seen in

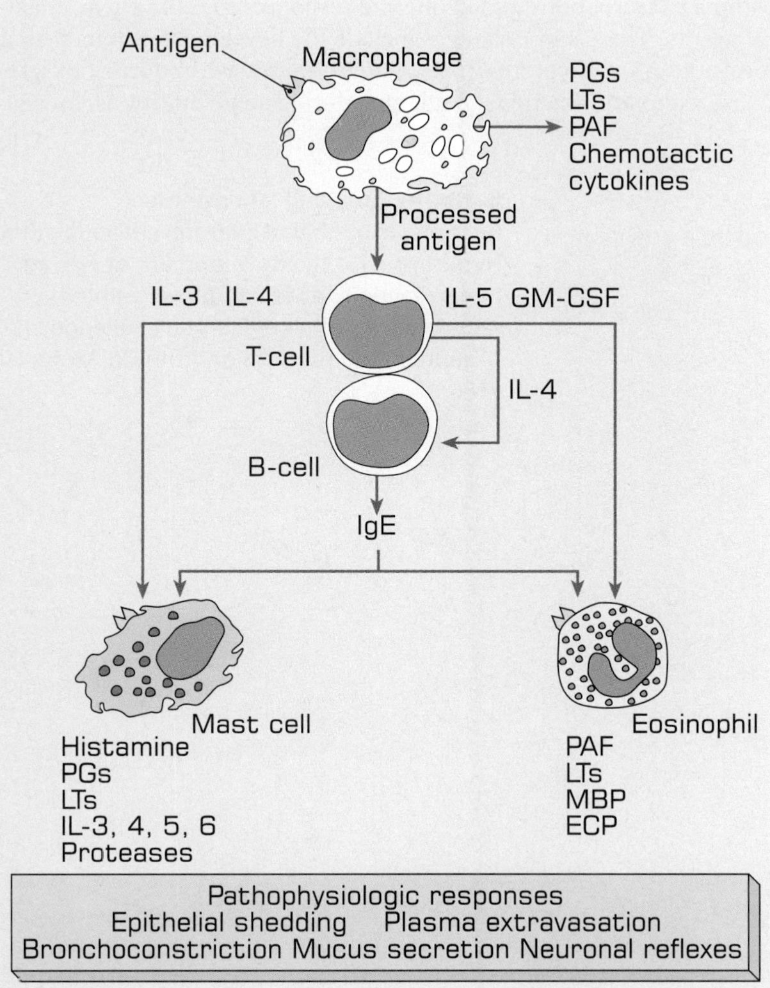

5.17 Model showing cells and mediators interacting to result in asthma pathophysiology. (Adapted with permission from Alabaster and Moore, 1993.)

asthma. Late-phase reactions have important implications for both the pathogenesis and therapy of asthma.

The term 'intrinsic' asthma has been applied to those in whom IgE allergy was not detectable by skin testing. However, a recent study documented increased serum IgE levels in a large asthmatic cohort, indicating that, regardless of age, asthma is 'almost always' associated with some type of IgE-related reaction. In certain patients, however, the specific IgE antibody involved is not detectable using conventional methodologies, such as skin or serum IgE antibody testing. Consequently, any differentiation between 'extrinsic' and 'intrinsic' asthma may relate more to our lack of ability to detect or identify specific IgE antibody involvement than to the triggering of asthma by external or internal factors. Therefore, all asthma may be considered intrinsic with extrinsic triggers. Even this differentiation, however, lacks adequate substantiation, and the use of the terms extrinsic and intrinsic to characterize asthma should be discontinued.

Viral respiratory infections also play a role in both provoking asthma exacerbations and in altering responses to other environmental agents. These latter changes include the development of increased levels of airway hyperreactivity, and an increased frequency of late-phase asthmatic reactions to allergen during acute infections. Indeed,

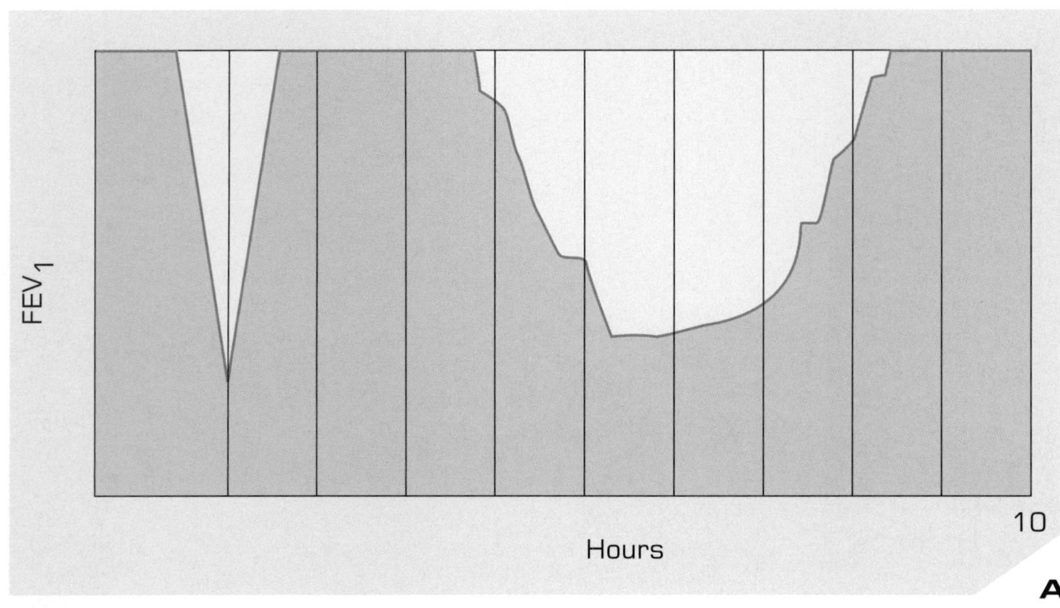

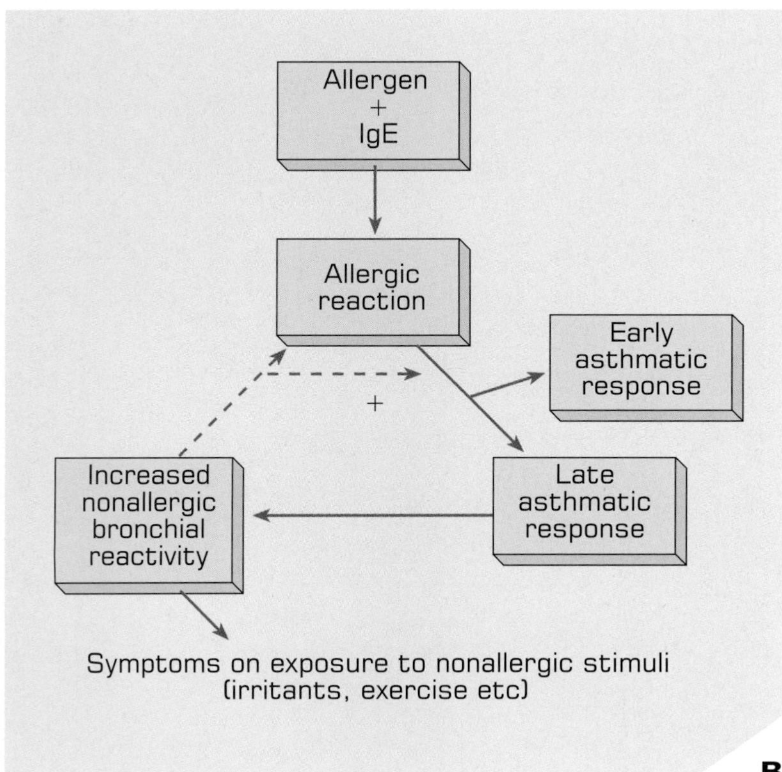

5.18 (A) Early and late asthmatic responses to inhaled allergen challenge. (B) Hypothesis for the development of airway hyperreactivity after late-phase asthmatic responses to inhaled allergen challenge (Adapted with permission from Cockroft, 1983).

the increases in airway hyperreactivity which follow a respiratory viral infection may persist for weeks beyond the infection. Possible contributors to these phenomena include direct epithelial damage, the production of virus-specific IgE antibodies, enhancement of the production of IgE antibodies specific for other antigens, and increases in the level of mediator release from inflammatory cells.

Viral infections which are clinically detectable only in the upper respiratory tract can be associated with bronchial hyperreactivity and small airway dysfunction. Viral infections account for up to 40% of wheezing episodes in young children during the fall and winter seasons. In children followed prospectively, between 6 and 11 episodes of virus-induced wheezing per 100 children were observed annually during the first 24 months of life. The spectrum of viruses which can cause wheezing in various age groups is shown in **5.19**. Respiratory syncytial virus, the main cause of infantile bronchiolitis, typically affects children under 3 years of age. In contrast, rhinovirus and *Mycoplasma pneumoniae* are the major causes of wheezing in older children and adults. Indeed, *M. pneumoniae* may cause more than 50% of wheezing episodes in adolescents. Parainfluenza virus types 1 and 3 together account for 26% of all virus-induced wheezing episodes, second only to respiratory syncytial virus in overall frequency.

Certain viruses, including respiratory syncytial and parainfluenza viruses, could also function as allergens by stimulating the formation of virus-specific IgE antibodies. A hypothetical model illustrating the induction of airway hyperreactivity by virus or allergen and specific IgE antibodies is presented in **5.20**. The mechanism involves airway inflammation, i.e., infiltration with inflammatory cells and the presence of inflammatory mediators in the lumen. Airway inflammation, which develops during the late allergic reaction, is considered the histologic correlate of airway hyperreactivity.

In addition to viruses and allergens, other environmental agents, including inhaled ozone, can induce airway inflammation and hyperreactivity. Once airway hyperreactivity is present, airway obstruction, and thus the common asthma symptoms of wheezing and dyspnea, can be triggered by subthreshold levels of exposure to non-specific environmental irritants, like cigarette smoke and SO_2.

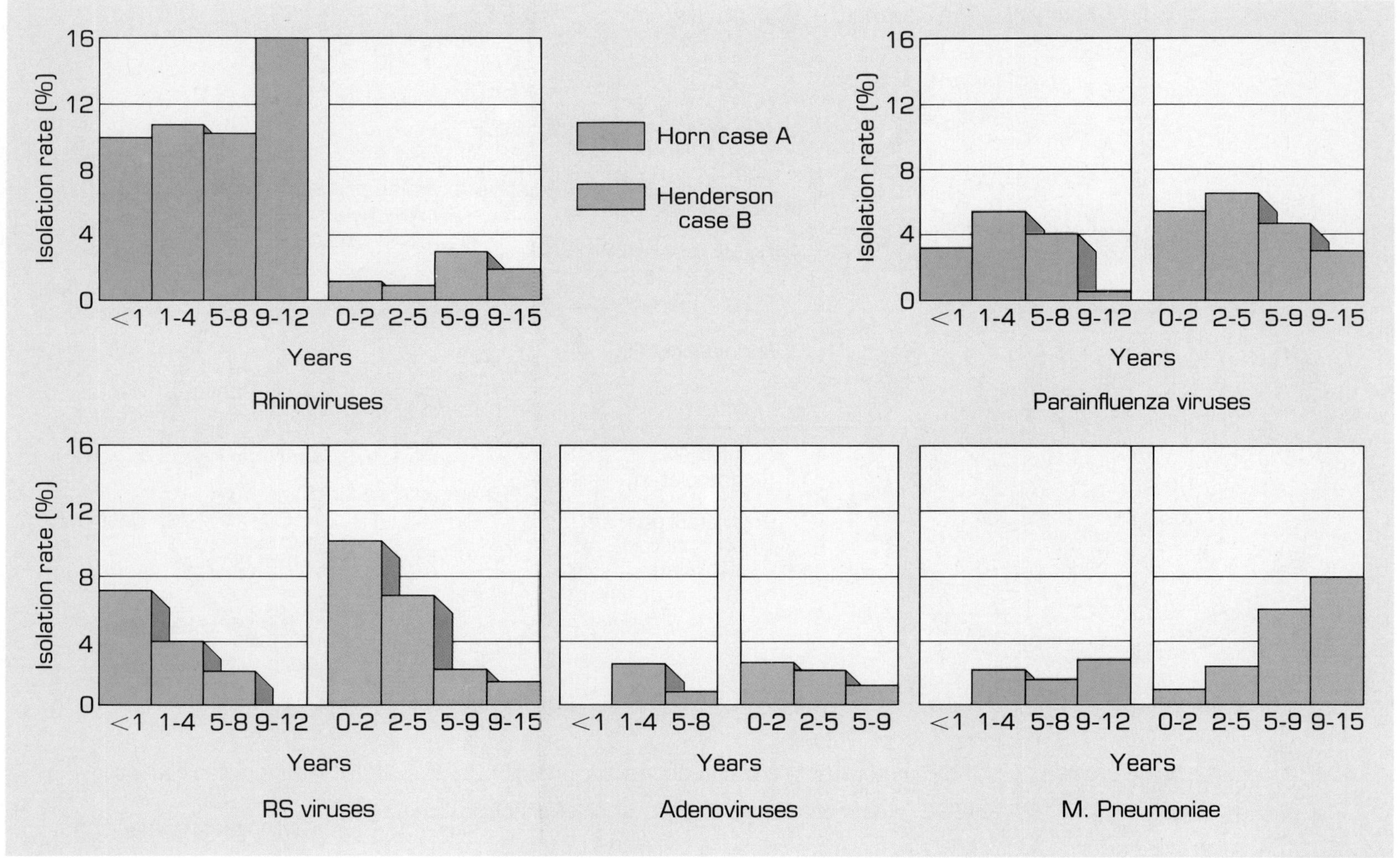

5.19 Isolation rate (%) in relation to age in years for rhinoviruses, parainfluenza viruses, respiratory syncytial (RS) viruses, adenoviruses, and *Mycoplasma* (*M.*) *pneumoniae* observed in two studies. (Adapted with permission from Horn, 1979, from Henderson, 1979, and from *Pediatric Clinics of North America*, **35**(5):1014, 1988.)

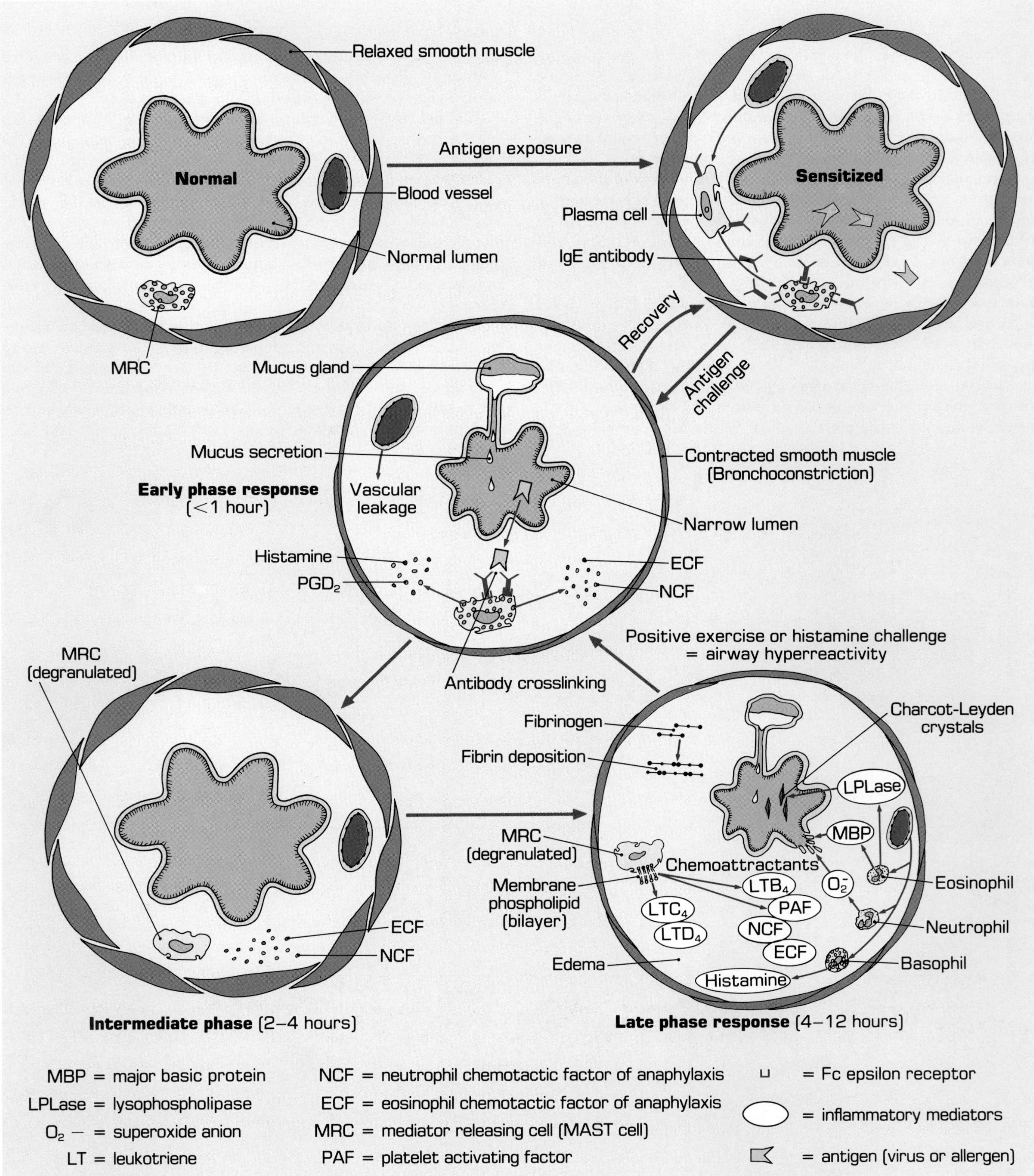

5.20 Hypothetical model illustrating the induction of airway hyperreactivity by virus or allergen-specific IgE antibodies. Note that airway hyperreactivity develops or increases after the late-phase response.

PATHOPHYSIOLOGY OF ACUTE EXACERBATIONS OF ASTHMA

The development of the typical symptoms of acute asthma (progressive worsening of cough, breathlessness, wheezing, and chest tightness) is accompanied by decreases in expiratory airflow rates. Bronchial smooth-muscle contraction is one of the primary factors contributing to the airway obstruction. Other contributory factors include mucosal edema and mucus plugging, which results in air trapping and hyperinflation. Physiologic changes which progress as the acute process worsens include both clinical and laboratory alterations. Clinically, patients with progressive airway obstruction use accessory muscles of respiration (sternocleidomastoid muscles) to maintain the state of hyperinflation. This, in turn, enables patients to maintain airway patency and thus adequate gas exchange. Indeed, the use of accessory muscles to breathe correlates very well with the severity of an episode of acute asthma, and is superior to dyspnea and wheezing as a sign of a severe episode.

The severity of acute asthma, however, is best assessed by pulmonary function testing. During acute asthma, progressive changes are noted in functional residual capacity (increased), FEV_1 (decreased), peak expiratory flow rate (decreased), and forced vital capacity (decreased). The latter change correlates with the degree of hyperinflation. Blood gas assessment may reveal hypoxemia because of mismatching of ventilation and perfusion. Hypocapnia (reduced arterial CO_2 levels) and respiratory alkalosis (increased pH) are the usual manifestations of early acute asthma, since alveolar ventilation is maintained at this stage. However, with more severe obstruction, ventilation is compromised and arterial CO_2 levels rise (hypercapnia) with decreased pH and respiratory acidosis. The latter finding signals the development of acute respiratory insufficiency and the presence of an FEV_1 which is less than 25% of predicted.

Other physiologic changes which occur in acute asthma include increased pulmonary vascular resistance, and an increased afterload on the left ventricle due to the high negative pleural pressures which result from lung hyperinflation. The clinical manifestation of these changes is the development of pulsus paradoxus, which is an exaggerated fall in systolic pressure during inspiration. Its presence correlates with an FEV_1 less than 50% of the predicted value for that patient.

DIAGNOSIS

In patients who present with respiratory distress or wheezing for the first time, a complete differential diagnosis of all causes of upper and lower airway obstructive processes must be undertaken. In the older child or adult with mild, infrequent episodes of wheezing that respond to bronchodilator therapy, asthma is readily diagnosed. However, with daily wheezing, frequent exacerbations, lack of response to bronchodilators, or poor growth, other diagnoses must be considered. These include chronic obstructive pulmonary disease, cystic fibrosis, α-1-antitrypsin deficiency, carcinoid syndrome, and an associated immunological deficiency (*see* Chapter 17).

Chronic obstructive pulmonary diseases, which include chronic bronchitis, emphysema, bronchiectasis, and bronchopulmonary dysplasia, are distinguished by their lack of significant reversibility with bronchodilator therapy. Cystic fibrosis, a multi-system disease with which airway hyperreactivity can be associated, may present with chronic cough, wheezing, and recurrent infections, especially sinusitis. Additionally, malabsorption with bulky, foul-smelling stools, failure to thrive, and clubbing of the nail beds are common. Indeed, clubbing is a very rare sign of chronic asthma and, if present in a wheezing patient, suggests another chronic pulmonary disease. α-1-Antitrypsin deficiency, an inherited autosomal-recessive disorder, is characterized by the onset of progressive emphysema in adults, especially those who smoke cigarettes, but may also manifest as hepatic disease in the neonate and young child.

In wheezing infants, the differential diagnosis includes disorders that are unique to that age group, especially bronchiolitis (**5.21**). In many infants, bronchiolitis is the initial manifestation of asthma and differentiation between the two is occasionally difficult. Even though these two diseases share common clinical manifestations, sequelae, and possible pathogeneses, the distinction between them remains clinically useful for the following reasons:

- Many children with bronchiolitis do not develop asthma and may be inappropriately labeled with the stigma of asthma.
- Children less than 2 years of age frequently do not respond to inhaled or injected bronchodilators.

Even though acute management is the same, the clinician generally should attempt to differentiate on clinical grounds between virus- and non-virus-induced wheezing episodes. If wheezing due to allergen or other inhalant exposure is suspected historically, an appropriate evaluation for allergen sensitivity and the subsequent application of avoidance techniques to prevent future exacerbations should ensue.

Status asthmaticus, a complication of asthma, is diagnosed by failure to improve significantly after appropriate bronchodilator therapy and indicates a need for hospitalization. This is manifested by post-therapy wheezing, elevations in respiratory rate, and abnormalities in the inspiratory:expiratory ratio. Progressive deterioration of respiratory function in the context of maximal medical therapy for status asthmaticus indicates impending respiratory failure, which progresses to respiratory failure if untreated. The diagnosis of impending respiratory failure is based on arterial blood gas findings of PaO_2 of <70 in 40% FiO_2, and $PaCO_2$ >45 (or an increasing $PaCO_2$ on serial blood gases) in the appropriate clinical setting.

If the diagnosis is unclear on clinical grounds, then specific laboratory studies must be performed to document asthma or rule out disorders that mimic it. An algorithm for diagnosing asthma is shown in **5.22**. Pulmonary function tests in asthmatic patients older than 5 years show airway obstruction at baseline or after methacholine challenge and, further, document reversibility of airway obstruction after administration of an aerosolized bronchodilator. In children younger than 5 years, or those such as the elderly in whom testing is unreliable, the diagnosis must be made solely on the basis of historical and physical findings, in conjunction with clinical response to bronchodilators. Lack of a prompt response to bronchodilator does not, however, eliminate asthma as a diagnostic consideration.

Patients who present with a history of isolated chronic cough or exercise-induced wheezing can be diagnosed by the reversibility of symptoms with a bronchodilator. When necessary, this impression can be confirmed by a positive pulmonary function or methacholine bronchoprovocation test. In patients who have sudden onset of wheezing and respiratory distress, the differential diagnosis for lower airway disorders includes respiratory infections, left ventricular failure, and foreign-body aspiration. Lower respiratory infections (pneumonia) generally produce fever and more localized findings of râles, decrease and change in quality of breath sounds, and egophony. A history of cardiac disease and auscultatory findings of diffuse crackles, basilar râles, and a third heart sound help to distinguish left ventricular failure with pulmonary edema from asthma.

In children, especially toddlers, aspiration of a foreign body that becomes lodged in a mainstem bronchus may produce wheezing which is at times partially responsive to bronchodilator therapy (**5.23**). The history of a choking episode and physical findings of unilateral wheezing and hyperresonance aid in distinguishing aspiration from asthma, but do not confirm the diagnosis. Airway compression by anomalous vessels or mass lesions is often distinguishable from bronchiolitis by virtue of absence of signs of infection, and from asthma by failure to respond to bronchodilators. Radiographic studies, such as barium swallow with fluoroscopy, can be very helpful in distinguishing between these entities (**5.24A**). Gastroesophageal reflux can be associated with asthma and is diagnosed by pH-probe testing or radiography (**5.24B**). Cough secondary to drugs (e.g., angiotensin-converting enzyme (ACE) inhibitors) should be considered in patients presenting with cough as the primary manifestation. Patients in whom the diagnosis is unclear should be referred to an asthma care specialist.

Pulmonary function tests are important in confirming suspected asthma. Between episodes of acute asthma, the findings depend on the chronicity and severity of the disease. Pulmonary function may be entirely normal in mild asthmatics, but acute airway obstruction can be induced by provocative methacholine inhalation. In contrast, marked reductions in expiratory flow rates may be present in severe asthmatics at baseline, and are characteristically observed to a greater degree during acute asthma. However, a decreased expiratory flow rate due to asthma, an obstructive lung disease, must be differentiated from that due to restrictive lung diseases, such as cystic fibrosis (**5.25A**).

Airway obstruction, when present, may or may not reverse with bronchodilator. If obstruction is detected, reversibility with bronchodilator, as illustrated conceptually in (**5.25B**), should be determined and used to guide the formulation of a therapeutic regimen. Bronchodilator effectiveness may relate to the relative contribution of smooth-muscle contraction versus inflammation as the cause of airway obstruction.

The clinician conducting an outpatient laboratory evaluation for asthma should always consider an immunologic etiology and include the appropriate allergy testing, so that potential inciting agents can be avoided. The most economic and reliable method is allergy skin testing, with serum specific IgE antibody tests serving as an alternative method when skin testing is contraindicated (*see* Chapter 3). IgE levels may be a useful adjunct in suggesting an allergic etiology. Additionally, sinus radiographs may be indicated in selected patients, since chronic sinusitis can exacerbate asthma (*see* Chapter 10).

DIFFERENTIATING FEATURES OF ASTHMA AND BRONCHIOLITIS IN CHILDREN

	Asthma	**Bronchiolitis**
Primary etiologies	Viruses, allergens, exercise, etc.	Respiratory syncytial virus
Age of onset	50% by 2 years of age 80% by 5 years of age	< 24 months
Recurrent wheezing	Yes (characteristic)	70% (2 episodes) 30% progress to asthma (3 episodes)
Onset of wheezing	Acute if allergic or exercise-induced	Insidious
Concomitant symptoms of upper respiratory infection	Yes, if infectious	Yes
Family history of allergy and asthma	Frequent	Infrequent in children with 2 episodes
Nasal eosinophilia	With allergic rhinitis	Absent
Chest auscultation	If viral, as in bronchiolitis Non-viral: high-pitched expiratory wheezes	Fine, sibilant râles, and coarse inspiratory and expiratory wheezes
Concomitant allergic manifestations	If allergic asthma	Usually absent
IgE level	Elevated	Normal
Responsive to bronchodilator	Yes (characteristic)	Unresponsive or partially responsive

5.21 Differentiating features of asthma and bronchiolitis in children. (With permission from Skoner *et al.*, 1987.)

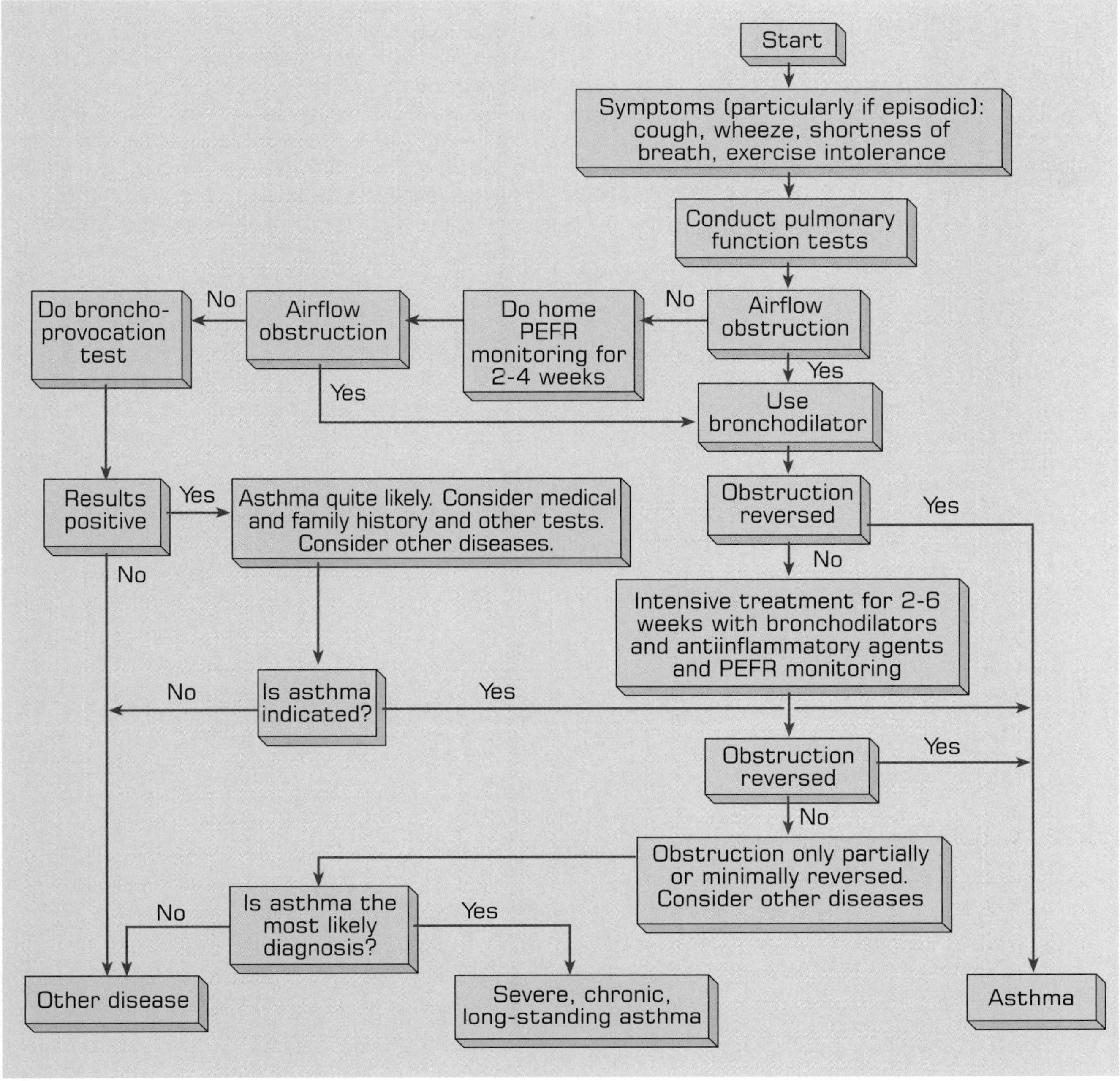

Start
Symptoms (particularly if episodic): cough, wheeze, shortness of breath, exercise intolerance
Conduct pulmonary function tests
Airflow obstruction
No
Yes
Do home PEFR monitoring for 2-4 weeks
Airflow obstruction
No
Yes
Do broncho-provocation test
Use bronchodilator
Results positive
Yes
No
Asthma quite likely. Consider medical and family history and other tests. Consider other diseases.
Obstruction reversed
Yes
No
Intensive treatment for 2-6 weeks with bronchodilators and antiinflammatory agents and PEFR monitoring
Is asthma indicated?
No
Yes
Obstruction reversed
Yes
No
Obstruction only partially or minimally reversed. Consider other diseases
Is asthma the most likely diagnosis?
No
Yes
Other disease
Severe, chronic, long-standing asthma
Asthma

5.22 Algorithm for diagnosing asthma.

Carrot
Right mainstem bronchus
Carina
Left mainstem bronchus

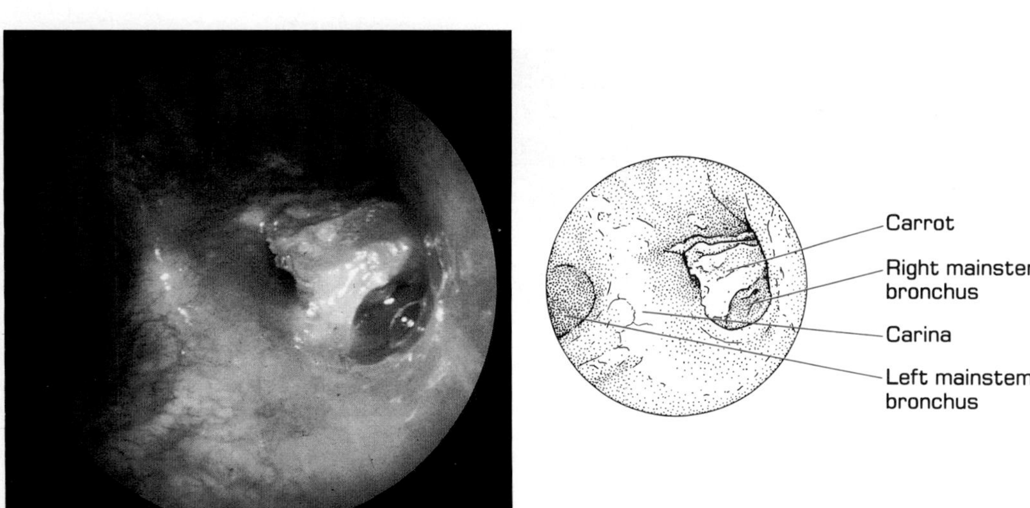

5.23 Piece of carrot lodged in right mainstem bronchus just below the carina, as visualized during bronchoscopy. Foreign bodies such as this can cause airway obstruction that is partially responsive to bronchodilator. (Courtesy of Dr Sylvan Stool, Children's Hospital of Pittsburgh.)

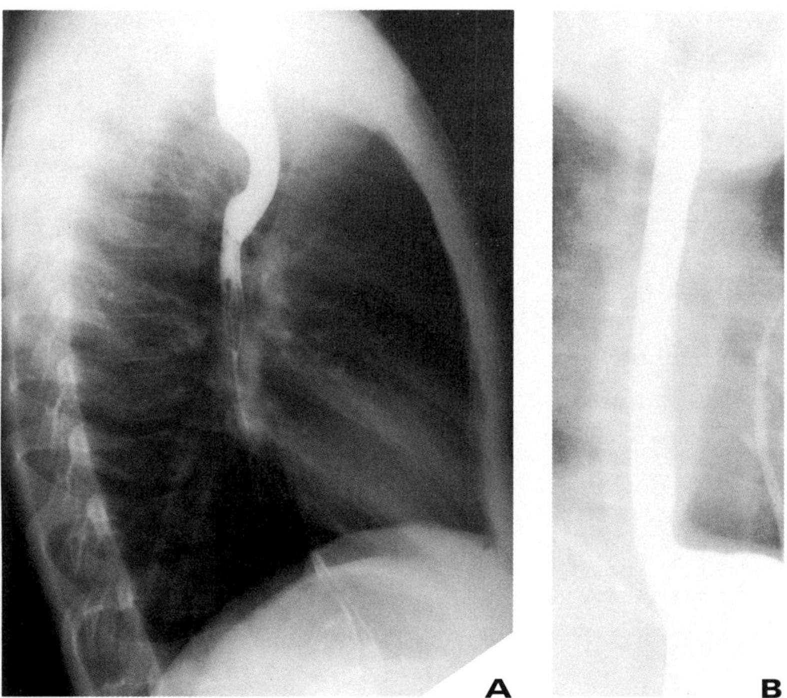

5.24 (A) Barium swallow (lateral chest radiograph) demonstrating upper airway compression by right-sided aortic arch with aberrant left subclavian and diverticulum at the left subclavian origin. Note the round indentation on the posterior wall of the esophagus and the anterior displacement and compression of the trachea, which can cause wheezing and mimic asthma. (B) Radiograph demonstrating gastroesophageal reflux. Note that the gastroesophageal sphincter is wide open and that the reflux of barium extends over the entire length of the esophagus. This can cause aspiration and wheezing, mimicking asthma. (Courtesy of Dr Beverly Newman, Children's Hospital of Pittsburgh.)

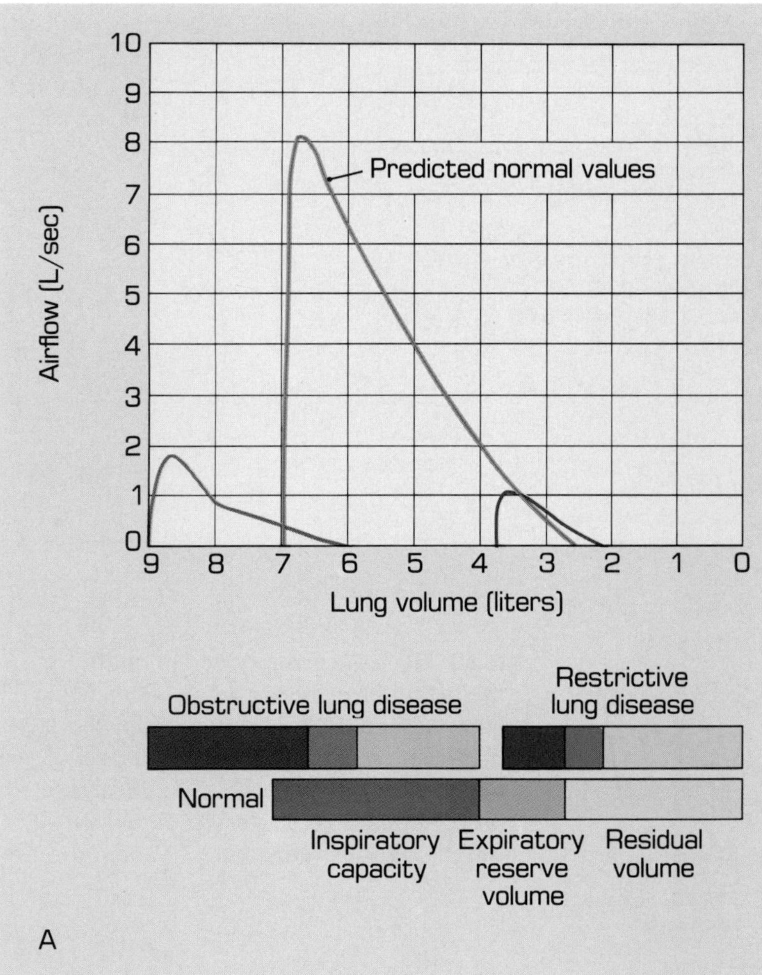

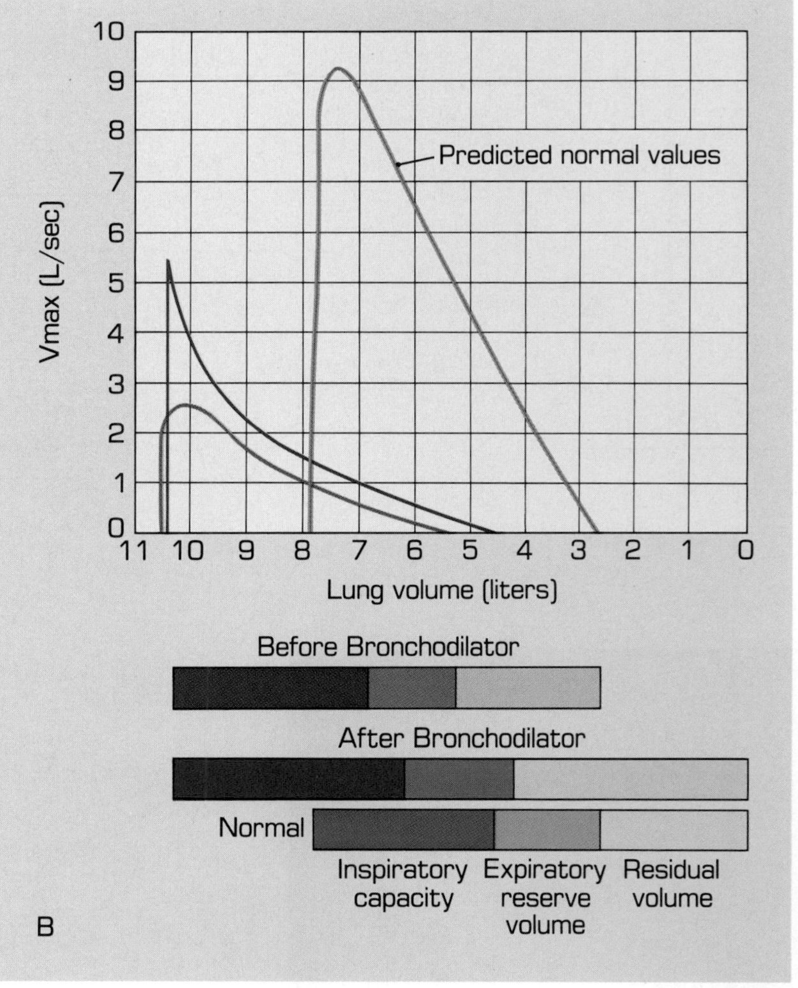

5.25 (A) Maximum expiratory flow rates are reduced in both obstructive lung diseases, such as asthma, and restrictive lung diseases. However, in asthma the airflow is limited at high lung volumes, in contrast to restrictive lung diseases, in which airflow is limited because the lung volume is decreased. (With permission from Cherniack, 1987, p. 91.) (B) Bronchoconstriction characteristic of hyperreactive airways is generally reversible. Indices of expiratory airflow in asthmatic patients thus improve after inhalation of a nebulized bronchodilator (e.g., a $beta_2$-adrenergic agonist). (With permission from Cherniack, 1987.)

Peripheral blood and sputum eosinophilia are usually present during recurrent and chronic asthma. Some clinicians, particularly those caring for adults, use the eosinophil count as a guide to therapy, since decreased counts generally accompany clinical improvement. The radiographic features of uncomplicated acute asthma include hyperinflation, peribronchial cuffing, and atelectasis. Arterial blood (5.26) usually shows hypoxemia, hypocarbia, and respiratory alkalosis, due to hyperventilation during the early stages of acute asthma. However, as the degree of airway obstruction increases and/or respiratory muscles tire, hypoxemia persists and carbon dioxide retention (hypercarbia) is detectable, resulting in a respiratory acidosis. This indicates impending respiratory failure.

Identification of a viral etiology using fluorescent antibody tests or enzyme-linked immunosorbent assays (ELISA) has little impact on acute therapy due to the paucity of available anti-viral medications, and should be limited to severely ill patients or the onset of an epidemic to document epidemiology.

TREATMENT

Asthma therapy is administered in several different settings, including those in outpatient (home/office), emergency department, and inpatient (hospital) facilities.

OUTPATIENT MANAGEMENT OF CHRONIC ASTHMA

The goals of effective outpatient asthma management are shown in 5.27. There are several general principles which should guide the clinician in providing asthma treatment. First, asthma is a chronic disease with periodic acute exacerbations. Second, treatment should be based upon an understanding of the pathophysiology of asthma, highlighted by the prophylactic use of environmental control measures and anti-inflammatory agents to treat the underlying inflammation, and the 'as needed' use of bronchodilator agents to treat the periodic acute bronchospasm. Four important components of outpatient asthma management have been identified – objective measures, environmental controls, asthma education, and pharmacologic therapy (5.28).

Objective measures

The two main objective measures of lung function are office-based spirometry and home-based peak expiratory flow-rate measurements. Pulmonary function studies by spirometry are essential in diagnosing asthma and in assessing asthma severity. The importance of obtaining these measurements is highlighted by the observation that the patient's symptoms and the physician's assessment of severity often do not correlate with the severity of airflow

BLOOD GAS CHANGES[a] – STATUS ASTHMATICUS

Severity	PO_2	PCO_2 pH	pH	Base excess
Mild	↓	↓	↑	Respiratory alkalosis
Moderate	↓↓	Normal	Normal	Normal
Severe	↓↓↓	↑	↓	Metabolic/respiratory acidosis

[a]↓ = low; ↑ = high.

5.26 Arterial blood-gas changes with increasing severity of airway obstruction and asthma.

THE GOALS OF EFFECTIVE OUTPATIENT ASTHMA MANAGEMENT

1. Maintenance of normal or near-normal pulmonary function rates
2. Maintenance of normal activity levels
3. Prevention of chronic or frequently recurring symptoms (e.g. night cough, exercise-induced symptoms)
4. Prevention of recurrent acute exacerbations of asthma
5. Avoidance of adverse effects from asthma medications

5.27 The goals of effective outpatient asthma management.

IMPORTANT COMPONENTS OF OUTPATIENT ASTHMA MANAGEMENT

1. The use of objective measures of lung function
2. Environmental measures to reduce exposure to allergens and irritants
3. Patient education
4. Pharmacologic therapy

5.28 Important components of outpatient asthma management.

obstruction. Office-based spirometry should be conducted in the initial evaluation of all patients with suspected asthma, and during subsequent evaluations on a periodic basis.

To assess the response to therapy in the office, emergency department, or hospital, either spirometry or peak expiratory flow-rate measurement can be used. Measurement of peak expiratory flow rates (PEFR) using a peak flow meter (**5.29A** and **5.29B**) should be used to monitor the course of asthma at home and the response to therapy in patients of 6 or more years of age. These values can provide valuable information to the managing clinician about asthma severity and the need to add or delete medications.

It is essential to provide teaching to patients for whom peak flow meters are prescribed, both on the proper use of the instrument and on the interpretation of values. For the latter, published predicted normal values for a given individual can be used. However, since the values for many patients are consistently higher or lower than predicted norms, establishing a 'personal best' PEFR value is an acceptable alternative. The patient and clinician then use this value as a standard in evaluating subsequent measurements. 'Personal best' PEFR values can be established by the performance of twice-daily PEFR measurements during a 'well' period, or during a period of maximum therapy. This value should be re-established on a yearly basis. PEFR values should be recorded in the morning and evening, both before and after use of any inhaled medications. Highly stable asthmatics may not need to continuously monitor PEFR, although the ability to detect the early onset of obstruction may be compromised under this condition.

Through the use of predicted norm or personal best values, PEFR zones should be developed. Green zones (80–100% of predicted or personal best) indicate normal values. Yellow zones (50–80%) signal caution and a possible need for a temporary increase in medication. Alternatively, an increase in prophylactic therapy may be indicated. Finally, a red zone (<50%) indicates a medical emergency, whereby an inhaled bronchodilator should be used immediately, and the clinician should be notified if the values do not improve and stay in the yellow or green zones (**5.30**). Transport to an emergency facility may be indicated if the response is inadequate. This also signals the need for a temporary increase in medication (systemic corticosteroids).

Environmental controls

The identification of asthma triggers is essential in the management of asthma. An evaluation for the presence of allergen-specific IgE antibodies is warranted in patients with moderate or severe asthma. This is usually accomplished with puncture or intradermal skin testing (*see* Chapter 3). *In vitro* tests, which provide the same information as skin tests, may also be used. However, these tests are usually less sensitive and more expensive. Testing for IgE to a panel of inhalant allergens is indicated, but routine testing for food allergies is not indicated. One possible exception is the infant or young child with asthma, who may be allergic and wheeze in association with ingestion of milk, soy, or (rarely) other foods, such as peanut, egg, or wheat (*see* Chapter 13). Food allergens are uncommon triggers of asthma symptoms in older children and adults. Allergy skin testing should be conducted and supervised by the clinician, who interprets the results in the context of the medical history and physical examination, and who recommends appropriate therapy. Therapy based upon skin tests or serum IgE assays alone, in the absence of a clinical evaluation (the so-called 'remote' care being popularized in some managed care environments), is not recommended.

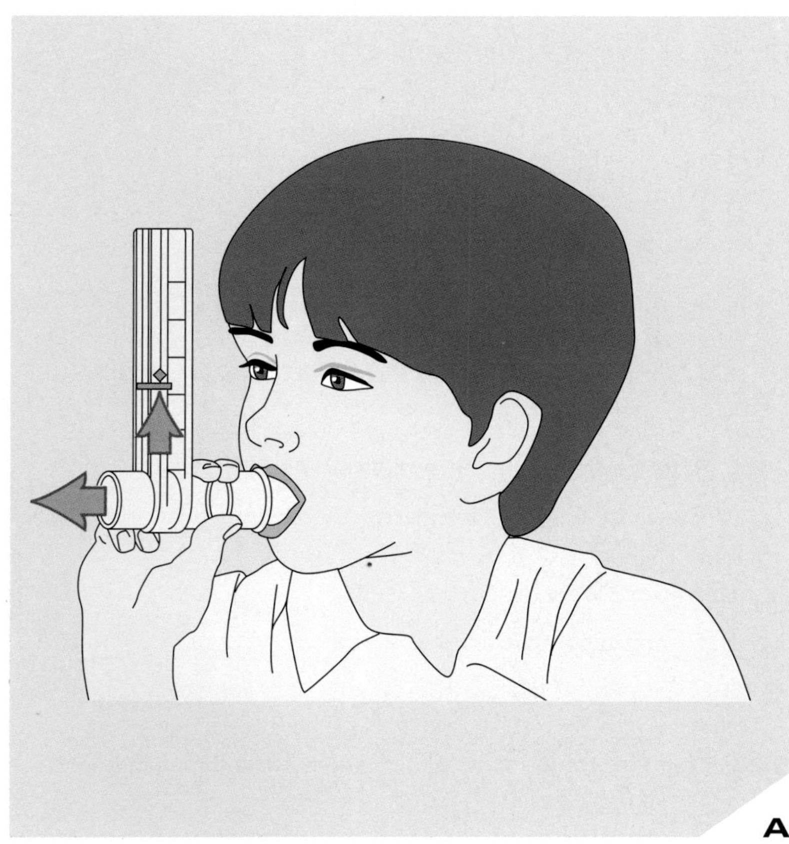

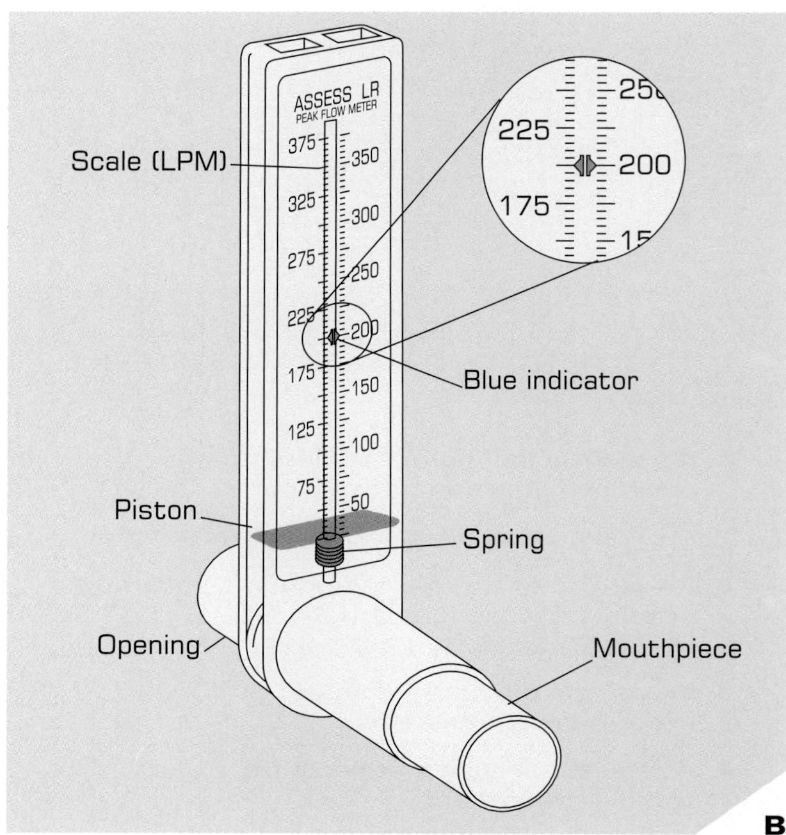

5.29 Example of (A) a patient using a peak flow meter, and (B) a typical peak flow meter used to monitor asthma severity.

After identification of the offending allergens, thorough environmental control measures should be implemented in the patient's living and working environments. This may include measures to control outdoor allergen exposure, such as staying indoors, with windows closed, in an air-conditioned environment (especially during midday and afternoon, when pollen and mold counts may be high), and reduction of indoor allergen exposure to molds, dust mites, cockroaches, and pet animal allergens. Indoor humidity levels should be maintained at 35–50%. Several other control measures may be particularly helpful, including air conditioning, and the use of central indoor air-cleaning devices, such as mechanical filters (high-efficiency particulate air or HEPA filter) and electrical filters (electrostatic precipitator). Vacuum sweepers have a tendency to mobilize fine respirable allergens, and provoke symptoms when used by dust-allergic people who should use a face mask, a central vacuum cleaner system with the collecting bag outside the home, or a cleaner fitted with a HEPA filter.

Non-allergen, indoor irritants which may also contribute to asthma exacerbations include tobacco smoke, smoke from wood-burning heating stoves, strong odors and sprays, and chemical air pollutants, especially ozone and sulphur dioxide. Exposure to these irritants should also be reduced.

If allergen and irritant avoidance is not possible, and the appropriate medications fail to control symptoms of allergic asthma, allergy immunotherapy should be considered. Allergy immunotherapy has been shown to reduce the symptoms of asthma associated with a variety of allergens, including house-dust, cat dander, grass pollen, and alternaria. Specific details of allergen immunotherapy are presented in Chapter 9. However, it is generally recommended that, if the patient's symptoms improve, monthly injections should continue for 3–5 years. On the other hand, if there is no improvement following two allergy seasons after reaching the maintenance levels of immunotherapy, it should be discontinued.

Parents should also be queried about day-care attendance in infants and toddlers, since it may result in repeated exposure to respiratory viruses, which are a major trigger of wheezing in this age group. Reduction in the frequency of upper respiratory infections caused by such viruses may result in a significant clinical improvement.

Asthma education

Asthma education and the formulation of a partnership between the patient, family, and physician are of paramount importance in managing asthma. Educational topics should include a definition of asthma, asthma triggers and how to avoid or control them, key points about signs and symptoms of asthma, characteristic changes in the airways of patients with asthma, the role of the different types of medications (anti-inflammatory, bronchodilator), treatment, and patient fears about medications. This should also include education on the correct use of inhalers, criteria for pre-medicating to prevent symptoms, the optimal use of home PEFR monitoring, and the provision of written plans on recommended treatments for daily therapy and episodic acute asthma exacerbations. Specific, individualized guidelines for seeking advice from the clinician or emergency department care should also be provided. Such asthma education has been shown to reduce the morbidity associated with asthma and to improve asthma control.

Pharmacologic therapy

In treating chronic asthma on an outpatient basis, the clinician must first classify the severity of the asthma as mild, moderate, or severe,

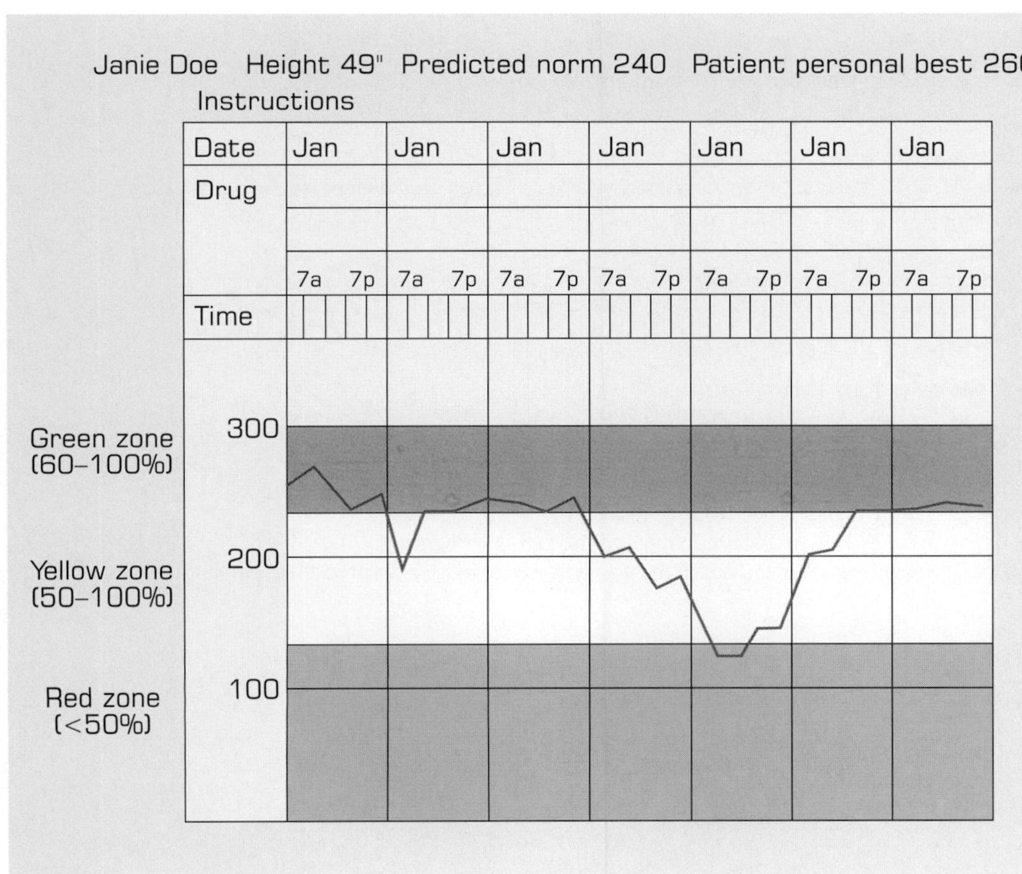

5.30 Typical peak flow meter diary. This patient dipped into the yellow zone on January 19, and recovered after use of a short-acting beta$_2$ agonist. The patient entered the red zone on January 22, and gradually improved after beginning therapy with systemic corticosteroids. (National Asthma Education Program Expert Panel Report, 1991.)

based upon guidelines which rely heavily on the frequency of symptoms (**5.31**). After classification, an incremental approach to treatment is recommended. This involves the initiation of a therapeutic regimen which is most appropriately matched to the patient's level of severity. If clinical improvement is not accomplished using that treatment, additional therapy is instituted until control of symptoms is achieved (**5.32A** and **5.32B**). After the goals of asthma therapy are achieved and there is a sustained clinical improvement, a step-down approach is used, where asthma medications are gradually withdrawn as tolerated. These therapy guidelines are detailed in two consensus reports: The National Heart, Lung and Blood Institute *Guidelines* (1991) that classified asthma as mild (episodic), moderate, and severe (**5.32A**), and the *International Consensus Report* (US Department of Health and Human Services, 1992) that classified asthma as mild, moderate (less severe), moderate (more severe), and severe (**5.32B**).

Therapy can be divided into several categories, including regimens that reverse symptoms (therapeutic for bronchospasm) and those which prevent symptoms (prophylactic against bronchospasm or inflammation) (**5.33**). The effects of various drug

CLINICAL CHARACTERISTICS	
Mild Asthma	
Symptoms	• Brief exacerbations no more than 1–2 times/week • Asymptomatic between exacerbations
Nocturnal Symptoms	• <1–2 times/month
PEFR	• PEFR > 80% of predicted (at baseline) when asymptomatic • Varies ≥20% when symptomatic
Spirometry	• Minimal or no evidence of airway obstruction • (Near) normal expiratory flow-volume curve • Normal lung volume • Significant (> 15%) reversibility of obstruction after inhaled bronchodilator
Moderate Asthma	
Symptoms	• Exacerbations 1–2 times/week • Cough & wheezing may be frequent between acute exacerbations if untreated
Nocturnal Symptoms	• 2–3 times/week
PEFR	• PEFR 60% to 80% of predicted at baseline; variability 20–30%
Spirometry	• Evidence of airway obstruction • FEV_1/FVC ratio < 70% • Significant (> 15%) reversibility of obstruction after inhaled bronchodilator
Severe Asthma	
Symptoms	• Daily wheezing, low-grade cough • E.R. visits > 3 times/year • Hospitalizations > 2 times/year
Nocturnal Symptoms	• Almost nightly interruption of sleep
PEFR	• PEFR > 60% of predicted at baseline; variability > 30%
Spirometry	• Substantial airway obstruction • Flow-volume loop shows marked concavity • Total lung capacity & residual volume may be increased • Incomplete reversibility of obstruction after inhaled bronchodilator

5.31 Guidelines for categorizing asthma severity as mild, moderate, and severe.

pretreatments on the model of IgE antibody-induced airway inflammation and hyperreactivity are shown in **5.34A** and **5.34B**. Since beta agonists are mainly bronchodilators, their therapeutic effects are mostly in the form of the reversal of bronchoconstriction during the early asthmatic response. They have virtually no effect on the late response and the resultant increases in airway inflammation and hyperreactivity. In contrast, corticosteroids, which inhibit phospholipase A_2 and the liberation of fatty acid-derived mediators (prostaglandins, platelet activating factor, leukotrienes), and cromolyn, which stabilizes mast cell membranes, inhibit the late response to allergens, reducing the resultant increases in airway inflammation and hyperreactivity. Cromolyn inhibits the early response as well, whereas the effect of steroids on the early response is probably only evident after prolonged use. The actions of anti-asthma drugs relevant to this model of asthma are shown in **5.15**.

Activities requiring strenuous exertion or exposure to cold air are often restricted or modified due to their propensity to induce bronchospasm. These factors may limit job opportunities and recreational sports for asthmatic patients, and they must be considered by

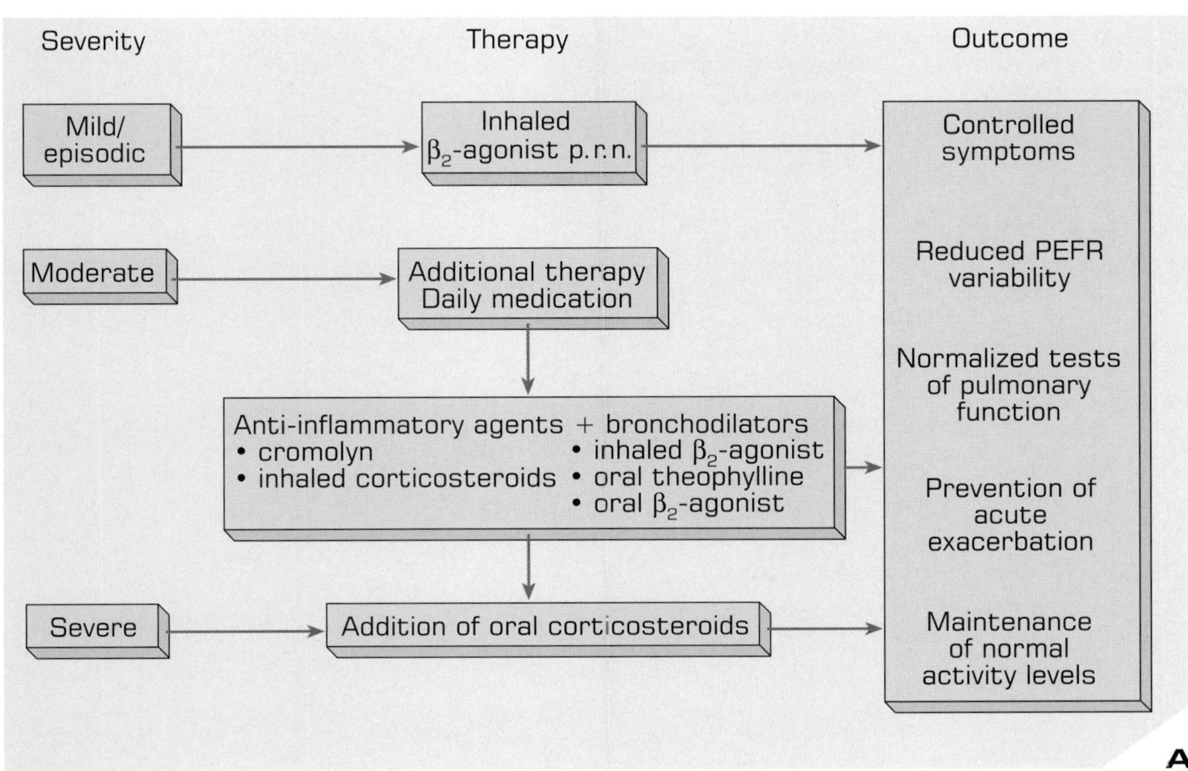

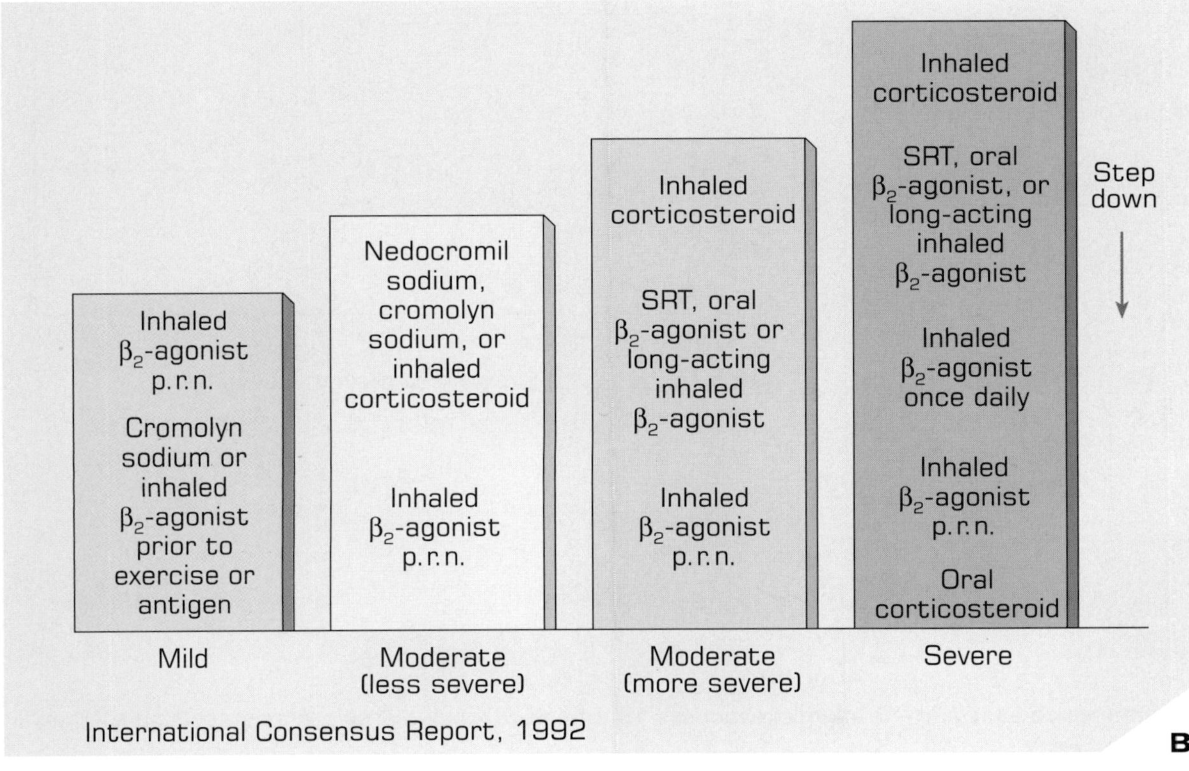

5.32 Stepwise approach to the pharmacologic therapy of asthma as proposed by the National Heart, Lung, and Blood Institute (A), and the International Consensus Report (B). Sustained release theophyllin (SRT) prescibed as needed (p.r.n.).

patients seeking employment and recreation. Exercise of short duration and low intensity (e.g., swimming) is less likely to induce wheezing than that of long duration and high intensity (e.g., distance-running, sprinting). However, asthmatics should be encouraged to pretreat exercise-induced asthma with a beta agonist or cromolyn metered-dose inhaler and participate only at the highest level of exertion which does not trigger bronchospasm. Exercise-induced asthma can be managed with premedication using either inhaled beta agonist or cromolyn sodium immediately before exercise.

Patients with asthma should be referred to an asthma specialist (allergist or pulmonologist) for pulmonary function studies, questions of differential diagnosis, evaluation of the role of allergy and irritants, consideration for allergy immunotherapy, or evaluation of the medication plan if the goals of therapy are not met.

TYPES OF ASTHMA THERAPY

Therapy	Reverse symptoms (therapeutic)	Prevent symptoms (prophylactic)
$Beta_2$ agonists	Yes	Yes
Theophylline	Yes	Yes
Inhaled cromolyn	No	Yes
Inhaled corticosteroids	No	Yes
Systemic corticosteroids	Yes	Yes[a]
Anti-cholinergics	Yes	Yes
Environmental controls	No	Yes
Allergy immunotherapy	No	Yes[b]

[a]Only if prophylactic therapy with inhaled corticosteroids is unsuccessful.
[b]Only for allergic asthma.

5.33 Types of asthma therapy.

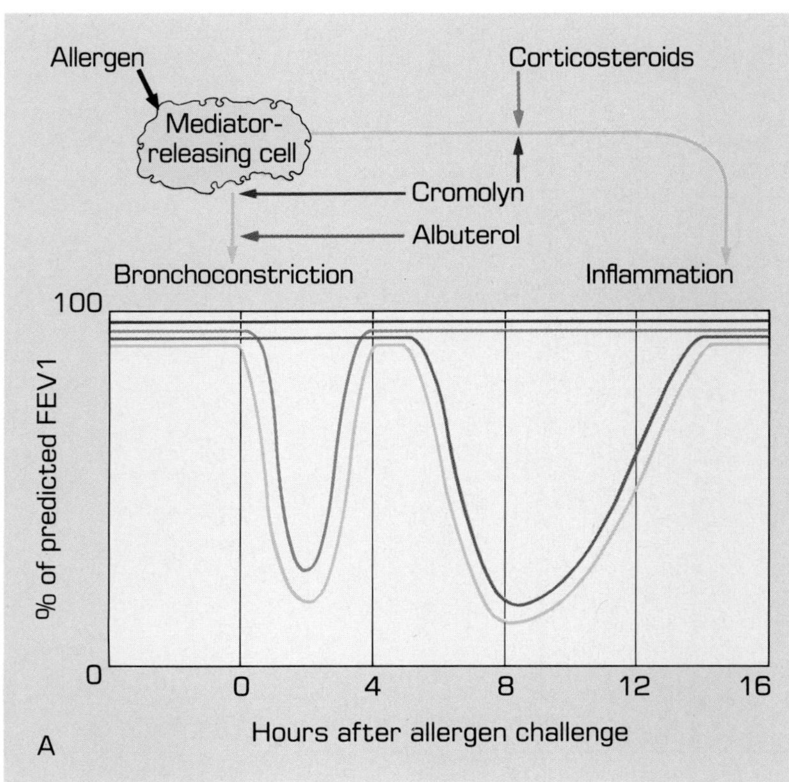

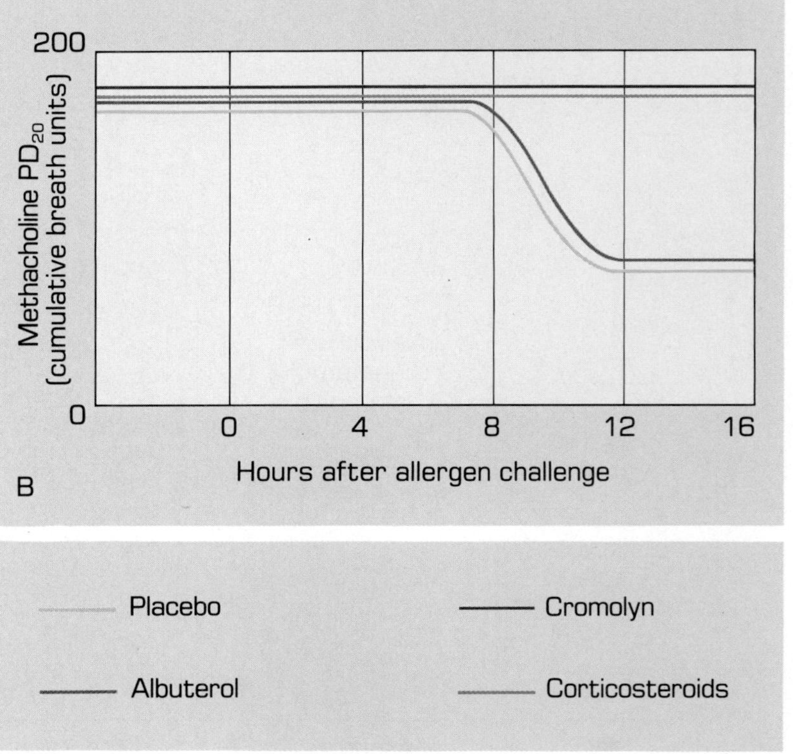

5.34 (A) Effects of inhaled drug pre-treatments on early and late allergic responses. (B) Effects of inhaled drug pre-treatments on allergen-induced increases in airway hyperresponsiveness.

SPECIFIC DRUGS

Bronchodilator drugs

Beta$_2$ agonist. The clinician must be cognizant of several important aspects of drug delivery and pharmacokinetics when employing inhaled bronchodilator therapy. Nebulized beta-adrenergic agents are an important component of asthma therapy and are the initial bronchodilator used for most asthmatics, except very young children. These agents can be administered by a metered-dose inhaler or aerosolized via a nebulizer with a portable air compressor. Their efficacy and immediate onset of action differentiate them from most other forms of asthma therapy, and ideally suit them to both outpatient and inpatient asthma therapy. The development of newer agents with longer durations of action and more selective beta2 receptor action has further solidified their role and enhanced their usefulness in asthma management (5.35).

When delivered by metered-dose inhaler, especially in children less than 5 years of age or the older adults who lack the coordination necessary for its use, the placement of a spacing device between the mouth and inhaler mouthpiece is advisable and efficacious (5.36). Some clinicians feel that the use of spacing devices is indicated in all asthmatics who use metered dose inhalers.

Beta$_2$-adrenergic agonists, which act through the relaxation of airway smooth muscle, are considered the treatment of choice for acute asthma exacerbations. Both oral and inhaled preparations are available. Inhaled, short-acting agents (e.g., albuterol) should be used every 4–6 hours on an as-needed basis for the treatment of acute bronchospasm. A newer agent, salmeterol, has a much longer duration of action (12 hours) and is indicated for the prevention of acute bronchospasm. Twice-daily administration makes this formulation convenient and useful, especially for the prevention of nocturnal asthma and asthma associated with exercise of long duration. However, due to the longer time until its onset of action (compared to albuterol), salmeterol should not be used as a bronchodilator to treat acute asthma. Sustained release, orally administered albuterol can also be useful under the same circumstances as salmeterol.

The side effects of beta$_2$ agonists can include tachycardia, tremor, headache, palpitations, and hypokalemia. The relatively greater beta$_2$ receptor selectivity of salmeterol (beta$_2$:beta$_1$ ratio = 85,000 versus 1375 for albuterol) has resulted in diminution of a number of these side effects. The regular use of inhaled short-acting beta$_2$ agonists has also been associated with increased bronchial hyperresponsiveness, diminished asthma control, and increased morbidity, although these findings are considered controversial.

Theophylline. Theophylline's bronchodilator effect was first described in 1920. The advent of sustained-release preparations in 1970 led to the convenient and widespread use of theophylline as a bronchodilator in the treatment of chronic asthma, especially nocturnal asthma. Theophylline has well-known bronchodilatory effects. Recently, it has been postulated that theophylline may also have anti-inflammatory properties, but further investigation of this possibility is necessary. This could potentially explain the reported steroid-sparing effect of theophylline. Although theophylline remains a useful maintenance medication in the treatment of chronic asthma, its use to treat acute asthma has decreased dramatically, due to the publication of studies demonstrating a lack of efficacy versus placebo in this setting.

ADRENERGIC AGONISTS USED IN THE TREATMENT OF ASTHMA

Agonist	Duration of action (hours)	Types of use[a] Prophylaxis E.I.B	Types of use[a] Prophylaxis Daily	Types of use[a] Therapy	Activity relative to epinephrine[b] Alpha	Activity relative to epinephrine[b] Beta$_1$	Activity relative to epinephrine[b] Beta$_2$
Epinephrine	1–2	-	-	+	E	E	E
Isoproterenol	2–3	-	-	+	E	E	E
Isoetharine	2–3	-	-	+	L	E	G
Metaproterenol	3–5	+	-	+	L	E	G
Terbutaline	4–6	+	-	+	L	E	G
Albuterol	4–6	+	-	+	L	E	G
Salmeterol	10–12	+	+	-	L	E	G

[a]Recommended types of use: prophylaxis – as needed to prevent exercise-induced bronchospasms or daily use to prevent wheezing; therapy – as needed to treat wheezing.
[b]E = Equivalent, G = Greater, L = Lesser.

5.35 Adrenergic agonists useful in the treatment of asthma.

The serum theophylline concentration that provides benefit without toxicity needs to be monitored in patients on chronic therapy or during hospitalization for status asthmaticus. Serum concentrations in the 5–15 µg/ml range are generally acceptable, and help patients avoid many of the undesirable dose-related side effects which can accompany higher concentrations (headaches, vomiting, seizures). Serum levels of theophylline are under the influence of a wide variety of factors (**5.37**), which necessitates frequent monitoring. These include febrile illnesses, diet, pregnancy, age, liver disease, congestive heart failure, and concomitant drug usage. Thus, an asthmatic with a stable therapeutic theophylline level who is placed on concomitant erythromycin or phenobarbital therapy develops altered theophylline metabolism and may experience symptoms related to toxic or subtherapeutic theophylline levels, respectively. Cigarette smoking increases metabolism of theophylline, whereas viral infection may enhance or retard its metabolism.

Gastrointestinal intolerance or exacerbation of gastroesophageal reflux has been noted in patients treated with theophylline and it can provoke a variety of symptoms related to the central nervous system. Many of the earlier studies linking theophylline to behavioral or learning difficulties have been compromised by design flaws or misinterpretation of study results. Indeed, recent studies have shown that theophylline lacks adverse effects on behavior and learning, but may have a transient caffeine-like effect on the central nervous system.

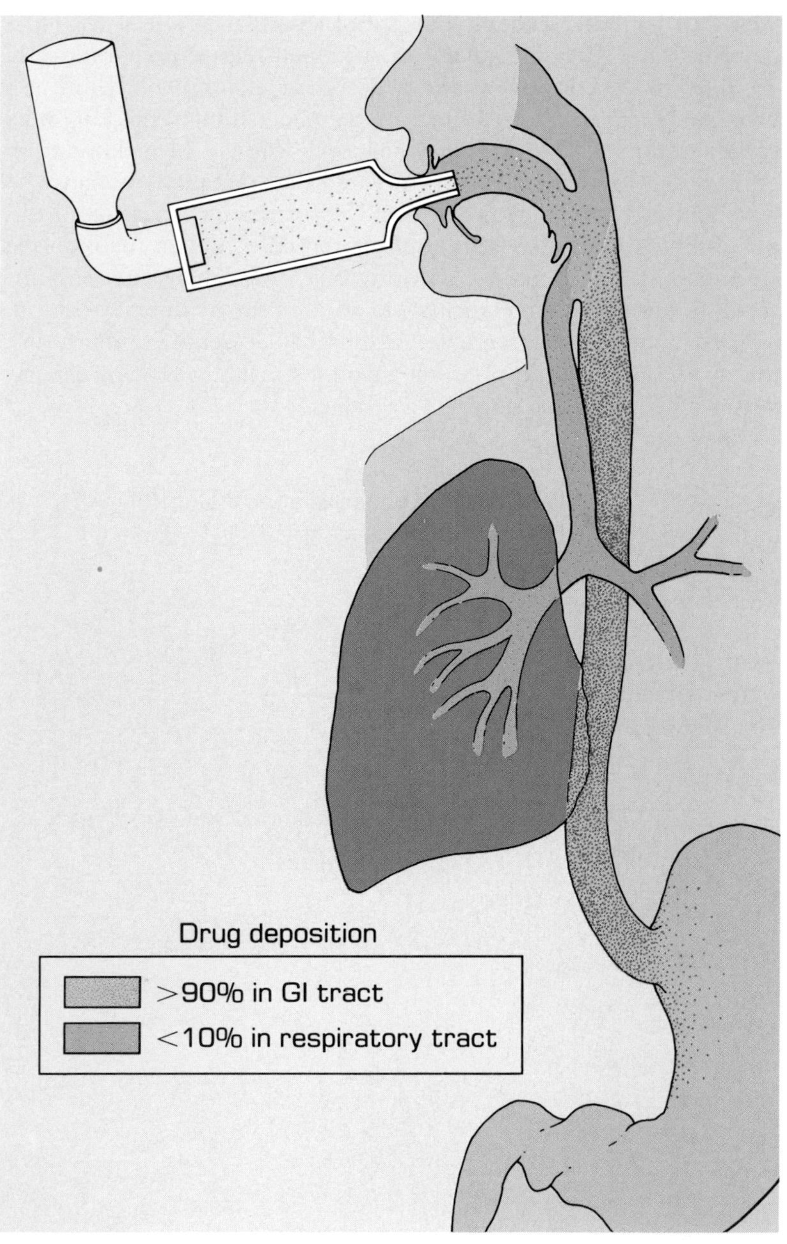

5.36 Illustration of a spacing device placed between the metered-dose inhaler and the mouthpiece. Its use lessens the need for coordination when using the metered-dose inhaler. Note that approximately 10% of the inhaled dose reaches the airways, while the remainder is deposited in the alimentary (GI) tract.

Anti-cholinergic. These agents, including ipratropium bromide and atropine, reduce mucus gland secretion and may induce bronchodilation by blocking cholinergic stimulation. In this regard, they are helpful ancillary medications for the treatment of asthma. Anti-cholinergic drugs are not anti-inflammatory, do not diminish bronchial hyperreactivity over time, and are not to be used as a primary medication for asthma treatment.

Anti-inflammatory drugs

Cromolyn sodium. For years, this agent was the only non-steroidal inhaled anti-inflammatory agent for asthma treatment. It is virtually devoid of side effects and is tolerated quite well by nearly all patients. It is thought to inhibit IgE-mediated release of inflammatory mediators from mast cells. Cromolyn inhibits early and late-phase allergen-induced lower airway obstruction, and prevents the acute obstruction that develops after exercise and exposure to cold, dry air. However, it does not reverse bronchospasm and is not to be used as a bronchodilator to treat acute asthma. Asthma patients may benefit from cromolyn, but some consider it more beneficial in mild, allergic asthma. It is available as a solution for aerosol nebulization and as a metered-dose inhaler. A trial of 4–6 weeks is recommended, since its onset of action is slow.

Nedocromil sodium. Nedocromil, available in a metered-dose inhaler formulation, is the newest non-steroidal anti-inflammatory agent to treat asthma. Like cromolyn, this agent is also virtually devoid of side effects. Nedocromil has been shown to reduce bronchial hyperresponsiveness and improve pulmonary function.

FACTORS INFLUENCING THEOPHYLLINE CLEARANCE

Factors	Decreased clearance	Increased clearance
Age	Prematures, neonates, age >50 years	Age 1–16 years
Weight	Obesity (in relation to total body weight)	
Diet	Dietary methylxanthines, high carbohydrates	Low carbohydrates, high protein, charcoal-broiled meats
Habits		Cigarette smoking (tobacco or marijuana)
Drugs	Troleandomycin Erythromycin Cimetidine Influenza vaccine	Phenytoin Phenobarbital Isoproterenol (intravenous) Terbutaline
Diseases	Cirrhosis Congestive heart failure Chronic obstructive pulmonary disease Acute pulmonary edema Acute viral illnesses	

5.37 Factors affecting theophylline clearance.

A particularly strong effect on asthmatic cough has been noted in several studies.

Corticosteroids. Orally administered or injected corticosteroids are indicated for the acute, short-term therapy of severe exacerbations. Systemic corticosteroid therapy is indicated in the management of acute asthma and is mandatory in the therapy of status asthmaticus. By appropriately timing the intervention with corticosteroids, the clinician may benefit the patient and reduce hospitalizations. Based on current medical literature, the times to initiate corticosteroid therapy in outpatient and inpatient asthma are shown in **5.38A**. Since the action of corticosteroids is dependent on cellular internalization (**5.38B**), therapy should be instituted promptly once an indication for use is established.

Typically, patients begin oral prednisone (2 mg/kg/day or maximum of 60 mg/day) at the onset of an acute exacerbation and continue the treatment for a total of 3–5 days. Oral preparations can also be used as alternate-day maintenance therapy for chronic, severe asthma. Although high-dose, short-term corticosteroid therapy is relatively safe in severe life-threatening disorders, chronic systemic administration in patients with severe asthma carries a significant risk for adverse effects, including growth suppression, adrenal suppression, osteoporosis, cataracts, weight gain, and hypertension. Complications which are detectable on physical examination include weight gain, 'moon-type' facies, hirsutism, polycythemia (red, ruddy complexion), and short stature (**5.39**). Such side effects of excessive steroid therapy for chronic asthma should be avoidable complications.

TIMING OF CORTICOSTEROID USE IN ASTHMA

Location	Stage of asthma	Steroid use
Hospital	Status asthmaticus	Yes
Emergency department	Acute asthma	Yes (early)[a]
Home	Chest symptoms	Yes
Home (recurrent asthma)	Start of URI[b]	Yes[c]
Home (not recurrent)	Start of URI[b]	No

[a] *N Eng J Med*, **314**:151, 1986.
[b] URI = upper respiratory infection.
[c] *Pediatr*, **81**:624–629, 1988.

A

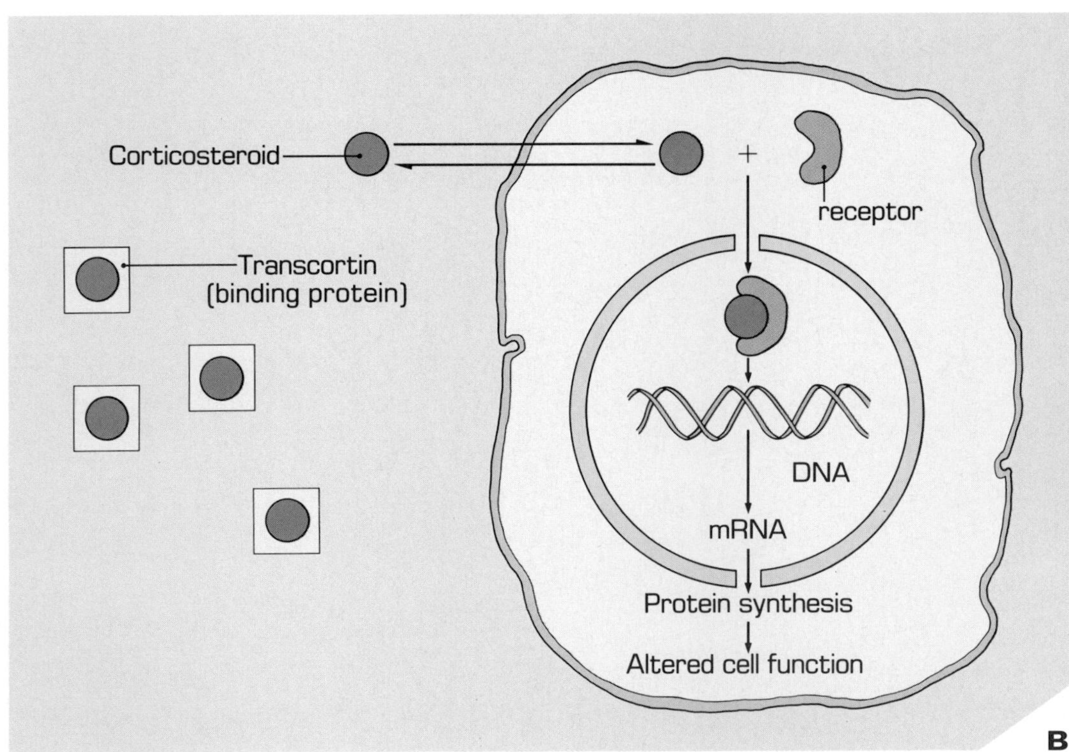

B

5.38 (A) Timing of corticosteroid use in asthma. (B) Proposed mode of action of corticosteroids. Note that corticosteroids bind to a cytosolic receptor and exert their effects by affecting protein synthesis, thus accounting for their delayed onset of action. (With permission from Kaliner, M, *J Allergy Clin Immunol*, **76**:321, 1985.)

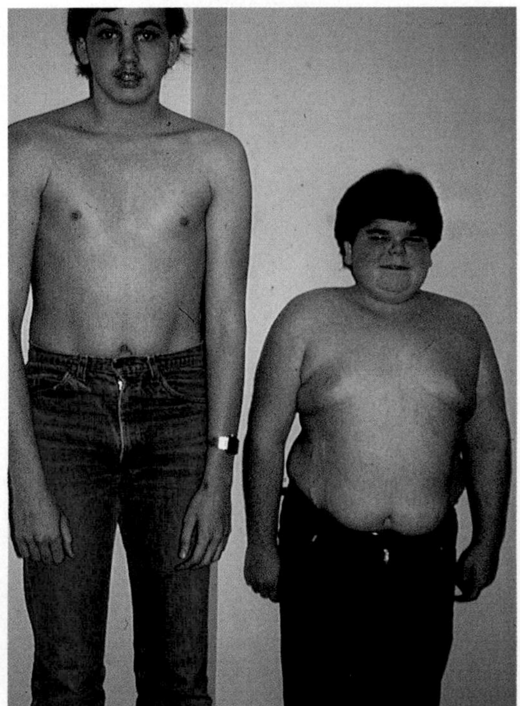

5.39 Short stature, a complication of corticosteroid therapy for chronic asthma, is illustrated by the 16-year-old steroid-dependent asthmatic next to a normal 16-year-old. (With permission from Skoner *et al.*, 1987).

Inhaled corticosteroids represent an important advance in the treatment of chronic asthma, and are safe and effective. Their potent anti-inflammatory effects are at least partially related to interference with the production of leukotrienes, prostaglandins, and cytokines. Use of these agents is associated with diminished bronchial hyperresponsiveness. Many of these agents can be used in children as young as 6 years of age. Immediate benefit may not be evident, since suppression of symptoms and improvement in PEFR are frequently not maximal until treatment has been administered for 1–4 weeks. Therefore, education about the relative onset of action and value of these agents, versus the more commonly used beta agonists, must be provided by the managing clinician.

Significant effects of inhaled corticosteroids on the hypothalamic–pituitary–adrenal axis do not occur when used in manufacturer-recommended doses, but can be seen when very high doses (1600–2600 µg/day) are administered. Effects on growth are generally not present at doses of less than 400 µg/day. However, doses of greater than 400 µg/day presumably carry a dose-dependent risk for adverse effects on growth, although little evidence to support this presumption is available. Some clinicians and guidelines advocate the use of a cut-off dose of 1000 µg/day, above which concern is enhanced and care by an asthma specialist is recommended. However, such effects can be minimized by the incorporation of spacers and mouth-rinsing techniques, which reduce the systemic absorption from the oral cavity and gastrointestinal tract.

Other. Other drugs, including troleandomycin (TAO), gold, and methotrexate, are available to treat asthma which is poorly responsive to more standard therapeutic regimens, including corticosteroids. However, in many instances, efficacy has not been unequivocally established, and their use remains experimental, controversial, and individualized.

OTHER THERAPY

Annual influenza-virus vaccination is recommended for adults and children with asthma severe enough to require regular medical follow-up or hospitalization.

HOME/EMERGENCY DEPARTMENT MANAGEMENT OF ASTHMA EXACERBATION

The guidelines for the management of childhood asthma exacerbations at home and in the emergency department are summarized in **5.40** and **5.41**, respectively.

HOSPITAL MANAGEMENT OF ASTHMA EXACERBATION

The guidelines for the management of childhood asthma exacerbations in the inpatient hospital are summarized in **5.42**. Status asthmaticus (poor response to Emergency Department treatment protocol) is treated with intravenous corticosteroids, oxygen, and a nebulized beta agonist on a regular, frequent (every 1–2 hours), or even continuous basis. Patients are weaned from it as they improve. If the patient has been on chronic maintenance theophylline therapy as an outpatient, then parenteral theophylline therapy should also be instituted. Most pediatric patients improve on this therapeutic regimen and are discharged within 3 days, but adults frequently respond less rapidly and require longer periods of hospitalization. In general, beta adrenergic dosing intervals of less than 2 hours require observation and monitoring in an intensive-care facility. A patient with status asthmaticus must be monitored closely during the first 6–12 hours of

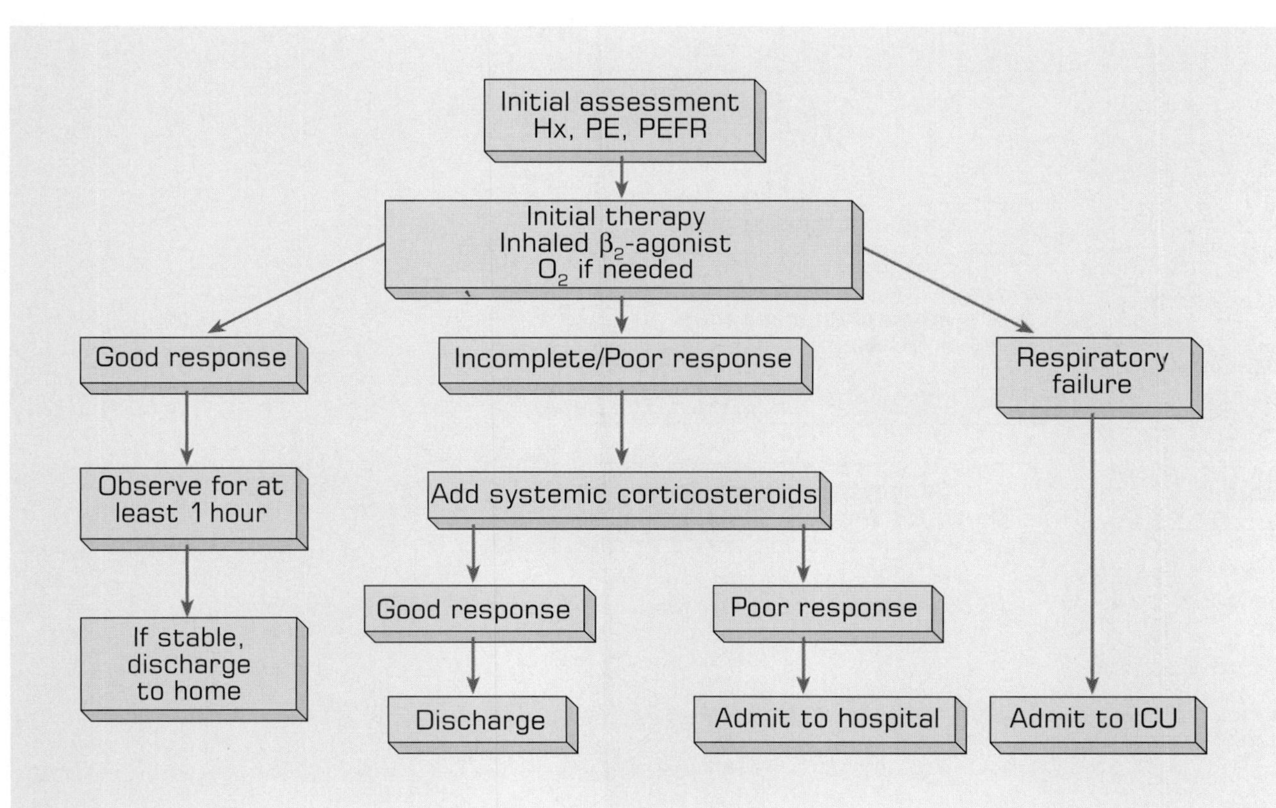

5.40 Emergency department management of acute asthma exacerbations in children.

hospitalization for impending respiratory failure, so that therapy to prevent progression to respiratory failure can be instituted.

Therapy for impending respiratory failure consists of the correction of acid–base imbalances in the setting of an intensive-care unit, where cardiac and respiratory function can be closely monitored. Intravenous isoproterenol has been used to treat pediatric patients, but should never be used in an asthmatic older than 16 years because of its cardiotoxicity. If respiratory failure supervenes despite intense medical management, artificial mechanical ventilation is indicated.

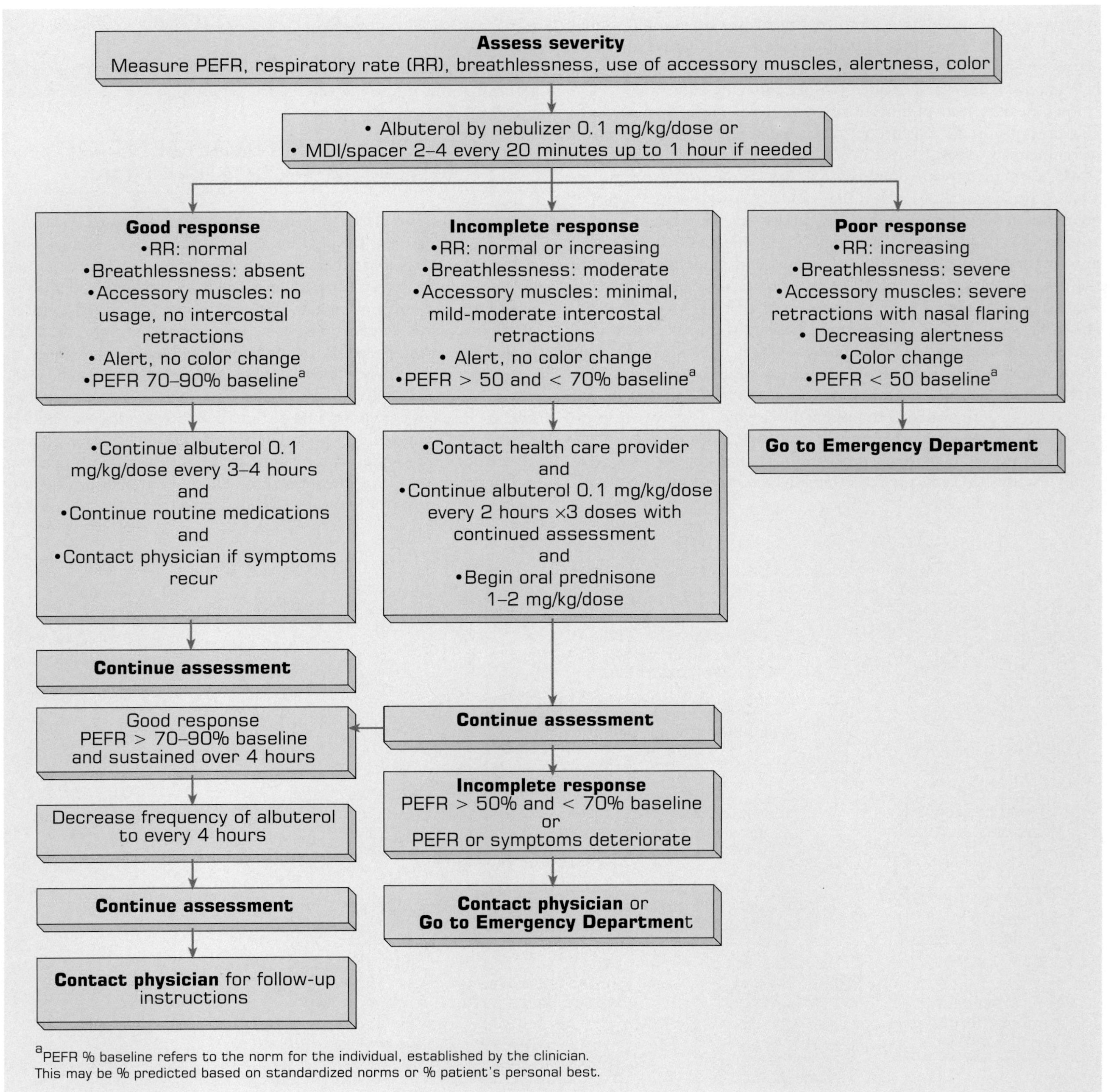

5.41 Home management of acute asthma exacerbations in children.

MANAGEMENT OF ASTHMA DURING PREGNANCY

It is essential that sufficient lung function and blood oxygenation be maintained during pregnancy, so that an adequate oxygen supply to the fetus is supplied. Increased perinatal mortality, increased prematurity, and low birth weight can all result from poorly controlled asthma. For most drugs used to treat asthma, there is little evidence to suggest an increased risk to the fetus. Exceptions include corticosteroids and epinephrine. Therapy with the lowest possible doses of the fewest possible medications should be the goal of treatment of asthma during pregnancy.

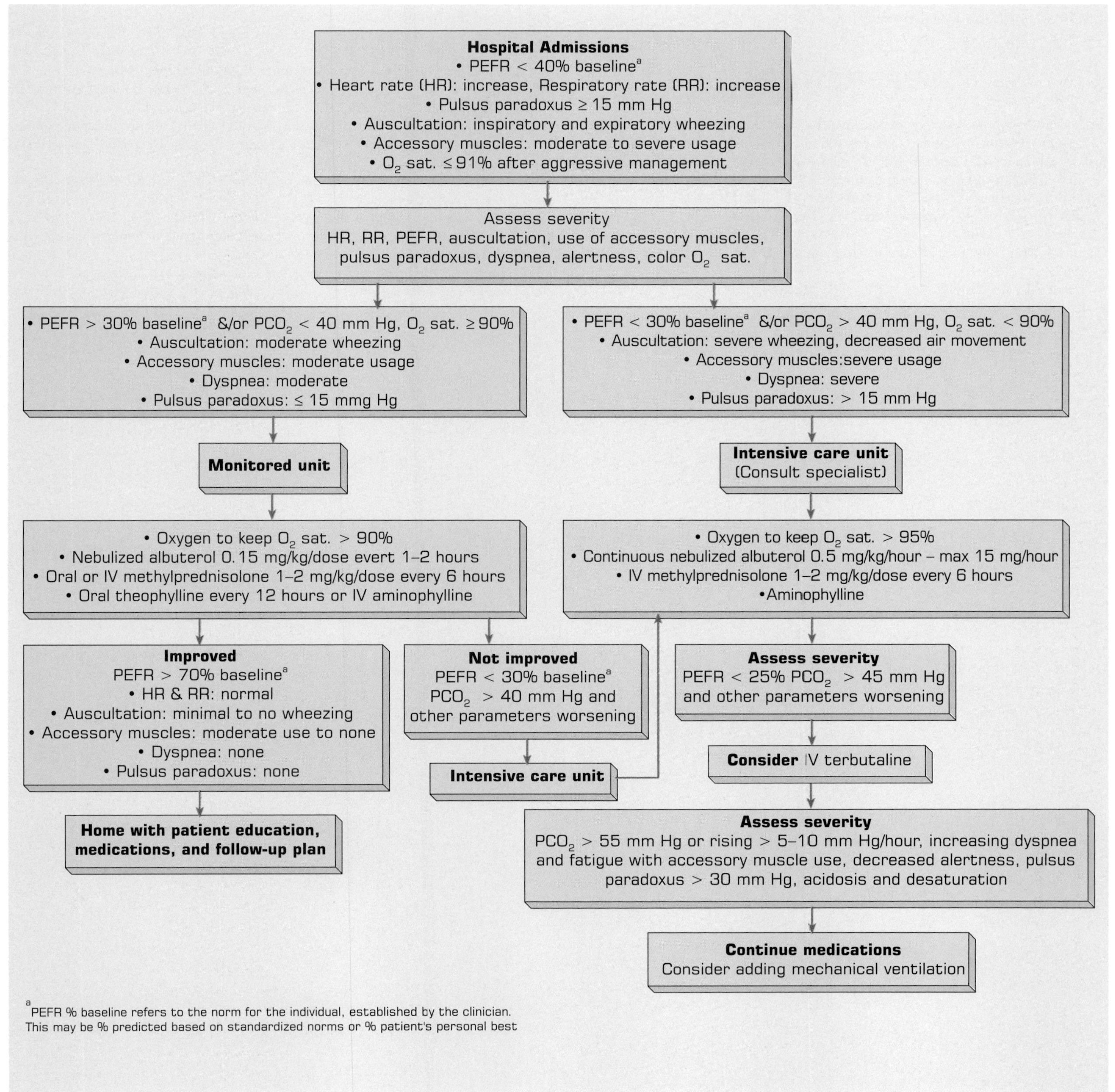

5.42 Hospital management of acute asthma exacerbations in children.

IDENTIFICATION OF PATIENTS AT RISK FOR ASTHMA-RELATED DEATH

Care of asthmatic patients should include the identification of patients at risk for asthma-related death. Clues include the presence of previous life-threatening exacerbations of asthma, the lack of adequate and ongoing medical care that provides appropriate follow-up and prophylactic therapy, and significant depression and/or psychosocial behavioral problems.

REFERENCES

Alabaster VA, Moore BA: New perspectives on basic mechanisms in lung disease – drug intervention in asthma – present and future. *Thorax*, **48**(2):176–182, 1993.

Broide DH, Paine M, Firestein G: Eosinophils express IL-5 and GM-CSF mRNA at sites of allergic inflammation in asthmatics. *J Clin Invest*, **90**:1414–1424, 1992.

Burrows B, Martinez FD, Halonen M, Barbee RA, Cline MG: Association of asthma with serum IgE levels and skin-test reactivity to allergens. *N Engl J Med*, **320**:271–277, 1989.

Cherniack RM: Continuity of care in asthma management. *Hosp Practice*, **Sept 15**, 1987.

Djukanovic R, Roche WR, Wilson JW, *et al.*: Mucosal inflammation in asthma. *Am Rev Respir Dis*, **142**:434–457, 1990.

Ellis EF: Asthma in childhood. *J Allergy Clin Immunol*, **72**:526–539, 1983.

Gurwitz D *et al.*: Increased incidence of bronchial reactivity in children with a history of bronchiolitis. *J Pediatr*, **98**:551–555, 1981.

Henderson FW *et al.*: *J Pediatr*, **95**:183–190, 1979.

Horn MEC *et al.*: *Thorax*, **34**:23–28, 1979.

Kaliner M: Mast cell mediators and asthma, in Herzog H, Perruchoud AP (eds): *Progress in Respiration Research – Asthma and Bronchial Hyperreactivity*, S. Karger, Basel, Switzerland, 1985.

Madonini E *et al.*: Seasonal increase of bronchial reactivity in allergic rhinitis. *J Allergy Clin Immunol*, **79**:358–363, 1987.

Middleton E, Reed CE, Ellis EF, Adkinson NF, Yunginger JW (eds): *Allergy: Principles and Practice*, The C.V. Mosby Company, St. Louis, 3rd edn, Volume II (Clinical Science), 1988.

National Heart, Lung, and Blood Institute: *National Asthma Education Program: Guidelines for the Diagnosis and Management of Asthma*, National Institutes of Health, Bethesda, MD, No. 91-3042, August, 1991.

Skoner D, Stillwagon P, Friedman R, Fireman P: Pediatric allergy and immunology, in Davis H, Zitelli B (eds), *Atlas of Pediatric Physical Diagnosis*, Gower Press, London, 1987.

Skoner DP, Caliguiri L: The wheezing infant, in P. Fireman (ed.): *Pediatric Allergic Disease*, W.B. Saunders, 1988.

Sly RM: Changing asthma mortality. *Ann Allergy*, **73**:260, 1994.

Taylor SM *et al.*: Airway reactivity in chronic obstructive pulmonary disease. *Am Rev Respir Dis*, **132**:30–35, 1985.

US Department of Health and Human Services: *International Consensus Report on Diagnosis and Management of Asthma*, Public Health Service, National Institutes of Health, Bethesda, MD, 1992.

CHAPTER 6

Occupational Allergies

Raymond G. Slavin

The work place is increasingly recognized as a fertile area for the production of human disease. Many of these occupational conditions are of interest to the allergist, particularly those involving the skin, nose, and lungs (**6.1**). Occupational disease of the skin may be of the allergic contact type, such as chromium sensitivity which affects cement workers, or of the primary irritant type caused by organic solvents, which affects automobile workers. The nose can be involved in an IgE-mediated allergic reaction to a specific allergen, such as wheat flour which affects bakers, or a non-specific, non-allergic reaction to an irritant such as coal dust, which affects miners. Among the occupational diseases that involve the lungs are the following: hypersensitivity pneumonitis (*see* Chapter 7), which afflicts farmers who have a sensitivity to thermophilic organisms present in moldy hay, fibrotic diseases (such as silicosis, asbestosis, and berylliosis), and asthma.

OCCUPATIONAL ASTHMA

Occupational asthma is a condition characterized by variable airway narrowing that is causally related to exposure to airborne dusts, gases, vapors, or fumes present in the working environment (Newman-Taylor, 1980). Though precise figures are difficult to obtain, it is estimated (many believe, underestimated) that occupational asthma affects 500,000 Americans, which is approximately 5% of the total asthmatic population. The difficulties confronting epidemiologists in search of statistics in this area are numerous. First, there is great variance in the incidence of occupational asthma in response to different substances. Of workers exposed to proteolytic enzymes, 10–40% become sensitive to them, while only 5% of workers exposed to Western Red Cedar dust develop occupational asthma. Variance also occurs within the same industry and even the same factory; this is largely due to varying work conditions, including ventilation. For example, textile workers involved in a dusty operation, such as the carding process, develop much higher rates of byssinosis than those in other areas of the textile plant. There is also a certain degree of self-determination involved in the varying asthma statistics. Those who develop asthma early in their careers are more likely to leave the setting and seek employment elsewhere. Finally, in a difficult economy in which jobs are relatively scarce, workers are less likely to complain about asthma for fear of losing their jobs. All these factors contribute to the precarious epidemiologic studies of occupational asthma.

OCCUPATIONAL DISEASES OF INTEREST TO ALLERGISTS

1. **Skin**
   Allergic contact – chromium
   Primary irritant – benzene
2. **Nose**
   Allergic – wheat flour
   Non-allergic – coal dust
3. **Lung**
   Hypersensitivity pneumonitis – moldy hay
   Fibrotic disease – silica, asbestos, beryllium
   Asthma – animal protein

6.1 Occupational diseases of importance to allergists.

CONTRIBUTING FACTORS

Several factors contribute to the development of occupational asthma. Within factories, the nature and concentration of inhaled substances are important. Agents of high molecular weight are more likely to sensitize workers. Low molecular weight substances with good haptenic properties have the ability to combine with carriers, such as serum proteins, and may also sensitize workers. In general, the higher the level of exposure to the sensitizing substance, the higher the prevalence of occupational asthma (**6.2** and **6.3**). Conditions within factories also play important roles. Industrial accidents or spills may expose a worker to increased levels of allergenic or irritating substances (**6.4**). Proper industrial hygiene includes monitoring of air, automation of industrial procedures, and provision of uniforms equipped with clean ventilation, disposable masks, and gloves (**6.5**). Certain host factors also contribute to the development of occupational asthma. The presence of pre-existing atopy increases the likelihood that a worker will develop an IgE-mediated reactivity to such agents as bacillus subtilis enzyme and locusts. Smoking has also been shown to increase the development of some sensitivities. Specific IgE antibody to tetrachlorophthalic anhydride, a substance found in plastics factories, is increased in smokers exposed to that substance.

An illustration of the various human responses to the same chemical in different forms is given in **6.6**. Exposure to trimellitic anhydride (TMA), an active chemical widely used in the production of plastics and epoxy resins, results in four different clinical syndromes (Paterson *et al.*, 1986).

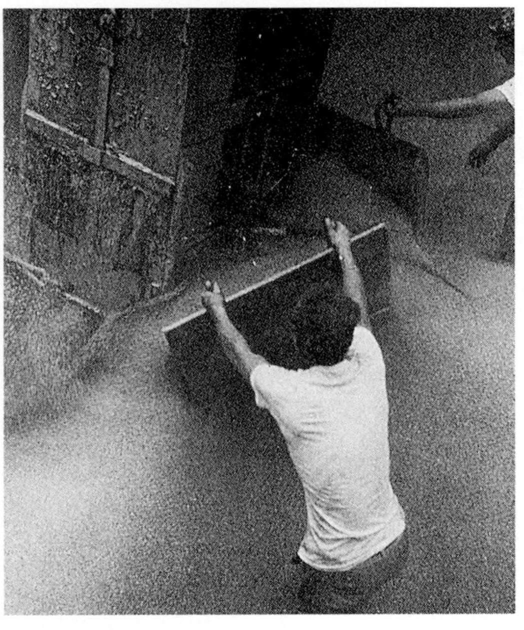

6.2 Workers loading grain aboard ships are exposed to a variety of bronchial irritants. (Reproduced with permission from Slavin, 1978.)

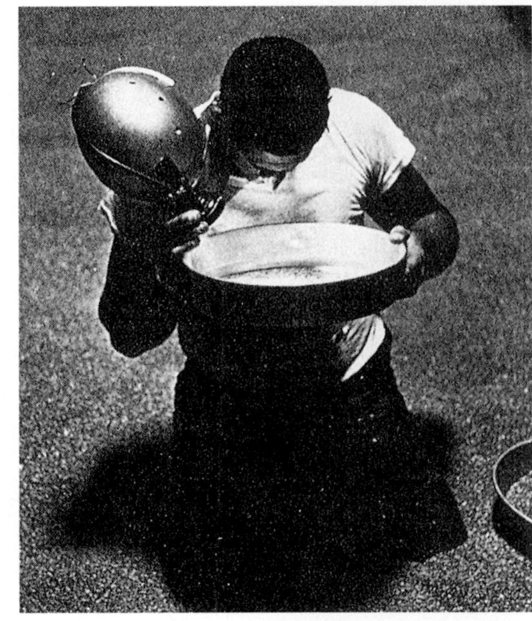

6.3 Corn inspector inhales dust while sifting grain, and can develop occupational asthma. (Reproduced with permission from Slavin, 1978.)

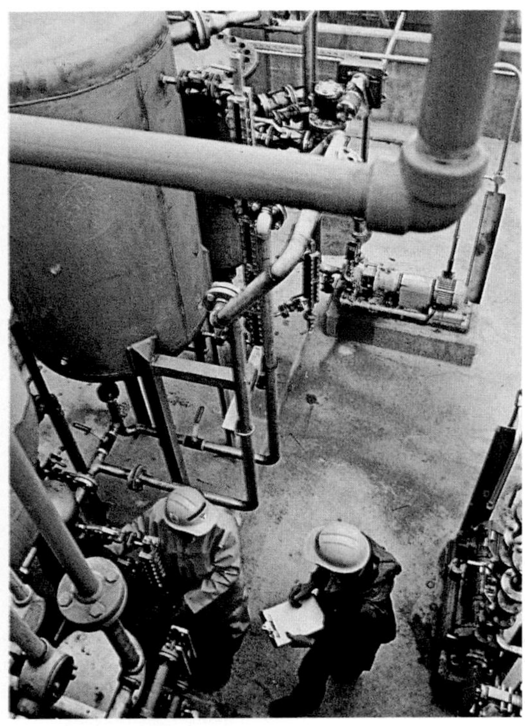

6.4 Isocyanate plant with evidence of reddish foam spill. (Courtesy of Dr Emil J. Bardana, Portland, Oregon.)

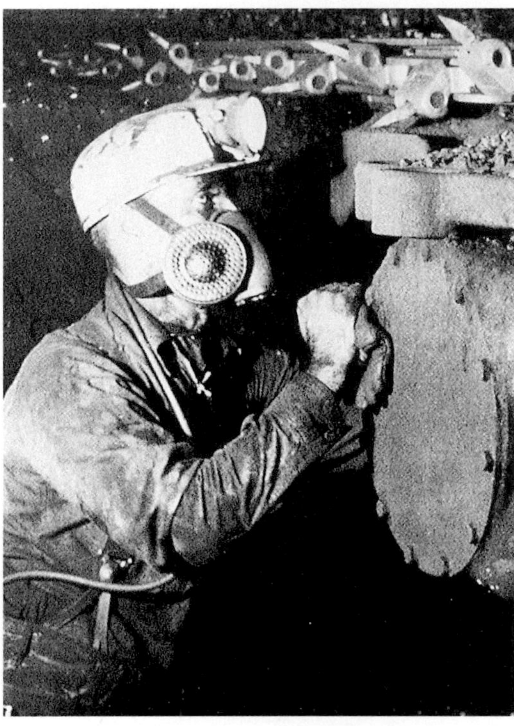

6.5 Sandblaster wearing respirator. (Courtesy of Dr Emil J. Bardana, Portland, Oregon.)

- Immediate rhinitis and asthma that appear clinically to be allergic in nature are correlated with the presence of IgE anti-TMA-hapten antibodies.
- Workers may also develop a late onset asthma with systemic symptoms such as achiness and fatigue. This has been termed 'TMA-flu' and is correlated with presence of IgG anti-TMA-hapten antibodies.
- A third reaction associated with high TMA exposure is a non-specific bronchial irritation marked by a cough. This condition is not accompanied by any significant immunologic changes.
- A fourth clinical syndrome found after exposure to TMA is associated with extensive pulmonary infiltrates that produce so-called 'white outs' on chest radiography. Hemoptysis, severe dyspnea, a restrictive lung picture, hypoxemia, and anemia are also seen. The condition is called the pulmonary disease–anemia syndrome. The immunologic characteristic is the presence of IgG antibody against the TMA hapten protein, and respiratory tract cells, particularly erythrocytes.

PATHOGENESIS OF OCCUPATIONAL ASTHMA

Occupational asthma may be classified in several ways. However, the pathogenesis is best understood when classified in terms of its basic mechanisms.

REFLEX BRONCHOCONSTRICTION

Workers who have pre-existing asthma or bronchitis may respond in a non-specific fashion to irritants, such as cold air, or inert particles, such as talc. Reflex bronchoconstriction results from the direct effect of such substances on irritant receptors in the bronchial wall.

ALLERGIC

Typical IgE-related allergic asthma often develops at the work place. 6.7 lists the clinical characteristics that might prompt a clinician to consider an immunologic basis for a patient's occupational asthma. Allergic asthma does not result from an initial exposure, as does reflex or inflammatory asthma. A period of sensitization must occur; this can vary from just a few weeks to as long as 20 years. In addition, only some, not all, exposed workers are affected. The incidence is generally low – it does not exceed the 20% of allergic patients found in the general population. Sensitivity to causative antigens increases with time; the longer the patient is exposed, the more severe the reaction. Moreover, in clinical testing through bronchoprovocation, as discussed later, a pulmonary reaction can be elicited with small amounts of the substance, amounts far smaller than those generally encountered in the work place. Finally, patients with allergic occupational asthma exhibit the phenomenon of immunologic memory, or anamnesis. If an individual who has developed sensitivity after a period of exposure to a given substance

CLINICAL SYNDROMES DUE TO TMA

TMA exposure	Clinical syndromes	Immunologic characteristics
Dust	Immediate rhinitis, asthma (TMA asthma)	IgE anti-TMA hapten
	Late asthma with systemic symptoms (TMA flu)	IgG anti-TMA hapten
	Cough; airway irritation	No antibody response
Fumes	Hemoptysis, pulmonary infiltrates, dyspnea (pulmonary disease–anemia syndrome)	Anti-hapten antibodies

6.6 Clinical syndromes related to TMA exposure.

CLINICAL CHARACTERISTICS OF ALLERGIC OCCUPATIONAL ASTHMA

1. Asthma appears only after repeated exposures
2. Only a proportion of exposed subjects are affected
3. Sensitivity increases with time
4. Reactions elicited by exposure to small amounts
5. Immunologic memory or anamnesis

6.7 Clinical characteristics of allergic occupational asthma.

is removed from that environment for a time and then reintroduced to it, asthma develops in a much shorter time than previously necessary.

Several allergens encountered at the work place can cause immunologically mediated occupational asthma. A partial list of these allergens with their associated occupations is given in **6.8**. Substances of high molecular weight are generally regarded as the strongest allergens. Indeed, it was once thought that most of the industrial materials inhaled by workers, such as gases, vapors, fumes, and mineral dusts, could not produce allergic reactions because of their small molecular weights. Strictly speaking, this is true, as the substances alone are not immunogenic. However, many of them are excellent haptens and when combined with tissue proteins, such as human serum albumin, form complexes that do stimulate immune responses.

INFLAMMATORY

A third category of occupational asthma resembles the IgE-mediated type, but no immune process has as yet been found with it. Hence, one can say only that it occurs because of irritation or inflammation in the lungs. A condition known as reactive airway dysfunction syndrome (RADS) is seen after exposure to high concentrations of irritant gases, such as ammonia, sulfur dioxide, or chlorine. It produces chemical pneumonitis and occasional wheezing, but should be distinguished from true occupational asthma. RADS follows a single, large exposure and the wheezing generally resolves spontaneously, although it may continue for several years.

Agents that cause irritative or inflammatory occupational asthma are listed in **6.9**. Isocyanates are active chemicals widely used in the manufacture of paints, varnishes, adhesives, and polyurethane foam. They include toluene diisocyanate (TDI), diphenylmethane diisocyanate (MDI), naphthalene diisocyanate (NDI), and hexamethylene diisocyanate (HDI). Specific IgE sensitivity occurs in only 5–10% of workers with TDI-induced asthma. There are some indications that, *in vitro*, TDI inhibits isoproterenol-stimulated cyclic AMP production. Since cyclic AMP inhibits mediator release from mast cells, the net result may be an increase in the release of mediators and consequently, asthma. Further investigations are required to clarify the pathogenesis of isocyanate-induced asthma.

SOME CAUSES OF ALLERGIC OCCUPATIONAL ASTHMA

Substance	Occupations	Substance	Occupations
High molecular weight		*Low molecular weight*	
Animal protein	Laboratory workers, veterinarians	Platinum	Jewelers, refiners
Papain	Brewers, lens workers	Trimellitic anhydride	Plastics workers, epoxy resin workers
Wheat flour	Bakers, millers	Phthalic anhydride	Plastics workers epoxy resin workers
Trypsin	Plastics workers, pharmaceutical workers		
Soybean dust	Farmers, food processors		
Vegetable gums	Printers, food workers		

6.8 High and low molecular weight substances that cause allergic occupational asthma.

SOME CAUSES OF NON-IMMUNOLOGIC (INFLAMMATORY) OCCUPATIONAL ASTHMA

Substance	Occupation
Isocyanates (TDI, MDI, NDI, HDI)	Automobile spray painters, foundry workers
Polyvinylchloride	Meat wrappers
Western Red Cedar	Sawmill workers, carpenters

6.9 Some substances that cause non-immunologic (inflammatory) occupational asthma.

Meat-wrappers asthma is associated with exposure to volatile pyrolysates that are generated when polyvinylchloride (PVC) soft-wrap film is thermally activated. Recently, it has been demonstrated that phthalic acid anhydride is among the pyrolized materials generated from thermally activated price labels.

Approximately 5% of the workers who are exposed to Western Red Cedar dust develop occupational asthma. The offending substance in Red Cedar dust appears to be plicatic acid, but only 30% of affected workers demonstrate an IgE antibody against a plicatic acid–human serum albumin conjugate. Non-immunologic factors obviously play important roles as well.

NON-SPECIFIC MEDIATOR-RELEASE

The final type of occupational asthma results from a direct histamine release that is not immunologically mediated. The best example is byssinosis, seen in the cotton, flax, and soft-hemp industries. The characteristics of byssinosis are listed in **6.10**. It is most prevalent among workers exposed to cotton in its initial processing stage, possibly because of the presence of a vegetable fiber called the bract that adheres to the cotton boll. This vegetable bract does have histamine-releasing properties *in vitro*. The symptoms of byssinosis are chest tightness, shortness of breath, coughing, and wheezing; these generally appear on the first working day of the week. On subsequent working days, as well as over the weekend, the worker is well. As the disease progresses, however, the symptoms extend into the rest of the week, ultimately becoming chronic even in the absence of exposure.

DIAGNOSIS

The standard approach to the diagnosis of occupational asthma is given in **6.11**. First, the clinician must ascertain whether the patient does, indeed, have bronchial asthma (the overall diagnosis of asthma is discussed in Chapter 5). Characteristic complaints include cough, tightness in the chest, shortness of breath, and wheezing. The diagnosis must be confirmed by spirometric testing, which demonstrates airflow obstruction. Reversibility of obstruction should also be shown after appropriate bronchodilator treatment. If there is no

FEATURES OF BYSSINOSIS

1. **People at risk**
   Cotton, flax, and soft-hemp workers engaged in carding, spinning and other dusty operations.
2. **Symptoms**
   Chest tightness, shortness of breath, coughing, and wheezing.
3. **Appearance of symptoms**
   Initially – the first work day of the week.
   Later – on subsequent work days.
   Eventually chronic symptoms in absence of exposure.

6.10 Clinical features of byssinosis.

DIAGNOSIS OF OCCUPATIONAL ASTHMA

1. **Confirm the presence of asthma**
   A. Spirometry
   B. Airway hyperresponsiveness
2. **Establish that an agent in the work place is causing asthma**
   A. History
   B. Skin and serologic tests
   C. Natural challenge
   D. Controlled bronchial challenge: non-specific, dusts, aerosol, vapors, and gases

6.11 Steps in the diagnosis of occupational asthma.

evidence of airway obstruction, it is imperative to demonstrate hyperresponsiveness by bronchoprovocation with an agent such as methacholine. This procedure is described in Chapter 3.

HISTORY AND PHYSICAL EXAMINATION

Once the diagnosis of asthma has been established, the next step is to demonstrate that the asthma is due to an occupational exposure. A detailed history must be taken of the patient's work environment. This must list not only the materials with which the patient works directly, but also other agents that are encountered in the work place. It is helpful to know if co-workers are similarly afflicted. There is generally a latent period from the first day that symptoms appear; this period can vary considerably from one month to 20 years. A tell-tale sign of occupational asthma is the improvement of symptoms over weekends, holidays, and vacations, with recurrence of symptoms upon return to the work place. The correlation of exposure with symptoms is promptly apparent. However, many substances that are encountered in the work place, particularly the low molecular weight compounds, give rise to delayed onset symptoms that may not appear until hours after exposure. Patients who work in such an environment have no symptoms during their working hours, but will complain of coughing, chest tightness, and wheezing at night.

Site visit

A site visit to the work area is of great value in terms of eliciting the exact cause of occupational allergic disease. The patient may be unaware of the substances to which he or she is exposed and may forget certain routine acts in relating their occupational history. Visiting the work site enables the physician to see the patient in action and to obtain a much more accurate picture of the types of exposure. The 1986 OHSA '*Right to Know*' Act makes it mandatory for industry to provide Material Safety Data Sheets, which give detailed information about the substances to which the workers are exposed, and the health effects of each.

SKIN AND SEROLOGIC TESTS

Following a careful history, appropriate diagnostic tests can be carried out. Skin tests or *in vitro* tests, such as the radioallergosorbent test (RAST) or enzyme-linked immunosorbent assay (ELISA), may be performed with extracts prepared from suspected substances in the work place. These tests are useful in detecting specific IgE antibody and suggest cause-and-effect relationships. Low molecular weight compounds must be attached to carrier proteins, such as human serum albumin, to perform these tests. Extracts of occupational antigens are prepared in several ways, summarized in **6.12**. First, the occupational dust is defatted by shaking it with ether and decanting the oily ether layer. The ether is allowed to evaporate and then extraction, with buffered saline and toluene, is carried out at room temperature for 72 hours with frequent agitation. Filtration is then performed through ordinary filter paper. The mixture is centrifuged and the supernatant fluid is dialyzed against a glycerinated, buffered saline–aqueous mixture for 24 hours. The solution is then concentrated by air drying in dialysis tubing. Scratch test materials eventually become approximately one-tenth of their original volume, while intradermal testing materials end up being used at their original volumes. The solution is then sterilized by filtering through millimicron filters into sterile vials.

PREPARATION OF OCCUPATIONAL ANTIGEN EXTRACTS

1. Defatting
2. Extraction
3. Filtration
4. Centrifugation
5. Dialysis
6. Concentration
7. Sterilization

6.12 Steps in the preparation of occupational allergen extracts.

PULMONARY FUNCTION STUDIES

Natural challenge

At some point, it may be helpful to obtain objective evidence that a patient's asthma is work-related. This is best done by an inhalation challenge, followed by measurements of pulmonary function. A natural challenge is performed by returning the patient to the work place and monitoring his or her symptoms and peak expiratory flow rates before and after a work shift. The changes in peak flow after one work shift are greatest when the patient has been away from work for a period of several days. Significant symptoms accompanied by changes in peak expiratory flow at work are highly suggestive that asthma is associated with the work place. However, occupational asthma cannot be excluded on the basis of negative findings from studying just one work shift. Though it is tedious and time-consuming, the worker may have to be monitored over longer periods of time with multiple recordings of peak expiratory flow rates to further test lung function. Peak expiratory flow is measured three times a day, upon waking, at work, and before bedtime, over a period of four weeks. At the same time, serial measurements of non-specific bronchial reactivity in response to methacoline or histamine are taken. A decrease in bronchial activity when away from the work place and an increase in bronchial reactivity upon return to work, together with a 20% fall in peak expiratory flow rate, is indicative of a causal relationship between the work environment and the asthma (**6.13**). Specific bronchial challenge is usually unnecessary in such cases.

Controlled laboratory challenge

A bronchial challenge, performed in a specialized laboratory with a specific suspected allergen from the work place, may be performed for several reasons. The first is to investigate previously unrecognized substances for their possible etiologic roles. The second is to separate out the offending substances from the often complex work environment. The third is to more accurately confirm the diagnosis of occupational asthma when questions of disability and liability are raised. The procedure is time-consuming and potentially dangerous, since severe asthma can be produced by excessive concentrations. Therefore, specific bronchial challenges should be performed only by trained professionals in specialized settings with resuscitation equipment. Challenges can be performed with dusts (**6.14**), nebulized aerosols, and vapors or gases.

In the case of IgE-mediated occupational agents, serial end-point skin titration should be performed with the aqueous extract. The starting inhaled dose should be the concentration that elicited a 2+ intradermal skin-test reaction.

In the case of non-IgE-mediated substances, a strong correlation has been found between the degree of non-specific bronchial

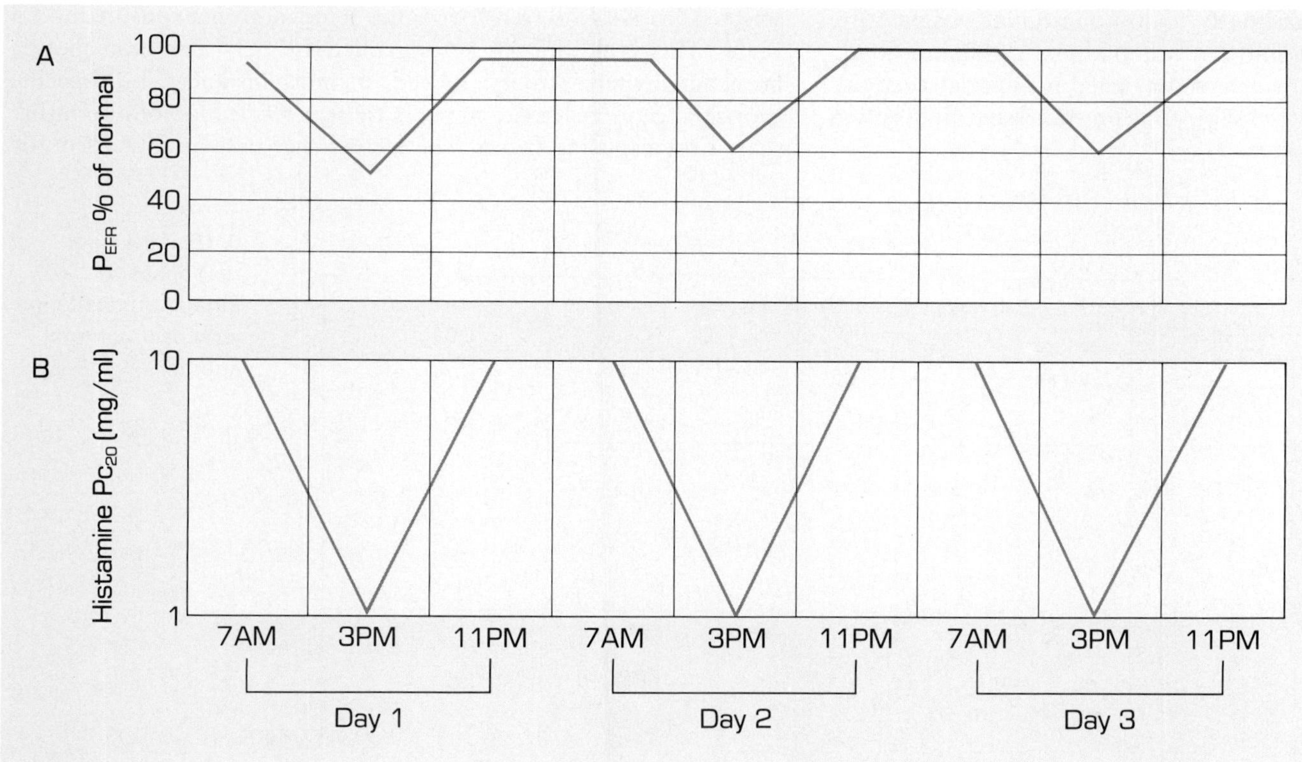

6.13 Results of a three-day monitoring of a patient with suspected occupational asthma. (A) On the initial day, the PEFR dropped by more than 20% while the patient was at work. It returned to normal that evening, and remained normal until the patient returned to work the next morning. (B) Bronchial reactivity, as measured by the response to inhaled histamine, increased at work (the amount of histamine needed to cause a 20% fall in pulmonary function decreased 10-fold). It returned to normal when the patient was away from work.

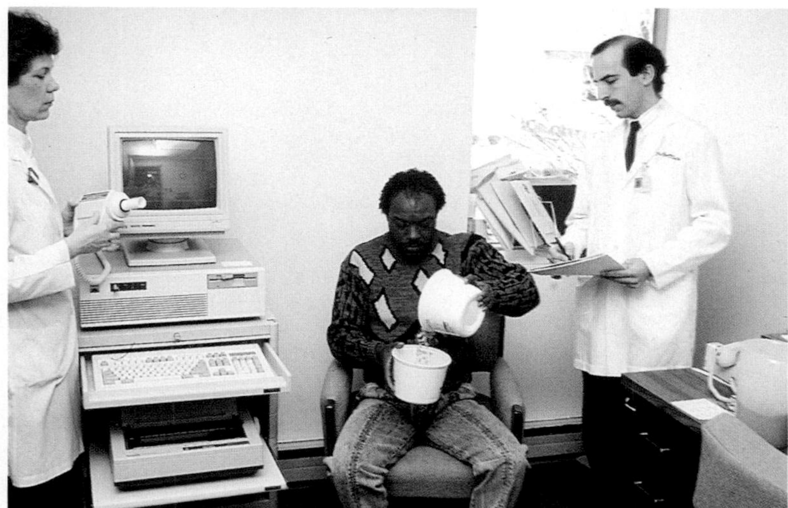

6.14 Bronchial challenge performed with dust in the laboratory setting. The patient is transferring dust from one container to another. The medical attendant is on the right and pulmonary function technician on the left.

reactivity and the initial dose of the offending agent with which to begin testing. If the response to methacholine or histamine is significant at low concentrations, the bronchial challenge should be administered with a small starting dose of the offending agent.

Airway responses to inhalation challenges with occupational agents are shown in **6.15**. They are similar to the reactions seen in challenges with naturally occurring substances, such as ragweed and mold (*see* Chapter 3), with two important differences. First, isolated late responses, particularly to low molecular weight substances, are much more common in occupational asthma. Second, there is a phenomenon of recurrent nocturnal asthmatic reactions that occur at approximately the same time on successive nights after a single exposure to an allergen.

PROGNOSIS

There have been several follow-up studies on occupational asthma, which indicate that even though the condition frequently improves, many patients with the disease do not completely recover after cessation of exposure. This has been shown to be true for the disease when it is associated with isocyanates, colophony, snowcrabs, and particularly for Western Red Cedar, in which more than 50% of affected workers fail to recover after removal from exposure for 3.5 years. This condition is accompanied by persistent non-specific bronchial hyperreactivity. Indeed, in most instances, non-specific bronchial hyperreactivity appears to be a result of exposure rather than a predisposing factor. The factors that unfavorably affect the

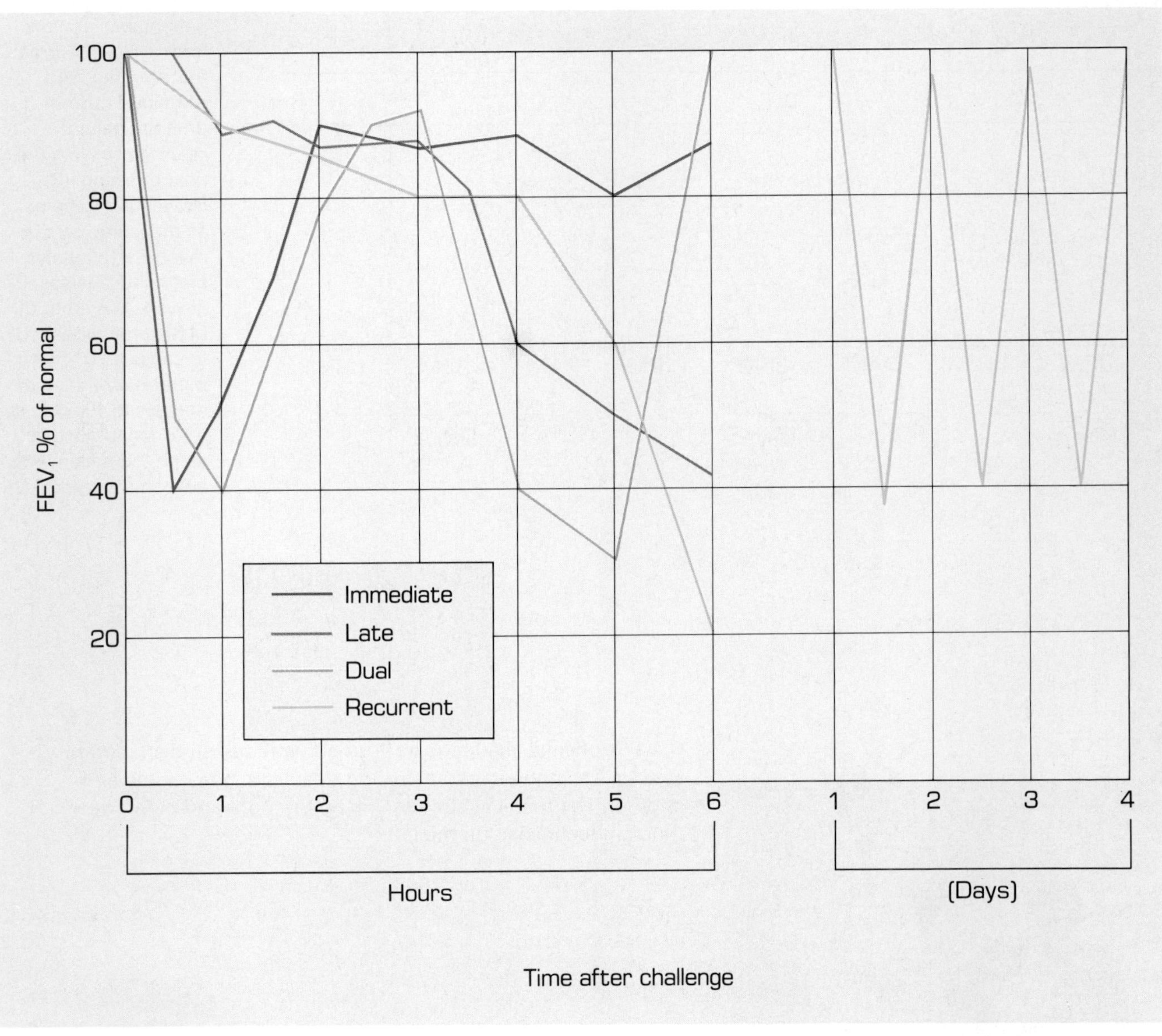

6.15 Airway responses to inhalation challenge with occupational agents.

prognosis and persistence of symptoms are given in **6.16**. The greater the length of exposure and the longer the duration of symptoms before the diagnosis is made, the worse is the prognosis and the greater the chance of persistent symptoms. The severity of asthma and the frequency of attacks also adversely affects prognosis, as do the baseline lung function measurements. Workers who demonstrate a dual bronchial response to the inhaled agent, that is, an early and late phase, and those with increased responses to inhaled methacholine or histamine, also have a worse prognosis and have an increased chance of persistent symptoms. It is evident from reviewing these factors that it is vital to diagnose occupational asthma early in its course and to remove the patient from the work environment as soon as possible.

MANAGEMENT

Occupational allergic diseases afford an opportunity to the clinician to practice preventive medicine, the most definitive approach to managing any disease.

Once the diagnosis of occupational asthma is made in a patient and the inciting agent identified, the worker's environment should be modified as much as possible (**6.17**). Improving ventilation and enclosing certain dusting operations may not only help presently affected employees, but also prevent the development of sensitivity in healthy workers. Protective devices, such as masks, respirators, gloves, and special clothing, may also be useful.

It has been suggested that screening applicants for jobs in which there is a possibility for work-place sensitization will decrease the incidence of occupational allergic disease. **6.18** indicates that this would be a very ineffective method. In this study (Platts-Mills *et al.*, 1987) on laboratory workers, rejecting the 71 out of the total of 179 workers who had positive skin tests to inhalants would have excluded only 66% of the workers who developed rhinitis and asthma on exposure to rats. Only 44% of those who developed rhinitis and asthma due to rats would have been excluded if the 41 workers with both a positive history and positive skin tests to inhalants had been rejected. In summary, many atopic people do not become allergic to rats, while a large number of rat-allergic patients were not previously atopic.

Pharmacologic treatment of occupational asthma is basically the same as that prescribed for other forms of asthma (*see* Chapter 5). This includes beta agonists, cromolyn sodium, and inhaled corticosteroids. Corticosteroids and cromolyn are particularly important in inhibiting the late-phase bronchial responses that are especially common in occupational asthma. Periodic medical surveillance should be mandated in environments where workers are exposed to agents known to cause occupational asthma. Such surveillance includes periodic skin testing, pulmonary function studies, and education of employees as to the nature of potential hazards in the work place. If all the measures, including environmental control, protection devices, and modest use of medications, are not successful, then the patient must be removed permanently from the hostile working environment.

FACTORS AFFECTING THE PROGNOSIS OF OCCUPATIONAL ASTHMA

1. Length of exposure
2. Duration of symptoms before diagnosis
3. Severity and frequency of attacks
4. Lung function
5. Dual bronchial response
6. Degree of bronchial hyperreactivity

6.16 Factors affecting the prognosis of occupational asthma.

OCCUPATIONAL ASTHMA: WHAT CAN BE DONE?

1. Environmental control – industrial hygiene
2. Protective devices
3. Medications – beta agonists, theophylline, cromolyn, corticosteroids
4. Periodic medical surveillance
5. Removal of the worker

6.17 Management of patients with occupational asthma.

ATOPY AMONG RAT-ALLERGIC LABORATORY WORKERS

	Rhinitis and asthma due to rats	Total workers
Atopic by history and skin test	8 of 18 (44%)	41 of 179
Atopic by skin test	12 of 18 (66%)	71 of 179

6.18 Prevalence of atopy among rat-allergic laboratory workers. (Adapted with permission from Platt-Mills *et al.*, 1987.)

Industry must take some responsibility for health of workers – **6.19** shows measures taken by the detergent industry which have essentially eliminated the entity of enzyme-induced asthma. Workers in particularly dusty parts of the plant were carefully instructed in the use of protective devices. An assay was developed for measuring concentrations of enzyme in the air, and periodic skin testing and pulmonary function measurements were performed. Finally, the basic manufacturing process was altered so as to encapsulate the proteolytic enzyme portion of the product.

ENVIRONMENTAL PLANT PRECAUTIONS

1. Enclosure of open operations
2. Automation of certain hand operations
3. Space suits with air supply
4. Disposable gloves and uniforms
5. Masks with cartridge and filters
6. Air monitoring
7. Spot checks of workers
8. Encapsulation of proteolytic enzymes

6.19 Precautionary measures for the prevention of occupational asthma.

OCCUPATIONAL RHINITIS

Occupational rhinitis is defined as the episodic work-related occurrence of sneezing, nasal discharge, and nasal obstruction. It often co-exists with occupational asthma. In general, nasal symptoms that follow contact with materials at work appear to parallel the time course of bronchial symptoms, and presumably result from the same sort of pathogenesis. As discussed previously, the mechanisms for occupational rhinitis are irritative, with examples being coal dust, talc, and cold air, and allergic due either to high or to low molecular weight substances.

Direct nasal challenge can be performed either naturally at the work place, or under controlled circumstances in the office or laboratory. Responses may be quantified by either symptom scores or rhinomanometry (**6.20**).

OCCUPATIONAL DERMATITIS

Occupational skin disorders are an important cause of morbidity and disability in the work place. Contact dermatitis makes up the vast majority of occupational skin disorders, with 80% being non-immunologic irritant contact dermatitis, and 20% being attributable to allergic etiologies, particularly Type IV delayed hypersensitivity (**6.21**).

SUMMARY

Occupational allergic diseases have become more common in the past decade and the incidence will probably increase as industries introduce more sensitizing agents. The primary role of the physician continues to be to insure the good health of patients and this concept should be expanded to include protecting the health of workers.

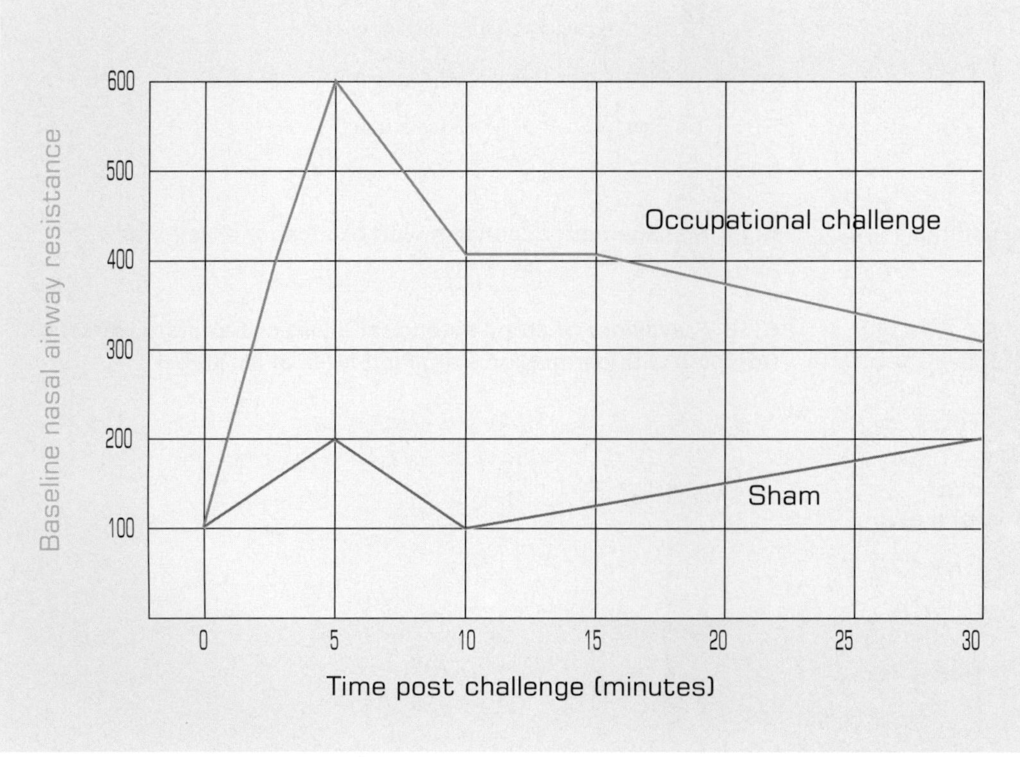

6.20 Nasal response to occupational challenge expressed as percent change from baseline.

OCCUPATIONAL ALLERGIC CONTACT DERMATITIS

Occupation	Sensitizer
Florist	Alstroemeria (Peruvian lily)
Nurse	Latex (rubber accelerators and anti-oxidants)
Cement maker	Chromate
Telephone lineman	Poison ivy (rhus)
Hairdresser	Paraphenylenediamine
Printer	Acrylics

6.21 Occupational allergic contact dermatitis.

REFERENCES

Chan-Yeung M, Lam S: Occupational asthma. *Amer Rev Resp Dis*, **133**:686, 1986.

Chan-Yeung M, Malo JL: Natural history of occupational asthma, in Chan-Yeung M, Malo JL, Bernstein DI (eds): *Asthma in the Workplace*, B.C. Dekker, Chapter 14, 1993.

Lopez M, Salvaggio JE: Diagnostic methods in occupational allergic lung disease. *Clin Rev Allergy*, **4**:289, 1986.

Newman-Taylor AJ: Occupational asthma. *Thorax*, **35**:241, 1980.

Platts-Mills TAE *et al.*: Occupational asthma and rhinitis related to laboratory rats; serum IgG and IgE antibodies to the rat urinary allergen. *J Allergy Clin Immunol*, 75:505, 1987.

Paterson BF, Patterson R, Grammer LC: Pathogenesis of occupational lung disease. *Clin Rev Allergy*, **4**:303, 1986.

Slavin RG: Asthma in adults III: Occupational asthma. *Hosp Pract*, **13**:133, 1978.

Terr AI: The atopic worker. *Clin Rev Allergy*, **4**:267, 1986.

CHAPTER 7

Hypersensitivity Pneumonitis

Raymond G. Slavin

The ready access to potent antigens, and the presence of large numbers of immunocompetent cells, including sensitized lymphocytes, macrophages, neutrophils, eosinophils, plasma cells, and mediator substances, all contribute to make the lung an important immunologic shock organ (**7.1**). In addition to these categories, some immunologic diseases, such as hypersensitivity pneumonitis, may represent a combination of immunologic responses.

While the present era of interest in hypersensitivity lung disease began more than 50 years ago, with the first description of Farmer's lung, a great deal of study and an increased awareness of hypersensitivity pneumonitis has been prompted recently by the availability of new immunologic techniques. These have aided, not only in the diagnosis, but also in a better definition of the pathogenesis.

Synonyms for hypersensitivity pneumonitis include pulmonary hypersensitivity syndrome and extrinsic allergic alveolitis. The latter term is perhaps the best and most descriptive. 'Extrinsic' refers to an exogenous antigen or allergen. 'Allergic' indicates that the disease has a hypersensitivity basis. 'Alveolitis' refers to that part of the lung that is most affected by this disease process. Whichever term is used, we are referring to the same underlying pathogenic entity – namely, a condition caused by sensitivity to organic dust inhalation.

EPIDEMIOLOGY

Several factors determine the nature of an individuals response to inhalation of organic dust (**7.2**). First is the basic immunologic reactivity of the host. An atopic or allergic individual typically responds to organic dust inhalation with the production of an IgE skin-sensitizing antibody. A non-allergic or non-atopic individual tends to respond to organic dust inhalation with the production of a precipitating antibody.

A second factor influencing the response is the nature and source of the antigen. Perhaps the most important is the particle size of the dust. The optimal size for penetration of the alveoli is 4–6 microns (μm). Particles larger than 10 μm are trapped in the upper airway and unable to reach the alveoli in amounts sufficient to cause injury.

A third factor determining the response to organic dust is the nature and circumstance of the exposure. An intense but intermittent exposure results in a clinical picture different from that of a less intense exposure of longer duration. A good example of this is the response to avian antigens. Intermittent, heavy exposure of short duration, such as experienced by a pigeon fancier who cleans out his coops twice a week, produces an acute form of hypersensitivity pneumonitis that is usually reversible. However, a part-time employee in a pet store may have more continuous exposure of relatively shorter duration, which results in a subacute, insidious form that is also usually reversible. Long-term exposure, such as experienced by an elderly house-bound woman, with two parakeets, may result in chronic, irreversible disease (**7.3**).

RESPONSIBLE ANTIGENS

A variety of antigens may result in hypersensitivity pneumonitis. As our awareness of the disease process increases and other forms of environmental exposure develop, the list continues to expand. **7.4** lists the general categories of antigens with examples of each.

THE LUNG AS AN IMMUNOLOGIC SHOCK ORGAN

Gell and Coombs classification	Immunologic characteristic	Pulmonary manifestation
Type I	IgE-mediated	Allergic bronchial asthma
Type II	Autoimmune, cytotoxic	Goodpasture's syndrome
Type III	Immune complex, precipitating antibody	Polyarteritis
Type IV	Lymphocyte, cell-mediated	Tuberculosis

7.1 The lung as an immunologic shock organ.

CLINICAL PRESENTATION

The clinical manifestations of hypersensitivity pneumonitis are essentially the same regardless of the offending antigen, but may vary depending on the intensity and frequency of exposure. 7.5 contrasts the features of the three forms of hypersensitivity pneumonitis defined in 7.3 (Stankus, 1988).

In the acute form associated with intermittent, intense antigen exposure, the main symptoms are fever, chills, cough, dyspnea, headache, body aches, and malaise, appearing 4–6 hours after organic dust inhalation. Remission of symptoms follows 12–18 hours later in the absence of further exposure.

Intermittent but longer term exposure results in the subacute form of hypersensitivity pneumonitis marked by progressively increasing fatigue, dyspnea, weight loss, and productive cough. Râles become more widespread.

In the chronic form caused by prolonged organic dust exposure, the symptoms seen in the subacute form progress resulting in pulmonary fibrosis and respiratory failure.

FACTORS DETERMINING RESPONSE TO ORGANIC DUST INHALATION

1. **Immunologic reactivity of host**

   Atopic, non-atopic

2. **Nature and source of antigen**

   Particle size, growth in airway

3. **Nature and circumstances of exposure**

   Intense and intermittent versus low-grade; chronic

7.2 Factors determining response to organic dust inhalation.

NATURE OF DISEASE RELATED TO EXPOSURE

Exposure	Example	Disease
Intermittent, short-term	Pigeon breeder	Acute – reversible
Intermittent, long-term	Pet store employee	Subacute – usually reversible
Long-term	Parakeet owner	Chronic – irreversible

7.3 Nature of disease with respect to type of exposure.

ANTIGENS RESPONSIBLE FOR HYPERSENSITIVITY PNEUMONITIS

Category of antigen	Disease
Thermophilic organisms	
Micropolyspora faeni	Farmer's lung
Thermoactinomyces sacchari	Bagassosis
Mold	
Aspergillus clavatus	Malt worker's lung
Penicillium roqueforti	Cheese worker's lung
Animal	
Bird protein	Pigeon breeder's lung
Gerbil protein	Gerbil keeper's lung
Amoeba (*Naegleria gruberi*)	Humidifier lung
Chemical	
Toluene diisocyanate	Bathtub finisher's lung

7.4 Antigens responsible for hypersensitivity pneumonitis.

TESTS

Radiographic findings

Chest radiographic findings may vary depending on the type or disease. The acute form of hypersensitivity pneumonitis is associated with bilateral, diffuse, finely granular infiltrates, characteristic of alveolar or interstitial pneumonitis. There is generally apical sparing (7.6). In addition, micronodular densities may appear on the radiograph with a patchy distribution (7.7). In the chronic form of hypersensitivity pneumonitis, the infiltrates become confluent and diffuse, interstitial fibrosis appears. As the disease advances, chest films show a progressive loss of volume that is associated with cardiac enlargement (7.8).

Pulmonary function studies

Pulmonary function studies in acute hypersensitivity pneumonitis reveal a restrictive type of ventilatory impairment associated with low vital capacity and low arterial oxygen saturation that falls further with exercise. In the subacute and chronic forms, obstructive defects are observed also.

CLINICAL PRESENTATION OF HYPERSENSITIVITY PNEUMONITIS

Features	Acute	Subacute	Chronic
Chills and fever	+		
Dyspnea	+	+	+
Cough	Non-productive	Productive	Productive
Malaise and myalagia	+	+	+
Weight loss		+	+
Râles	Bibasilar	Widespread	Widespread
Chest radiograph	Nodular infiltrates	Nodular infiltrates	Pulmonary fibrosis
Precipitins	+	+	+
Pulmonary function	Restrictive	Restrictive and obstructive	Restrictive and obstructive
Reversible	Yes	Yes	No

7.5 Clinical presentation of hypersensitivity pneumonitis.

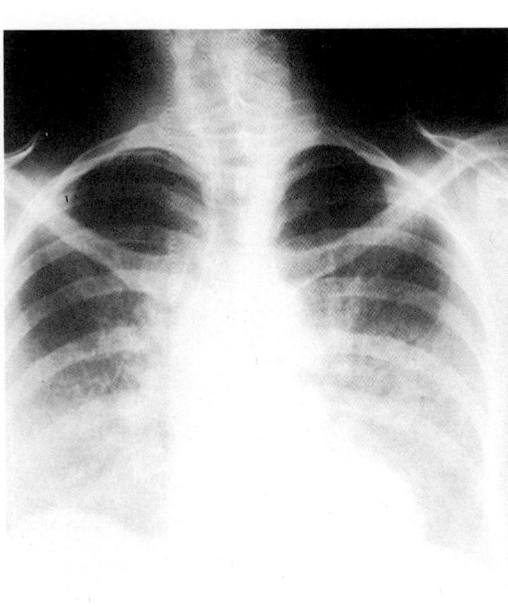

7.6 Chest radiograph showing diffuse, bilateral, finely granular infiltrates characteristic of alveolar or interstitial pneumonitis. Note the sparing of upper lung fields.

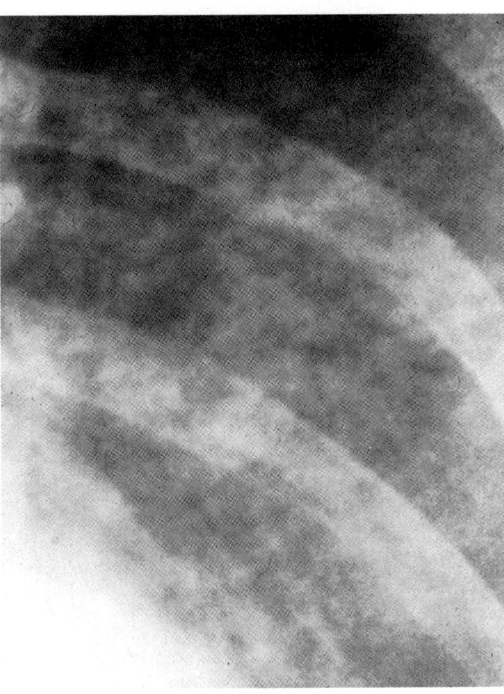

7.7 Magnified view of chest radiograph demonstrating patchy micronodular densities.

Bronchoprovocation tests

Bronchoprovocation tests may be helpful when the specific diagnosis is in doubt because of the relevance of the particular exposure. Under carefully controlled conditions, an aqueous extract of the antigen in question is delivered to the bronchi. A positive result is identified by temperature elevation, chills, cough, dyspnea, leukocytosis, and changes in pulmonary function after 4–6 hours (**7.9**). Provocative bronchial challenges should not be performed on a routine basis and must be used with great caution because of their possible severe systemic effects, including cough, fever, and dyspnea.

PATHOLOGIC PICTURE

The findings of hypersensitivity pneumonitis upon performance of a lung biopsy vary, depending on the stage of the disease. Initially, there is patchy interstitial and peribronchial inflammation with a predominance of lymphocytes and plasma cells (**7.10** and **7.11**). Frequently, macrophages with foamy cytoplasm and giant cells are seen (**7.12**). In the subacute stage, non-caseating granulomas, which progress in the chronic stage to interstitial fibrosis, appear (**7.13**).

PATHOGENESIS

Serum-precipitating antibody directed against the offending antigen is considered an immunologic hallmark of hypersensitivity pneumonitis (**7.14**). It was believed for some time that the Type III immune response marked by the presence of immune complexes played a major role in the pathogenesis of hypersensitivity pneumonitis. A good deal of evidence, as presented in **7.15**, disputes this. Precipitating antibody is generally seen in hypersensitivity pneumonitis, but is certainly not pathognomonic of the disease since as many as 50% of exposed but asymptomatic individuals have titers as high as symptomatic individuals. Experimental models of hypersensitivity pneumonitis have been created in the guinea pig, rabbit, mouse, and monkey. After immunization, which results in production of serum-precipitating antibody alone, transfer of serum to unaffected animals followed by an appropriate inhalation challenge does not result in disease production. When hypersensitivity pneumonitis patients are challenged with antigen inhalation, serum complement does not decrease, and finally, vasculitis is not ordinarily seen upon lung biopsy of hypersensitivity pneumonitis,

It now appears that cellular immune responses constitute the primary mechanism for lung injury seen in hypersensitivity pneumonitis. **7.16** summarizes the evidence for the vital contribution of Type IV immune response. In a rabbit model of hypersensitivity pneumonitis, acute disease is better correlated with immunization procedures favoring cell-mediated hypersensitivity than with the presence of serum-precipitating antibody. Pigeon breeders with symptomatic disease demonstrate *in vitro* proliferation of lymphocytes and production of macrophage-migration inhibition factor in response to pigeon antigen, in contrast to asymptomatic breeders with precipitins who show no such reactivity. As previously noted, the lung biopsies of patients with hypersensitivity pneumonitis shows large numbers of lymphocytes and non-caseating granulomas, both of which are compatible with a cell-mediated immune

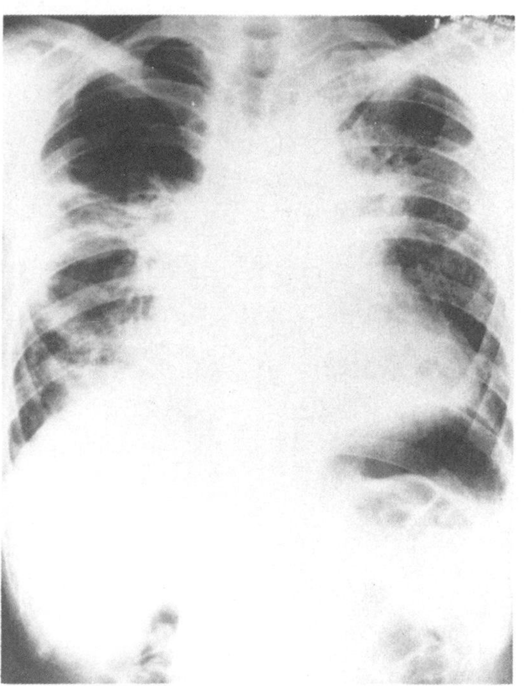

7.8 Chest radiograph of chronic bagassosis, showing extensive fibrosis and bullous emphysema. (Courtesy of Dr John Salvaggio, Tulane University School of Medicine.)

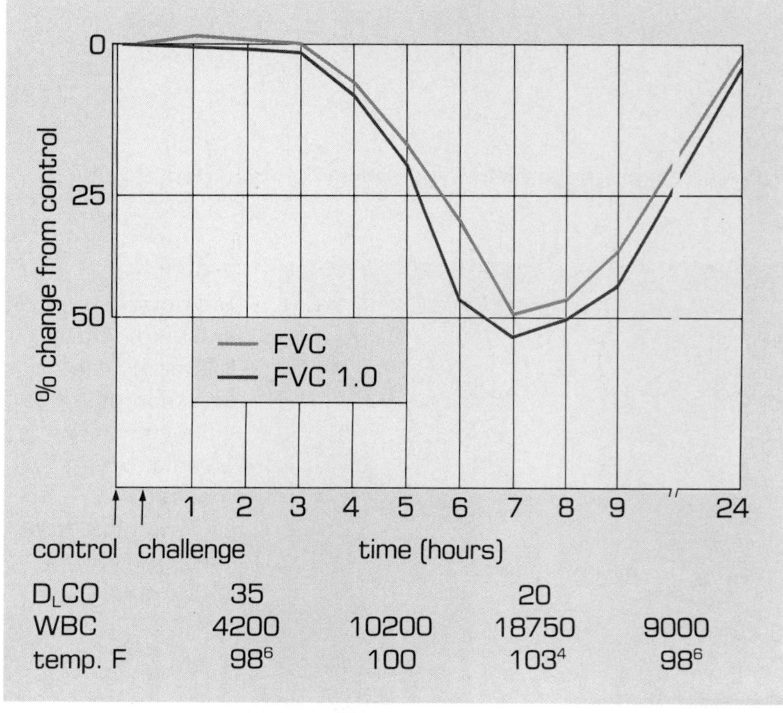

7.9 Bronchial challenge results from aqueous extract inhalation in a case of hypersensitivity pneumonitis. (Reproduced with permission from Fink, 1993.)

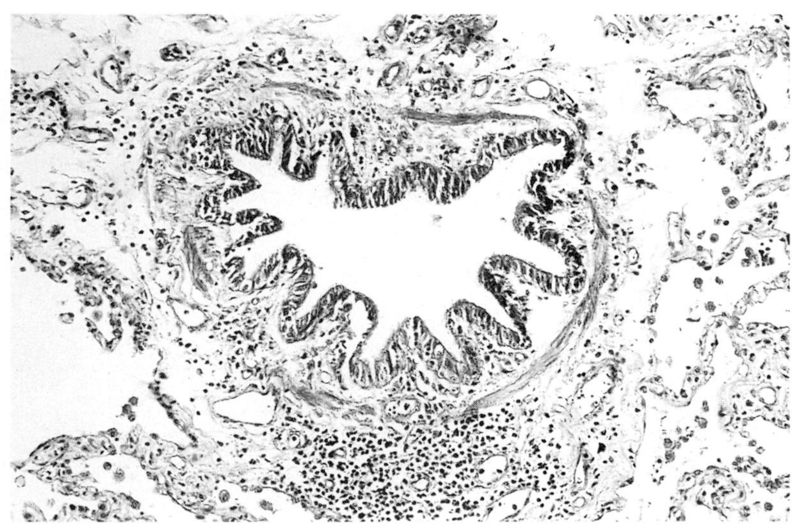

7.10 Peribronchial infiltration of lymphocytes and plasma cells. (Courtesy of Dr Carlos Bedrossian, St. Louis University School of Medicine.)

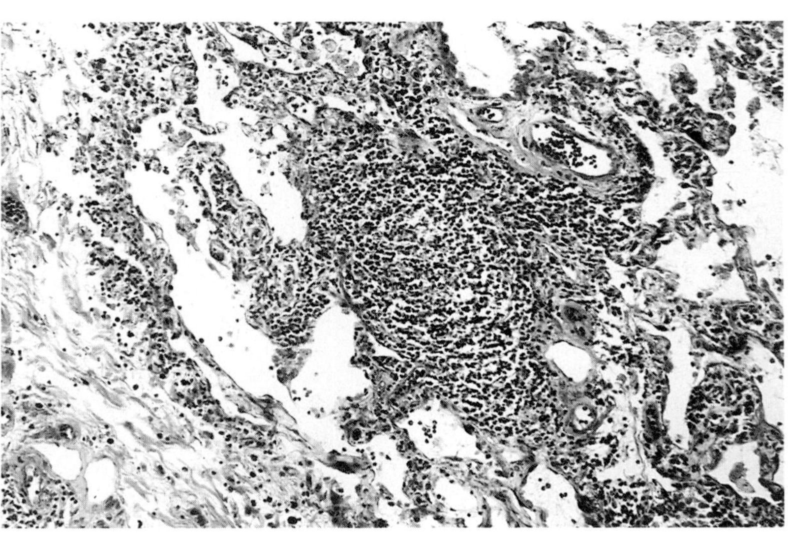

7.11 Interstitial infiltrate of lymphocytes and plasma cells around distal air spaces. (Courtesy of Dr Carlos Bedrossian, St. Louis University School of Medicine.)

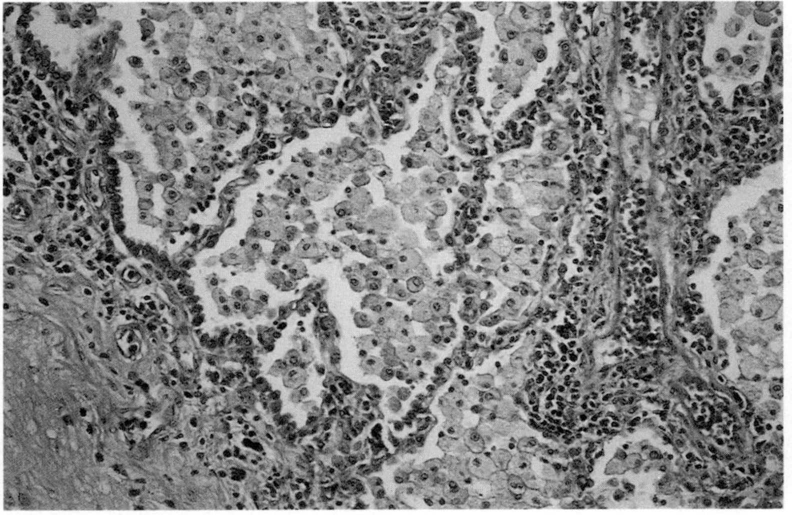

7.12 Lymphocytic and plasma cell infiltration of alveolar walls. The alveoli are filled with foamy macrophages. (Courtesy of Dr Carlos Bedrossian, St. Louis University School of Medicine.)

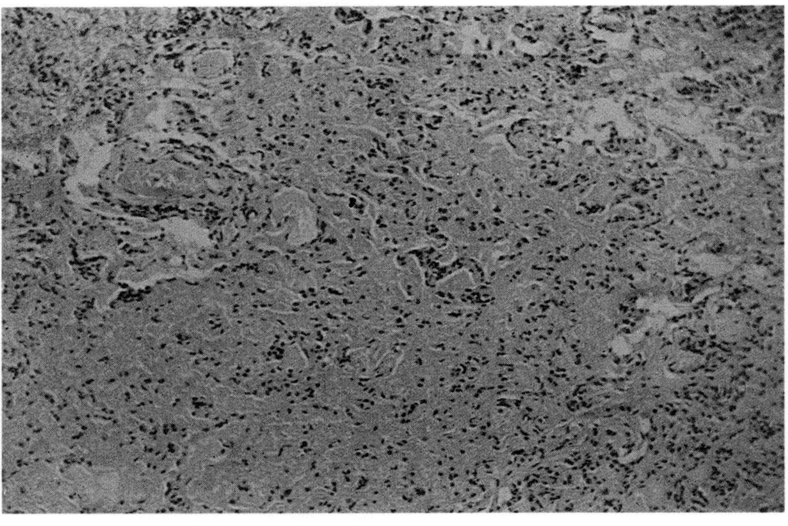

7.13 End stage of hypersensitivity pneumonitis, showing dense fibrosis.

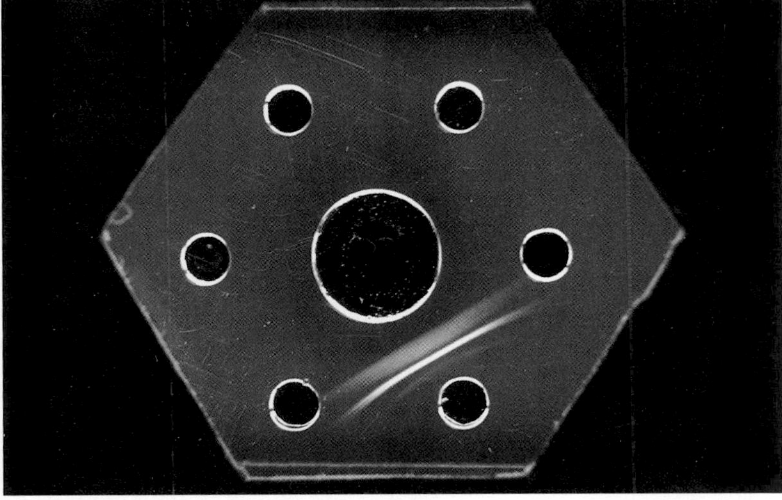

7.14 Double gel diffusion plate showing positive precipitin bands between patient serum (center well) and pigeon serum. Two other hypersensitivity pneumonitis antigens are negative.

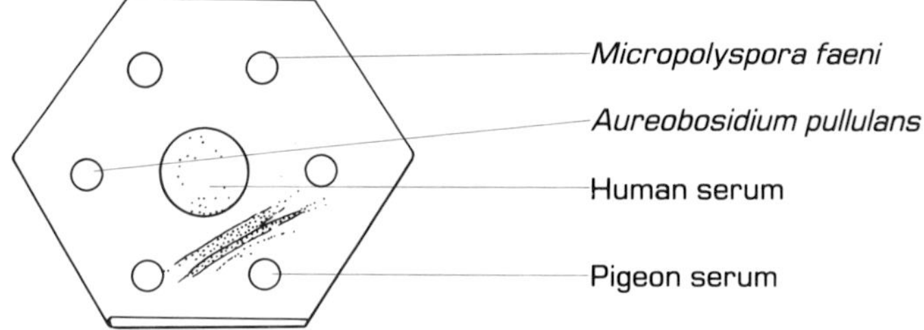

response. Finally, bronchoalveolar lavage fluid from patients with chronic hypersensitivity pneumonitis contains large numbers of lymphocytes, the majority of which are T-lymphocytes. Further analysis reveals that the predominant T-cell subset is the T8 positive or T-suppressor cell. Lavage fluid also contains significantly increased levels of total protein, IgG and IgM. C_4 and C_6 levels in lavage fluid are similar to controls, indicating that there is no direct evidence of local, complement-mediated reactions.

One recent study has shown a marked increase, on the order of 1000-fold, in numbers of mast cells in lavage fluid of hypersensitivity pneumonitis. The investigators suggest that mast cell degranulation is important in regulating the number of immune and inflammatory cells in the lung, and that a late-phase reaction initiated by antigen-induced mast cell degranulation may be important in the pathogenesis of hypersensitivity pneumonitis.

7.17 depicts the suggested pathogenesis of hypersensitivity

EVIDENCE AGAINST TYPE III AS THE MOST IMPORTANT IMMUNE RESPONSE IN HYPERSENSITIVITY PNEUMONITIS

1. Precipitating antibody is present in 50% of exposed but asymptomatic individuals.
2. Serum alone cannot transfer disease from affected to unaffected experimental animals.
3. Serum complement does not decrease when hypersensitivity pneumonitis patients are given inhalation challenge with antigen.
4. Vasculitis is not seen on lung biopsy.

7.15 Evidence against Type III as the most important immune response in hypersensitivity pneumonitis.

EVIDENCE FOR TYPE IV AS THE MOST IMPORTANT IMMUNE RESPONSE IN HYPERSENSITIVITY PNEUMONITIS

1. In experimental animals, development of hypersensitivity pneumonitis is better correlated with cell-mediated immunity.
2. *In vitro* lymphocyte proliferation to antigen.
3. *In vitro* production of macrophage-migration inhibitor factor.
4. Large numbers of lymphocytes and non-caseating granulomas seen on lung biopsy.
5. Bronchoalveolar lavage fluid shows large numbers of lymphocytes with activated T-suppressor cells being predominant.

7.16 Evidence for Type IV as the most important immune response in hypersensitivity pneumonitis.

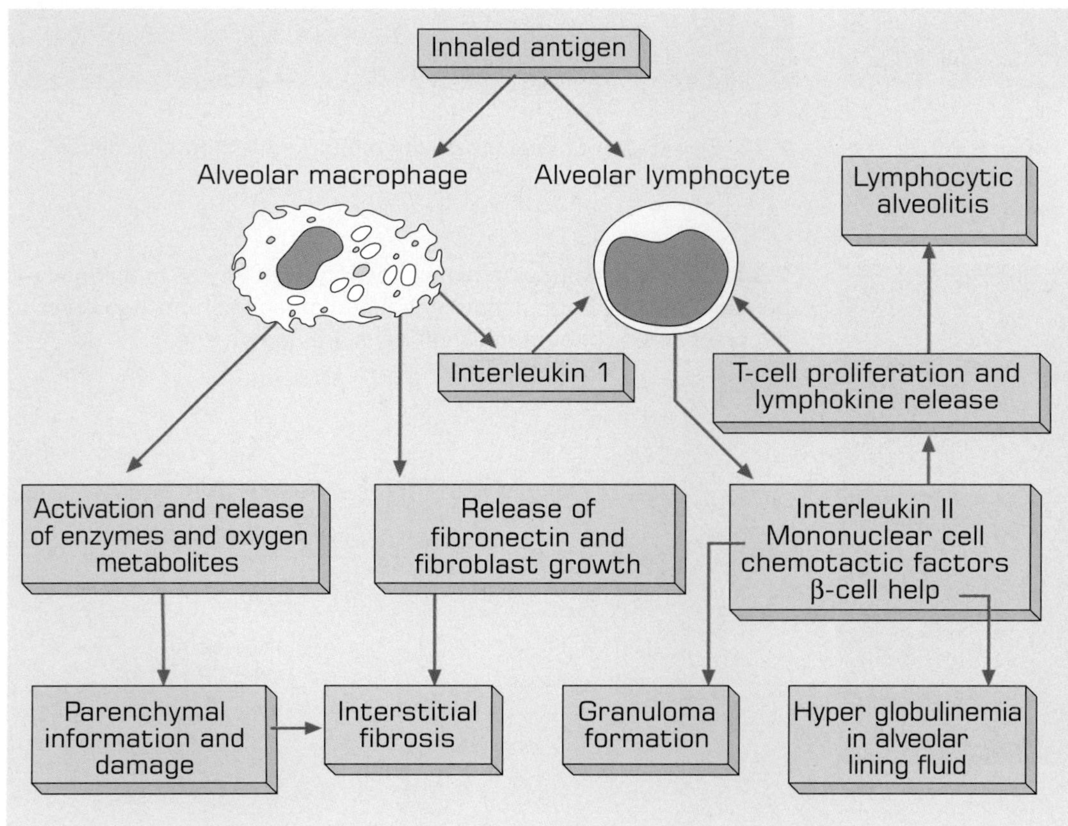

7.17 Suggested pathogenesis of hypersensitivity pneumonitis. (Reproduced with permission from Stankus, 1988.)

pneumonitis. It combines a non-immunologic pathway (macrophage activation resulting in a release of enzymes, oxygen metabolites, fibronectin, and fibroblast growth factor) with an immunologic pathway (interleukins resulting in T-cell proliferation and lymphokine release).

DIAGNOSIS OF HYPERSENSITIVITY PNEUMONITIS

1. Recurrent pneumonitis, interstitial pneumonitis, or pulmonary fibrosis.
2. Onset of signs and symptoms 4–6 hours after exposure with remission on avoidance.
3. Typical chest radiograph finding.
4. Pulmonary function test showing restrictive pattern.
5. Serum-precipitating antibody.
6. Bronchial challenge.
7. Bronchoalveolar lavage.
8. Lung biopsy.

7.18 Diagnosis of hypersensitivity pneumonitis.

DIAGNOSIS

The diagnosis of hypersensitivity pneumonitis is summarized in **7.18**. The diagnostic index of suspicion should be kept high and the disease should be strongly suspected in any case of recurrent pneumonitis, interstitial pneumonitis, or pulmonary fibrosis. A careful history should elicit the signs and symptoms of the disease in association with exposure and remission on avoidance. A chest radiograph taken at the acute stage shows diffuse, finely granular infiltrates confined to the lower lung field (*see* **7.6**). A restrictive pattern is seen on pulmonary function testing, as are serum precipitins against the offending antigen. The history, chest radiograph, pulmonary function testing, and serum precipitin should offer presumptive evidence of hypersensitivity pneumonitis. Only in unusual circumstances does one have to resort to bronchial challenge, bronchoalveolar lavage, or lung biopsy.

DIFFERENTIAL DIAGNOSIS

A number of pulmonary illnesses must be ruled out when considering the diagnosis of hypersensitivity pneumonitis. A disease which is often confused in the clinician's mind with hypersensitivity pneumonitis is allergic bronchopulmonary aspergillosis. **7.19** summarizes the rather clear distinction between these two entities. Sarcoidosis is an interstitial lung disease that may be confused with hypersensitivity pneumonitis. One distinguishing characteristic is seen on bronchoalveolar lavage. As already stated, the lavage of hypersensitivity pneumonitis shows a preponderance of T8 positive suppressor lymphocytes. Lavage of sarcoidosis patients reveals a preponderance of T4 positive helper cells.

DIFFERENTIAL CHARACTERISTICS OF EXTRINSIC ALLERGIC ALVEOLITIS (HYPERSENSITIVITY PNEUMONITIS) AND ALLERGIC BRONCHOPULMONARY ASPERGILLOSIS

	Extrinsic allergic alveolitis	Allergic bronchopulmonary aspergillosis
Basic nature of patient	Non-atopic	Atopic
Physical examination	±	Wheezing
Skin test	±[a]	Dual positivity
Radiography	Pulmonary infiltrates (interstitial)	Pulmonary infiltrates (lobar)
Complications	Pulmonary fibrosis	Atelectasis, bronchiectasis
Blood count	Normal or leukocytosis	Eosinophilia
Sputum	Normal	Eosinophilia, mycelia
IgE	Normal	Elevated
Pulmonary function	Restrictive	Obstructive (restrictive late in course)
Antibody	Precipitating (IgG)	Precipitating (IgG) and non-precipitating (IgE)
Proposed immunologic basis	Immune complexes and delayed hypersensitivity (Types III and IV)	Immediate hypersensitivity and immune complexes (Types III and IV)

[a]Positive reaction is immediate and late in some patients with pigeon breeder's lung.

7.19 Differential characteristics of extrinsic allergic alveolitis (hypersensitivity pneumonitis) and allergic bronchopulmonary aspergillosis. (Reproduced with permission from Slavin, 1983.)

PREVENTION AND TREATMENT

Clearly, the most important aspect in the management of hypersensitivity pneumonitis is recognition and avoidance of the causative antigen. Once the disease is suspected, a careful environmental survey of the patient's occupational, home, and vocational life must be carried out to search for the presence of offending antigens. When the disease is diagnosed and the antigens recognized the definitive therapy is early avoidance. Hypersensitivity pneumonitis may be an ultimately fatal disease due to progressive respiratory insufficiency. A general approach to the prevention of hypersensitivity pneumonitis is given in 7.20. A number of interventions decrease the formation of antigens in conducive environments. For example, the growth of thermophilic actinomycete spores in compost can be suppressed by treatment with a 1% solution of propionic acid. Water that remains for long periods of time in older air conditioning or humidification units may become a fertile source for the growth of thermophilic organisms. Therefore, the water needs to be changed and the unit cleaned on a regular basis. Contaminated ventilation systems have to be thoroughly cleaned and replaced. Blowing cool air through stored hay helps to prevent the growth of mold. Harvesting crops when the moisture content is low also results in less exposure to organic dusts.

In occupational situations where organic-dust generation is inevitable, every effort should be made to reduce the worker's exposure. In enclosed spaces, extremely dusty materials should be handled mechanically. Materials such as sugar cane should be stored outside and cattle fed outside as much as possible, so that the associated organic dusts can be diluted by the ambient air.

In terms of removal of dusts from the air, improved ventilation may aid considerably. Electrostatic air purifiers may be of help in instances where the concentration of dust is not too great. The use of personal dust respirators or masks is limited because of their inconvenience. A Type IIB filter is quite effective in filtering small particles, but causes so much resistance to the flow of air that people hard at work are unable to wear it. An airstream helmet in which an electrical pump blows air through a filter and into the breathing zone is heavy and uncomfortable to wear. Even the best device only has a maximum filtering capacity of 99% for fine particles. The remaining 1% can produce new attacks in highly sensitive individuals. When the disease is not yet manifest, even a filter with 95% filtering capacity is adequate. Good results have been reported with a 3M disposable mask. Model 8719 (**7.21**). When the above environmental control measures cannot be carried out or are inadequate, the patient should be removed from that work area. This may entail a change in the work place or type of work or, in extreme cases, a change in occupation. It is not known how long or what level of exposure is required to produce irreversible pulmonary changes. It would be fair to say that if the diffusing capacity has not returned to normal within 3 months, the individual should be advised to leave that particular work place.

The treatment of hypersensitivity pneumonitis is summarized in **7.22**. In many cases, no treatment is necessary other than avoidance of the causative antigen. Corticosteroid therapy can, however, greatly accelerate the clinical improvement and should be considered for very ill patients with gross radiographic or physiologic abnormalities, such as hypoxemia. Oral prednisone in an initial daily dose of 40–60 mg is usually adequate and should be continued until there is significant improvement in clinical, radiographic, and pulmonary function tests. Prednisone may then be slowly tapered until the resolution of clinical and radiologic signs is complete. The total duration of therapy is generally no more than 4–6 weeks, providing exposure to the antigen is prevented. It must be emphasized and re-emphasized to the patient that corticosteroids are not a substitute for antigen identification and avoidance.

In cases of severe hypoxemia in the acute stage, oxygen should be administered in amounts sufficient to keep the partial pressure of oxygen (PaO_2) between 60–100 mm Hg. Other supportive measures include antitussives and antipyretics. On occasion, despite the physician's best efforts, the patient may elect to return to the same work place or occupation. In these instances, long-term continuous administration of corticosteroids may be called for. One should

PREVENTION OF HYPERSENSITIVITY PNEUMONITIS

1. **Decrease formation of antigens**
   — Add chemicals to prevent growth.
   — Change water frequently in humidification or air-conditioning units.
   — Use storage dryers on hay and straw.
   — Harvest crops when moisture content is low.
2. **Decrease exposure to organic dust**
   — Mechanically handle dusty materials within closed spaces.
   — Remove dusts from ambient air.
   — Wear personal respirators or masks.
3. **Remove worker from disease-producing environment**

7.20 Prevention of hypersensitivity pneumonitis. (Reproduced with permission from Terho, 1982.)

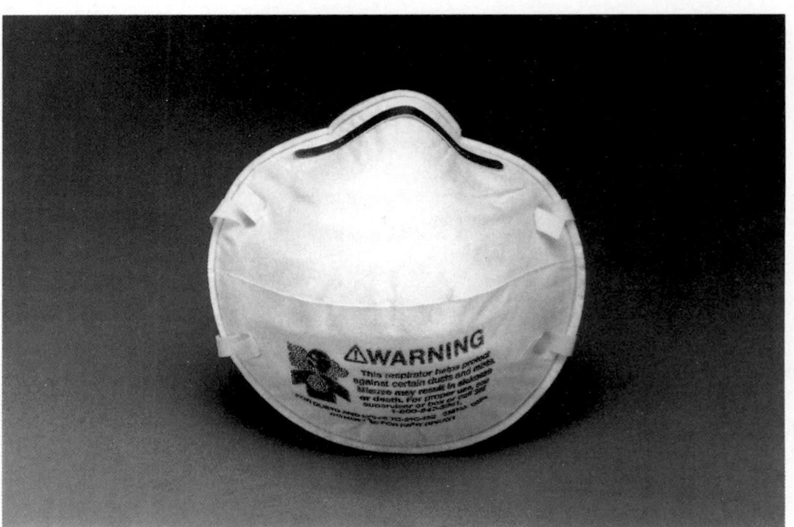

7.21 A 3M disposable mask. Model 8710, found to be useful in prevention of hypersensitivity pneumonitis. (Courtesy of 3M Center, St. Paul, MN.)

strive for an alternate-day program utilizing the lowest dose that still controls the patient's symptoms. The chronic form of hypersensitivity pneumonitis develops insidiously and occurs either after repeated acute episodes or as a result of long-term, low-grade exposure. A therapeutic trial of steroids can be given, but should be continued only if the radiographic findings and the physiologic testing indicate a beneficial response.

TREATMENT OF HYPERSENSITIVITY PNEUMONITIS

Acute form
— Remove patient from exposure - may entail hospitalization.
— Administer oxygen.
— Prescribe oral prednisone 40–60 mg/day with slow taper.
— Use supportive measures - rest, antitussives, antipyretics.

Repeated acute or subacute form
— Decrease exposure as much as possible.
— Administer long-term corticosteroids emphasizing alternate-day therapy.

Chronic form
— Trial with corticosteroids but continue only if radiographic findings and physiologic testing indicate a response.

7.22 Treatment of hypersensitivity pneumonitis. (Reproduced with permission from Slavin, 1988.)

REFERENCES

Fink JN: Hypersensitivity pneumonitis, in Middleton E Jr, Reed CE, Ellis EF, Adkinson NF Jr, Yunginger JW (eds): *Allergy: Principles and Practice*, C.V. Mosby, St Louis, 1993.

Slavin RG: Allergic bronchopulmonary aspergillosis, in Middleton E Jr, Reed CE, Ellis EF (eds): *Allergy: Principles and Practice*, C.V. Mosby, St Louis, Chapter 49, 1983.

Slavin RG: Hypersensitivity pneumonitis, in Lichtenstein LM, Fauci AS (eds): *Current Therapy in Allergy, Immunology and Rheumatology*, C.V. Mosby, St Louis, 1988.

Stankus RP, DeShazo RD: Hypersensitivity pneumonitis, in Schwartz MI, King TE, Jr (eds): *Interstitial Lung Disease*, B.C. Decker, 1988.

Terho EO: Extrinsic allergic alveolitis: management of established cases. *Eur J Resp Dis*, **123**:101, 1982.

CHAPTER 8

Allergic Bronchopulmonary Aspergillosis

Raymond G. Slavin

Allergic bronchopulmonary aspergillosis (ABPA) is a hypersensitivity response in the lung to the genus of mold *Aspergillus*. *Aspergillus* is a hardy and ubiquitous organism that thrives on a substrate with low moisture content. It has been identified in such diverse areas as fertile soil, air, decaying vegetation, swimming pool water, and flour. In addition it is one of the most commonly cultured molds from houses and is particularly prevalent in basements, crawl spaces, bedding, and housedust. *Aspergillus fumigatus* is the most common species of this mold affected man and while the respiratory tract is the most frequent site of infection, other tissues may also be involved, such as the sinuses, bones, skin, and meninges.

The five types of lung disease that are caused by *Aspergillus* are seen in **8.1**. The conditions are varied and illustrate how the same organism can elicit different clinical responses, depending on the degree of exposure and the nature of the host.

Disseminated or invasive aspergillosis is seen in individuals with an immune response that has been compromised, either naturally, through the development of an underlying primary disease such as leukemia, or iatrogenically, through immunosuppressive drugs taken to prevent homograft rejections. It is associated with invasion of the bronchial wall resulting in a definite bronchitis, and is often accompanied by pneumonia, mycotic abscesses, and systemic spread.

Aspergilloma or mycetoma is the most common form of aspergillosis and consists of superficial invasion of an anatomic abnormality such as a bronchogenic cyst or a bronchiectatic cavity.

Bronchial asthma may result from an IgE-mediated response to *Aspergillus* much like the allergic response to other molds or pollen.

Extrinsic allergic alveolitis or hypersensitivity pneumonitis may present as so-called Malt worker's lung due to a sensitivity to *Aspergillus clavatus* growing in the moldy barley on the floors of breweries. Allergic alveolitis is discussed in detail in Chapter 7 of this atlas.

Allergic bronchopulmonary aspergillosis is a condition first described in 1952 and characterized by pulmonary eosinophilia associated with pulmonary infiltrates, and eosinophilia both in peripheral blood and sputum (Hinson, 1952).

CLINICAL CHARACTERISTICS OF ABPA

The diagnostic criteria for ABPA are seen in **8.2**. The presence of seven major criteria makes the diagnosis highly likely with all eight making it a certainty.

MAJOR CRITERIA

Symptoms

Patients with allergic aspergillosis are almost always atopic and have a history of bronchial asthma. A good clinical clue to the diagnosis is an asthmatic who has been under good control but who then develops worsening asthma that is often steroid dependent with recurrent pulmonary infiltrates. Patients often complain of anorexia, headache, general aches and pains, loss of energy, and temperature elevation. The disease tends to affect the younger age group, with most cases occurring in patients under the age of 40. Most often, no clear relationship can be established between a history of exposure to moldy vegetative matter and the onset of symptoms. In the majority of patients there are general signs of airway obstruction with crepitant rales localized over areas of pulmonary infiltration.

Skin tests

Peripheral eosinophil levels are generally over $1000/mm^3$ and levels greater than $3000/mm^3$ are not unusual. A positive wheal and erythema reaction to an *Aspergillus* skin test is a necessary finding in ABPA (**8.3**). A negative skin test, for all intents and purposes, rules out the diagnosis. On the other hand, a positive skin test indicates only the presence of IgE antibody to *Aspergillus* and is not absolutely diagnostic of allergic aspergillosis. Twenty-five percent of bronchial asthmatics are skin-test positive to *Aspergillus fumigatus*.

PULMONARY DISEASE DUE TO *ASPERGILLUS*

1. Disseminated aspergillosis
2. Aspergilloma or mycetoma
3. Bronchial asthma
4. Extrinsic allergic alveolitis (Malt worker's lung)
5. Allergic bronchopulmonary aspergillosis

8.1 Pulmonary diseases due to *Aspergillus*.

DIAGNOSTIC CRITERIA FOR ALLERGIC ASPERGILLOSIS

Major criteria

1. Episodic bronchial obstruction
2. Peripheral blood eosinophilia
3. Positive immediate skin reactivity
4. Serum-precipitating antibodies
5. Elevated serum IgE
6. Elevated IgG and IgE anti-*Aspergillus* antibodies
7. History of pulmonary infiltrates
8. Central bronchiectasis

Minor criteria

1. *Aspergillus fumigatus* positive sputum culture
2. History of expectorating brown plugs or flecks
3. Arthus (late) skin reactivity

8.2 Diagnostic criteria for allergic aspergillosis (modified from Rosenberg, 1977).

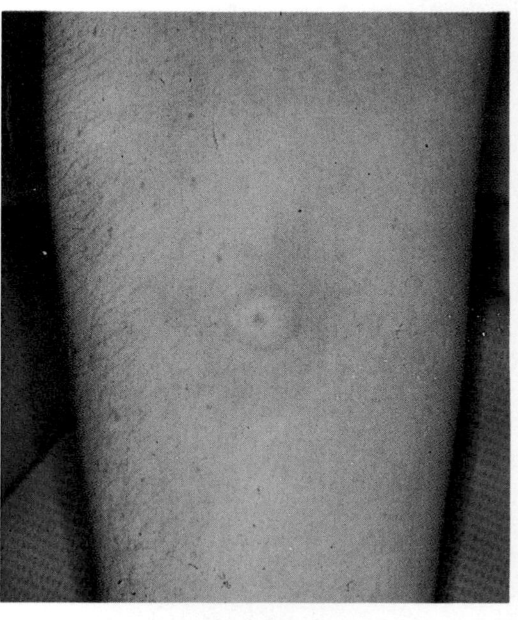

8.3 A positive wheal and flare reaction occurring 15 minutes after a prick test with 1,000 aqueous solution of *Aspergillus fumigatus* in a patient with ABPA.

Blood tests

Precipitating antibody of the IgG type to *Aspergillus fumigatus* is present in the serum of 69% of patients with allergic aspergillosis (**8.4**). When the serum is concentrated three to four fold, the percentage of positive precipitin reactions increases to well over 90%. As in the case of immediate skin reactions, the presence of precipitating antibody to *Aspergillus fumigatus* is not absolutely diagnostic of allergic aspergillosis, for it has been demonstrated in 9% of hospitalized patients, 27% of patients with Farmer's lung, and practically all patients with aspergilloma.

In allergic aspergillosis, serum IgE levels are markedly elevated, generally being over 1000ng/ml and reaching levels as high as 78,000 ng/ml. This is significantly higher than in uncomplicated, allergic bronchial asthma. The majority of total serum IgE is not directed to *Aspergillus fumigatus*, indicating that nonspecific stimulation of the IgE system is occurring. IgE and IgG antibody levels against *Aspergillus fumigatus*, as determined by either radioimmunassay or enzyme-linked immunosorbent assay techniques, have been shown to be significantly higher in allergic aspergillosis than in uncomplicated allergic asthmatics. They may be particularly important in differentiating patients with ABPA from asthmatics who have positive skin tests and positive precipitins to *Aspergillus fumigatus*.

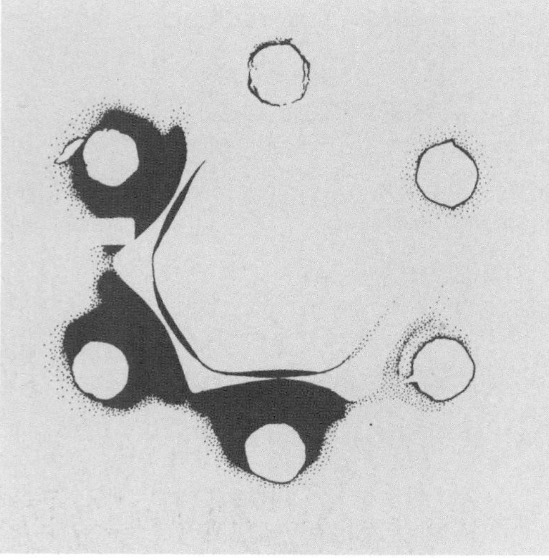

8.4 *Aspergillus fumigatus* 10mg/ml is placed in the center well. Normal serum is in the top well. Sera from a patient with ABPA are placed in the other wells with dates indicating when the sera were drawn. With time and clinical improvement, the precipitin band diminishes. The large indistinct precipitin band appearing close to and curving around the well in which the test serum is placed, represents a reaction between serum C-reactive protein and a somatic polysaccharide substance in certain Aspergillus extracts. It is of no immunologic significance. (Reproduced with permission from Slavin, 1970.)

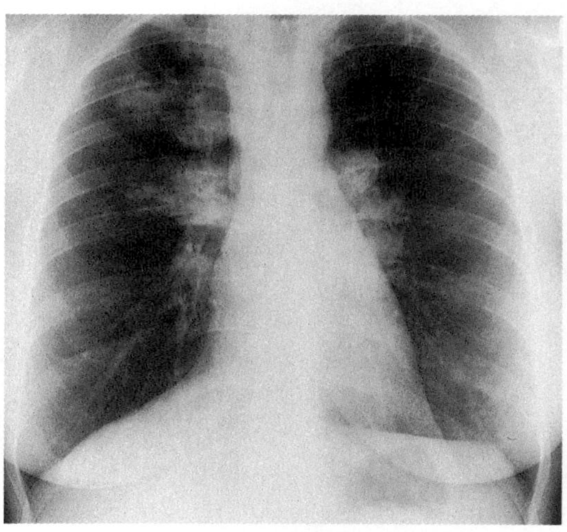

8.5 Multiple nodular densities at both hilar areas and right upper lobe in a patient with ABPA.

Radiographic findings

A variety of radiographic abnormalities have been described in ABPA. Most frequently seen is a large homogeneous shadow or shadows without fissure displacement, which usually appear in the upper lobes (**8.5**). The shadow may be patchy, triangular, lobar, or oblong, and it frequently shifts from one site to another (**8.6**). Another frequently seen abnormality is a 'tramline' shadow, which consists of two parallel hairline shadows extending out from the hilum in the direction of the bronchi (**8.7**). This is thought to represent bronchial wall edema. Ring shadows consisting of hair-like rings indicate thick-walled, empty bronchi (**8.8**). Another common radiographic finding in allergic aspergillosis is atelectasis of a segment, a lobe, or the whole lung due to mucus-plug occlusion (**8.9**).

It is important to realize that an inconspicuous radiographic appearance can represent extensive tissue damage. The diagnosis of ABPA can be suspected from such a modest finding as a tramline shadow or by residual damage such as a shrunken upper lobe.

In the patient with ABPA, an extremely distinctive bronchogram is seen in the form of cylindrical, or, more often saccular, bronchiectasis involving the proximal or central bronchi with normal filling of the distal or peripheral bronchi (**8.10**). This suggests a local toxic reaction in the bronchial wall resulting from the presence of the fungus, rather than the usual sequence of events leading to ordinary bronchiectasis; that is, bronchial obstruction, atelectasis, and infection. Tomography has been shown to be quite satisfactory for the identification of central bronchiectasis and should be considered

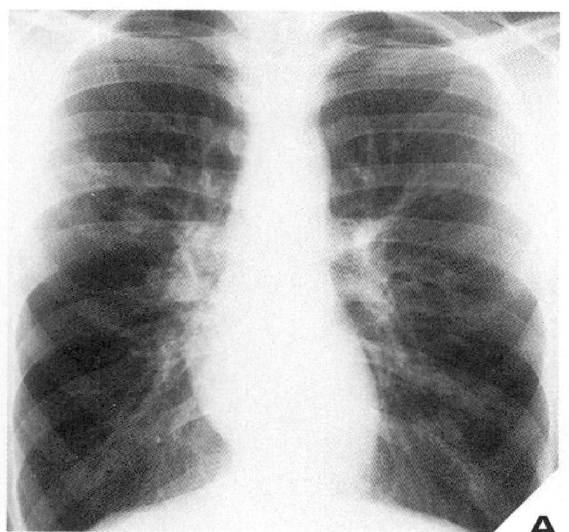

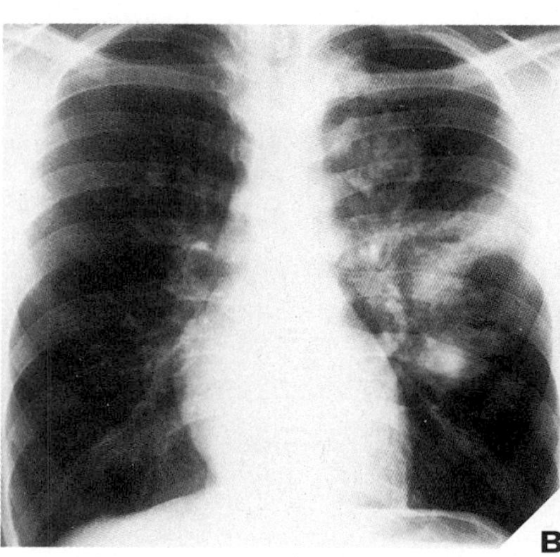

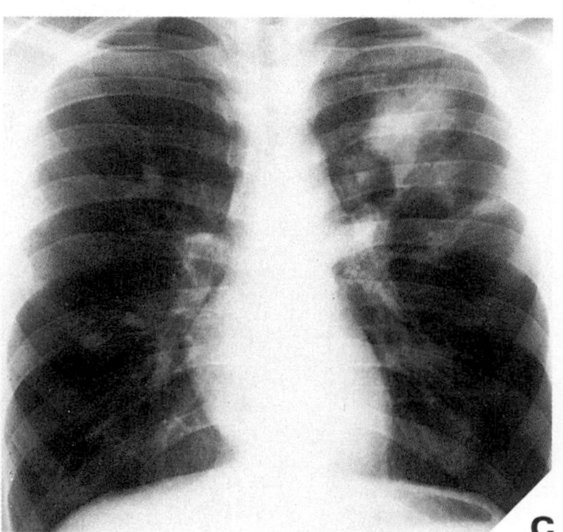

8.6 Chest radiographs demonstrating fleeting infiltrates in the case of ABPA. (A) Soft nodular infiltrates in the right upper lobe suggest tuberculosis. (B) Fourteen days later, there is some clearing on the right with a new infiltrate present in the left midlung field. (C) Ten days later, the left midlung has cleared but a new infiltrate is present in the upper lobe. (Reproduced with permission from Slavin, 1985.)

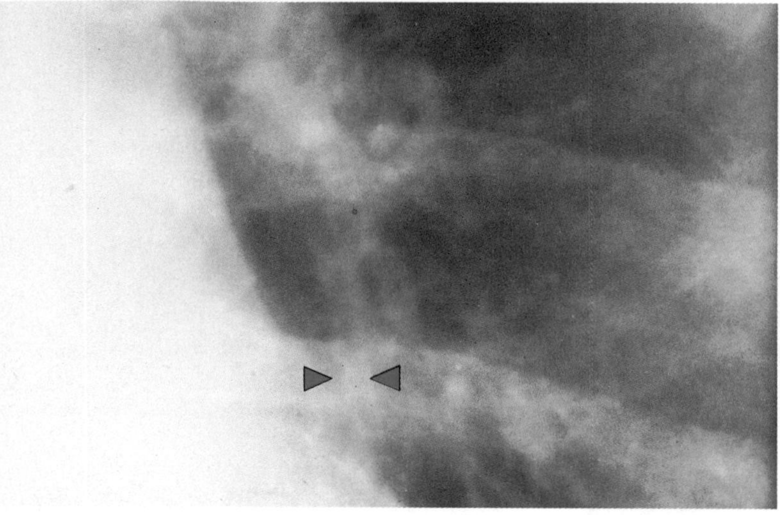

8.7 Chest radiograph of a patient with ABPA. Arrows point to 'tramline' shadows, indicative of edema of the bronchial wall. (Reproduced with permission from Slavin, 1983.)

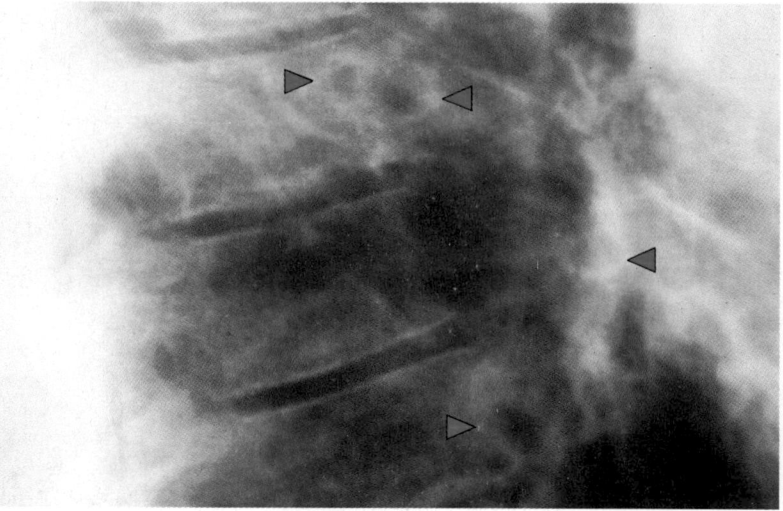

8.8 Chest radiograph of a patient with ABPA. Arrows point to ring shadows, indicative of thick-walled, empty bronchi. (Reproduced with permission from Slavin, 1983.)

particularly in the pediatric age group, where general anesthesia is required for bronchography. A computerized tomography (CT) scan of the chest is probably the most useful noninvasive technique for the diagnosis of bronchiectasis in ABPA (**8.11**).

Minor criteria

The majority of patients with ABPA produce hard, solid sputum plugs of different size, shapes, and colors, ranging from green to brown or beige. Fungal mycelia with large numbers of eosinophils

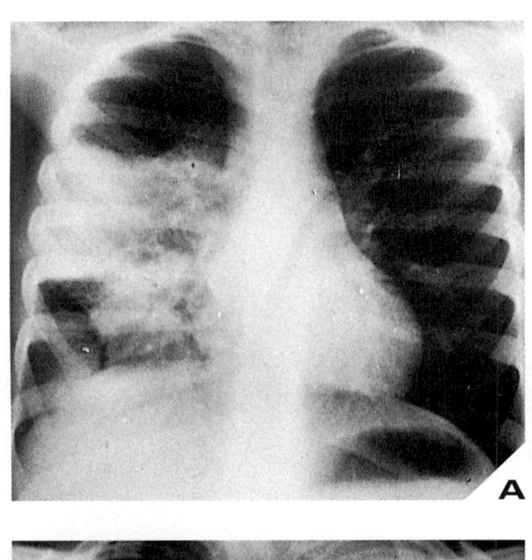

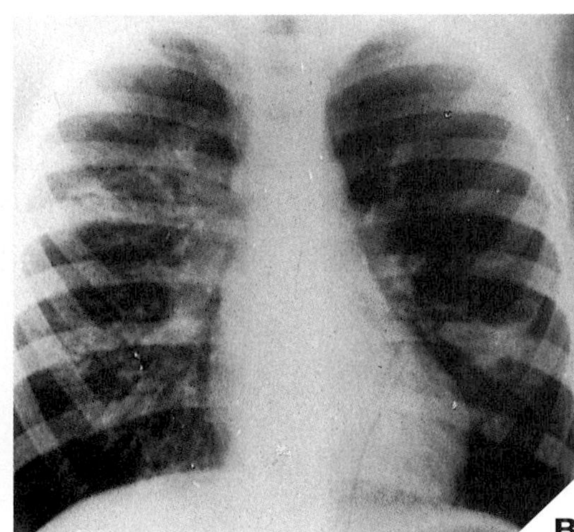

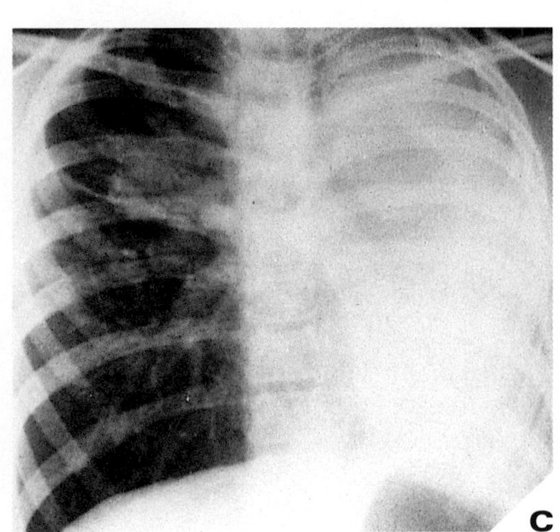

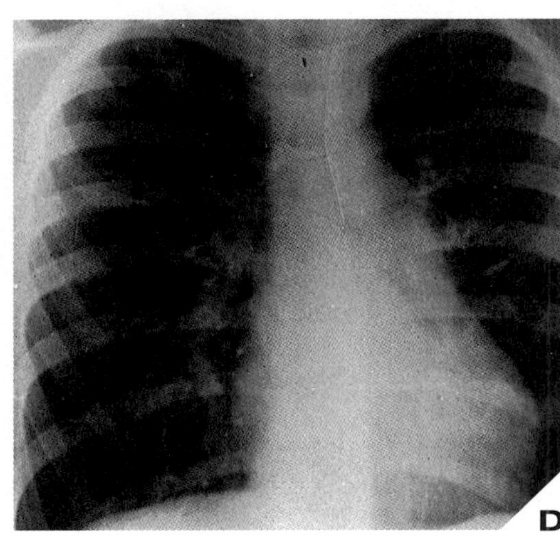

8.9 Chest radiographs of a nine year old girl with ABPA. (A) Right middle and right lower lobe consolidations are seen. (B) General involvement of all lobes on the right with left upper lobe and left lingular involvement five months later. (C) After interval of one to one and one-half years, there is a right upper lobe infiltrate with atelectasis and total collapse of the left lung with herniation across the middle. (D) Six weeks after institution of therapy, infiltrates have cleared but dilated bronchi are seen. (Reproduced with permission from Slavin, 1970.)

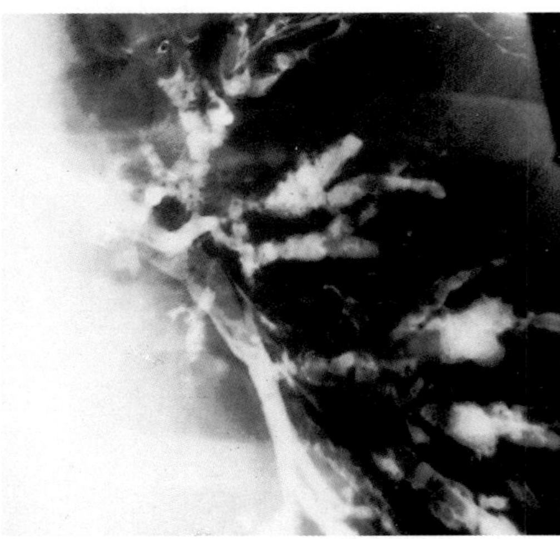

8.10 Bronchogram of a patient with ABPA, showing saccular proximal involvement with peripheral sparing. (Reproduced with permission from Slavin, 1983.)

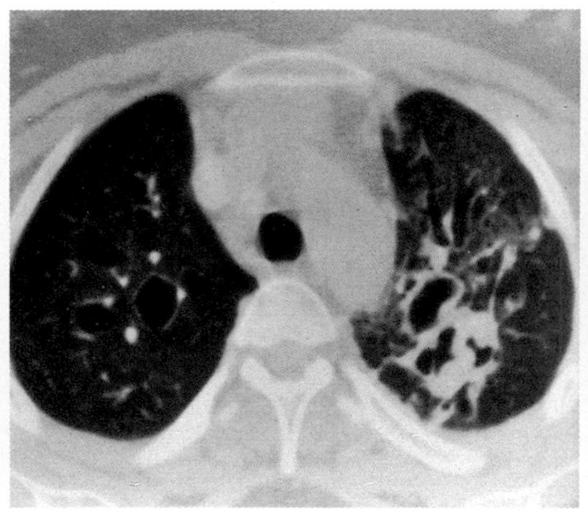

8.11 CT scan of the chest in a patient with ABPA. Dilated bronchi are seen bilaterally with a marked inflammatory response in the left posterior lung field.

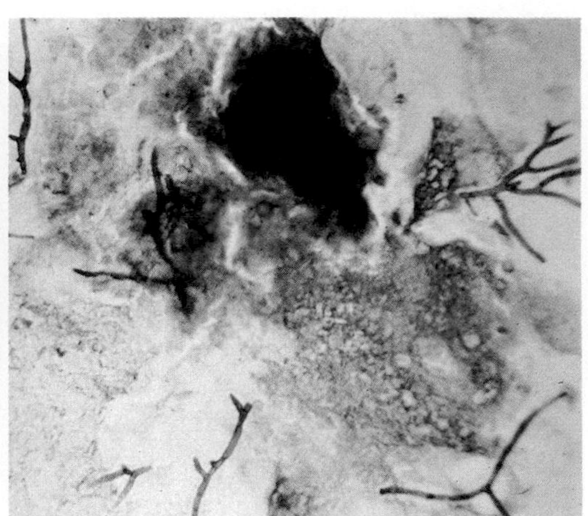

8.12 Sputum smear of patient with ABPA showing eosinophils with good preservation of cytoplasm. Gomorimethenamine silver-Giemsa counterstain (Reproduced with permission from Slavin, 1970.)

are frequently seen on direct examination of the plugs (**8.12**). Good preservation of cytoplasm, indicating active growth of the fungus, is an important feature. This contrasts with the dead mycelia, devoid of cytoplasm, seen in patients with aspergilloma. A positive sputum culture for *Aspergillus* is not necessarily diagnostic of aspergillosis as the organism is commonly inhaled and expectorated by the population at large.

Intradermal testing with the protein fraction of *Aspergillus fumigatus* results in a dual skin-test reaction in practically all patients with allergic aspergillosis. In the dual skin-test reaction, the immediate wheal and erythema response (see **8.3**) appears in 10 to 15 minutes and subsides over the next two hours. Then, at three to four hours, erythems and poorly defined edema begin at the skin-test test, reaching a peak at eight hours (**8.13**) and resolving within 24 hours. Skin biopsy of a positive, late reaction shows the presence of IgG, IgM, IgA, and the C3 component of complement.

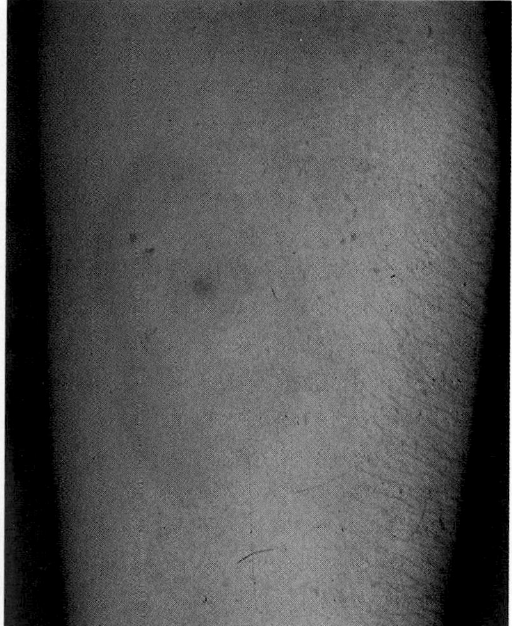

8.13 The peak at eight hours of the Arthus (late) reaction showing erythema and poorly defined edema at the site of a intradermal 1:10,000 *Aspergillus fumigatus* skin test.

OTHER TESTS

Pulmonary function

In allergic aspergillosis, pulmonary function testing during clinical flares shows significant decline in total lung capacity, vital capacity, forced expiratory volume in one second (FEV1), and carbon monoxide (CO) diffusion (DLCO). The decrease in DCLO is due to the presence of bronchiectasis; it is a very important index of disease severity as uncomplicated bronchial asthma is associated with a normal DLCO. The abnormal pulmonary function tests return to baseline with remission, and most patients who receive proper treatment after diagnosis do not suffer significant functional deterioration. The end or fibrotic stage of ABPA, as seen in patients who have not been treated early enough or appropriately, is characterized by irreversible obstruction and restriction.

Bronchial challenge

Patients with allergic aspergillosis will respond to a bronchial challenge with *Aspergillus fumigatus* in much the same way as to a skin test. After an immediate fall in FEV1 and subsequent clearing, a late asthmatic reaction occurs at four to six hours that is associated with fever and leukocytosis. Beta agonists will block the immediate reaction, corticosteroids will prevent the late reaction, and comolyn will block both the immediate and late responses (**8.14**).

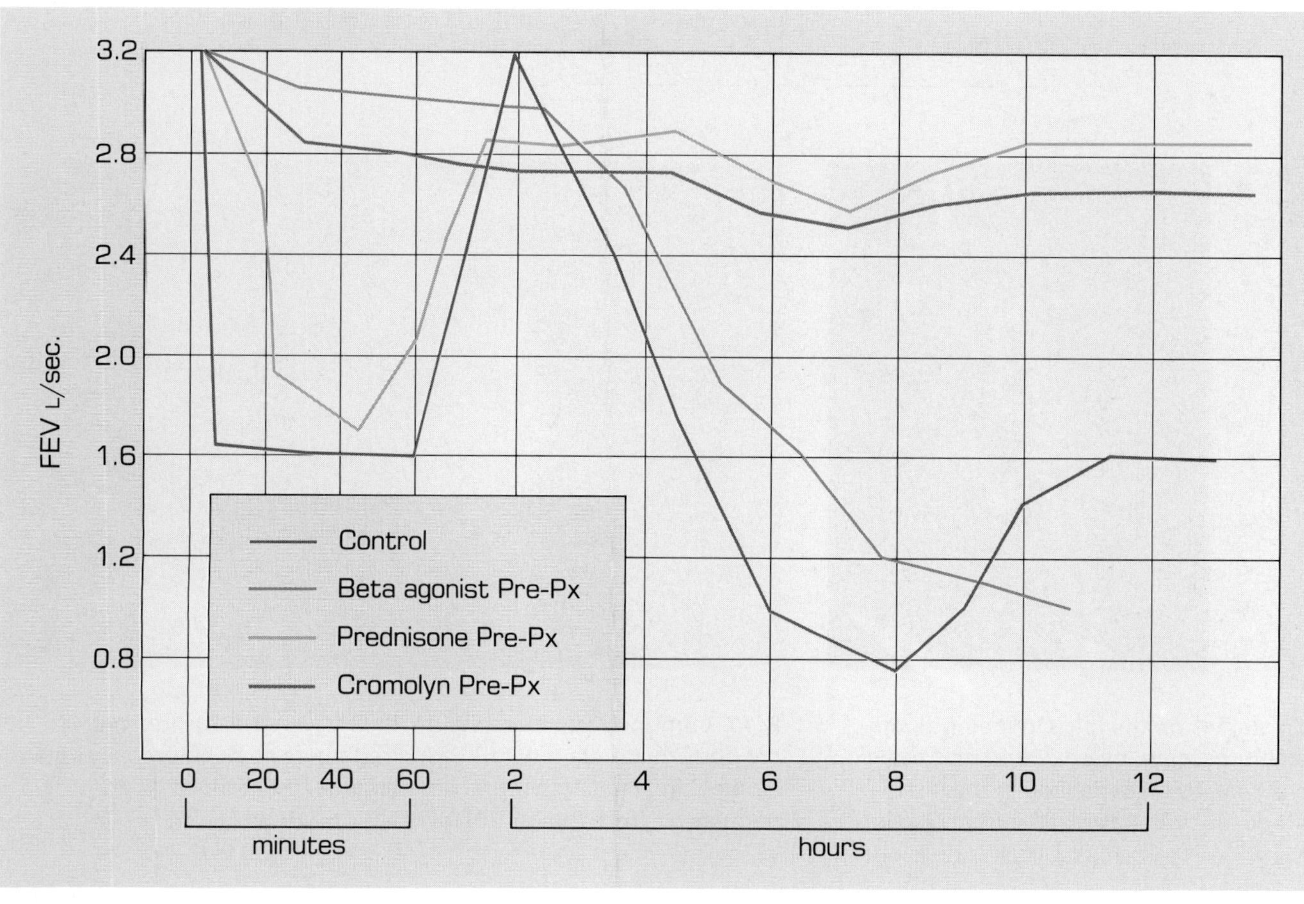

8.14 The dual phase bronchial response in ABPA with the effects of cromolyn sodium, prednisone, and beta agonists.

Lung biopsy

Tissue obtained by lung biopsy of patients with ABPA, shows largely bronchocentric involvement with little in the way of vasculitis. The bronchial wall is infiltrated by mixed inflammatory cells, primarily eosinophils and mononuclear cells. Bronchi are dilated and frequently filled with inspissated mucus and exudate. In areas of lung parenchyma, one sees prominent eosinophilic infiltration with evidence of major, basic protein in eosinophils (8.15) and deposited in tissues (8.16). By special immunochemical staining, small fragments of septate hyphae of *Aspergillus* may be seen in the parenchyma (8.17). In areas of extreme consolidation, chronic inflammatory cells are seen with granuloma formation. There is a significant increase in activated T cells with an approximate two-to-one, helper-to-suppressor ratio.

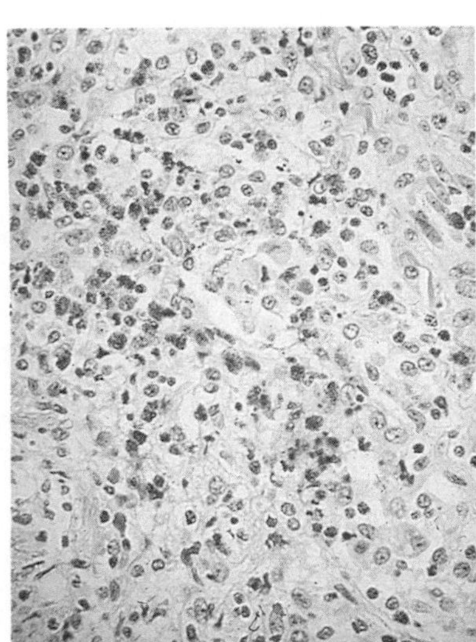
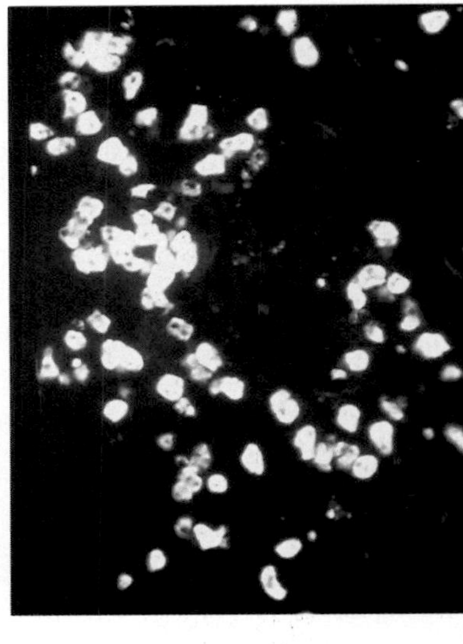

8.15 Lung biopsy of a patient with ABPA. Hematoxylin and eosin stain is on the left. On the right, the same section is stained with flourescein-labeled, anti-major basic protein antibody. Positive staining corresponds to eosinophils (×400). (Reproduced with permission from Slavin, 1988.)

PATHOGENESIS

Based on the clinical and pathologic features, one can postulate as to the pathogenesis of ABPA. The disease process begins with the inhalation and trapping of the short-chained spores of *Aspergillus fumigatus* in the viscid secretions contained in the constricted airway of the asthmatic patient. The size of the spores and the broad temperature range at which *Aspergillus fumigatus* grows makes this organism uniquely suited for colonization of a human bronchial tree. Most other fungal spores will not survive at normal, human body temperature, but *Aspergillus fumigatus* germinates and forms mycelia in the bronchi. Allergic aspergillosis is clearly distinguished from other hypersensitivity responses to inhaled allergens, in that the allergen actively grows in the respiratory tract and continually sheds soluble and particulate antigens in the large, subsegmental bronchi. The marked inflammatory reaction that occurs in the airway wall, perhaps potentiated by IgG anti-*Aspergillus* antibody, enables soluble *Aspergillus fumigatus* antigen and mycelia fragments to penetrate and deposit in the lung parenchyma. Here, IgE anti-*Aspergillus* antibody and *Aspergillus* antigen combine to cause mast cell degranulation. Among the mast cell products is eosinophil chemotactic factor of anaphylaxis (ECF-A), the release of which calls forth the tissue infiltration of eosinophils. Major basic protein from the eosinophils causes marked tissue damage. A significant increase of activated T cells, particularly in the helper cells, explains the presence of such cell-mediated immune tissue responses as granuloma formation. A practical approach to the

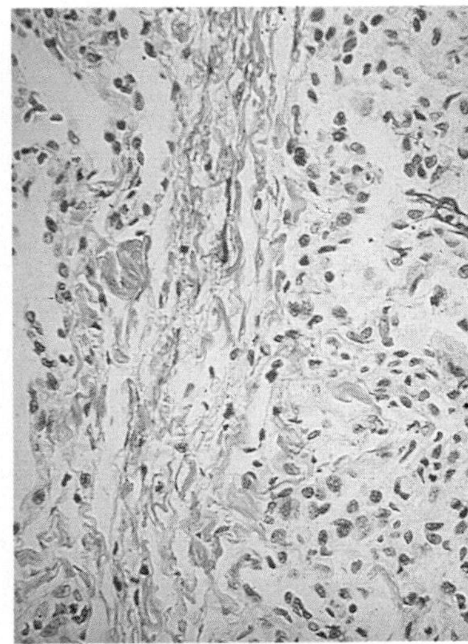
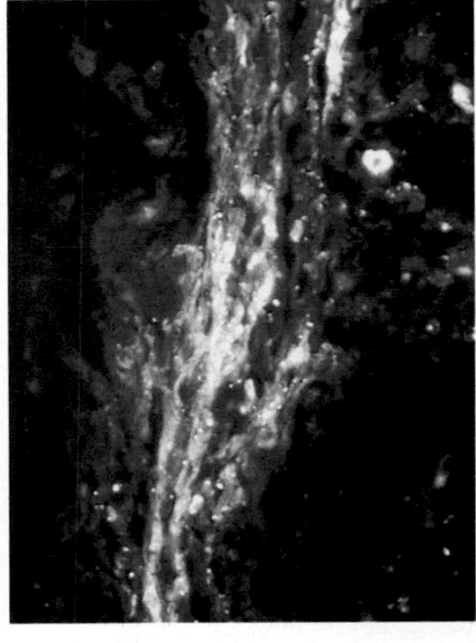

8.16 Hematoxylin and eosin stain is on the left. On the right, the same section is stained with fluorescein-labeled, anti-major basic protein. Major basic protein is seen to be deposited in the inter lobular septum (×400). (Reproduced with permission from Slavin, 1988.)

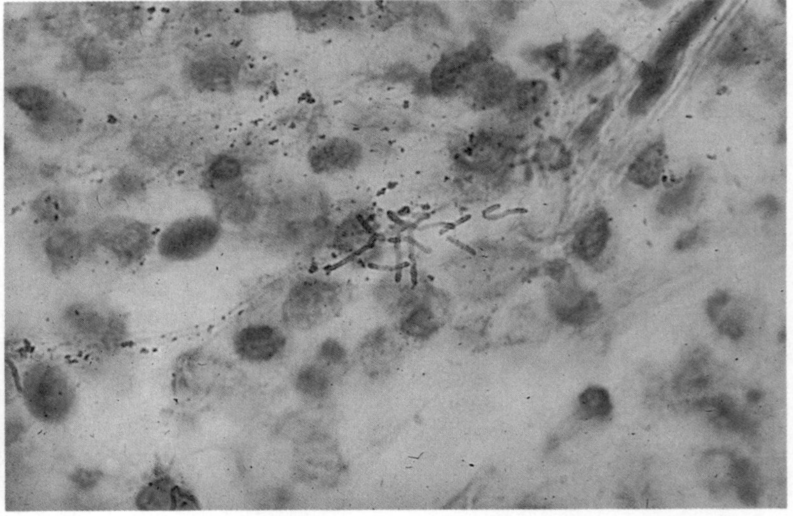

8.17 Immunoperoxidase stain with anti-*Aspergillus fumigatus* antibody in a patient with ABPA. Fragments of dichotomous septate hyphae are seen in the lung parenchyma. (Reproduced with permission from Slavin, 1988.)

diagnosis of ABPA would be to perform a skin test to *Aspergillus* on any patient with a history of pulmonary infiltrates and asthma. If the skin test were positive, then serum would be checked for total IgE and precipitins to *Aspergillus fumigatus*. In questionable cases, bronchograms, tomograms, or CT scans would be obtained to confirm a diagnosis. **8.18** depicts in a flow diagram a diagnostic approach to allergic aspergillosis. The new hybridoma technology and subsequent availability of monoclonal antibodies has afforded the opportunity to obtain purified antigens of aspergillus. These purified antigens should improve the immunodiagnosis of allergic aspergillosis and lead to a better understanding of the pathogenesis of this disease.

Staging of allergic aspergillosis has been suggested to provide an index of disease severity and progression (Patterson, 1982) (**8.19**). The first or acute stage is associated with full blown disease and a good response to corticosteroids. In the second or remission stage, the patient is free of significant disease. The third or exacerbative stage is associated with recurrent flares of ABPA. In the fourth stage, asthma becomes more severe and is steroid dependent; recurrent flares of ABPA also occur. The fifth or end stage is marked by irreversible, obstructive, and fibrotic pulmonary function changes, carrying a poor prognosis.

DIFFERENTIAL DIAGNOSIS

A number of medical conditions may be associated with asthma and pulmonary infiltrates (**8.20**). The primary diagnostic considerations are bacterial pneumonia, carcinoma, and tuberculosis. The frequently seen radiographic findings in allergic aspergillosis of upper lobe shrinkage and cavitation are particularly suggestive of tuberculosis. Appropriate bacterial study can rule this out.

Mucoid impaction of bronchi is associated with obstruction of proximal bronchi by large plugs of inspissated mucus and exudate. A large percentage of patients have asthma or chronic bronchitis with

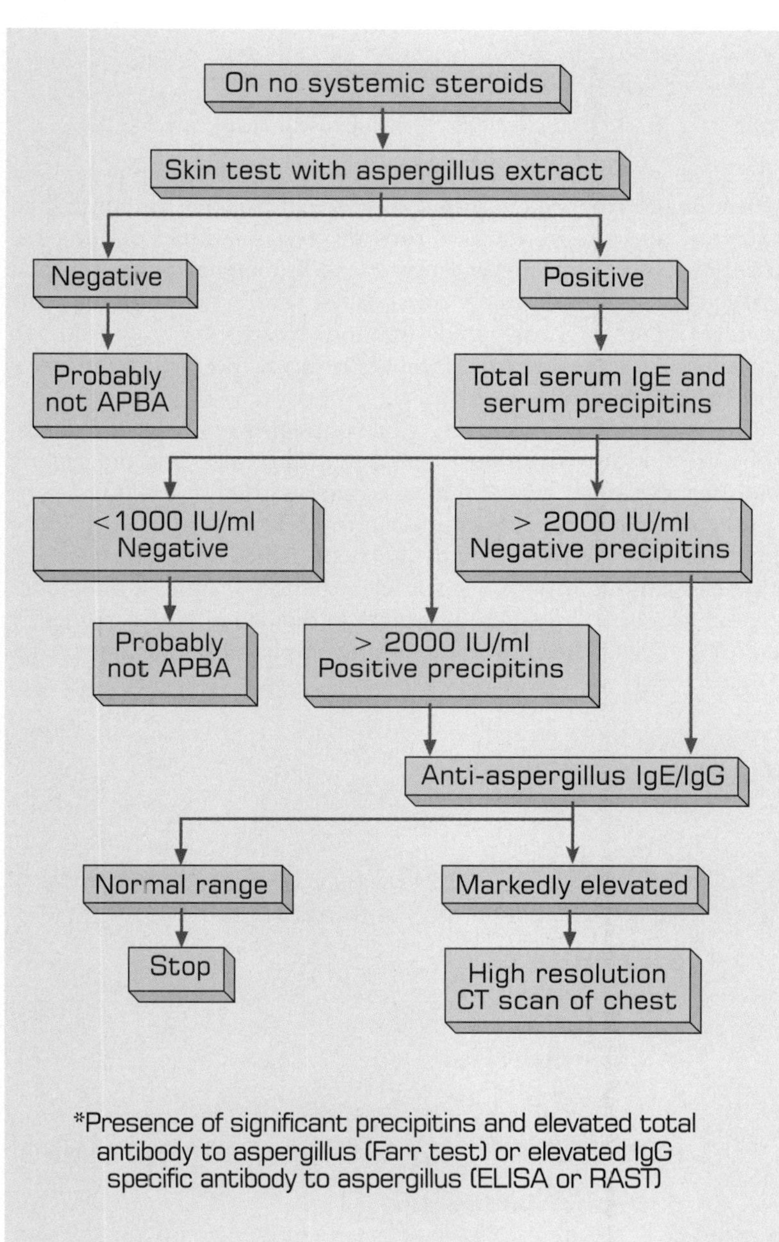

8.18 Asthma, eosinophilia, and transient pulmonary infiltrates.

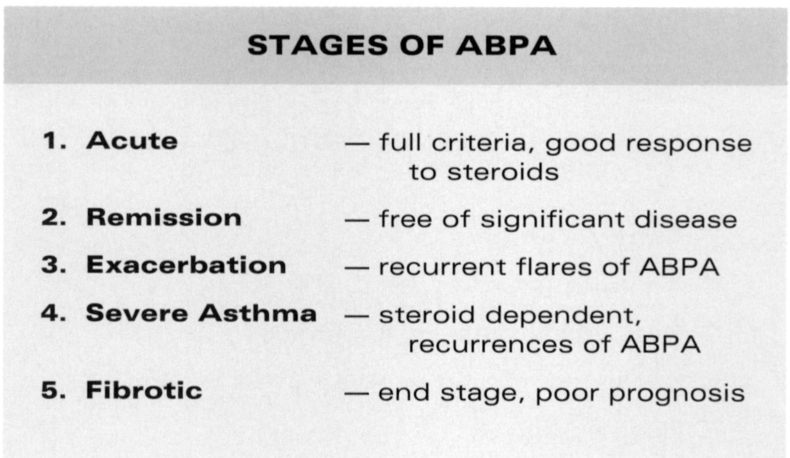

STAGES OF ABPA

1. **Acute**	— full criteria, good response to steroids
2. **Remission**	— free of significant disease
3. **Exacerbation**	— recurrent flares of ABPA
4. **Severe Asthma**	— steroid dependent, recurrences of ABPA
5. **Fibrotic**	— end stage, poor prognosis

8.19 Stages of ABPA. (Adapted with permission from Patterson, 1982.)

DIFFERENTIAL DIAGNOSIS OF ABPA

1. Bacterial penumonia
2. Carcinoma
3. Tuberculosis
4. Mucoid impaction
5. Eosinophilic pneumonia
6. Bronchocentric granulomatosis

8.20 Differential diagnosis of ABPA.

eosinophilia. Fungal hyphae are generally not identified with mucus plugs, and there is usually no evidence of *Aspergillus* hypersensitivity. Corticosteroids are rarely of benefit in mucoid impaction, in contrast to the favorable response they elicit in patients who suffer from allergic aspergillosis.

Eosinophilic pneumonia, also called pulmonary eosinophilia or the PIE syndrome (pulmonary infiltrate with eosinophilia), consists of migratory pulmonary infiltrates, which are usually accompanied by an excess of eosinophils in the peripheral blood. Cough, anorexia, and weight loss are noted. A peripheral density adjacent to the pleura with a clear central zone is a characteristic radiographic finding. This has been described as a photographic negative of pulmonary edema. Etiologic factors include chemicals, helminths, and fungi. When an etiologic diagnosis is not found, the condition is termed cryptogenic or idiopathic pulmonary eosinophilia. Characteristics include predominance in females, and marked eosinophilia, with less cough, sputum, and airway obstruction.

Bronchocentric granulomatosis is associated with asthma, mucoid impaction, and the presence of noninvasive fungi. The distinctive pathologic lesion is the replacement of bronchial epithelium by granulation tissue.

Association with cystic fibrosis

The incidence of allergic aspergillosis in patients with cystic fibrosis is markedly increased, on the order of 10 to 12%. The diagnosis of ABPA is particularly difficult to make because of the similarities of the two diseases (**8.21**). In cystic fibrosis there is an increased incidence of atopy, asthma, positive skin tests and precipitins to *Aspergillus fumigatus* , positive sputum cultures for *Aspergillus fumigatus*, increased serum IgE, radiographic changes of hyperinflation, peribronchial inflammatory changes, mucoid impaction, atelectasis, predominant upper lobe infiltrates, and bronchiectasis. The diagnosis of ABPA may be suggested if peripheral blood eosinophils are markedly increased (above 25%), if the serum IgE is greatly elevated to levels above 1000 ng/ml, if the IgE and IgG anti-*Aspergillus* are significantly elevated and if pulmonary infiltrates do not respond to antibiotics, are transient, and resolve with corticosteroids.

SIMILARITIES OF ABPA AND CYSTIC FIBROSIS

1. Atopy
2. Asthma
3. Positive skin test to *Aspergillus fumigatus*
4. Positive precipitin to *Aspergillus fumigatus*
5. Elevated IgE
6. Pulmonary infiltrates
7. Bronchiectasis

8.21 Similarities of ABPA and cystic fibrosis.

TREATMENT

The basic aim of therapy in ABPA is to break the vicious cycle in which fungus, trapped in viscid secretions contained in the constricted asthmatic airway, continues to provide large quantities of antigenic material. The clinical presentation of ABPA may be quite subtle and a paucity of symptoms may be associated with quite profound tissue damage. Therefore, early and strenuous treatment is important to prevent the inexorable consequences of bronchiectasis, pulmonary fibrosis, and cor pulmonale.

Without question, the cornerstone of treatment is corticosteroids. They are the only drug with consistent clinical and radiographic improvement and a concomitant decrease in total serum IgE.

The overall therapeutic approach to ABPA is seen in **8.22**. Once the diagnosis of ABPA is made, corticosteroids must be given in a large enough quantity over a sufficient period of time. A daily dose of prednisone, 60 mg/kg body weight in divided doses, is frequently required to clear the chest radiograph completely in the adult. After

THERAPY OF ABPA

1. **Corticosteroids**
   - Initial dose - 60 mg prednisone per day in divided doses (30 to 45 mg in children)
   - After radiographic clearing - 0.5 mg/kg body weight in single daily dose for two weeks
   - Gradual taper to 0.25 mg/kg body weight over six-week period
   - Switch to 0.50 mg/kg body weight every other day for six weeks
   - Gradual taper over another three-month period
2. **Bronchodilators**
   - Theophyllines, beta agonists
3. **Fluids**
   - Avoidance of ice
4. **Expectorants**
   - Potassium iodide, guaifenesin
5. **Physical therapy and postural drainage**
6. **Bronchial lavage**
7. **In difficult cases, consider itraconazole**

8.22 Therapy of ABPA.

radiographic clearing, a single daily dose of 0.5 mg/kg of body weight is given for two weeks. At this point, there is a gradual taper to 0.25 mg/kg body weight over a six-week period. The dose is then switched to 0.5 mg/kg body weight every other day for another six weeks and then gradually tapered over a three-month period. In total, the steroid treatment is given over approximately a seven-month period. During this period, monthly serum IgE levels are obtained. A decrease from the initial, markedly elevated level is always seen. A rise in the serial IgE level, subsequently tested on a monthly basis, should prompt an increase in steroid therapy.

Because of the known beneficial effects of corticosteroids, other important aspects of therapy are often forgotten. Effective removal of fungus from the airway is vital and therefore, attention to bronchial toilet is extremely important. Bronchodilator therapy must be continued throughout the course of therapy. Particularly in the acute phase, effort should be made to remove the viscid secretions with oral fluids, to avoid ice that may cause reflux bronchospasm, to use expectorants such as potassium iodide or guafenesin, and to employ aggressive physical therapy and postural drainage (**8.23**). In stubborn cases, bronchial lavage may have to be used. There have been promising reports on the effectiveness of itraconazole, an oral fungal agent, on decreasing the fungal burden in allergic aspergillosis. Expectoration of the nidus of infection will hopefully prevent permanent anatomical, bronchial damage. The majority of patients who receive an early diagnosis and proper treatment will show no significant functional deterioration as determined by pulmonary function testing.

REFERENCES

Greenberger PA. Allergic bronchopulmonary aspergillosis, in Middleton E Jr., Reed CE, Ellis EF, Adkinson NF Jr., Yunginger JW, Busse WW (eds): *Allergy; Principles and Practice*, CV Mosby, 1993 chapter 53.

Hinson KFW, Moon AJ, Plummer NS: Bronchopulmonary aspergillosis: a review and report of eight new cases. *Thorax* 1952; **7**:317.

Knutsen AP and Slavin RG: Allergic bronchopulmonary mycosis complicating cystic fibrosis. *Sem Res Infect* 1992; **7**:172 .

Patterson R, Greenberger PA, Radin RG, Roberts M: Allergic bronchopulmonary aspergillosis: staging as an aid to management. *Ann Int Med* 1982; **96**:286.

Rosenberg M, Patterson P, Mintzer R et al: Clinical and immunologic criteria for the diagnosis of allergic bronchopulmonary aspergillosis. *Ann Int Med* 1977; **86**:405.

Slavin RG: Allergic bronchopulmonary aspergillosis. *Clin Rev Allergy* 1985; **3**:167.

Slavin RG, Bedrossian CW, Hutcheson PS et al: A pathologic study of allergic bronchopulmonary aspergillosis. *J Allergy Clin Immunol* 1988; **81**:718.

Slavin RG, Laird TS, Cherry JD: Allergic bronchopulmonary aspergillosis in a child. *J Ped* 1970; **76**:416.

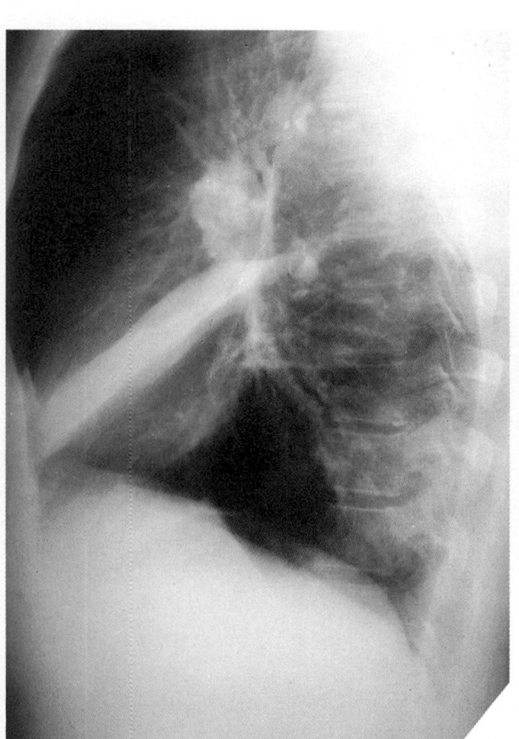

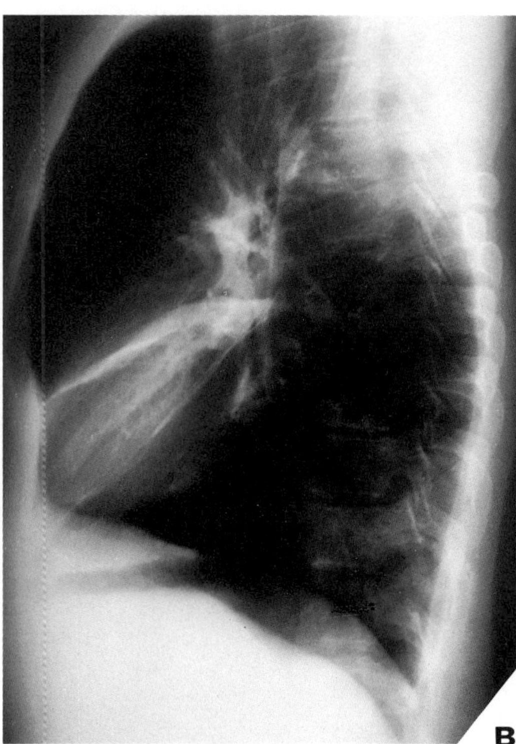

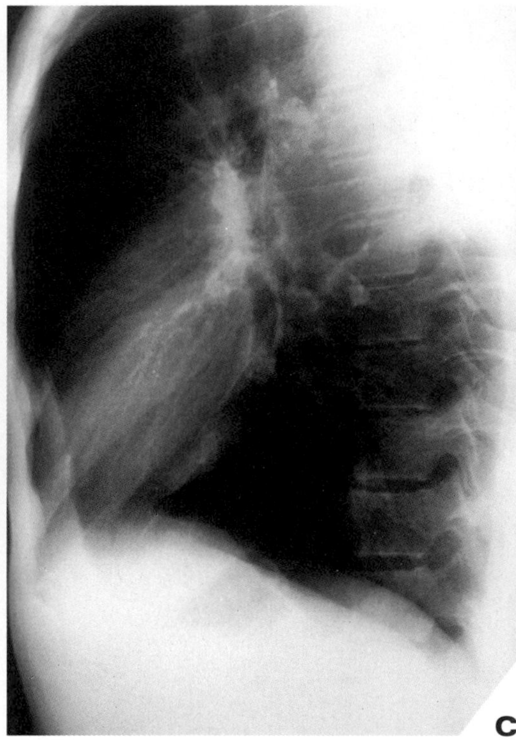

8.23 Chest radiographs (left lateral) illustrating the rapid clearing of the pneumonia and atelectasis of ABPA following corticosteroids, bronchodilators, physiotherapy, and postural drainage. (A) On admission, left lower lobe pneumonia and right middle lobe atelectasis. (B) Less than 24 hours later, there is clearing of the infiltrate, with improvement in the atelectasis. (C) One day later, both the infiltrate and atelectasis have resolved. (Reproduced with permission from Slavin, 1988.)

CHAPTER 9

Allergic Rhinitis

Philip Fireman

Allergic rhinitis is the most common allergic disease, affecting over 20 million people in the United States and many more world-wide. Although not life-threatening, this frequent illness causes considerable morbidity and results in expenditure of many millions of dollars in health care and loss of millions of working and school days.

Allergic rhinitis is provoked by exposure to antigenic environmental factors with resultant sneezing, nasal pruritus, rhinorrhea, nasal mucosal edema, and subsequent nasal obstruction. Symptoms can be episodic or perennial; when symptoms recur annually during certain months, the syndrome is called seasonal allergic rhinitis (**9.1**). Typically, seasonal allergic rhinitis does not develop until after the patient has been sensitized by two or more seasons. It is frequently referred to as 'hay fever' or 'summer cold', but these descriptive terms are misleading and should be discarded because fever is not a symptom of allergic rhinitis, and the common cold virus is not the etiology. Perennial allergic rhinitis can be constant or recurrent and it occurs year round. It can also be associated with seasonal exacerbations.

EPIDEMIOLOGY

The prevalence of allergic rhinitis in the general population is about 10%, with peak incidence in the post-adolescent teenage child. It increases during childhood from less than 1% in infancy to 5% between 5–9 years' old, 10% during adolescence, and finally to 15% after adolescence (**9.2**). Prevalence of allergic rhinitis remains constant in young adults, but gradually declines during the later years. Although allergic rhinitis is more common among young boys than girls, there is little sex difference after adolescence. Race and socio-economics are not major factors in the expression of this condition.

ALLERGIC RHINITIS

1. **Seasonal**
   - Episodic
   - Occurs annually
2. **Perennial**
   - Constant
   - Occurs continually through the year

9.1 Classification of allergic rhinitis. Seasonal allergic rhinitis ('hay fever') recurs annually during certain months, and is caused by pollens, fungi, or other allergens. Perennial allergic rhinitis, persistent year-round, is usually associated with indoor as well as outdoor aero-allergens.

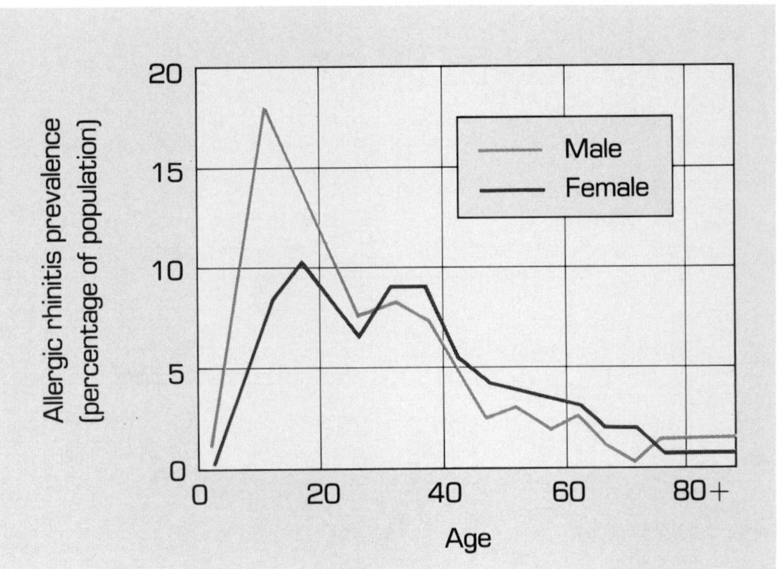

9.2 Prevalence of allergic rhinitis. Peak incidence of allergic rhinitis occurs in the post-adolescent patient. Since IgE antibodies do not traverse the placenta, infants are not born with allergic rhinitis, but acquire the syndrome after exposure to allergens during the first several years of life. The prevalence stabilizes during the adult years and gradually decreases during middle and advanced age. (Modified with permission from Weeke, 1987.)

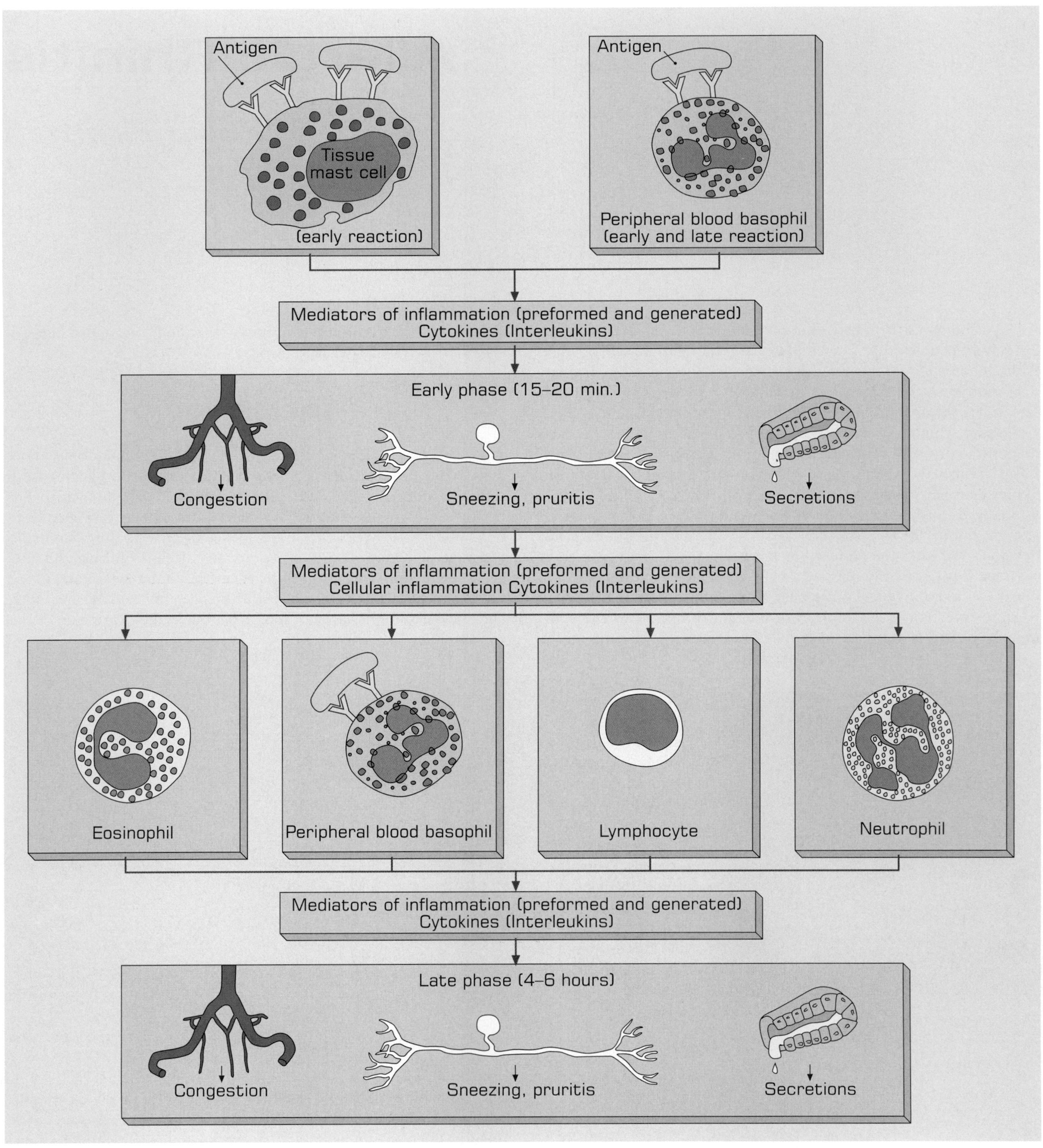

9.3 Mechanism of allergic reaction in allergic rhinitis. On re-exposure to an antigen to which the patient has been sensitized, the mast cells and basophils are activated, releasing a variety of inflammatory mediators and cytokines (interleukins). Collectively, these substances provoke the end organ changes recognized as the early and late-phase allergic reactions. The late reaction, arising 4–6 hours after the initial immediate response, appears to be mediated by the basophils alone. The mast cells and basophils both play a role in the initial reaction.

The familial nature of allergic rhinitis and its association with asthma and atopic dermatitis have been recognized for years. It is inherited as an autosomal trait and its immunogenetics have been the subject of several studies. Increased serum levels of IgE have been observed in patients with allergic rhinitis and their affected family members, suggesting a genetic influence in IgE synthesis. Several studies indicate that allergic rhinitis due to ragweed and IgE responses to purified ragweed antigen E are linked to a histocompatibility locus antigen (HLA) haplotype in successive generations of families with allergic rhinitis. Others have reported a correlation between haplotype HLA-A7 and increased production of IgE antibodies to purified ragweed antigen (Ra5) in patients sensitive to this allergen. A specific immune response (Ir) gene in allergic rhinitis awaits demonstration.

IMMUNOPATHOPHYSIOLOGY

Allergic rhinitis, along with allergic asthma, atopic dermatitis, and allergic urticaria, are described immunologically as hypersensitivity syndromes which are mediated in large part by IgE antibodies. After inhalation of an allergen, IgE antibodies are synthesized by plasma cells in lymphoid tissues adjacent to nasal mucosa and other portions of the respiratory tract. These IgE antibodies are also found in nasal secretions and sera. The Fc portions of the IgE antibodies bind to high-affinity receptors on the membranes of the tissue mast cells and circulating blood basophils, sensitizing these cells. During sensitization, there is no overt deleterious reaction. Upon subsequent challenge, allergen combines with its specific IgE antibody on the sensitized mast cells and basophils with resulting cell activation (9.3). The interaction of the allergen and IgE at the cell membranes releases preformed mediators and generates new mediators of inflammation, which manifest the early and late-phase allergic reactions. As illustrated in 9.3, these mediators initiate the inflammation with resultant increased vascular permeability, local edema, and eosinophil-laden secretions. The early allergic reaction occurs in minutes after allergen exposure. Approximately 50% of allergic rhinitis patients also manifest late-phase IgE allergy with prolonged tissue inflammation, peaking 4–6 hours after allergen exposure. In addition to these mediators, cytokines (including interleukins and other cellular-derived factors) are generated during this inflammatory response. Their specific roles and sequence of generation and action await delineation.

The immunologic effectors of allergic rhinitis are IgE antibodies; however, the mediators are responsible for the pathophysiology. Mediators of inflammation, including histamine, prostaglandin D_2 (PGD_2), leukotrienes and kinins, have been demonstrated in nasal secretions following specific allergen intranasal provocative challenge (9.4). Increased levels of histamine, as well as serine esterases, including tryptase, are found in nasal secretions during both the immediate (early) and late phase. The leukotrienes, formerly designated as slow-reacting substance of anaphylaxis (SRS-A), and kinins, including bradykinin, are also found in nasal secretions after allergen challenges. In contrast, PGD_2 is found in nasal secretions during the immediate but not during the late phase. Since this mediator is produced by mast cells and not basophils, it has been suggested that mast cells and basophils are involved in the early reaction, whereas basophils primarily contribute to the late phase. The

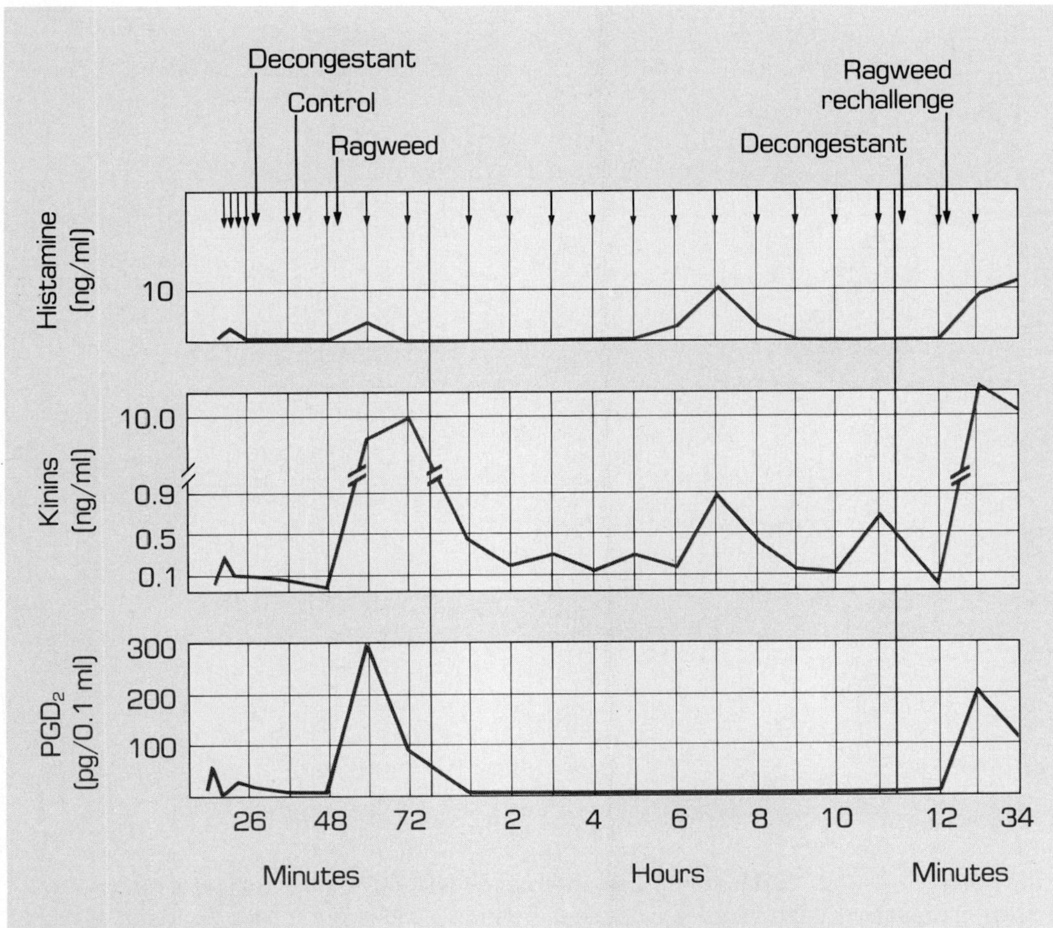

9.4 Profile of selected mediators present in nasal secretions collected by nasal wash from allergic rhinitis patients during early, late, and rechallenge responses to ragweed allergen. The time of each nasal wash is indicated by an arrow. Pretreatment with decongestants is necessary, since there are some mediators present in the nasal washes after the initial challenges. Histamine, kinins, tryptase, and prostaglandin D_2 (PGD_2) are present within in minutes (early-phase) of challenge with the ragweed allergen. In these experiments, without additional allergen, histamine and kinins reappear in nasal washes 2–8 hours after the initial exposure (late-phase). Note that PGD_2 is not present in secretions during the late-phase reaction. Upon subsequent re-exposure to the allergen during rechallenge, there are prompt increases in these mediators in nasal washes. These data help explain the almost continual (daily) symptoms that many allergic rhinitis patients experience.

function of eosinophils, attracted by the mediator eosinophil chemotactic factor of anaphylaxis (ECF-A), has yet to be defined clearly. A modulatory role for eosinophils has been suggested because the enzymes histaminase and arylsulfatase, which inactivate histamine and leukotrienes, respectively, are abundant in these cells. In addition, phospholipase, which inactivates platelet-activating factor (PAF) released from mast cells, is found in the eosinophils. Major basic protein, a product of eosinophils, as well as eosinophil cationic protein and eosinophil neurotoxin, may promote inflammation, cytotoxicity, and participate in the allergic reaction. The participation of neurohumors and vasoactive peptides seems likely, but their role needs definition.

Allergic rhinitis adversely affects normal nasal function which, besides its role as an airway **9.5**(A), includes filtration of particulate matter from inspired air, humidification of air, olfaction, and phonation **9.5**(B). The patient with allergic rhinitis not only has compromised nasal function, but also other portions of the contiguous respiratory tract, including the eustachian tube, sinuses, and bronchi, can be affected (**9.6**). Allergen-provoked eustachian tube obstruction has been detected not only after intranasal provocation, but also during seasonal, natural pollen exposure (*see* Chapter 11). Allergen, methacholine, or histamine bronchial challenge provokes lower airway obstruction (i.e., asthma) in 30% or patients with allergic rhinitis (*see* Chapter 5). That allergic rhinitis contributes to the pathogenesis of sinusitis has also been suggested (*see* Chapter 10).

CLINICAL PRESENTATION

Seasonal allergic rhinitis begins with frequent sneezing, nasal pruritus, and clear rhinorrhea, and then progresses to nasal obstruction (**9.7**). Perennial allergic rhinitis tends to manifest more stuffiness. Patients emphasize early morning and late evening symptoms, and nasal obstruction may interrupt sleep. They also complain of itching of the eyes, throat, ears, and nose (**9.8**). To relieve the nasal itch, some children may press the palm or arm upward against the nose in an 'allergic salute' (**9.9**). Constant rubbing of the itchy nose may produce a transverse nasal crease, a horizontal groove across the lower third of the nose (**9.10**). With nasal obstruction, the patient becomes a mouth breather, so snoring is a night-time symptom (**9.11**). Mouth breathing may contribute to orofacial dental abnormalities that require orthodontic procedures, but this has not been established definitely.

Seasonal allergic rhinitis is frequently accompanied by allergic conjunctivitis (*see* Chapter 12). When symptoms of nasal obstruction are severe, adjacent sinuses may be involved, causing facial discomfort or headaches. Patients with eustachian tube dysfunction complain of fullness or popping sounds in the ears. Hearing loss in a child with perennial allergic rhinitis suggests a conductive hearing deficit associated with otitis media with effusion (*see* Chapter 11). Loss of sense of smell and taste is also described. A few patients may complain of generalized malaise, irritability, and fatigue, which may be related to interrupted sleep.

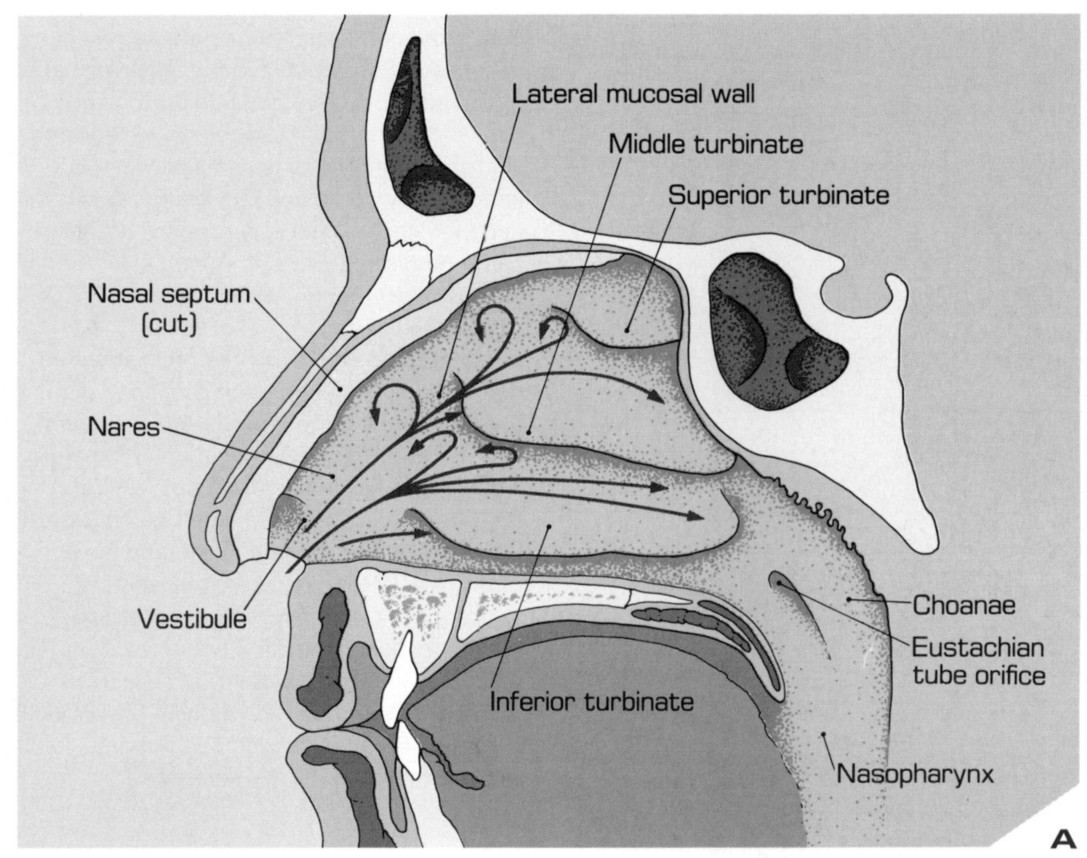

NASAL FUNCTION: IMPORTANT ASPECTS

1. Passage of air
2. Humidification
3. Warming of air
4. Filtering of air
5. Mucociliary action
6. Olfaction
7. Phonation

B

9.5 (A) Schematic representation of the inside of the nose, illustrating how the inspired air, after entering the nose, circulates over, under, and around the inferior, middle, and superior nasal turbinates. This pattern of circulation enables the nasal mucosa to more effectively filter, humidify, and warm the air. (B) Major aspects of nasal function.

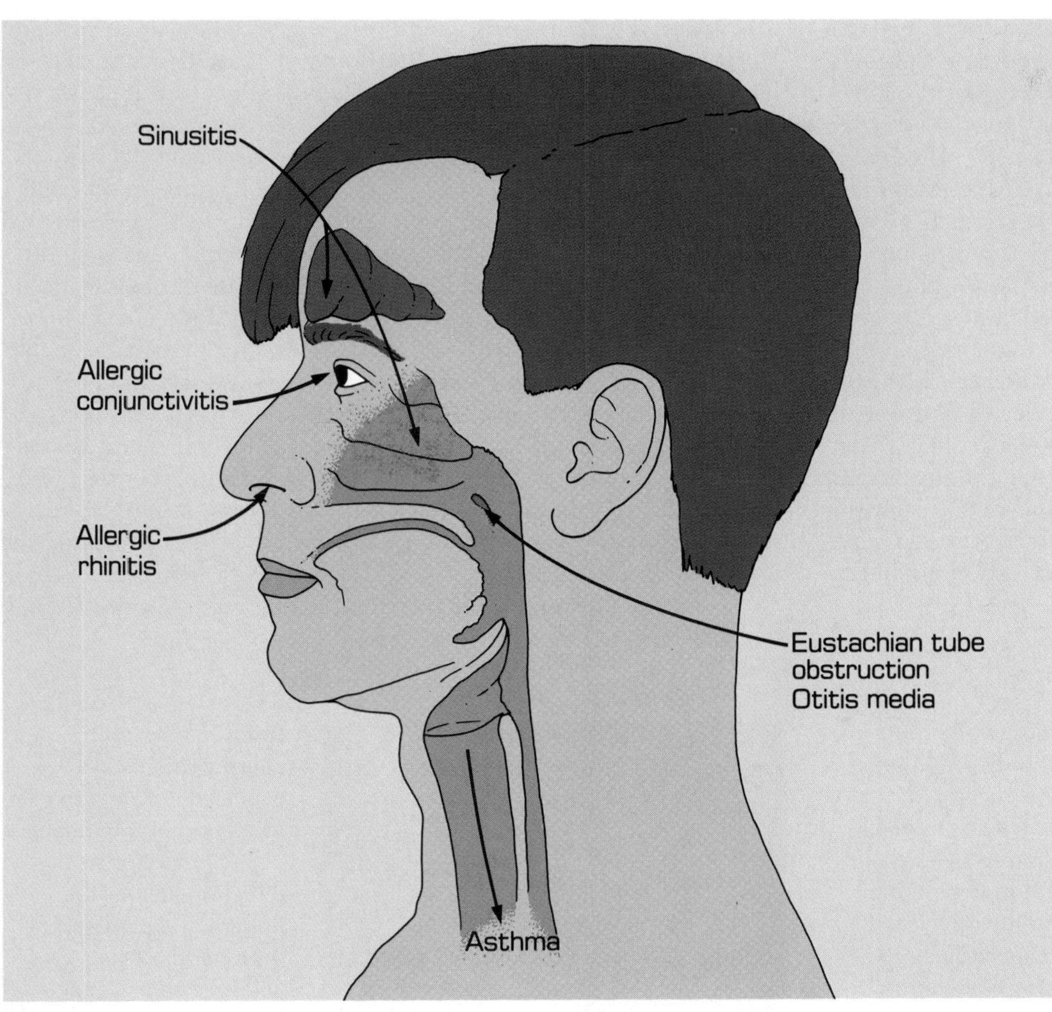

9.6 Diagram depicting the clinical conditions that can be associated with allergic rhinitis due to their continuous anatomic relationships within the respiratory tract. When evaluating a possible case of allergic rhinitis, the clinician should thoroughly examine all respiratory organs and related anatomic structures.

ALLERGIC RHINITIS: SYMPTOMS, PATHOPHYSIOLOGY, AND EFFECTOR MEDIATORS

Symptoms	Pathophysiology	Effector mediators
Tickling, itchiness, nose rubbing, allergic 'salute'	Pruritus	Histamine, prostaglandins
Sneezing	Sneezing	Histamine, leukotrienes
Nasal congestion, stuffy nose, mouth breathing, snoring	Mucosal edema, increased vascular permeability	Histamine, leukotrienes, bradykinin, PAF
Runny nose, post-nasal drip, throat clearing	Rhinorrhea, mucus secretion	Histamine, leukotrienes

9.7 Symptoms of allergic rhinitis as related to their pathophysiology and involved mediators of inflammation.

Patients with seasonal pollinosis describe increased symptoms as the season progresses, especially on dry, windy days; symptoms may continue well beyond the season. Repeated exposure to allergens increases nasal reactivity and 'primes' nasal mucosa, so that ordinarily innocuous concentrations of allergens and other environmental factors provoke symptoms. The pattern of symptoms helps distinguish seasonal from perennial allergic rhinitis. In subtropical climates, a seasonal aero-allergen exposure pattern may not be obvious, since pollen seasons extend for many months and fungi can be airborne year round. In much of the United States, however, trees pollinate in spring, grasses in late spring and summer, and ragweed during late summer and early fall (*see* Chapter 2). The arid southwestern US was traditionally pollen free, but the advent of irrigation and increased vegetation has changed the ecology. Even though airborne pollens spread for miles, increased concentrations are noted in areas of high plant density, with frequent complaints of more symptoms. If there is direct contact with considerable amounts of pollen, patients can have angioedema, especially of the eyes and throat.

Patients with perennial symptoms are more of a diagnostic challenge. Continuous exposure to home or occupational factors induces perennial symptoms, because congestion of the mucosal tissues does not return to normal during the few hours free of allergen exposure. In these patients, non-allergenic aerosolized irritants, such as cigarette smoke, fumes, industrial pollutants, and cosmetics, provoke increased symptoms. Additional non-allergenic factors include changes in barometric pressure, temperature, and humidity.

Examination of nasal mucosa requires the use of a nasal speculum with an appropriate light source (**9.12**). Although fiberoptic rhinoscopy is not needed for most cases, it can be a valuable adjunct in a more thorough inspection of the nose and nasopharynx (**9.13**). With development of nasal allergy, clear nasal secretions are evident. The mucosa appears pale, boggy, blue–gray, and edematous without much erythema (**9.14**). The turbinates become swollen and obstruct the nasal airway. When this occurs, it may be necessary to shrink the mucosa with a vasoconstrictor to document nasal polyps, which occur in 10–15% of adult patients (**9.15**). Conjunctival edema and hyperemia, along with Dennie's lines

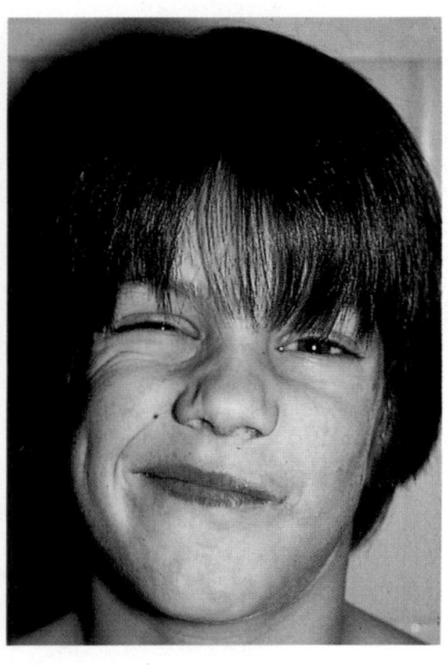

9.8 Nasal itching in patients with allergic rhinitis frequently causes facial grimacing and twitching. These symptoms are not only recognized by family and friends, but may be quite obvious during the physical examination. (Reproduced with permission from Zitelli and Davis, 1987.)

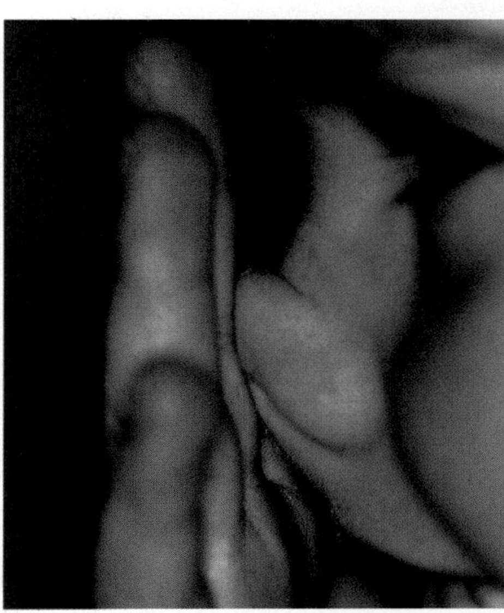

9.9 Children with allergic rhinitis are especially prone to forcibly rubbing their noses in an upward direction, using the fingers and palms of their hands. This 'allergic' salute may become a habit, and is frequently noted by parents. (Reproduced with permission from Zitelli and Davis, 1987.)

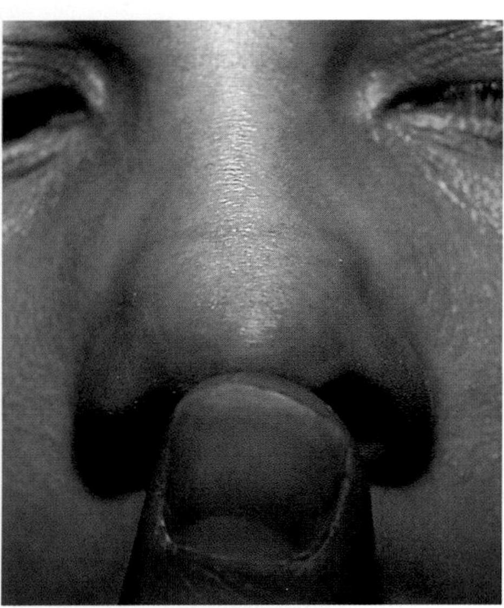

9.10 The chronic rubbing upward of the nose often results in a nasal crease in patients with allergic rhinitis. (Reproduced with permission from Zitelli and Davis, 1987.)

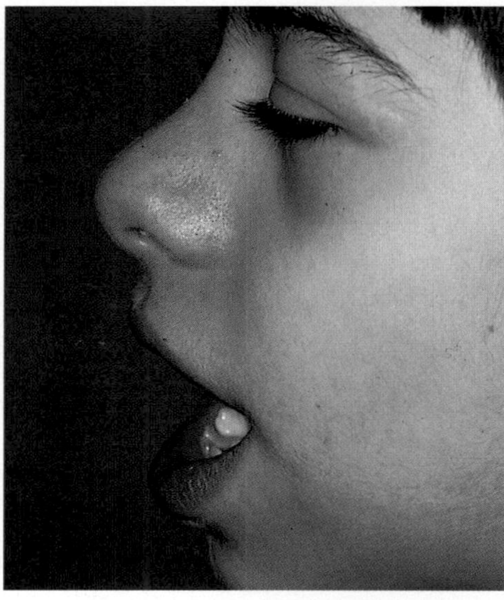

9.11 Open-mouthed breathing is typical in patients with long-standing chronic allergic rhinitis. This is similar to the appearance of patients with adenoidal hypertrophy causing posterior pharyngeal nasal obstruction. (Reproduced with permission from Zitelli and Davis, 1987.)

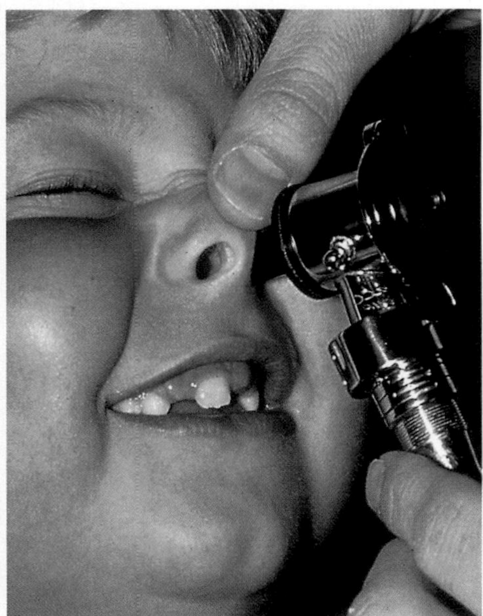

9.12 Inspection of the nasal mucosa. An illuminated nasal speculum is inserted into the nares for magnified visualization of the anterior nasal structures. This allows the clinician to view the anterior nares, and to inspect the middle turbinate. The speculum must be directed to allow visualization of the inferior or superior turbinate. This mode of examination does not allow visualization of the anterior or posterior nasopharynx. (Reproduced with permission from Zitelli and Davis, 1987.)

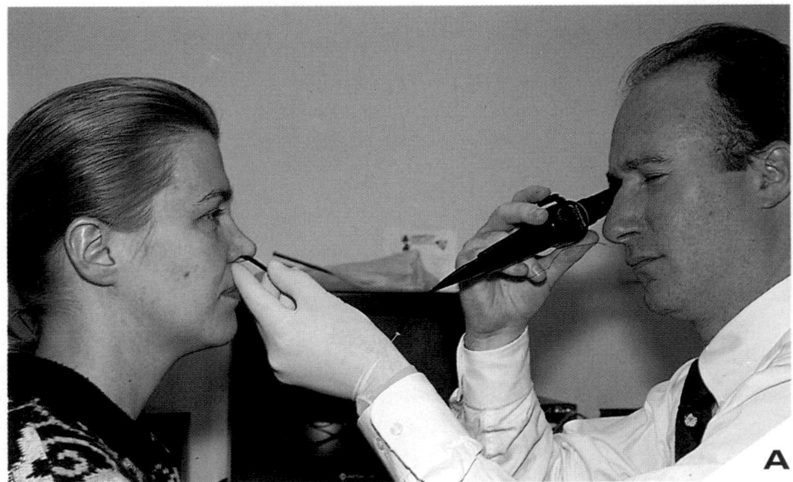

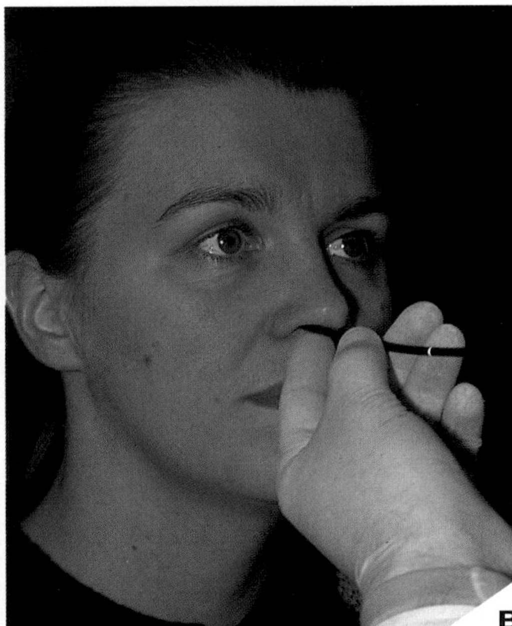

9.13 (A) Lateral and (B) frontal view of the fiberoptic rhinoscopic procedure which can be utilized for a more thorough examination of the nares, especially the anterior and posterior nasopharynx, which cannot be seen with a speculum. This examination also provides magnification of the nasal structures.

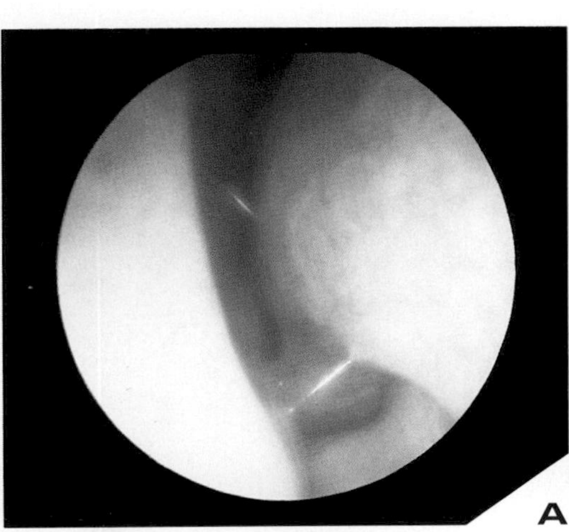

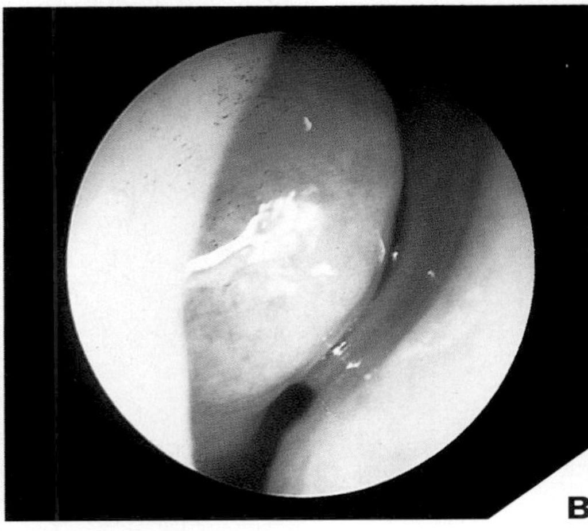

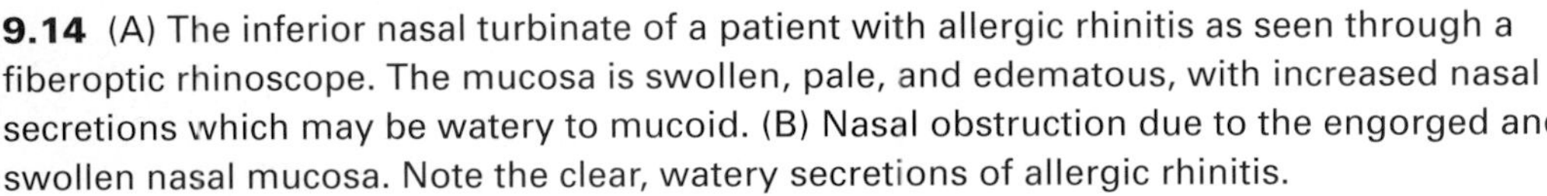

9.14 (A) The inferior nasal turbinate of a patient with allergic rhinitis as seen through a fiberoptic rhinoscope. The mucosa is swollen, pale, and edematous, with increased nasal secretions which may be watery to mucoid. (B) Nasal obstruction due to the engorged and swollen nasal mucosa. Note the clear, watery secretions of allergic rhinitis.

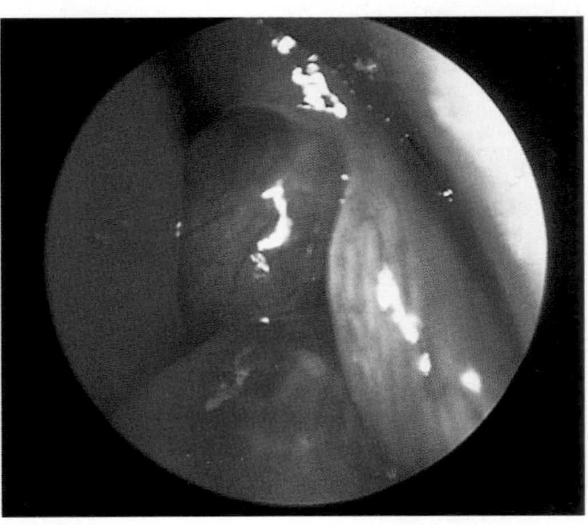

9.15 Appearance of nasal polyps on rhinoscopy. They are pale, bluish-gray, and almost gelatinous. These polyps, which obstruct the nasal airway, are best seen after application of a vasoconstrictor to shrink the nasal mucosa. (Photo courtesy of Dr Sylvan Stool, Department of Otolaryngology, University of Pittsburgh School of Medicine.)

(**9.16**), are frequent findings. Allergic rhinitis patients with considerable nasal obstruction and venous congestion, particularly children, demonstrate edema and darkening of the tissues beneath the eyes (**9.17**). These so-called 'allergic shiners' are not pathognomonic for allergic rhinitis; they can also be seen in patients with recurrent nasal and sinus congestion of any cause.

DIAGNOSIS

Analysis of cytology of expelled nasal secretions or scrapings of nasal mucosa obtained with a flexible plastic nasal probe can help in the differential diagnosis of selected patients with recurrent rhinitis. Expelled nasal secretions during exacerbation of allergic rhinitis contain increased eosinophils of more than 3% on stained smears (**9.18**). Nasal eosinophilia may not be evident during a superimposed infection or during steroid therapy. Increased nasal mucosal basophils (**9.19**), mast cells, and eosinophils are found in nasal scrapings not only from allergic rhinitis, but also from nonallergic eosinophilic rhinitis and primary nasal mastocytosis. The cytology of bacterial or viral infections shows a predominance of polymorphonuclear leukocytes (**9.20**).

Laboratory confirmation of the presence of IgE antibodies to specific allergens is often helpful in confirming the clinical diagnosis of allergic rhinitis and in reinforcing patient compliance (*see* Chapter 3). Testing should be performed when a seasonal pattern is not evident. Skin testing with the suspected allergens is mandatory in all patients prior to immunotherapy (hyposensitization) with allergen extracts, because the intensity of the skin reaction helps determine the initial treatment dose. End-point titration has been suggested as a guide for the initial dosage. However, this author does not recommend it, because it is expensive and lacks sufficient controlled data to document its validity. Clinicians should be selective; only common allergens of clinical relevance should be selected on the basis of prevalence in the patient's environment (*see* Chapter 2). The most useful allergens in the study of allergic rhinitis are the inhalants, especially the pollens, the molds (fungi), house dust, and animal products (**9.21**). Food testing is infrequently indicated.

The *in vitro* serum immunoassay (RAST, FAST, and ELISA) tests for assessing the presence of serum IgE antibodies to various

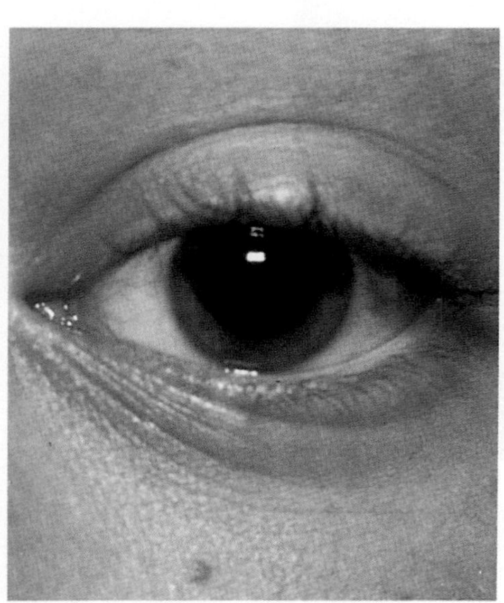

9.16 Dennie's lines on lower eyelid of a patient with allergic rhinoconjunctivitis. These lines originate at the inner canthus, and traverse one-half to one-third the length of the lower lid in an arc nearly parallel with its margin. (Reproduced with permission from Zitelli and Davis, 1987.)

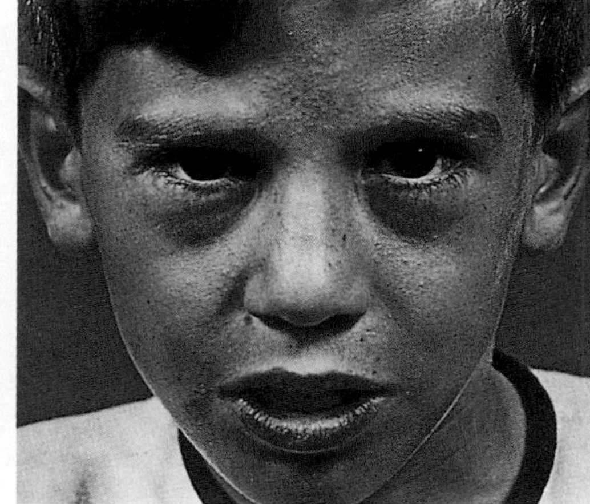

9.17 Suborbital venous congestion, edema, and darkening of the tissues under the eyes. This condition is frequently seen in patients with chronic allergic rhinitis and is referred to as an 'allergic shiner'. This patient's allergic rhinitis obstructed nasal breathing, resulting in open-mouthed breathing. (Photo courtesy of Dr Meyer B. Marks, Division of Pediatric Allergy and Immunology, University of Miami School of Medicine.)

allergens are 20% less sensitive than skin tests, and their increased cost is another disadvantage. Only rarely are IgE antibodies present in nasal secretions, and yet not detected in serum or evident by skin testing. The *in vitro* cytotoxic serum leukocyte test with foods and other allergens is unproven and not recommended.

A nasal provocation test performed by introducing the allergen into the nostril of the allergic patient elicits local pruritus, sneezing, rhinorrhea, and edema. The sublingual challenge with allergen is not a useful diagnostic test for allergic rhinitis. The provoked nasal obstruction can be measured by rhinomanometry. There are two

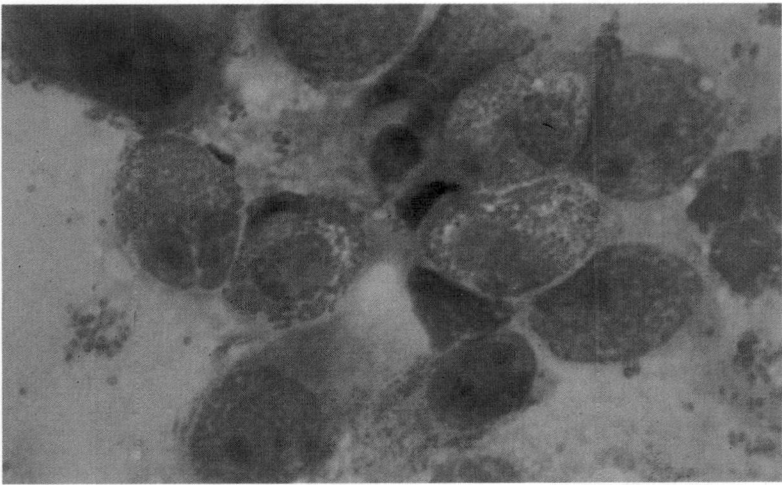

9.18 Nasal secretions obtained from a patient with allergic rhinitis, stained with Wright's stain. This high-power photomicrograph shows typical eosinophils, with red-staining granules, among the blue-staining nasal epithelial cells. (Courtesy of Drs. A. Jalowaryski and E. Meltzer, Division of Allergy and Immunology, University of California, San Diego.)

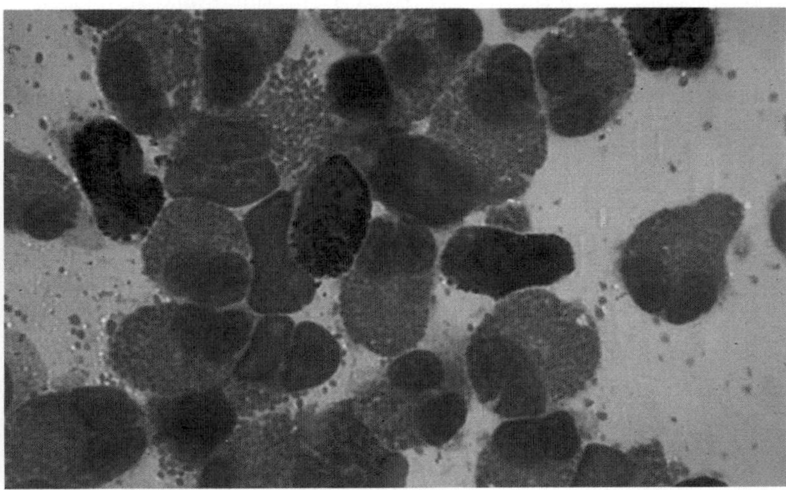

9.19 Nasal scrapings from a patient with allergic rhinitis. Obtained by using a flexible plastic probe, this material was spread on a microscope slide and stained with Wright's stain. This high-power photomicrograph shows several basophilic leukocytes, with their dark-blue cytoplasmic granules, among a cluster of eosinophilic leukocytes, with reddish cytoplasmic granules. (Courtesy of Drs. A. Jalowaryski and E. Meltzer, Division of Allergy and Immunology, University of California, San Diego.)

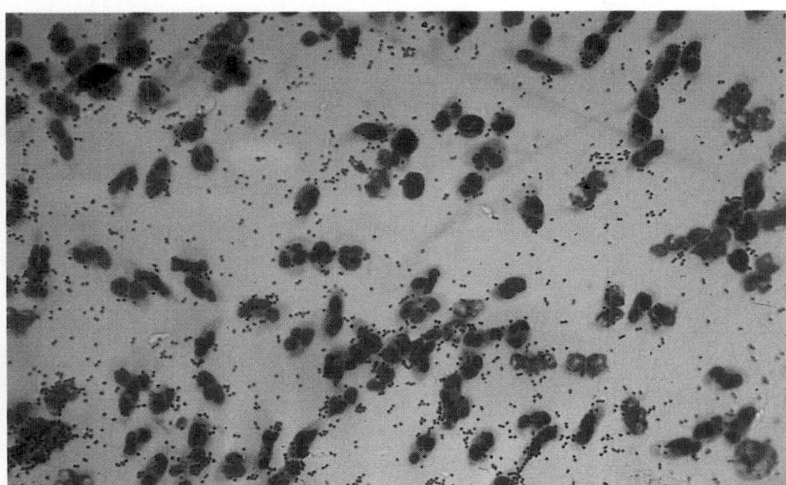

9.20 Nasal secretions photographed at low power from a patient with nasal infection. Typically, one sees many polymorphonuclear leukocytes, as well as bacteria, without any eosinophils. Viral rhinitis can also involve many polymorphonuclear leukocytes. (Courtesy of Drs. A. Jalowaryski and E. Meltzer, Division of Allergy and Immunology, University of California, San Diego.)

SELECTED INHALANT ALLERGENS USEFUL IN EVALUATION AND TESTING FOR ALLERGIC RHINITIS

Pollens (vary with geographical area)

— Weeds (ragweed, plantain, etc.)

— Grasses (Timothy, rye, etc.)

— Trees (oak, maple, etc.)

Fungi (molds)

— Seasonal (*Alternaria*, etc.)

— Storage (*Aspergillus*, etc.)

Animal products

— House-dust mites (cuticle, feces)

— Dogs, cats (dander, saliva)

— Birds (feathers, droppings)

9.21 Selected inhalant allergens useful in the evaluation and testing of allergic rhinitis.

approaches, anterior and posterior, to the measurement of air pressure and flow relationships in the nose [*Figures* **9.22**(*A*) and **9.22**(*B*)]. Anterior rhinomanometry requires minimum patient cooperation, but is compromised by the normal nasal cycling phenomenon in which air flow is predominant in one nostril for 2–3 hours and then alternates to the other side (**9.23**). This requires measurement of the resistance of both nostrils or of total nasal airway resistance. Alternatively, posterior rhinomanometry measures posterior pharyngeal pressure via an oral tube as nasal air flow is being monitored using a tightly fitting facial mask over the nose. However, 10% of adults cannot perform this test. Posterior rhinomanometry requires a storage oscilloscope because it is necessary to establish that an artifact-free pressure-flow curve has been achieved before nasal resistance measurements can be made. The development of computer-assisted rhinomanometry has now made this a fast accurate system. While it seems likely that rhinomanometry will be utilized more widely in the future, it has not yet been standardized for routine clinical practice.

DIFFERENTIAL DIAGNOSIS

Patients who present to the clinician with complaints of rhinorrhea and nasal obstruction may have symptoms not only due to allergy, but also to a variety of other conditions, including infections, structural changes, drug reactions, neoplasms, or foreign bodies (**9.24**). At its onset, an upper respiratory viral infection, with its clear,

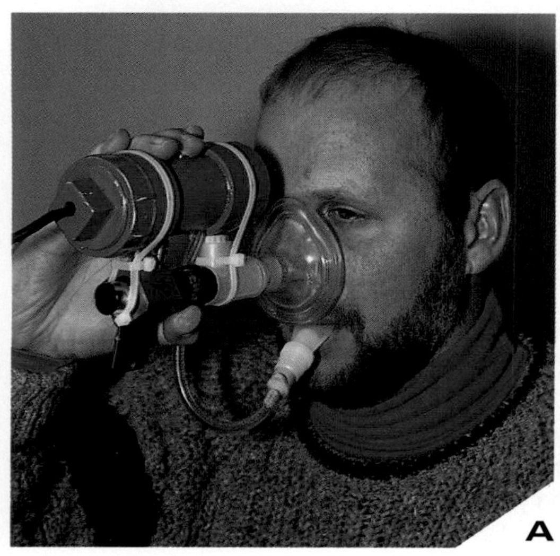

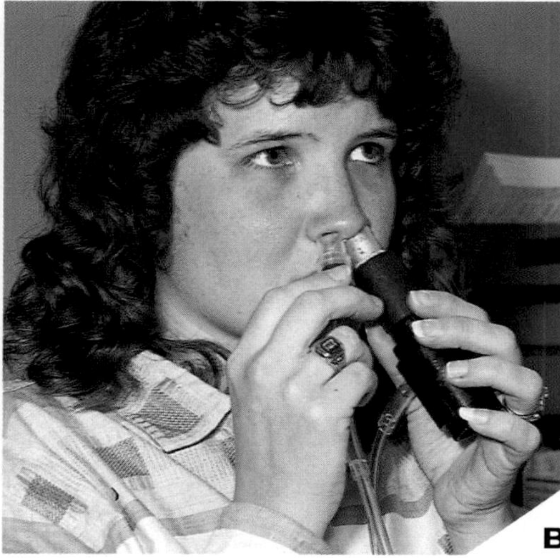

9.22 (A) Posterior rhinomanometry utilizes a face mask which fits securely around the nose. Nasal airflow is measured via a transducer attached to the nasal face mask. Nasopharyngeal pressure is measured via a plastic mouthpiece held securely between the teeth, with the lips closed. Nasal resistance is calculated from the airflow and pressure measurements which can be monitored and calculated with computer assistance. (B) Anterior rhinomanometry utilizes a system whereby nasal airflow is measured in one naris, while nasal pressure is measured in the other.

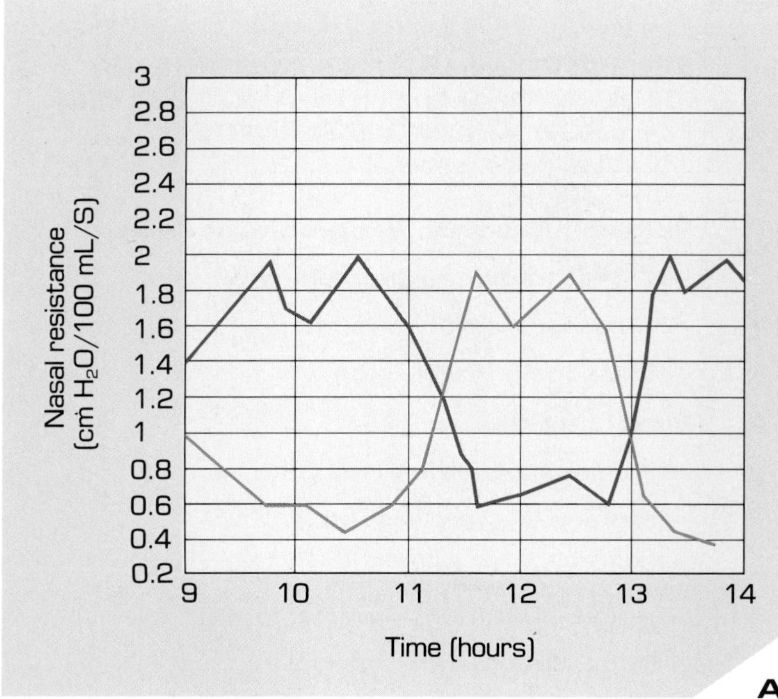

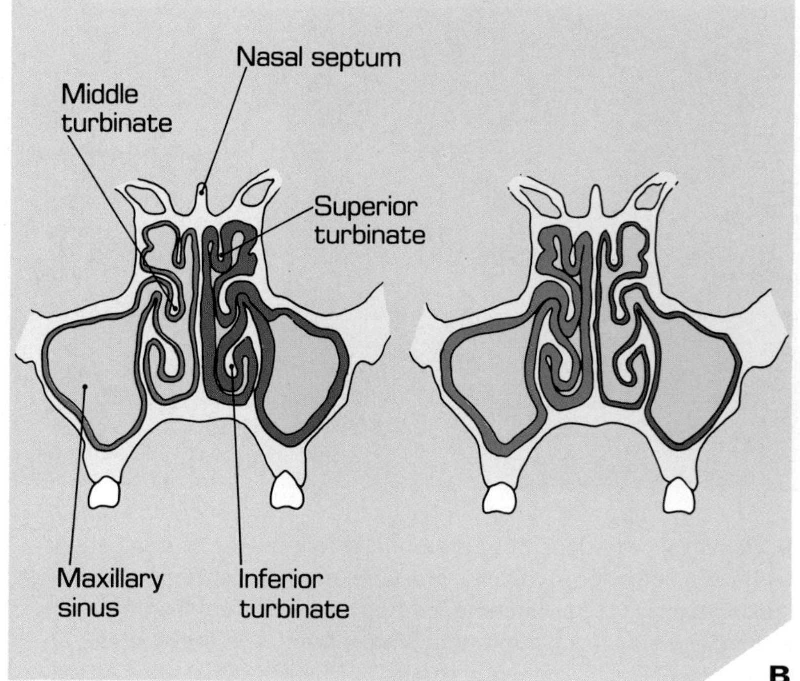

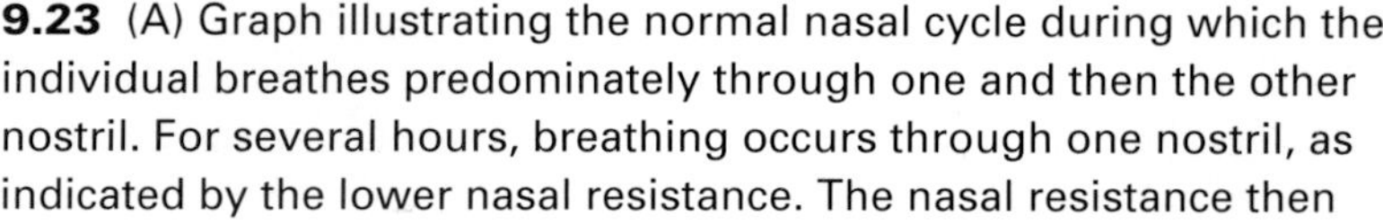
9.23 (A) Graph illustrating the normal nasal cycle during which the individual breathes predominately through one and then the other nostril. For several hours, breathing occurs through one nostril, as indicated by the lower nasal resistance. The nasal resistance then increases in that nostril, but decreases in the other, as the breathing cycles to the second nostril. (B) The alternating change in nasal airflow is accompanied by a functionally decreased nasal airway in one naris, and an increased airway in the other.

watery rhinorrhea and sneezing, resembles allergic rhinitis (9.25). Redness of the nasal mucosa is characteristic and, after several days, the purulent nasal discharge indicates infection. Demonstration of the predominance of neutrophils on a smear of nasal secretions (*see* 9.20) confirms this impression, but remember that nasal infections can be superimposed on allergic rhinitis.

Obstructions

Nasal obstruction and purulent rhinorrhea can also occur with foreign objects in the nares (9.26), but the unilateral symptoms differentiate this from allergic or infectious rhinitis. Beside nasal polyps (*see* 9.15), causes of unilateral nasal obstruction include deviation of the nasal septum (9.27) or neoplasm; both are detectable on

DIFFERENTIAL DIAGNOSIS OF CHRONIC RHINITIS AND NASAL OBSTRUCTION	
Rhinitis	**Other causes of nasal obstruction**
1. Allergic rhinitis: seasonal or perennial	1. Rhinosinusitis
2. Infectious rhinitis: chronic or acute (frequent recurrences)	2. Anatomical abnormality (e.g., deviated septum, enlarged adenoids)
3. Obstructive foreign body	3. Nasal polyps
4. Rhinitis secondary to topical decongestants, rhinitis medicamentosa	4. Tumor (e.g., angiofibroma)
5. Non-allergic rhinitis with eosinophilia (NARES)	5. Cerebrospinal fluid leakage secondary to perforation of the cribriform plate by fracture or tumor
6. Non-allergic vasomotor rhinitis (cholinergic)	6. Granulomatous disorders (e.g., Wegener's granulomatosis, sarcoidosis)
7. Hormonal rhinitis: pregnancy or hypothyroidism	
8. Atrophic rhinitis	

9.24 Differential diagnosis of chronic rhinitis and nasal obstruction.

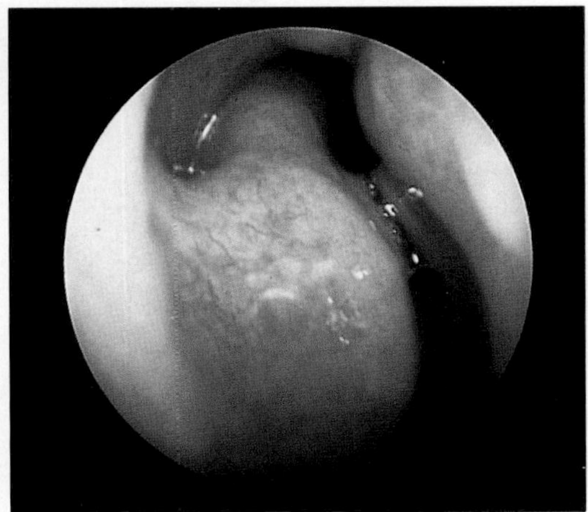

9.25 Clear, watery nasal secretions with swollen, reddish turbinates seen via fiberoptic rhinoscopy in a patient during the first few days of a viral rhinitis. Often the secretions become mucopurulent after several days.

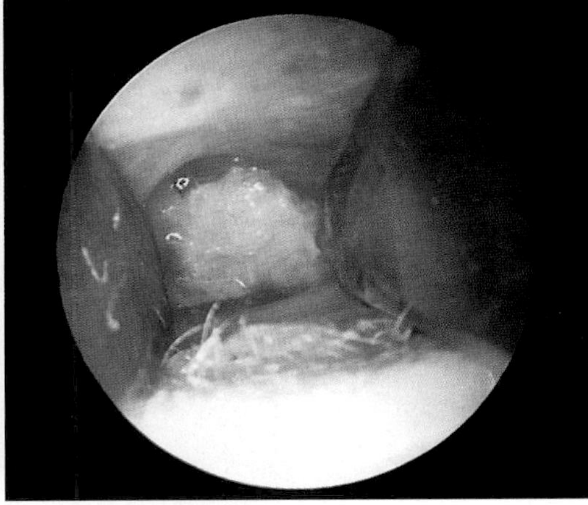

9.26 Yellow plastic foam lodged in a child's naris. This foreign body, which caused unilateral nasal obstruction and a mucopurulent discharge, could not be seen until a speculum was introduced into the nares to inspect the mucosa. (Photo courtesy of Dr. Sylvan Stool, Department of Otolaryngology, University of Pittsburgh School of Medicine.)

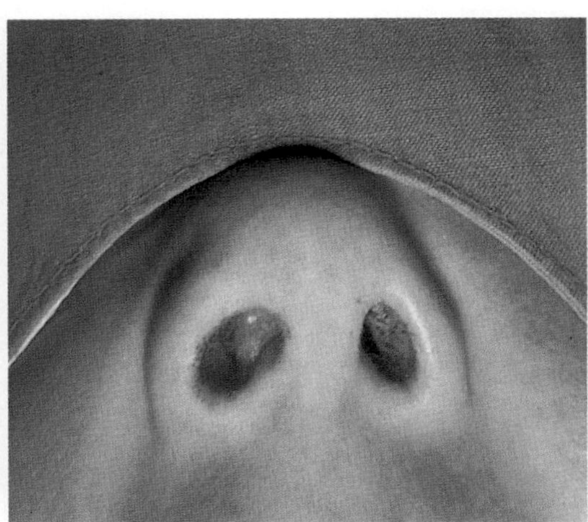

9.27 Deviation of the nasal septum. This condition can be seen on visual inspection of the nose. It frequently causes unilateral nasal obstruction. If severe, it can be corrected surgically. (Photo courtesy of Dr Sylvan Stool, Department of Otolaryngology, University of Pittsburgh School of Medicine.)

visual examination. Drugs such as reserpine can simulate allergic rhinitis and withdrawal establishes this diagnosis. The most common drug rhinopathy is rhinitis medicamentosa following administration of topical vasoconstrictors for more than 3–5 days. The mucosa becomes red and irritated, or pale and edematous. Other causes of nasal congestion include pregnancy, hypothyroidism, and non-allergic perennial rhinitis.

Allergic and non-allergic perennial rhinitis

The differential diagnosis between allergic and non-allergic perennial rhinitis can often be difficult. Non-allergic perennial rhinitis is more common in adults, and no immunologic etiology can be implicated. Allergy testing does not reveal a specific cause for the symptoms. In non-allergic rhinitis, the edematous mucous membranes are often pale with watery secretions, but contain no eosinophils. When eosinophilia is present, the syndrome is diagnosed as non-allergic rhinitis with eosinophilia (NARES). Vasomotor rhinitis is a vague category of chronic non-allergic nasal disease typically seen in adult women. These patients seem to have unusual awareness of their symptoms and complain of over-responsiveness of the nose to minimal changes of temperature, humidity, and odors. Immunotherapy (hyposensitization) is not to be used in these diseases, and drug therapy with antihistamine decongestants controls the symptoms inconsistently. Intranasal ipratropium or steroids may benefit some of these patients. A comparison of these different types of rhinitis is made in **9.28**.

COMPARISON OF ALLERGIC AND NON-ALLERGIC RHINITIS

	Allergic	**Non-Allergic**	
History		**NARES**	**Vasomotor**
Occurrence:	Seasonal, perennial	Perennial	Perennial
Age:	Children, adults	Mostly adults	Mostly adults
Sex:	Male, female	Male, female	Mostly female
Physical exam			
Edema:	Moderate, marked	Moderate	Moderate
Secretions:	Watery	Watery	Mucoid, watery
Lab tests			
Nasal eosinophils:	Common	Common	Coincidental
Allergen tests:	Positive	Coincidental	Coincidental
Therapy			
Antihistamines:	Beneficial	Rarely help	Rarely help
Decongestants:	Helpful	Sometimes help	Sometimes help
Steroids:	Beneficial	Helpful	Rarely help
Cromolyn:	Beneficial	Not helpful	Not helful
Ipratropium:	Not helpful	Not studied	Helpful
Immunotherapy:	Beneficial	Not indicated	Not indicated

9.28 Comparison of allergic and non-allergic rhinitis, including non-allergic rhinitis with eosinophilia (NARES) and vasomotor rhinitis.

THERAPY

Successful therapy of allergic rhinitis involves three general considerations (**9.29**):

- Identification and avoidance of the specific allergens and contributory factors.
- Pharmacologic management both to reduce and prevent symptoms.
- Immunotherapy to alter the patient's response to the allergen.

IDENTIFICATION AND AVOIDANCE

When feasible, avoidance of the allergen is the single best therapy for allergic rhinitis. Elimination of animal dander by elimination of a feather pillow or removal of a pet from the house may provide significant relief. Avoidance of more ubiquitous allergens, such as dusts, molds, and pollens, is much more difficult. House-dust mite control measures, particularly in the patient's bedroom, should include the use of airtight mattresses and box spring covers, and removal of dust collectors, such as stuffed toys, bookshelves, drapery, and hair carpet underpads wherever possible. Thorough weekly cleaning and vacuuming can reduce house dust. Electrostatic precipitrons installed in central forced-air heating and cooling systems can reduce house dust, pollens, and other airborne particles. HEPA filters are most effective, but are more expensive. Because single-room electrostatic precipitron units are less effective and may generate irritating ozone, they are not recommended. High temperatures, such as hot water (>130°F) during washing, decrease the house-dust mite antigen. This also occurs on exposure to sunlight for several hours. The role of denaturing agents, such as tannic acid, and acaricides, such as benzyl benzoate, in the management of house-dust mite allergy still requires better definition.

Patients who are very sensitive to grass pollens should try to avoid increased exposure during gardening, grass cutting, and camping. Room air-conditioners, which recirculate the air, can also effectively reduce pollen in a closed bedroom. Mold-sensitive patients should be instructed that seasonal outdoor molds thrive in compost, dead leaves, and cut vegetation. Damp basements and wallpaper, as well as bathrooms, are often sources of storage molds—reduction of moisture eliminates mold proliferation. If moisture cannot be eliminated, mold retardants can be incorporated into house paints. Molds in damp basements can be reduced by aerosolized paraformaldehyde or other antifungals.

THERAPY OF ALLERGIC RHINITIS: GENERAL CONSIDERATIONS

1. **Avoidance**
   Specific allergens
   Non-specific factors
2. **Pharmacologic management**
   Reverse symptoms
   Prevent symptoms
3. **Immunotherapy (hyposensitization)**
   Prevent symptoms

9.29 Major facets of therapy for allergic rhinitis.

Environmental control measures frequently require that patients modify their life-styles. Unfortunately, many patients do not have the enthusiasm, resources, or motivation to carry out avoidance procedures to better control their symptoms. The availability of effective modalities, as described below, provides additional therapeutic options (9.30).

PHARMACOLOGIC MANAGEMENT

Since most patients cannot completely avoid allergens, their symptoms are treated with drugs. Antihistamines are preferred for treating mild-to-moderatre allergic rhinitis. The antihistamines work by competing with histamine for the H_1 receptors carried on a variety

ALLERGIC RHINITIS: MANAGEMENT AND THERAPEUTIC OPTIONS

Management	Examples	Advantages	Disadvantages
Environmental control	Removal of dust, pet hair, dander, feathers, etc.	Few or no side effects; moderate expense	Labor intensive; poor compliance
Antihistamines	Chlorpheniramine, terfenadine, loratadine cetirizine	Orally active; relief of nasal and ocular symptoms with a single agent; relief of pruritus, sneezing	Side effects vary; little relief of nasal obstruction; terfenadine, astemizole, and loratidine are non-sedating, but expensive
Topical decongestants	Phenylephrine, oxymetazoline	Rapid relief of obstruction	Rebound congestion; rhinitis medicamentosa
Oral decongestants	Pseudoephedrine	Relief of obstruction	Tachyphylaxis; sympathomimetic side effects; risky for certain conditions
Topical steroids	Beclomethasone, flunisolide, triamcinolone, budesonide fluticasone	Few known side effects; relief of pruritus, sneezing, obstruction, secretions	Expensive; stinging and dryness can occur with some agents; parental resistance to steroid use; takes several days to two weeks to work
Systemic steroids	Prednisone	Effective in severe rhinitis	Risks almost always exceed benefits achieved with topical steroids (intranasal)
Cromolyn sodium		Few known side effects; relief of symptoms by prevention of mast cell degranulation	Expensive; may be needed as often as 4–6 times a day; best used before season
Immunotherapy		Most effective in seasonal allergic rhinitis; usually reduces medication requirements	Expensive and time-consuming; potential for severe reactions

9.30 Management and therapeutic options in allergic rhinitis, (Adapted with permission from Salter and Kaliner, 1989.)

of endothelial, epithelial, and tissue-cell membranes. There are several groups of antihistamines, which differ from each other in chemical structure and in action. Since the efficacy of one may diminish after months or years of use, a patient may eventually require another antihistamine from a different group. Therefore, the clinician should become familiar with representative antihistamines. The effectiveness of antihistamines, such as chlorpheniramine or any of its several equivalents, can be offset by their side effects, which include drowsiness, headache, and restlessness. Patients who become drowsy after taking antihistamines should be warned against driving an automobile or operating machinery. They are candidates for terfenadine, astemizone, or loratadine, newer non-sedating antihistamines, which do not cross the blood–brain barrier. Astemizole has a longer duration of action than terfenadine or loratadine, and is used once daily (which is also the dose for loratadine).

9.31 lists selected antihistamine formulations and dosages. There are two major groups, sedating (classical or first generation) and non-sedating antihistamines (second generation). These antihistamines have important drug interactions. The sedating antihistamines, which cross the blood–brain barrier, can potentiate the effects of psychotropic and sedative medications, such as barbiturates, narcotics, and diazepan, as well as alcohol; therefore, these are contraindicated in many skilled occupations, such as pilots, drivers, etc. Rarely, the second-generation H_1-antagonists, terfenadine and astemizole, may cause fatal or near-fatal cardiovascular events through overdosage. Concomitant administration of terfenadine or astemizole with antifungal medications, such as ketoconazole or itraconazole, or with macrolide antibiotics, such as erythromycin, clarithromycin, or troleandomycin, or other medications that inhibit the hepatic oxygenase P-450 cytochrome system may prolong the cardiac QTc interval or cause ventricular tachycardia (torsade de

FORMULATIONS AND DOSAGES OF REPRESENTATIVE H_1-RECEPTOR ANTAGONISTS

H_1-receptor antagonist	Formulation	Recommended dose[a]
First generation		
Chlorpheniramine	Tablets: 4 mg, 8 mg[b], 12 mg[b] Syrup: 2.5 mg/5 ml Parenteral solution: 10 mg/ml	Adult: 8–12 mg 2 × day[c] Child: 0.35 mg/kg/24 hr
Hydroxyzine	Capsules: 25 mg, 50 mg Syrup: 10 mg/5 ml	Adult: 25–50 mg 2 × day (or once a day, at bedtime) Child: 2 mg/kg/24 hr
Diphenhydramine	Capsules: 25 mg, 50 mg Elixir: 12.5 mg/5 ml Syrup: 6.25 mg/5 ml Parenteral solution: 50 mg/ml	Adult: 25–50 mg 3 × day Child: 5 mg/kg/24 hr
Second generation		
Terfenadine	Tablets: 60 mg, 120 mg[d] Suspension: 30 mg/5 ml[d]	Adult: 60 mg 2 × day or 120 mg/day Child: 3–6 yr, 15 mg 2 × day; 7–12 yr, 30 mg 2 × day
Astemizole	Tablets: 10 mg Suspension: 10 mg/5 ml[d]	Adult: 10 mg/day Child: 0.2 mg/kg/day
Loratadine	Tablets: 10 mg Syrup: 1 mg/ml[d]	Adult: 10 mg/day Child: 2–12 yr, 5 mg/day; >12 yr and >30 kg, 10 mg/day
Cetirizine[d]	Tablets: 10 mg	Adult: 5–10 mg/day

[a]The dose for a child should be given if the patient weighs 40 kg (90 lb) or less.
[b]A tablet of this size is a timed-release formulation.
[c]The timed-release formulation should be given.
[d]Not approved for use in the United States at time of publication.

9.31 Formulations and dosages of representative H_1-receptor antagonists.

pointes). Such abnormal cardiac events have not been described for loratadine or cetirizine. Since terfenadine, astemizole, and loratadine are metabolized in the liver, these medications should be used with caution, with reduced dosages for patients with liver disease.

When nasal obstruction by secretions is prominent, an oral alpha-adrenergic decongestant, such as phenylephrine, phenylpropanolamine, or cyclopentamine, should be used individually or in combination with an antihistamine. To ascertain the most effective preparation, it may be necessary to employ one or more trials of an antihistamine or antihistamine–decongestant combination. Topical nasal alpha-adrenergic vasoconstrictors usually provide prompt symptomatic relief, but should not be used for more than several days. Many patients, after 7–10 days of treatment, develop so-called rebound vasodilation and, at times, habituation. It is necessary to discontinue nose drops to relieve this rhinitis medicamentosa.

If symptoms cannot be controlled with antihistamines, decongestants, and avoidance, then intranasal topical steroid therapy with beclomethasone, flunisolide, fluticasone, triamcinolone, or budesonide is appropriate. These agents are rapidly metabolized, with few side effects. Oral or parenteral corticosteroids are usually contraindicated. Topical agents achieve better compliance in adults than in children, perhaps because adults better tolerate the intranasal aerosol delivery system. Another useful intranasal topical aerosol is cromolyn, which inhibits mediator release from mast cells. It has gained widespread acceptance in recent years, and though less effective than steroids, should be considered in patients who require continuous, long-term therapy. It has fewer side effects than steroids. These intranasal anti-inflammatory medications and their recommended dosages are listed in 9.32.

INTRANASAL ANTI-INFLAMMATORY MEDICATIONS FOR ALLERGIC RHINITIS

Product	Formulation	Dosage
Steroids		
Beclomethasone	Aqueous MDI[a]	6 yrs and older: 1 or 2 sprays/nostril 2 times a day 12 yrs and older: 1 spray/nostril 2–4 times a day 6 to 12 years: 1 spray/nostril 3 times a day
Budesonide	MDI[a]	6 yrs and older: 4 sprays/ nostril once a day or 2 sprays/nostril 2 times a day
Flunisolide	Aqueous	12 yrs and older: 2 sprays/nostril once a day
Fluticasone	Aqueous	12 yrs and older: 2 sprays/nostril once a day
Triamcinolone	MDI[a]	
Cromolyn	Aqueous	6 yrs and older: 1 spray/nostril 3–4 times a day

[a]MDI, metered-dose inhaler.

9.32 Intranasal anti-inflammatory medications for allergic rhinitis.

IMMUNOTHERAPY

When symptomatic drug therapy and avoidance cannot control symptoms, immunotherapy (hyposensitization) should be considered. Several double-blind, controlled studies have shown immunotherapy to be 80% effective in reducing the symptoms of seasonal (**9.33**), as well as perennial allergic rhinitis. The patient's symptoms should closely correlate with the presence of specific IgE antibodies. Positive allergy tests that do not confirm the clinical presentation are false-positive reactions, and contribute to unnecessary and unsuccessful immunotherapy.

After the decision is made to initiate immunotherapy, the magnitude of the local skin reaction should be a guide to determining the initiating dose of allergen. This author does not agree with suggestions that immunotherapy can be initiated based on the results of *in vitro* serum IgE antibody. Not only does this hypothesis lack adequate documentation and clinical confirmation, but it also promotes provision of clinical care by non-physician health providers who do not see or examine the patient. End-point titration skin testing has also been recommended as a guide for initiation of immunotherapy, but this adds significantly to the cost of skin testing and requires more controlled documentation prior to acceptance.

The clinician begins with relatively weak subcutaneous injections of aqueous or alum-precipitated solutions of allergens. These are gradually increased in volume and concentration to the maximally tolerated dose as indicated by a moderate local reaction. A typical treatment protocol is outlined in **9.34.** It is imperative that the treatment does not induce systemic symptoms or provoke exacerbation of allergic rhinitis. After reaching the maximally tolerated dose, the time interval between injections is gradually increased

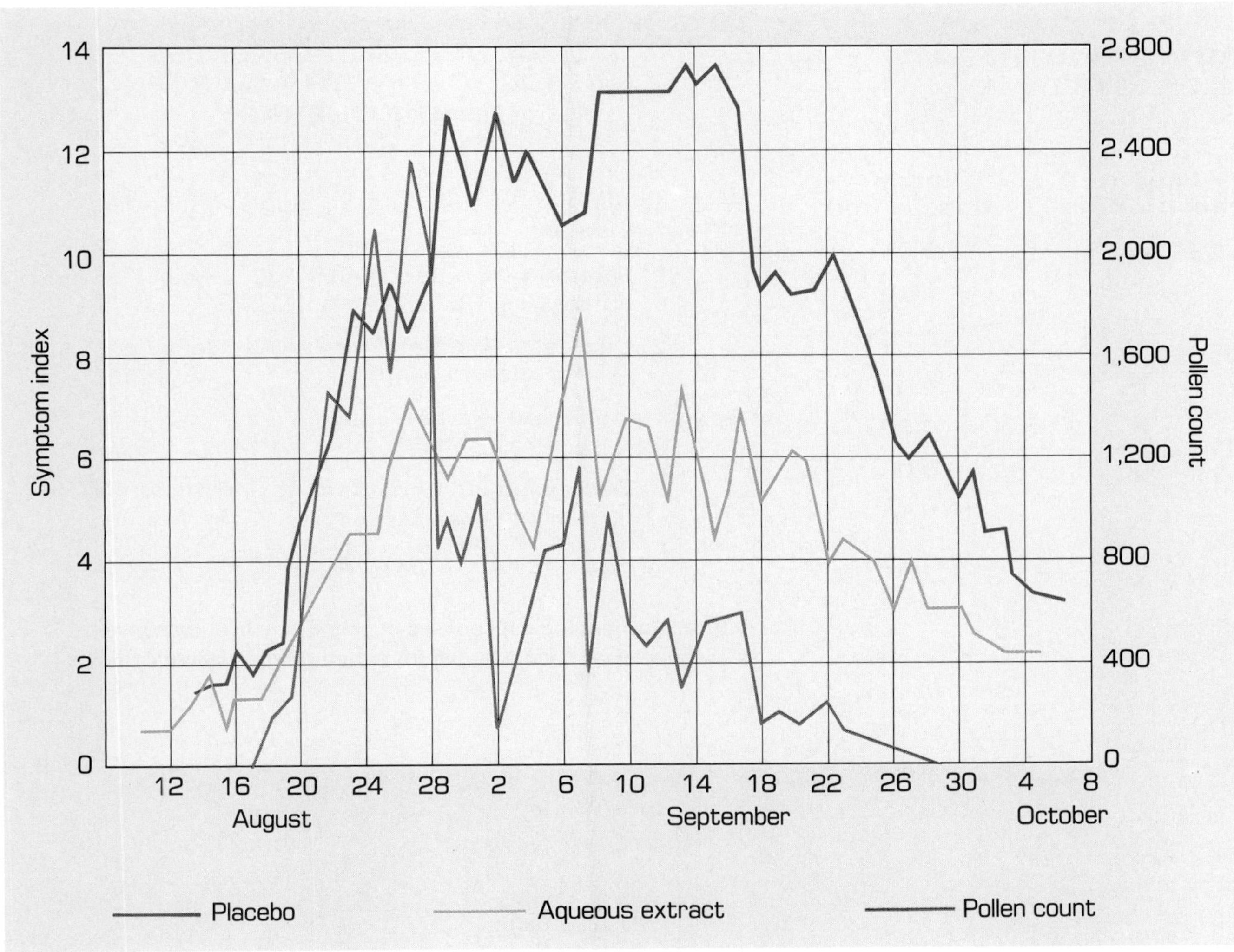

9.33 Typical results of several immunotherapy studies in patients with allergic rhinitis to ragweed pollen. Note the reduction of symptoms with aqueous extract immunotherapy as compared to placebo treatment. Also note the persistence of symptoms in allergic rhinitis patients for several weeks after subsidence of the pollen counts. (Modified with permission from Norman, 1980.)

from weekly to biweekly to monthly. Treatment is given perennially for several years. 9.35 outlines several potential mechanisms behind immunotherapy, though it is not known precisely how immunotherapy promotes clinical improvement in allergic rhinitis.

Immunotherapy may be expected to provide significant clinical improvement in more than 80% of patients with pollen-induced allergic rhinitis. If improvement is not obtained after a 2-year trial, the patient should be re-evaluated and discontinuation of immunotherapy should be considered. The duration of immunotherapy injections in patients who achieve clinical benefits is dependent on the patient's overall clinical response. In response to clinical improvement, the patient should be given the opportunity to stop treatment after approximately 3–5 years of injections. Many children with allergic rhinitis tend to improve with age and time. They are not 'growing out' of the allergy, because improvement is not related to physical growth, but to an as yet undefined age-related phenomenon.

There is no place for immunotherapy with allergens that can be easily removed or avoided. This is especially true for food allergens. The use of animal danders for immunotherapy should be limited to those individuals, such as veterinarians, who cannot avoid exposure to animal allergens.

It has been claimed that immunotherapy in children for seasonal allergic rhinitis may reduce their chances of developing pollen-induced asthma, but this hypothesis is open to many questions and needs to be substantiated. In general, patients with seasonal allergic rhinitis are more responsive to immunotherapy than those with perennial allergic rhinitis. The factors responsible for clinical improvement are multiple. Certain patients have exacerbations of symptoms after a spontaneous or induced remission for several seasons, and immunotherapy can be reinstituted without complication. In general, the prognosis for allergic rhinitis is better than that for non-allergic rhinitis.

PERENNIAL IMMUNOTHERAPY DOSAGE SCHEDULE

Interval (date)	Allergen concentration	Volume dosage (ml)
Weekly	1:10,000[a]	0.05
"		0.10
"		0.20
"		0.40
"		0.50
"	1:1000	0.05
"		0.10
"		0.20
"		0.40
"		0.50

Progress from
1:100
↓
1:10 in similar sequence[b]

[a]Very sensitive patients should begin at 1:100,000; this situation is rare.
[b]When maximum tolerated allergen dose is achieved, begin q 2 weeks then gradually advance q 3 weeks and ultimately q 4 weeks.

9.34 Typical treatment schedule for perennial allergen injection immunotherapy of allergic rhinitis.

IMMUNOLOGIC RESPONSES ASSOCIATED WITH ALLERGEN IMMUNOTHERAPY

1. Allergen-specific blocking (IgG) antibodies increase
2. Rise and then decrease in IgE-specific antibodies
3. Decreased basophil histamine release in response to allergen
4. Increased allergen specific suppressor T-cells
5. Decreased lymphocyte-cytokine response to allergen

9.35 Immunologic responses or changes in host response associated with the allergen immunotherapy of allergic rhinitis.

REFERENCES

Druce HM: Allergic and non-allergic rhinitis, in Middleton E, Reed CE, Ellis EF, Yunningen JW, Busse WW (eds): *Allergy; Principles and Practice,* Mosby, St. Louis, p. 1433, 1993.

Fireman P: Allergic rhinitis, in Bluestone CD, Stool SE (eds): *Pediatric Otolaryngology*, W.B. Saunders, Philadelphia, pp 793–804, 1990.

Fireman P: Nasal provocation testing: an objective assessment for nasal and eustachian tube obstruction. *J Allergy Clin Immunol*, **8**:953–970, 1988.

Naclerio RM, Proud D, Togias AG, *et al.*: Inflammation mediators in late antigen-induced rhinitis. *N Engl J Med*, **313**:65, 1985.

Norman PS: An overview of immunotherapy: implications for the future. *J Allergy Clin Immunol*, **65**:87, 1980.

Simmons FER: Allergic rhinitis: recent advances. *Pediatr Clin North Am*, Saunders, Philadelphia, **35**:1053, 1988.

Simmons FER, Simmons JK: Antihistamine therapy. *N Engl J Med*, **330**:1662, 1994.

Slater JE, Kaliner MA: Allergic rhinitis. *Am J Asthma Allergy*, **2**:101–106, 1989.

CHAPTER 10

Sinusitis

Raymond G. Slavin

Infection of the paranasal sinuses is an extremely common and often unappreciated medical condition in both children and adults. Statistics derived from the US Department of Health and Human Services indicate the prevalence of chronic sinusitis in 1981 to be greater than 31 million people. In this chapter, we discuss the structure and function of the paranasal sinuses, how they protect themselves from infection, and how general and local conditions may predispose an individual to sinusitis. The clinical presentation of sinusitis may be quite subtle and, therefore, the clinician must have a high diagnostic index of suspicion. In this chapter, clinical symptoms, physical findings, and diagnostic aids, particularly radiography, are placed in perspective. Appropriate medical therapy, including antibiotics, is generally effective in treating sinusitis, but in resistant cases, surgical intervention is necessary, and a variety of operative procedures are described. Finally, a complication of sinusitis, namely bronchial asthma, is discussed.

STRUCTURE AND FUNCTION

The paranasal sinuses are four paired structures that surround the nasal cavities (**10.1**). On the lateral side of the nose, each sinus has an opening or ostium through which drainage occurs. The anatomy of the maxillary sinus is pertinent in terms of its high incidence as a site of infection. As can be seen in **10.2**, the floor of the maxillary sinus is part of the tooth-bearing area of the maxilla and is below

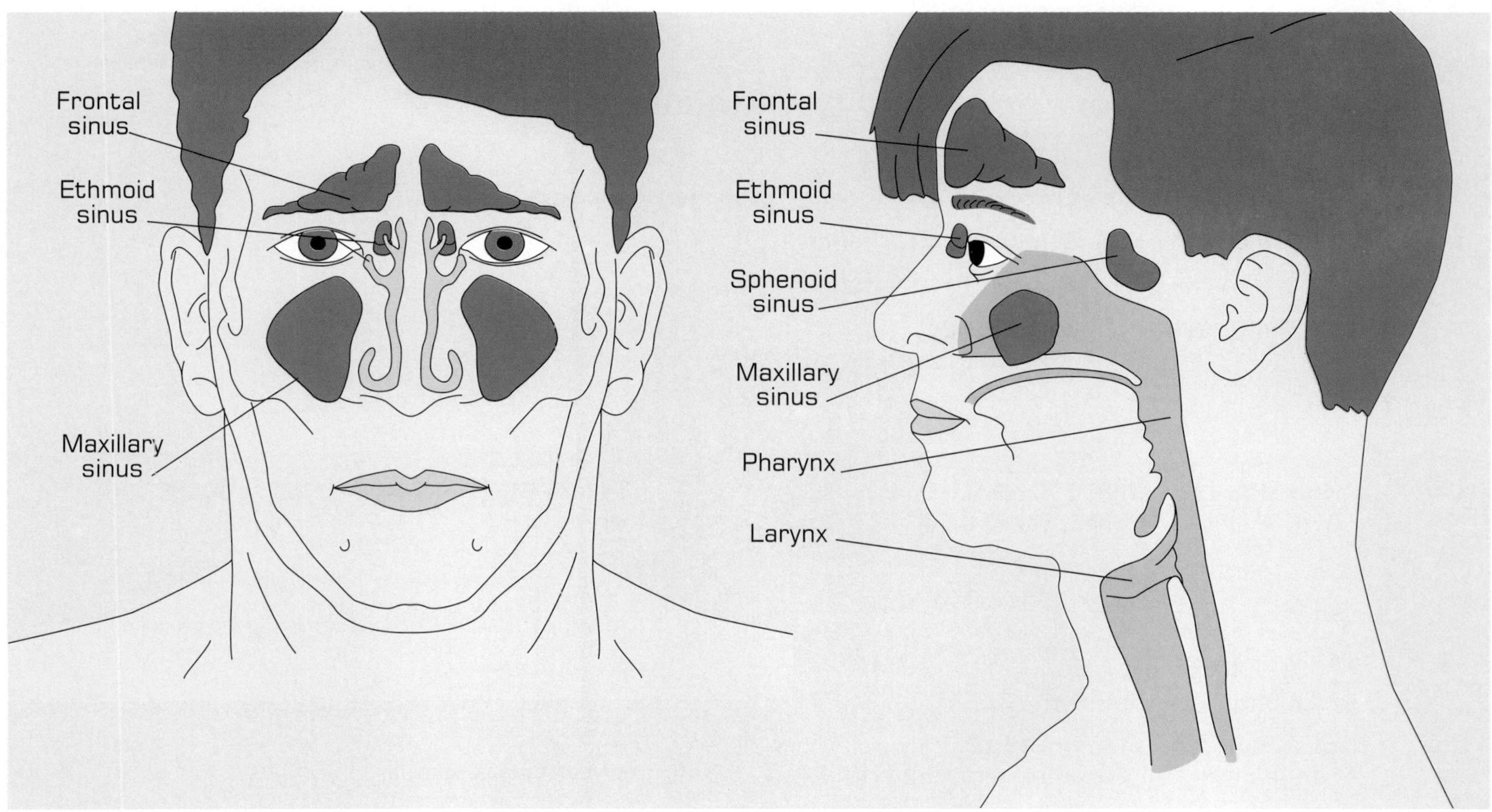

10.1 Frontal and lateral views of the head showing placement of the paranasal sinuses.

the floor of the nasal cavity in adults. The maxillary sinus ostium opens into the middle meatus between the middle and inferior turbinates and is located in a superior, rather than dependent, position on the nasal lateral wall. Thus, drainage from the maxillary sinus is anatomically inhibited.

The paranasal sinuses form as invaginations of the mucous membrane of the nasal cavity, so the mucous lining of the sinuses contains the same ciliated pseudostratified columnar epithelium, with goblet cells, as the nose.

10.3 shows the development of the paranasal sinuses. Especially important in terms of the diagnosis of sinusitis in children is the fact that the maxillary and ethmoid sinuses are radiographically evident in infancy.

The precise functions of the paranasal sinuses are not clear. Some suggestions have included roles in olfaction, voice response, production of protective mucus, dampening of sudden pressure changes in the nose during respiration, and lessening of skull weight (10.4).

PROTECTION AGAINST INFECTION

While secretory immunoglobulins and lysosomes play some role in the protection of the sinuses against infection, the major defense mechanism is an active mucociliary apparatus (10.5). Microorganisms and foreign particles that escape the filtering mechanism in the nose are trapped in the mucus of the sinuses. The underlying cilia then propel the mucus blanket or layer out of the sinus cavity

10.2 Sagittal section through a cadaver head showing the maxillary ostium on the medial wall of the maxillary sinus above its floor. (Courtesy of Dr. Margaret H. Cooper, St. Louis University School of Medicine.)

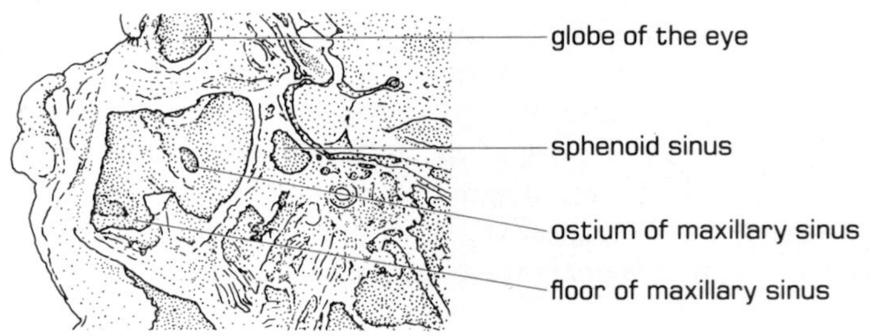

DEVELOPMENT OF THE PARANASAL SINUSES

	Anatomic appearance	Radiographic appearance
Maxillary	3rd to 5th prenatal month	Infancy
Ethmoid	3rd to 5th prenatal month	Infancy
Frontal	6th to 12th postnatal month	3rd to 7th year of life
Sphenoid	3rd year of life	9th year of life

10.3 Development of the paranasal sinuses.

POSSIBLE FUNCTIONS OF THE PARANASAL SINUSES

1. Olfaction
2. Voice response
3. Production of protective mucus
4. Dampening of sudden pressure changes in nose during respiration
5. Lessen skull weight

10.4 Possible functions of the paranasal sinuses.

PROTECTION AGAINST SINUSITIS

1. Mucus of the proper viscosity
2. Adequate numbers of actively beating cilia
3. Patent ostia

10.5 Protection against sinusitis.

through the ostium. Bacterial infection occurs when this self-cleansing mechanism becomes impaired. Mucus accumulates, stagnates, and becomes infected by relatively harmless, opportunistic bacteria that are normally present in the nose. Retention of secretions in the paranasal sinuses may be due to several different factors:

- Swelling of the mucous membrane of the nose leading to reduced patency of ostia.
- A quantitative reduction of cilia, retardation of ciliary movement, and insufficient coordination of cilia followed by reduced transport capacity.
- Overproduction of nasal secretions.

Patency of the ostium is the most important factor in the development of sinusitis. Decrease in size of the ostium results in a decline in sinus emptying time and gas exchange, thus leading to decreased oxygen tension, which in turn favors bacterial growth and purulence.

Returning now to the previous discussion of paranasal sinus anatomy, it is easy to see why maxillary sinusitis is so common. As noted, the base of the maxillary sinus (**10.2**) is below the floor of the nasal cavity in adults. The ostium, through which the maxillary sinus drains, is located in a superior position. Therefore, for discharge to occur into the nose in an upright position, the cilia of the maxillary sinus must move the mucous layer in a cephalid direction, against the force of gravity, to the draining ostium.

Given the mechanism that protects the sinuses against infection, it is now appropriate to look at **10.6** for a list of those conditions that may predispose an individual to sinusitis. Heading the list of local conditions are upper respiratory infection and allergic rhinitis. Both of these conditions result in edema of the nasal mucosa and obstruction of the ostium, with a decrease in sinus ciliary action. Mucus accumulates in the sinuses, and the stage is set for secondary bacterial infection and the conversion of mucus into mucopus. Mucopus further impairs ciliary function and increases the swelling around the ostium when it discharges into the nose, thus perpetuating a vicious cycle. There are also systemic factors that further serve to predispose an individual to sinusitis, such as cystic fibrosis.

MICROBIOLOGY OF SINUSITIS

Knowledge of the microbiologic picture in sinusitis (*see* **10.7**) has come from aseptic aspirates obtained by direct antral puncture or direct sampling during surgery. Nasal smears and cultures are so

FACTORS PREDISPOSING TO SINUSITIS

Local	Systemic
Upper respiratory infection	Immune deficiency
Allergic rhinitis	Cystic fibrosis
Overuse of topical decongestants	Bronchiectasis
Hypertrophied adenoids	Dysmotile cilia syndrome
Deviated nasal septum	
Nasal polyps	
Tumors	
Foreign bodies	
Swimming and diving	
Cigarette smoking	
Barotrauma	
Dental extraction and/or injections	

10.6 Factors predisposing a person to sinusitis (Slavin, 1988).

MICROBIOLOGY OF SINUSITIS

Acute	Chronic
Streptococcus pneumoniae	*Anaerobic streptococcus*
Haemophilus influenzae	*Bacteroides*
Branhamella catarrhalis	*Veillomella*
	Corynebacterium
	Staphylococcus aureus

10.7 Microbiology of sinusitis.

contaminated that they do not afford a meaningful picture of the microbiology of the sinuses.

DIAGNOSIS

The clinical presentation of sinusitis may be quite subtle; therefore, the clinician must maintain a high index of diagnostic suspicion. **10.8** shows the ways in which the diagnosis of sinusitis may be made.

Sinus infections are arbitrarily characterized by their duration as acute (up to three weeks), subacute (up to three months), and chronic (greater than three months). **10.9** displays the presenting findings in acute and chronic sinusitis.

DIAGNOSIS OF SINUSITIS

1, History
2. Physical examination
3. Nasal secretions
4. Fiberoptic rhinopharyngoscopy
5. Radiograph
6. CT scan
7. Ultrasound

10.8 Seven ways to diagnose sinusitis.

PRESENTING FINDINGS IN SINUSITIS

Acute	Chronic
Nasal obstruction	Nasal obstruction
Purulent nasal drainage	Purulent nasal and/or paranasal drainage
Fever	Coexistent otitis media (in children)
Facial pain	Hyposmia
	Fetid breath
	Sore throat
	Malaise
	Cough
	Wheeze

10.9 Presenting findings in sinusitis.

HISTORY AND PHYSICAL EXAMINATION

The most important clinical clue to the diagnosis of acute sinusitis is the failure of symptoms to resolve after a typical cold. The patient will note that nasal discharge that had previously been clear becomes yellow and green. Fever persists, chills may develop, and pain, more severe on bending or straining, is often felt in the cheek. On physical examination, thick purulent green or deep-yellow secretions are seen, most often in the middle meatus, which is the draining site of the maxillary sinus.

If mucopus is not evacuated, then acute sinusitis may enter a subacute or chronic phase. A patient's lack of pain or systemic symptoms makes the diagnosis of chronic sinusitis difficult for the physician to make on history alone. The patient with chronic sinusitis generally presents with nasal stuffiness, hyposmia, purulent nasal and postnasal secretions, sore throat, fetid breath, and malaise. On physical examination, an edematous and hyperemic nasal mucosa is generally bathed in mucopus.

DIAGNOSTIC TECHNIQUES

Nasal secretions

While nasal culture does not give an appropriate picture of the organisms responsible for sinusitis, microscopic examination of nasal secretions demonstrates sheets of polymorphonuclear neutrophils and bacteria. The recently introduced technique of fiberoptic nasopharyngoscopy (**10.10–10.12**) affords a splendid opportunity for better visualization of the draining ostia of infected sinuses and for obtaining specimens for culture.

Radiograph

The most common used adjunct in the diagnosis of sinusitis is radiography. The occipitomental, or Waters', view, with the head

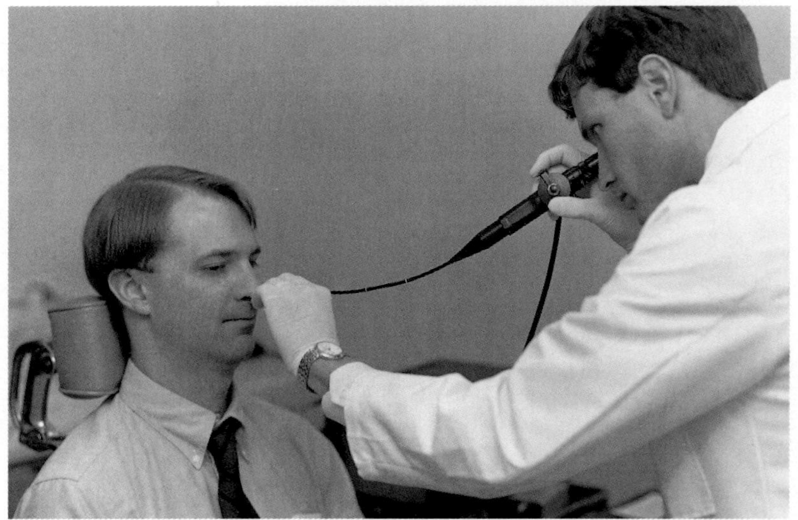

10.10 The fiberoptic nasopharyngoscope being inserted.

slightly tilted back, affords the best sight of the maxillary sinuses. The occipitofrontal, or Caldwell, view demonstrates both the ethmoid and frontal sinuses. The sphenoid sinus is seen on the lateral view. A normal Waters' view is shown in **10.13**, demonstrating the total radiolucency of the maxillary sinuses with a thin

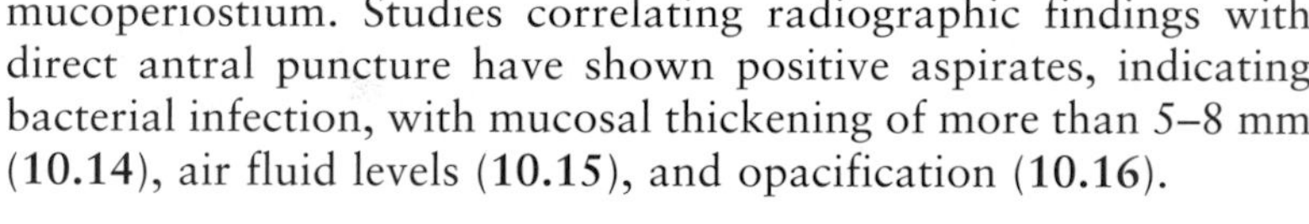

mucoperiostium. Studies correlating radiographic findings with direct antral puncture have shown positive aspirates, indicating bacterial infection, with mucosal thickening of more than 5–8 mm (**10.14**), air fluid levels (**10.15**), and opacification (**10.16**).

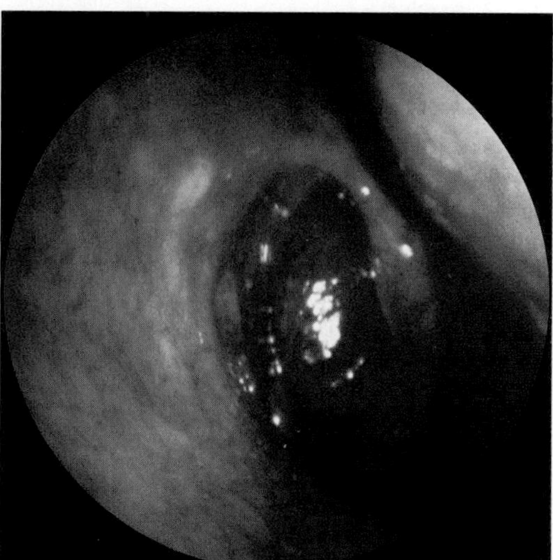

10.11 Endoscopic view of the left nostril. A large polyp arising from the hiatus semilunaris fills the anterior portion of the left middle meatus. (Courtesy of Dr David W. Kennedy, University of Pennsylvania.)

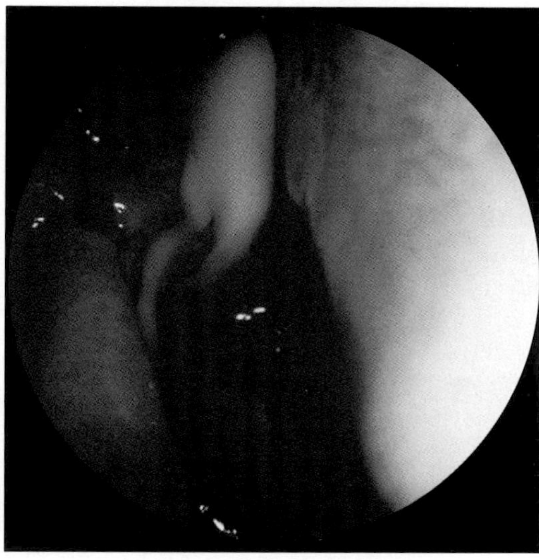

10.12 Endoscopic view of the left sphenoethmoidal recess. Pus is seen draining from the area of the sphenoid sinus ostium. (Courtesy of Dr David W. Kennedy, University of Pennsylvania.)

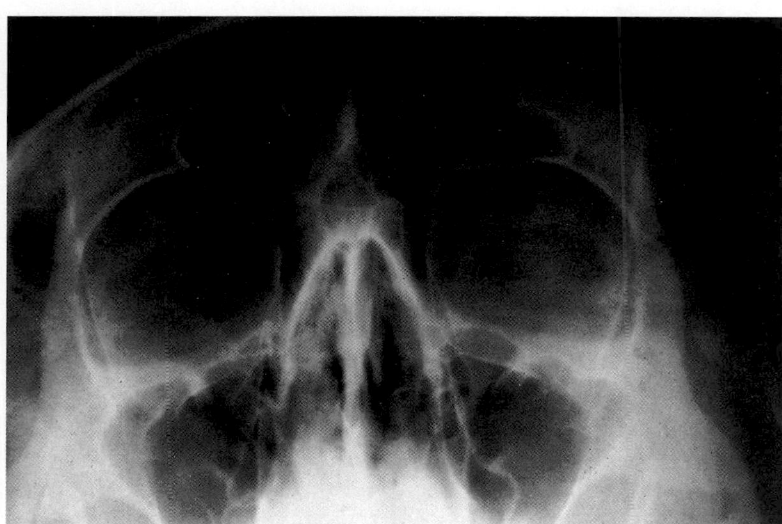

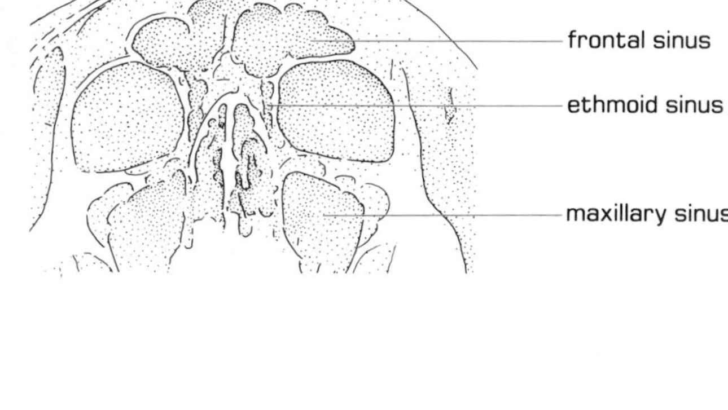

10.13 Waters' view of the paranasal sinuses. The maxillary sinuses are radiolucent and the mucoperiostium is thin.

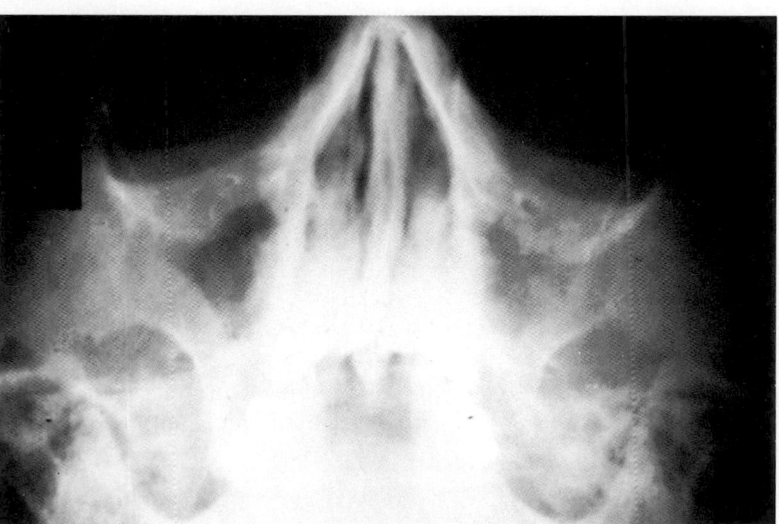

10.14 Waters' view of the sinuses. There is marked mucoperiostial thickening of both maxillary sinuses.

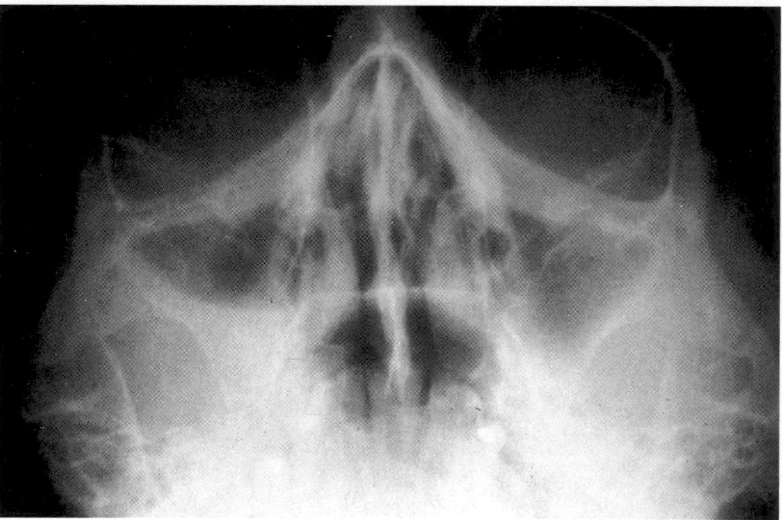

10.15 Waters' view of the sinuses. An air fluid level is seen in the right maxillary sinus.

Special mention should be made of sinus radiographs in children. Contrary to earlier belief, crying is not a cause of abnormal maxillary sinus radiographs in children older than one year of age; over that age, abnormal sinus radiographs are generally related to infection of the sinuses (Kovatch *et al.*, 1984).

Computed tomography (CT)

It has been suggested that pluridirectional tomography can delineate sinus disease more clearly than can plain radiography, revealing the extent of disease and bony destruction, and distinguishing opacification from membrane thickening (**10.17**). CT scans of patients with normal sinus radiographs often show areas of anterior ethmoidal disease (**10.18**). A four-slice coronal CT scan of the sinuses has been shown to be extremely effective in demonstrating sinusitis. The cost has been reduced so dramatically that, in the future, it will undoubtedly replace plain radiography in the diagnosis of sinusitis (**10.19**).

Ultrasonography

This technique, also termed ultrasound, has several significant advantages. It is relatively rapid and painless to perform, and it utilizes non-ionizing radiation. It has been found to be particularly useful in adults to diagnose fluid in the maxillary sinuses (**10.20**). However, it has some prohibitive disadvantages as well. Significant mucosal thickening may not be picked up by ultrasonography, and several studies have shown that this technique yields a high degree of false-positive and false-negative results. At the present time, ultrasound is not considered to be sufficiently accurate to be used as a substitute for radiography in diagnosing sinusitis.

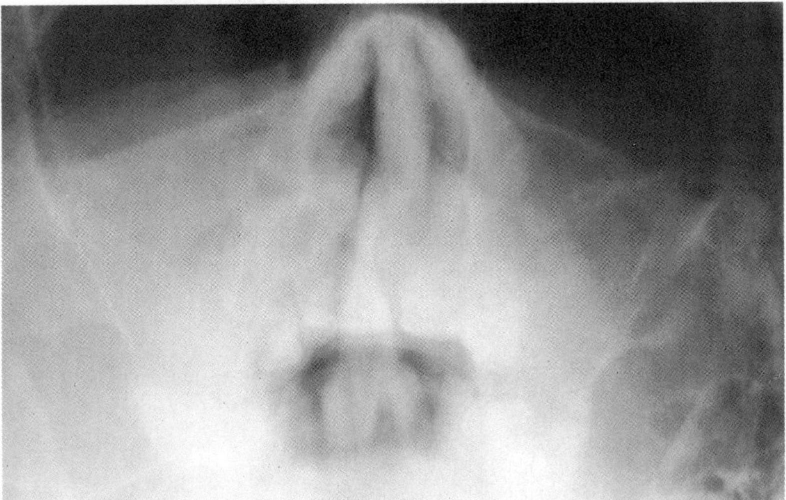

10.16 Waters' view of the sinuses. Both maxillary sinuses are opacified.

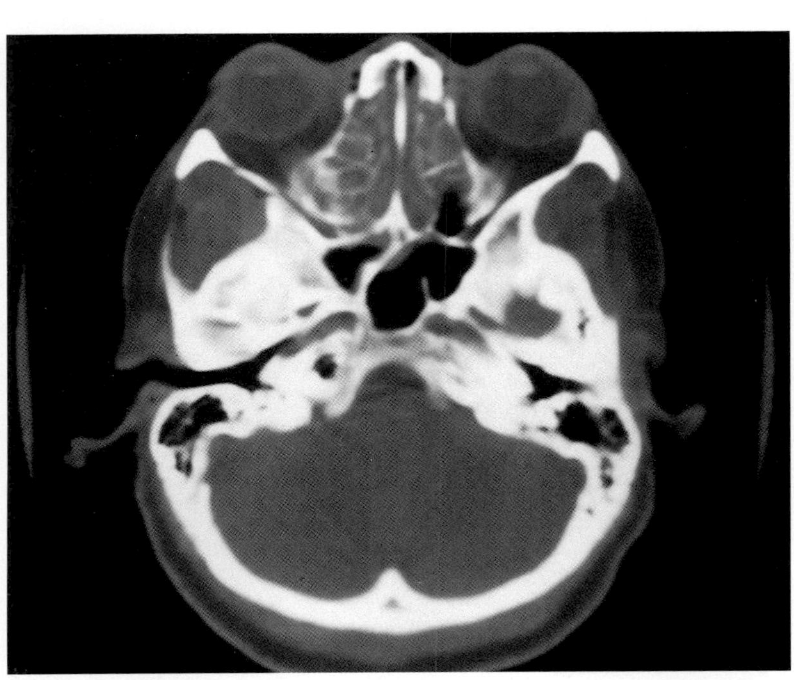

10.17 Transaxial CT scan. Both ethmoid sinuses are opacified.

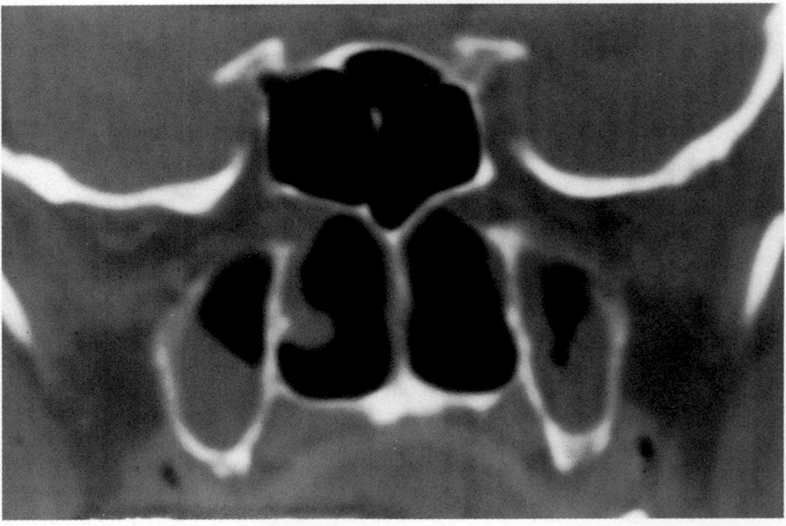

10.18 Coronal CT scan showing air fluid level in right maxillary sinus and marked mucoperiosteal thickening in the left maxillary sinus.

INDICATIONS FOR SINUS CT

1. Failure to respond to therapy
2. Negative radiographs despite persistent signs and symptoms
3. Demonstration of anatomic abnormalities
4. Localizing disease for possible surgery
5. Evaluation of infectious complications

10.19 Indications for sinus CT.

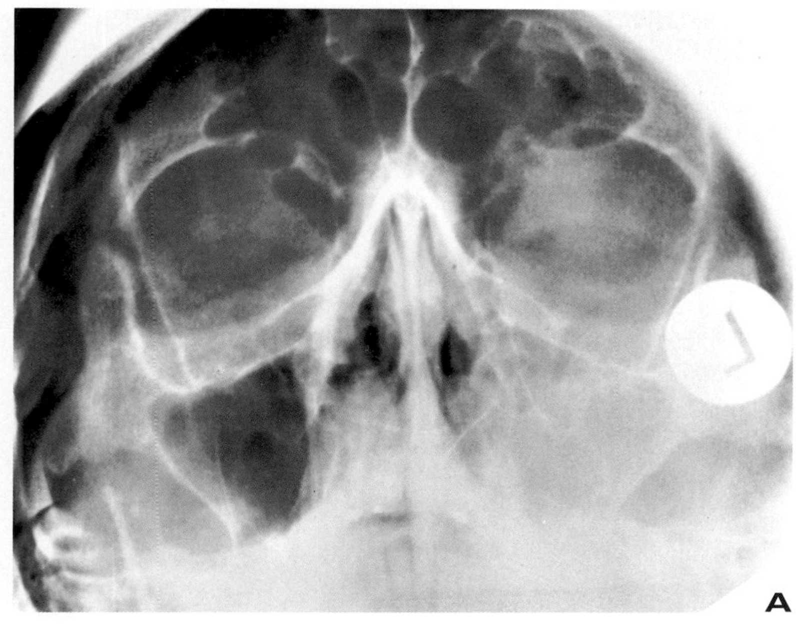

10.20 Radiograph and ultrasound tracings from a 36-year-old male patient with symptoms of facial pain, tenderness to touch on left side of cheek, and purulent discharge. (A) The radiograph shows a normal right maxillary antrum and an opacified left maxillary antrum. A-mode ultrasound tracings performed on the same day show (B) normal right maxillary sinus echoes and (C) the presence of an abnormal back-wall echo from the left maxillary sinus, indicating the presence of fluid. (Courtesy of Dr Howard M. Druce.)

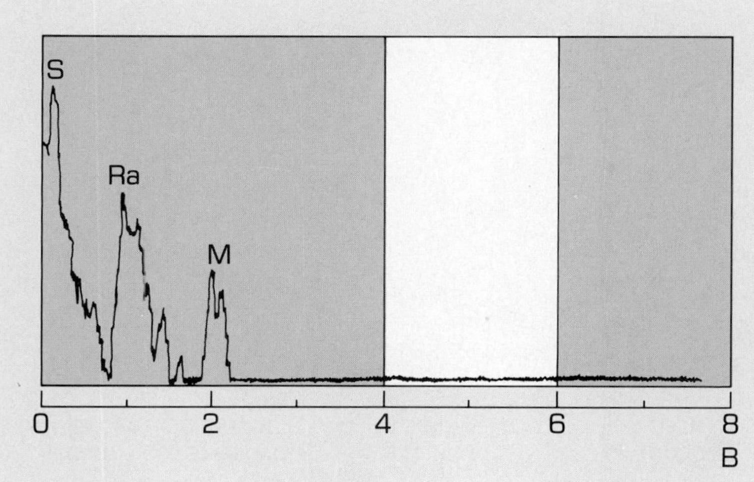

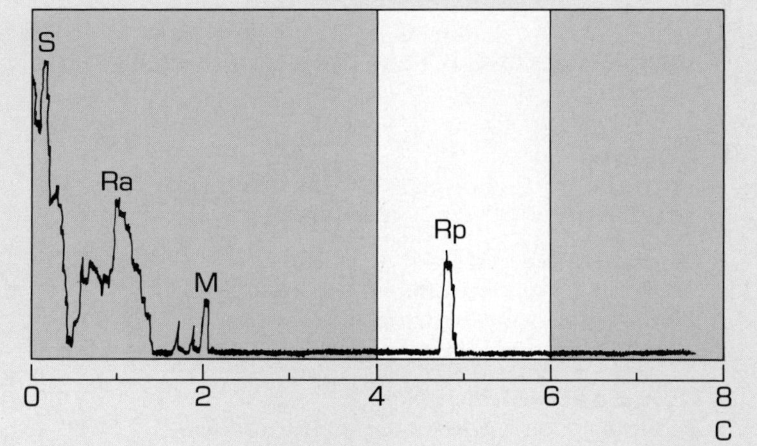

S = Sending pulse; through skin and muscle tissue

Ra = Recessus anterior; the anterior wall of the sinus cavity

M = Mucosa

Rp = Recessus posterior; the back wall of the sinus cavity

Ancillary laboratory tests

For resistant chronic sinusitis, other diagnostic tests must be considered. Humoral immune deficiency can be diagnosed by quantitation of serum immunoglobulins, specific antibody responses, and IgG subclasses. Underlying allergy can be determined by appropriate skin testing. Information on the causative pathogens of chronic sinusitis can only be gained by sinus aspirates, not by nasopharyngeal culture (**10.21**).

MEDICAL TREATMENT

Medical therapy of sinusitis includes analgesics, topical or oral decongestants, hot washcloths to the nasal area, steam inhalation, fluids, and antibiotics for the control of infection (**10.22**). Topical decongestants may help greatly in promoting sinus drainage, but may cause the so-called rebound phenomenon if used chronically. In this situation, the medication causes immediate vasoconstriction. After this subsides, the resultant vasodilation and consequent nasal congestion may exceed that which was present initially. Longer-acting preparations used in the prescribed fashion at 12 hour intervals do not cause the vasodilating rebound phenomenon over several days' usage. In some cases of hyperplastic rhinosinusitis, topical or systemic corticosteroids over a short period of time may be indicated. The antibiotic of choice for treatment of acute or chronic sinusitis is ampicillin or amoxicillin, for two reasons: first, the organisms responsible for both acute and chronic sinusitis are sensitive to these drugs; second, adequate mucosal and sinus fluid levels of these antibiotics is obtained. Trimethoprim with sulfamethoxazole may be used in cases of penicillin sensitivity. In many instances, bacteria responsible for sinusitis have become resistant to penicillin and cephalosporins by producing beta-lactamase enzymes that destroy the beta-lactam nucleus of these antibiotics. Clavulanic acid, an inhibitor of the beta-lactamase enzyme, has been introduced in

ANCILLARY LABORATORY TESTS FOR CHRONIC SINUSITIS

1. **Immunologic studies**

   Quantitative immunoglobulins

   Specific antibody responses: diphtheria, tetanus, pneumococcus

   IgG subclasses
2. **Allergy skin tests**
3. **Bacteriologic studies: antral puncture**

10.21 Ancillary laboratory tests for chronic sinusitis.

MEDICAL TREATMENT OF SINUSITIS

1. **Analgesics**
   Non-specific – fluids, rest, steam inhalation, hot washcloths to nasal area
2. **Decongestants**
   Topical – oxymetazoline, phenylephrine
   Oral – pseudoephedrine, phenylpropanolamine, phenylephrine
3. **Corticosteroids**
   Topical – beclomethasone, flunisolide, budesonide, fluticasone
   Oral – prednisone
4. **Antibiotics**
   Ampicillin or amoxicillin.
   Trimethoprim with sulfamethoxazole (in cases of penicillin sensitivity)

10.22 Medical treatment of sinusitis (Slavin, 1988).

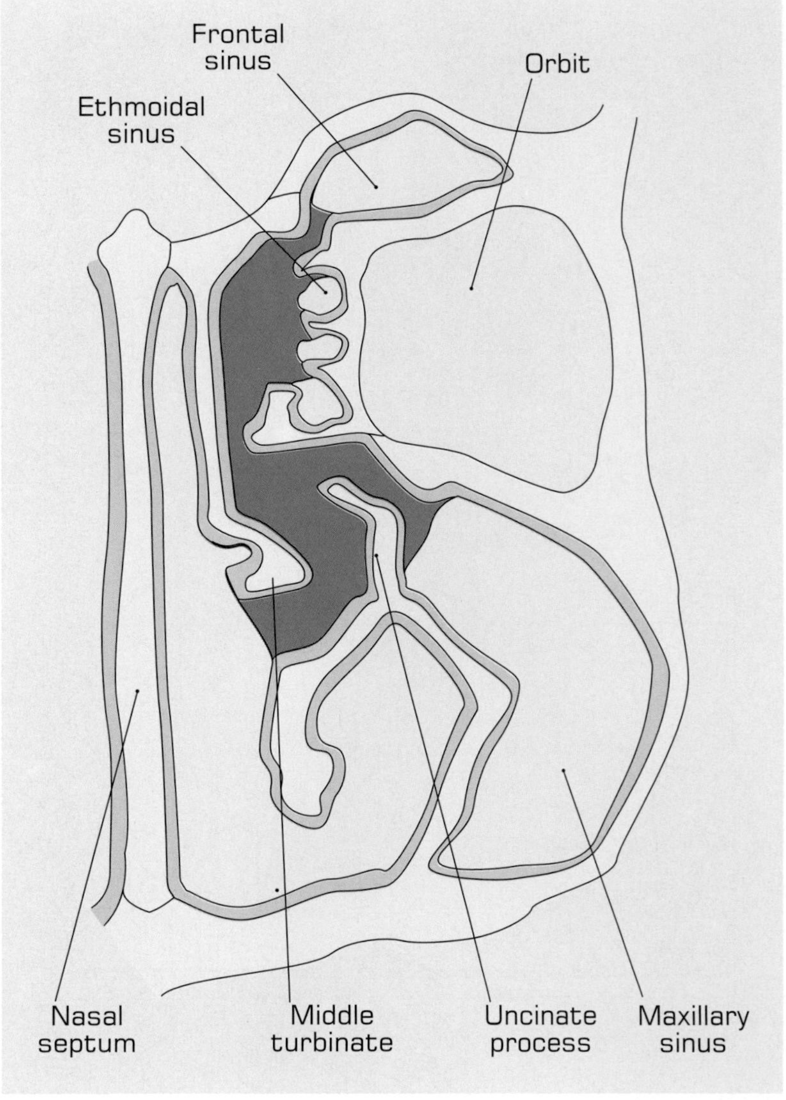

10.23 Coronal view showing osteomeatal unit (shaded dark pink) in relation to other structures. Blockage in this area leads to infection in frontal and maxillary sinuses.

combination with amoxicillin. Other antibiotics useful in infections due to beta-lactamase producing organisms are cefuroxime, cefprozil, clarithromycin, azithromycin, and loracarbef. The duration of treatment is as important as the choice of antibiotics: chronic recurrence of sinusitis is extremely high if therapy is for less than 3–4 weeks. Since the introduction of antibiotics, infectious complications of sinusitis (e.g., cellulitis, orbital abscess, cavernous sinus thrombosis, epidural or subepidural abscess, and osteomyelitis) have decreased markedly to the point of being rare.

SURGICAL TREATMENT

Persistent or recurrent episodes of sinusitis, despite appropriate medical therapy, necessitate consideration of surgical intervention. The tasks of the otolaryngologist are to relieve the obstruction of the ostia, resect inflamed or infected tissues, and provide an airway with drainage for all nasal and sinus compartments. A variety of surgical procedures have been utilized for the treatment of sinusitis, but functional endoscopic surgery has emerged as the technique of choice in most instances. The usefulness of the technique is predicated on the evidence that the middle meatus–anterior ethmoid complex (osteomeatal unit) is heavily involved in the pathogenesis of sinusitis (**10.23**). Infection generally begins in the ethmoid sinuses and persists if therapy is directed at other paranasal sinuses only. The availability of endoscopes with a variety of angles of view has greatly expanded the usefulness of this technique. Its advantage is that minimal trauma to the normal nasal sinus structures occurs with the conservative removal of disease, resulting in a quicker and more complete return to the natural physiology and mucociliary clearance and function of the sinuses.

An overall approach to the management of sinusitis is given in the flow diagram (**10.24**).

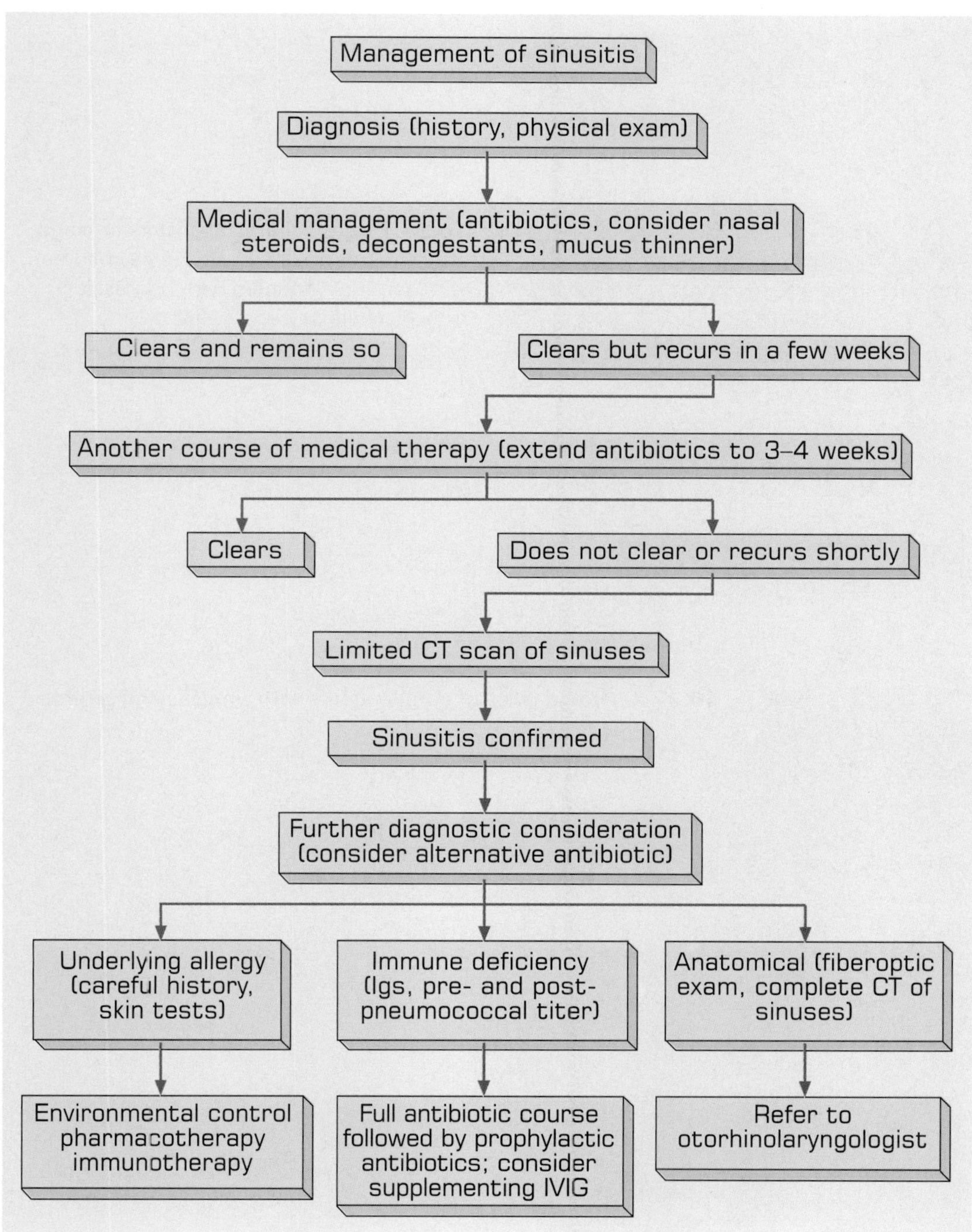

10.24 Management of sinusitis.

SINUSITIS AND ASTHMA

The relationship of nasal and paranasal sinus disease to bronchial asthma has been recognized for many years. Numerous observations have been made of the increased incidence of radiographically demonstrated sinusitis in both childhood and adult asthmatics (10.25). This, however, does not necessarily mean that there is a cause-and-effect relationship. A large number of studies performed both in experimental animals and humans have demonstrated that reflex bronchoconstriction can result from stimulation of receptors in the nose and nasopharynx. This could account for the clinical association of sinusitis and asthma.

This association has been examined both in children and adults. Rachelefsky *et al.* (1984), in a study of 48 children with sinusitis

ASSOCIATION OF SINUSITIS AND ASTHMA

Investigator	Year	Population	Percentage of radiograph abnormalities
Welle	1936	Adults	60
Berman	1974	Adults	52
Adinoff	1983	Children	52
Zimmerman	1987	Children	31
Fuller	1990	Children	75

10.25 Association of sinusitis and asthma.

DISEASE CHARACTERISTICS BEFORE AND AFTER TREATMENT FOR SINUSITIS IN 48 CHILDREN WITH ASTHMA

Characteristic	Before (%)	After (%)
Cough	100	29
Wheeze	100	15
Normal PFT	0	67
Bronchodilator use	100	21

10.26 Disease characteristics before and after treatment for sinusitis in 48 children with asthma. (Adapted with permission from Rachelefsky *et al.*, 1984.)

CHARACTERISTICS OF ADULT PATIENTS WITH SINUSITIS AND ASTHMA

1. Sinusitis preceded asthma in more than 90%.
2. Two-thirds were non-atopic based on history and skin tests.
3. More than half were aspirin sensitive.
4. More than half were receiving corticosteroids.
5. Two-thirds noted improvement in their asthmatic state after medical and/or surgical treatment of sinusitis.

10.27 Characteristics of adult patients with sinusitis and asthma.

and asthma, showed that 70% were able to discontinue taking bronchodilators after resolution of their sinusitis through antimicrobial therapy (**10.26**).

Our own studies have dealt largely with an adult population. Characteristics of adult patients with sinus disease and asthma are seen in **10.27**. In the great majority of cases, asthma historically followed the occurrence of sinusitis. Most of the patients were non-atopic and more than half were sensitive to aspirin. A clinical clue to the association of sinusitis and asthma is steroid dependency, and this should prompt the clinician to consider underlying sinusitis.

EFFECTS 5 YEARS AFTER SINUS SURGERY ON CLINICAL SYMPTOMATOLOGY IN ADULTS WITH SINUSITIS AND ASTHMA

Symptom improvement	Decrease in asthma medication
Asthma, 60%	60%
Nasal and/or sinus, 81%	

10.28 Effects 5 years after sinus surgery on clinical symptomatology in adults with sinusitis and asthma (Mings *et al.*, 1988).

Following surgical therapy for medically resistant sinusitis, 60% of the patients noted improvement in their asthmatic state, with 81% experiencing improvement in their nasal and/or sinus symptoms. Also, 60% were able to decrease asthma medications, including systemic corticosteroids (**10.28**).

In summary, there is no question as to the increased co-existence of sinusitis and bronchial asthma. There does seem to be suggestive evidence, both in children and adults, that medical or surgical therapy of sinusitis results in significant improvement in the asthmatic state. In any instance of corticosteroid-dependent asthma, consideration should be given to underlying sinusitis.

REFERENCES

Friedman WH, Slavin RG: Diagnosis and medical and surgical treatment of sinusitis in adults. *Clin Rev Allergy,* **2**:409, 1984.

Kennedy DW: Functional endoscopic sinus surgery. *Arch Otolaryng*, **111**:576, 1985.

Kovatch AL, Wald ER, Ledesma-Medina J. *et al.*: Maxillary sinus radiographs in children with non-respiratory complaints. *Pediatrics*, **73**:306, 1984.

Mings R, Friedman WH, Linford P, Slavin RG: Five-year follow-up of the effects of bilateral intranasal sphenoethmoidectomy in patients with sinusitis and asthma. *Am J Rhinol*, **71**:123, 1988

Rachelefsky GS, Katz RM, Siegel SC: Chronic sinus disease with associated reactive airway disease in children. *Pediatrics*, **73**:526, 1984.

Slavin RG: Relationship of nasal disease and sinusitis to bronchial asthma. *Ann. Allergy*, **49**:76, 1982.

Slavin RG: Nasal polyps and sinusitis, in Middleton E Jr, Reed CE, Ellis EF, Adkinson NF Jr, Yuninger JW (eds): *Allergy: Principles and Practice*, C.V. Mosby, St Louis, Chapter 54, 1988.

CHAPTER 11

Otitis Media

Philip Fireman

Otitis media is a very common disease characterized by an acute or chronic inflammation of the middle-ear mucosa, and is frequently associated with an upper respiratory tract infection. It is often followed by the development of an effusion within the middle ear. Otitis media with effusion (OME) may be a recurrent or chronic condition and is frequently recognized as a sequela of acute otitis media. OME may also be diagnosed on routine examination as an occult condition, perhaps following a subclinical or protracted inflammation of the middle ear. It occurs most commonly in infants and children under 4 years of age, but can be a problem in all age groups. Many synonyms have been used during the past 50 years to designate OME, including serous otitis media, secretory otitis media, mucoid otitis, 'glue ear', non-suppurative otitis media, catarrhal otitis, tubotympanic catarrh, and allergic otitis media. These descriptive terms have created much confusion. It is difficult to determine by history and visual inspection of the tympanic membrane alone the specific characteristics of a middle-ear effusion. Without a diagnostic aspiration, the clinician cannot be certain whether the fluid is serous, mucoid, or purulent, nor can the microbial characteristics of an effusion be identified. Since a diagnostic tympanocentesis is not currently recommended for most patients at the time of initial diagnosis, the generic OME is preferred. The other descriptive terms are not popular at this time since they may mislead the clinician in understanding the pathogenesis and potential etiology of the middle-ear disease.

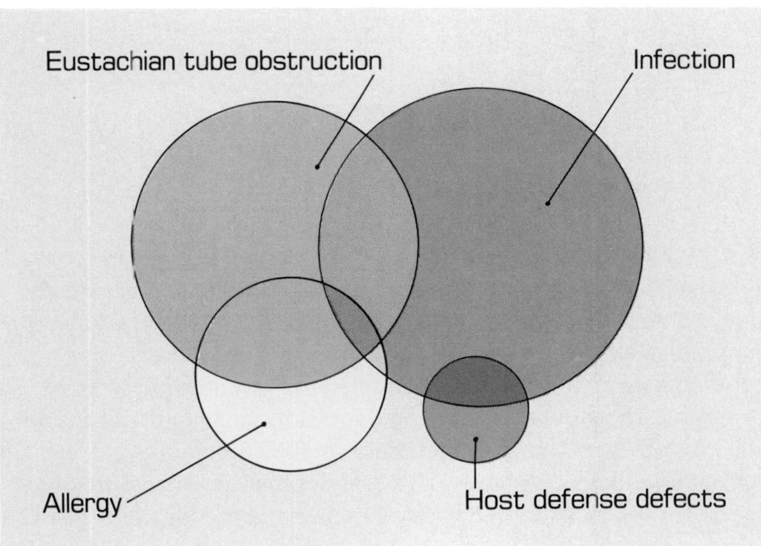

11.1 Indication of the proposed interaction between infection, eustachian tube obstruction, allergy, and host–defense defects in the pathogenesis of OME.

OTITIS MEDIA AND ALLERGY

The possibility that allergy contributes to otitis media is not a new concept; its role has been suggested for years. Therefore, this disease is of considerable interest to allergists. If a causal relationship between allergy and middle-ear disease were to be established then one would expect that anti-allergic therapy would reduce the morbidity associated with the otitis. Such therapy might be able to prevent hearing losses and delays in verbal communication that have resulted in infants and children from the presence of fluid in the middle-ear cavity. This chapter reviews the history, physical findings, and laboratory studies associated with otitis media and develops the concept that otitis media is due to several factors. As illustrated in **11.1**, not only infection and eustachian tube dysfunction, but also allergy and host-defense defects must be considered in middle-ear disease.

PATHOPHYSIOLOGY

STRUCTURE AND FUNCTION

OME appears to be related to abnormal functioning of the eustachian tube. Understanding and diagnosing this disease requires familiarity with the anatomy and physiology of the upper airway, which is made up of the nasal cavity, nasopharynx, eustachian tube, middle ear, and mastoid air cells (**11.2A**). The eustachian tube provides an anatomic communication between the nasopharynx and the middle ear and is in a unique position to effect changes in the middle ear secondary to reactions in the nose. In relation to the middle ear and the nasopharynx, the eustachian tube may be considered to be analogous in part to the bronchial tree in relation to the lung and nasopharynx. Like mucosa elsewhere in the respiratory tract, the mucosa lining the eustachian tube contains mucus-producing cells, ciliated cells, plasma cells, and mast cells. Unlike the bronchial tree, the eustachian tube is usually collapsed and thus closed to the nasopharynx and its contents (**11.2B**). Active opening of the

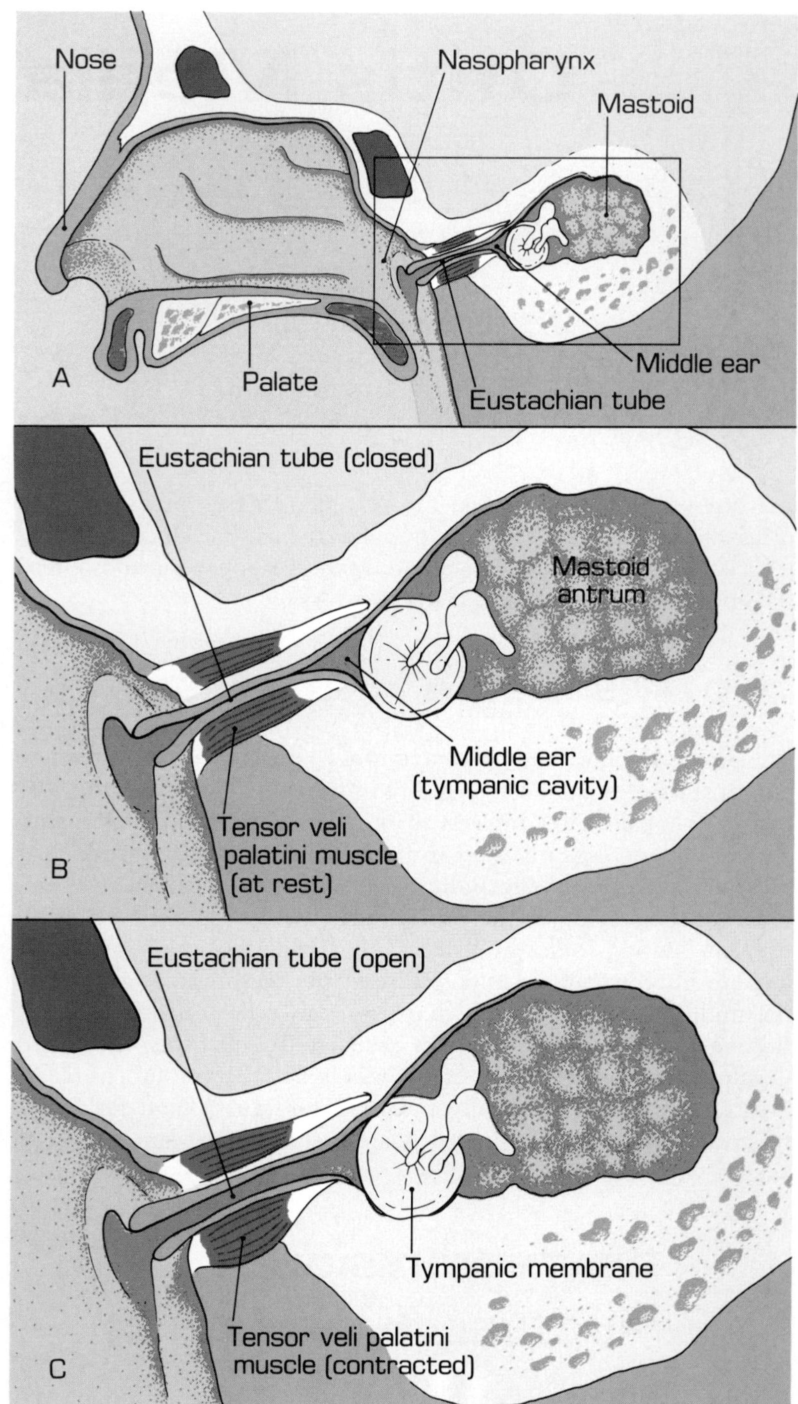

11.2 (A) The upper respiratory tract. The insert demonstrates the eustachian tube as an airway that provides an anatomic communication between the nasopharynx and the middle ear. (B) Enlargement of the insert from **11.2A**, showing the role of the eustachian tube in ventilating the middle ear. Tubal function is governed in part by the tensor veli palatini muscle. With the muscle at rest, the tube is almost always closed. (C) The tube opens when the muscle contracts during swallowing, yawning, crying, or sneezing. Obstruction of the tube plays a central role in the pathogenesis of otitis media. (Adapted with permission from Fireman, 1987.)

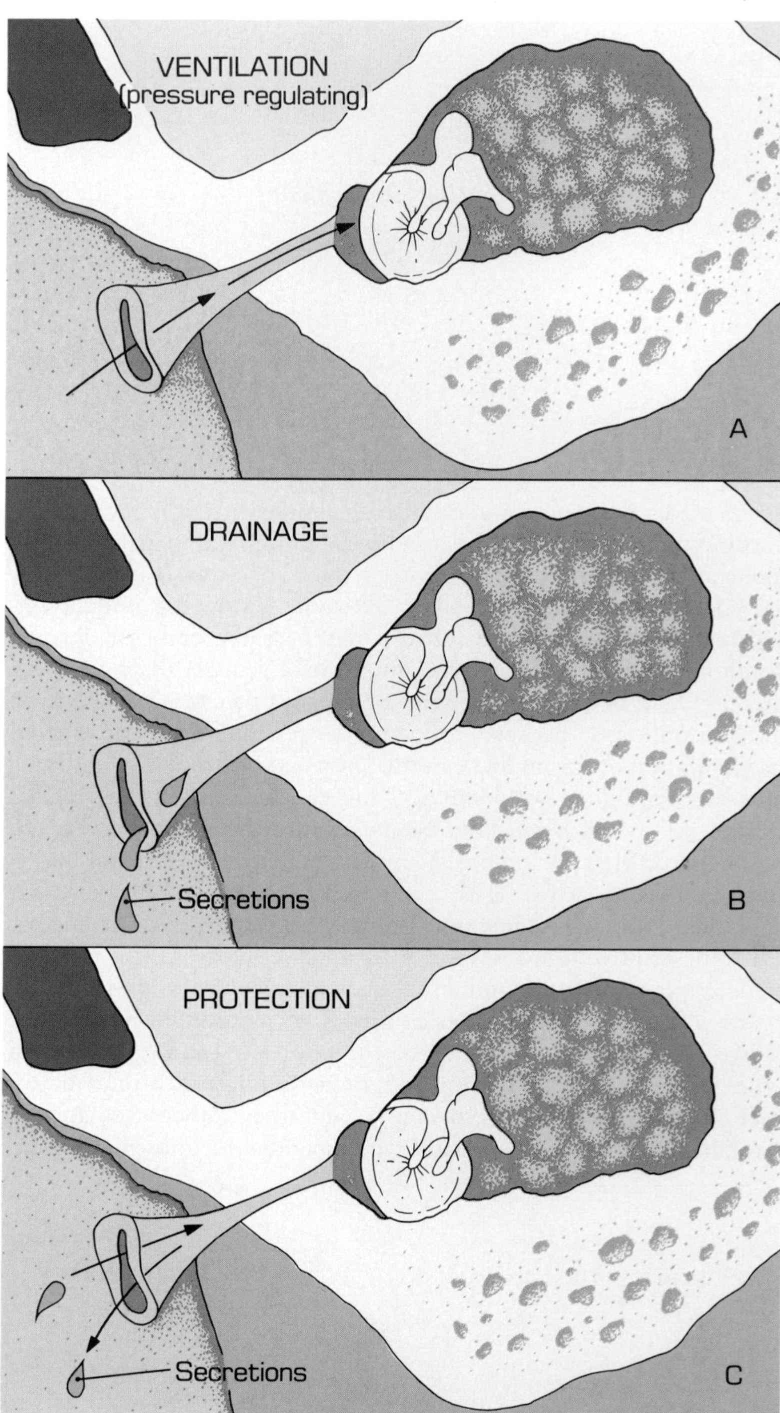

11.3 Physiologic functions of the eustachian tube as related to the middle ear. (A) Ventilation of the middle ear regulates pressure and equilibrates the middle-ear pressure with atmospheric pressure. (B) The tube allows for drainage and clearance of middle-ear secretions, and (C) protects the middle ear from nasopharyngeal secretions. These functions are analogous to those of the bronchial tree. Like other respiratory tract mucosa, the lining of the eustachian tubes contains mast cells, lymphocytes, macrophages, and plasma cells. (Adapted with permission from Bluestone, 1988.)

eustachian tube is accomplished by contraction of the tensor veli palatini (TVP) muscle during swallowing, yawning, crying, or sneezing (**11.2C**). In this regard, the eustachian tube, like the bronchial airway, serves several physiologic functions – protection, drainage, and ventilation: protection from nasopharyngeal secretions, drainage into the nasopharynx of secretions produced within the middle ear, and ventilation of the middle ear to equilibrate air pressure with atmospheric pressure and to replenish oxygen that has been absorbed (**11.3**).

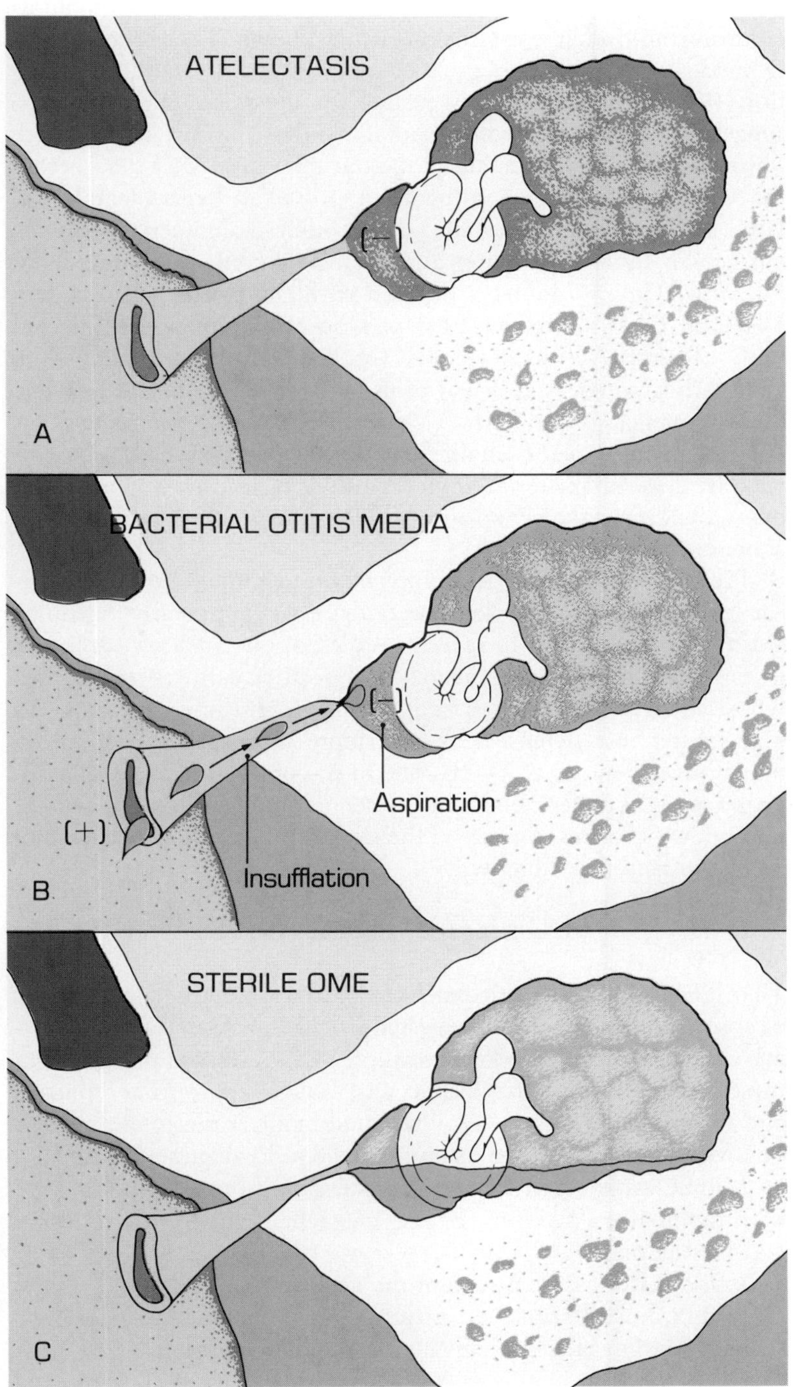

11.4 As in the lungs, interference with any of the functions of the eustachian tubes may predispose to (A) atelectasis, (B) infection and bacterial otitis media, and (C) resultant otitis media with effusion (OME). (Adapted with permission from Bluestone, 1988.)

PATHOGENESIS

In normal tubal function, intermittent opening of the tube maintains near-ambient pressure in the middle-ear cavity. It is suspected that in cases in which active swallowings are inadequate to overcome tubal resistance, the tube remains persistently collapsed, resulting in progressively negative middle-ear pressure. This type of ventilation appears to be common in children, since moderate-to-high negative middle-ear pressures have been identified by tympanometry in many children who are apparently normal. However, periodic or persistently high negative pressure may be pathologic and has been associated with abnormal function of the eustachian tube. Persistently high negative middle-ear pressure with severe retraction of the tympanic membrane has been termed atelectasis of the tympanic membrane and results in acute otitis media. If effective ventilation does not occur because of persistent eustachian tube obstruction, transudation of sterile middle-ear effusion into the tympanum can result, as a consequence of the constant absorption of oxygen by the middle-ear epithelium. Since tubal opening is possible in a middle ear with effusion, aspiration of nasopharyngeal secretions might occur, thus creating the clinical condition in which persistent effusion and recurrent acute otitis media occur together. Thus, abnormal eustachian tube function may predispose the middle ear to atelectasis, infection, or effusion (**11.4**).

EUSTACHIAN TUBE OBSTRUCTION

Two types of eustachian tube obstruction could result in acute or chronic OME – mechanical or functional. **11.5** shows a classification of common conditions associated with eustachian tube obstruction. Intrinsic mechanical obstruction may result from the inflammation of infection or allergy, whereas extrinsic obstruction may result from enlarged adenoids or tumors. Experimentally, allergic rhinitis provoked in patients with a history of allergy has been associated with the development of eustachian tube obstruction. This obstruction, related to edema and inflammation of the posterior nasopharynx, could be both extrinsic and intrinsic. A persistent collapse of the eustachian tube during swallowing may result in functional obstruction, which appears to be related to increased tubal compliance, an inefficient active opening mechanism by the TVP muscle, or both. Functional eustachian tube obstruction is common in infants and younger children, since the amount and stiffness of the cartilage support of the eustachian tube are less than in older children and adults. Also, there appears to be marked age differences in the angulation of the craniofacial base, which renders the TVP muscle less efficient before puberty. The pathogenesis of OME in infants and children with cleft palate is related to a functional obstruction of the eustachian tube.

ETIOLOGY

As illustrated in **11.1**, bacterial infection and eustachian tube dysfunction are the best understood etiologies. In addition, allergies, host-defense defects, or immune deficiencies may participate either directly or indirectly in the development of OME.

INFECTION AND OME

Bacteria have been cultured from 70% of middle-ear effusions in children with acute otitis media and have been shown to be similar to those found in the nasopharynx (**11.6**). *Streptococcus pneumoniae* have been cultured from approximately 30% and is clearly the most common infectious agent in all age groups. *Haemophilus influenzae*, non-typable, have been found in approximately 20% of the ear effusions. About 30% of these *H. influenzae* were beta-lactamase producing and the percentage of this amoxicillin-resistant organism has gradually increased over the last several years. In the past, the incidence of *Moraxella catarrhalis* had been about 5% but it is now 12%. About 75% of *M. catarrhalis* strains produced beta-lactamase. The emergence of these amoxicillin-resistant, beta-lactamase producing organisms associated with OME in 15–20% of children with ear disease has had an important impact on the choice of antibiotics for therapy. The frequency of Group A beta-hemolytic *Streptococcus* was 3% and *Staphylococcus aureus* was present in less than 2%.

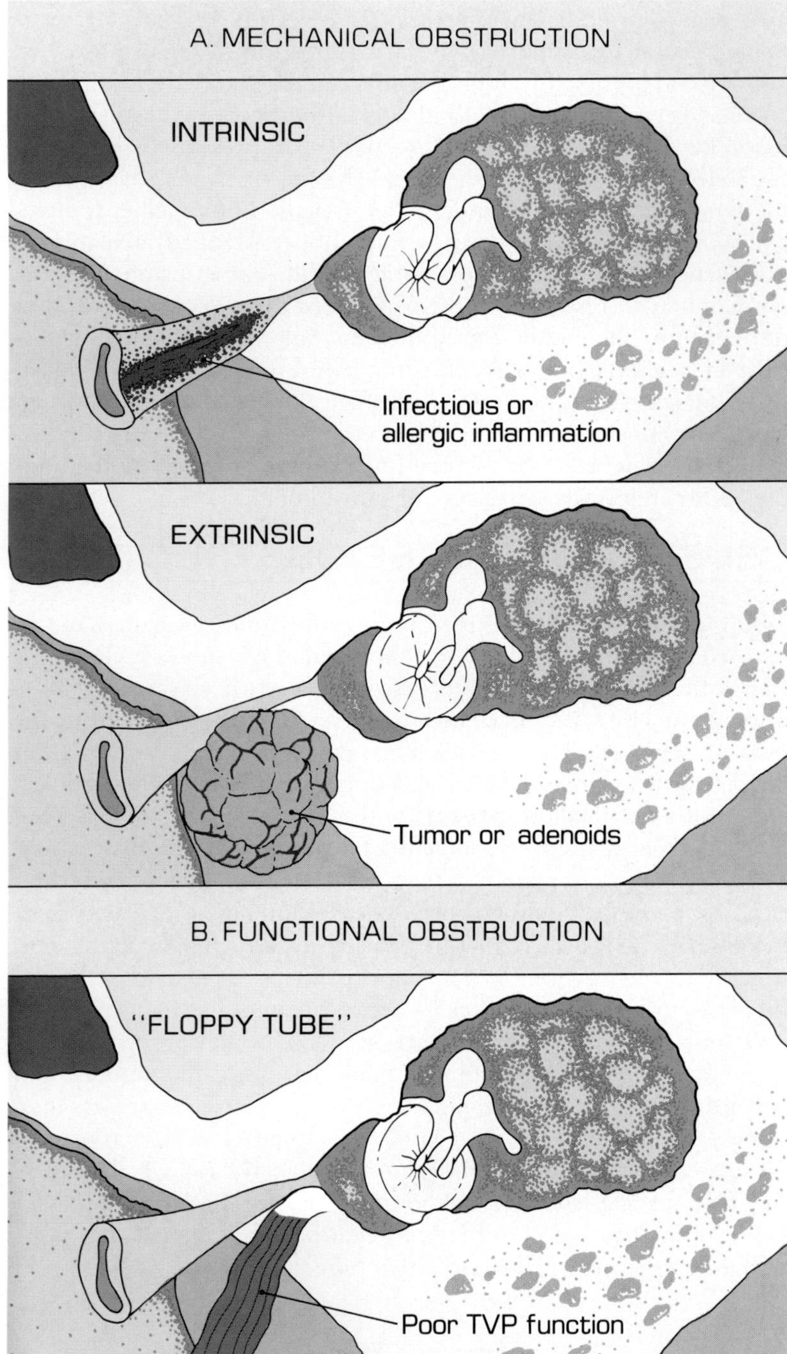

11.5 Pathophysiology of eustachian tube dysfunction, showing that the tube may be abnormally patent or obstructed. This illustrates several types of eustachian tube obstructions that contribute to OME. (A) Mechanical obstruction may be either intrinsic, due to inflammation produced by infection or allergy, or extrinsic, produced by peritubular conditions such as enlarged adenoids or tumors. (B) Functional obstruction, which is common in infants, is due to poor TVP muscle function or increased tubal compliance. (Adapted with permission from Bluestone, 1988.)

Anaerobic bacteria and viruses have been cultured infrequently from middle ear aspirates of children who have acute otitis media, but viral antigens have been identified using immune assays in 10–20% of middle-ear effusions. Why viruses have been difficult to culture from middle-ear effusions is not known. That bacterial otitis media is secondary to a preceding viral upper respiratory infections (URI), which resulted in eustachian tube obstruction, has been suggested by the observations that children have a more severe obstruction of the eustachian tube during a viral URI than before the URI. Rhinovirus or influenza A provoked experimental viral URI in susceptible normal young adult volunteers produced eustachian tube obstruction and negative middle-ear pressures in 70–80%. Those volunteers infected with rhinovirus had less than 5% mild OME, whereas 20% of susceptible volunteers infected with influenza A virus developed OME. One subject developed an acute otitis, whose middle-ear effusion aspirate contained genomic DNA sequences of influenza A virus and *S. pneumoniae* bacteria (as detected by polymeric chain-reaction analysis), even though this aspirate grew no bacterial or viral pathogens in culture. In addition, many children have symptoms of URI prior to their symptoms of acute otitis media.

Previously, it had been assumed incorrectly that chronic middle-ear effusions were sterile, especially after apparently adequate antimicrobial therapy. In several studies, about 50% of the chronic, persistent middle-ear effusions had positive cultures for bacteria whose microbiology was similar to that found in acute otitis. An inadequate host defense can contribute to recurrent respiratory infections as well as to OME. The most common of these unusual problems is IgA deficiency, but other immunoglobulin or cellular immunodeficiencies, as well as the immotile cilia syndrome, cannot be overlooked (*see* Chapter 17).

ALLERGY AND OME

That IgE-mediated allergic reactions participate in the pathogenesis of chronic OME has been suggested by clinical observations reporting a higher prevalence of chronic OME in allergic patients, but these studies were retrospective and lacked appropriate controls and experimental design. As illustrated in **11.7**, the role of allergy in OME may involve one or more of the following mechanisms:

- Middle-ear mucosa functioning as a target organ.
- Inflammatory swelling of the eustachian tube with resultant obstruction.
- Inflammatory obstruction of the nose and nasopharynx.
- Reflux, insufflation, or aspiration of bacteria-laden allergic nasopharyngeal secretions into the middle-ear cavity.

The last three mechanisms would be associated with abnormal function of the eustachian tube. Although histamine and other mediators of inflammation are present in middle-ear effusions, there is little evidence that the middle-ear mucosa functions as the allergic 'shock organ' via IgE antibody and allergen reaction.

There appears, however, to be a relation between upper respiratory tract infections as well as with allergy and eustachian tube dysfunction. A prospective study of children with recurrent or chronic middle-ear disease and functional obstruction of the eustachian tube showed more severe obstruction (mechanical) of the tube when an upper respiratory tract infection developed. A similar relationship has been reported between upper respiratory tract allergy and eustachian tube obstruction in a series of provocative, intranasal, allergen-inhalation challenge studies by our group at the Children's Hospital of Pittsburgh.

Nasal obstruction may also be involved in the pathogenesis of OME. Swallowing when the nose is obstructed (inflammation or obstructive adenoids) creates a closed nasopharyngeal chamber. During swallowing, an initial positive nasopharyngeal air pressure is followed by a negative pressure phase within the closed system. There are two possible effects of these pressures on a pliant tube – with positive nasopharyngeal pressure, secretions might be insufflated into the middle ear, especially when the middle ear has a high negative pressure; or with negative nasopharyngeal pressures, such a tube could be prevented from opening and become further functionally obstructed. This has been termed the 'Toynbee phenomenon'.

The following sequence of events is postulated to occur in patients who have respiratory allergy and otitis media (**11.8**). Most likely, a basic eustachian tube dysfunction is present in certain infants and children whose tubal function becomes compromised in the presence of upper respiratory tract allergy, similar to eustachian tube obstruction caused by an upper respiratory tract infection.

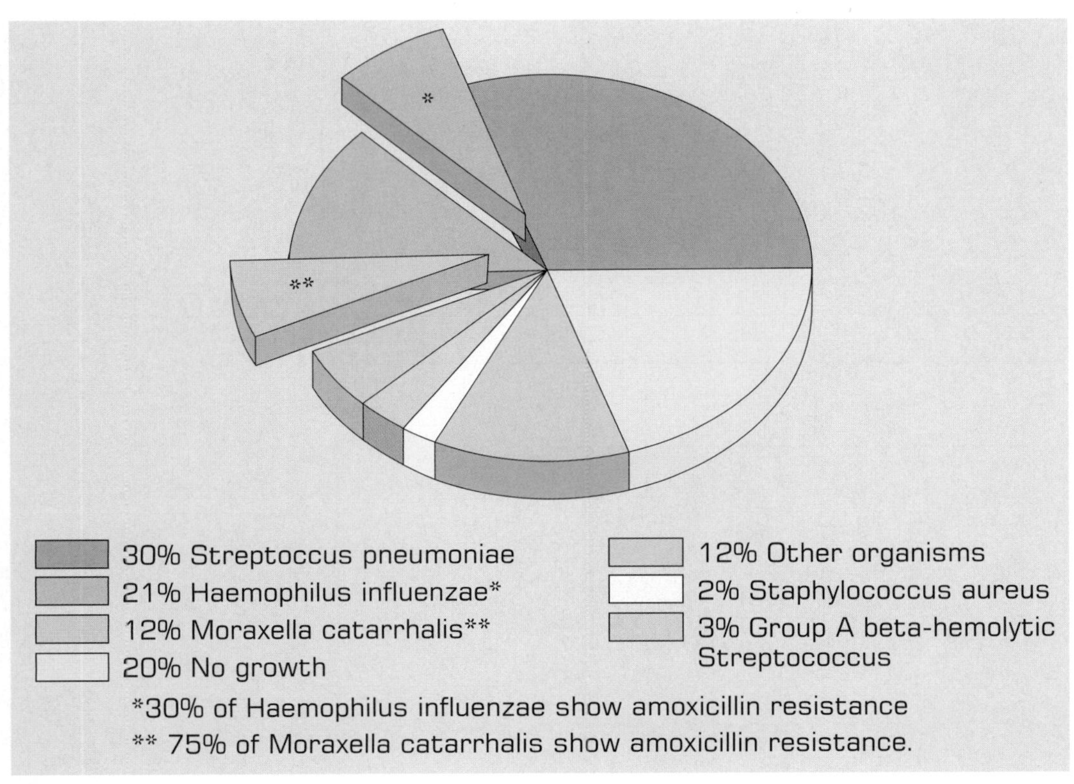

11.6 The percentage of bacteria cultured from middle-ear effusions of children with otitis media at the time of tympanocentesis. *Streptococcus pneumoniae* and *Haemophilus influenzae* account for more than 50% of the bacteria. Amoxicillin-resistant *H. influenzae* and *Moraxella catarrhalis* are present in effusions of 15–20% of children with OME.

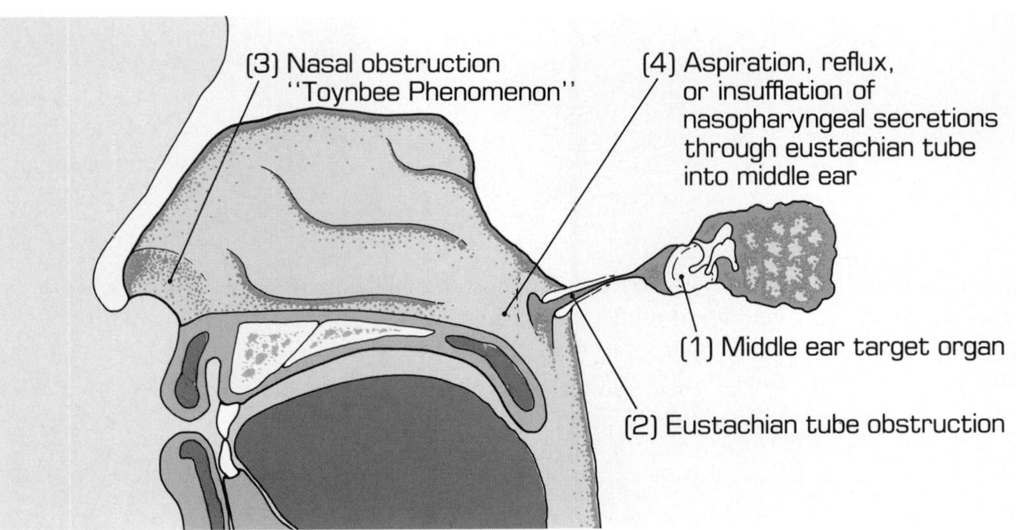

11.7 The four possible mechanisms involving allergy in the pathogenesis of OME. (Adapted with permission from Bluestone, 1988.)

Upper respiratory tract allergy may cause some intrinsic as well as extrinsic mechanical obstruction in patients who have normal eustachian tube function, but their normal active opening mechanism, i.e., TVP muscle pull, is able to overcome the obstruction. Therefore, patients who have functional obstruction due to poor muscular opening would be at highest risk for developing sufficient mechanical obstruction to give rise to middle-ear disease. Many children, as part of normal development, have difficulty actively opening their eustachian tubes; they are the population most at risk for manifesting OME.

DIAGNOSIS OF OTITIS MEDIA

HISTORY

The earliest signs of otitis media are most frequently ear pain and discomfort, which may be difficult to discern in a child who is too young to speak. The child may be irritable and pull on the affected ear. There may be an associated conductive hearing deficit that, if not recognized or if neglected, may predispose the child to subsequent speech pathology.

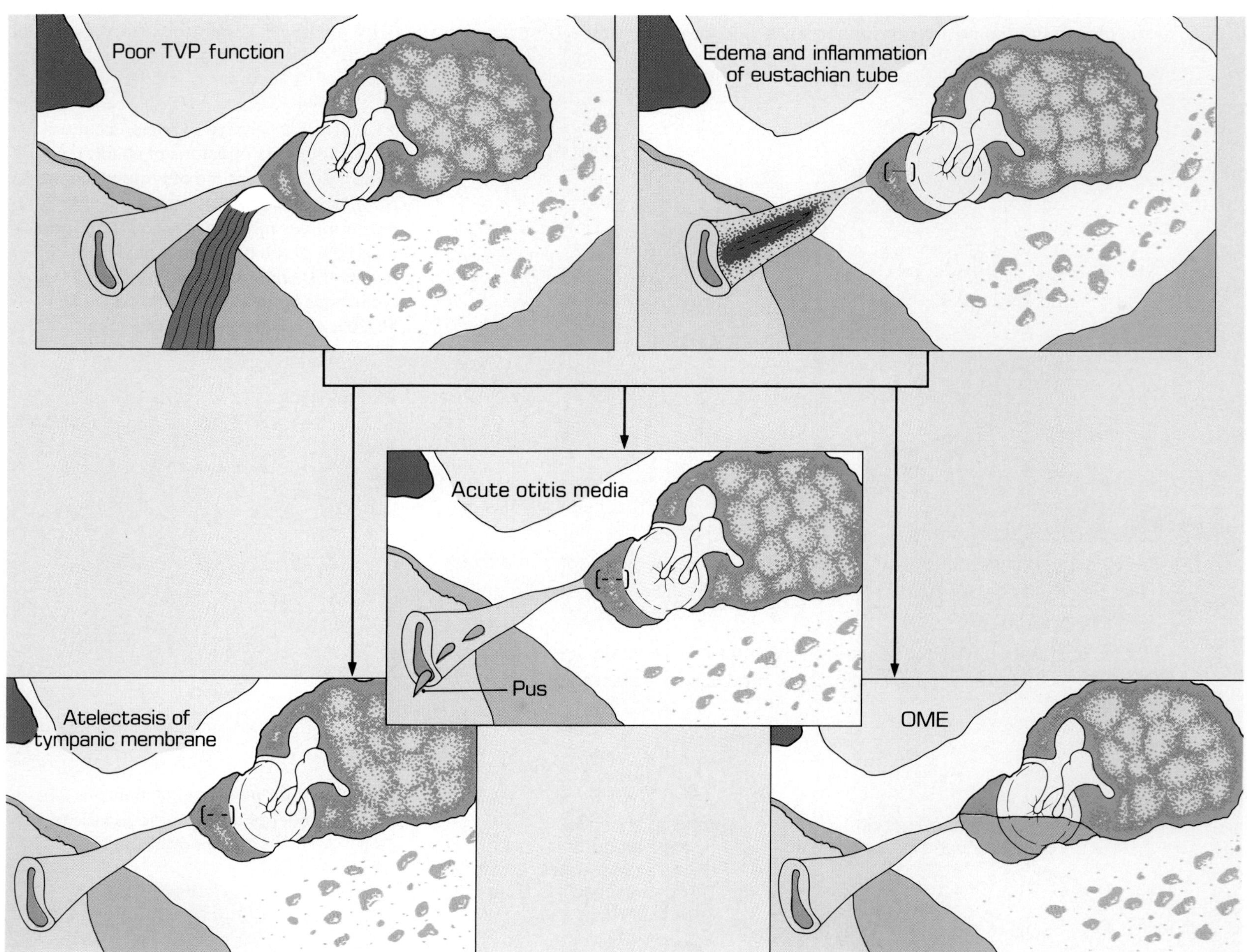

11.8 Two major causes of eustachian tube obstruction (ETO) are poor TVP function and edema of the tubal and nasopharyngeal mucosa (secondary to allergic inflammation). This schema shows how the allergy-produced inflammation may contribute to the failure of the tube to open and permit collection of fluid in the middle ear, leading to otitis media. The tube's relative shortness in children predisposes them to OME. (Adapted with permission from Bluestone, 1988.)

OME WITH ALLERGIC RHINITIS

Most children with otitis media have an associated rhinitis, and it is important to decide whether the rhinitis is infectious or allergic (**11.9A** and **11.9B**). The differentiation between infection and perennial allergic rhinitis can be difficult. Symptoms of an upper respiratory infection, such as fever and malaise with profuse acute rhinorrhea, would suggest an infection. The presence of a similar acute illness in immediate family members or contacts would also indicate an infection. Of course, a purulent rhinorrhea or pharyngitis would suggest an infection. A prolonged or recurrent seasonal rhinitis with itching and sneezing would suggest an allergic basis, as would bilateral red, itchy, swollen, non-purulent inflammation of the eyes, all of which are manifestations of allergic rhinoconjunctivitis (*see* Chapter 9).

Even if eustachian tube obstruction is minimal, patients with allergic rhinitis may have mild symptoms of eustachian tube dysfunction, such as 'popping' and 'snapping' sounds in the ear. These symptoms may be aggravated during airplane travel. Many of the patients experience these symptoms and go on to have more problems, such as hearing loss, ear discomfort, tinnitus, and, rarely, vertigo, during the worst periods of their allergic rhinitis. These symptoms may not be manifest in the non-verbal child. A family history of allergy along with a seasonal runny nose or a constant 'cold' should raise suspicions of an allergic diathesis. Other allergic conditions associated with allergic rhinitis include atopic dermatitis and allergic asthma. Seasonal allergic rhinitis occurs episodically, most typically in temperate North America during the grass and ragweed pollen seasons, whereas perennial allergic rhinitis evokes symptoms all year and can be due to non-seasonal allergens present in the home, especially the bedroom, or the workplace. These include house dust, dust mites, storage mold spores, animal products, or occupational allergens.

DIAGNOSTIC TECHNIQUES

Pneumatic otoscopy

Recognition of OME during the physical examination requires the use of the pneumatic otoscope (**11.10**). The allergist must choose the correct size speculum to fit each patient's ear canal. It is necessary to obtain a good pneumatic seal during an otoscopic examination to ascertain motility of the tympanic membrane by the gentle application of air pressure via the hand-held bulb. The technique and findings of pneumatic otoscopy are shown in **11.11**. The loss of normal movement of the eardrum during this procedure indicates loss of compliance of the eardrum either due to middle-ear effusion behind the drum or to increased stiffness because of scarring or thickening of an inflamed eardrum.

Otoscopic inspection requires visualization of the tympanic membrane and, frequently, cerumen may have to be removed from

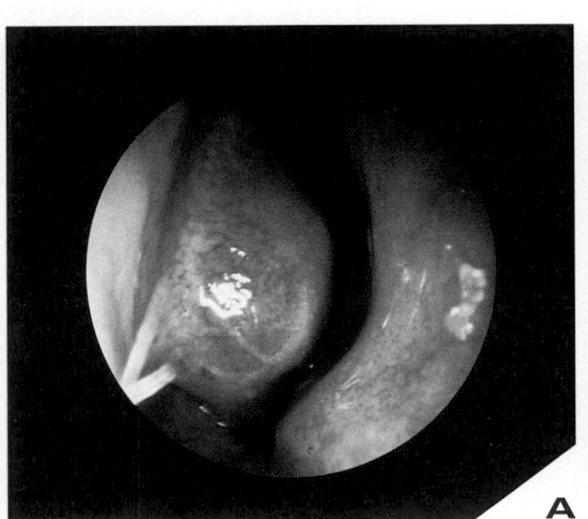

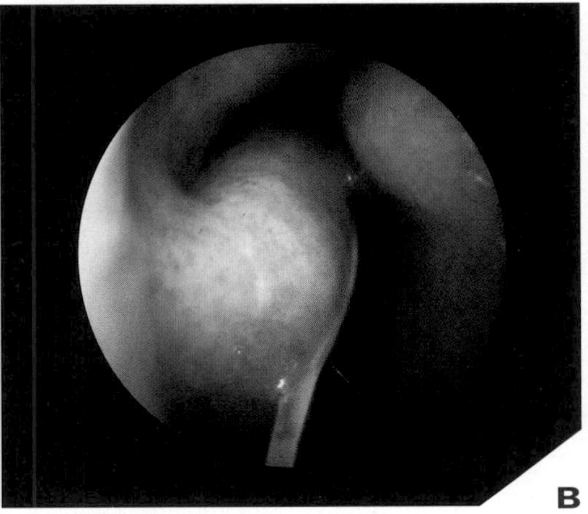

11.9 Otitis media is frequently associated with rhinitis. (A) Photograph of nasal mucosa taken via a rhinoscope, from a child with infections rhinitis. (B) Photograph of nasal mucosa from a child with allergic rhinitis.

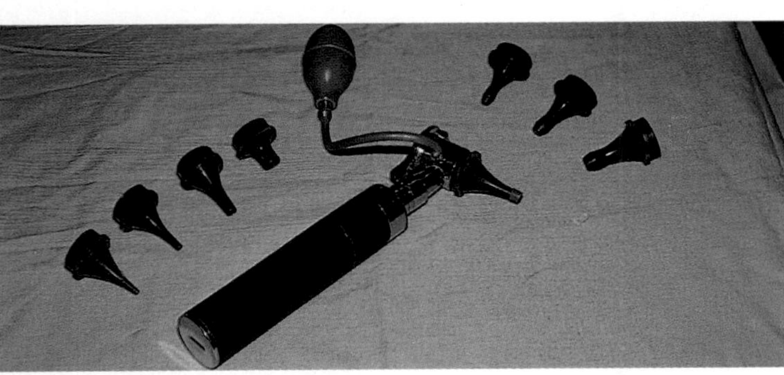

11.10 Pneumatic otoscopy. This procedure requires the proper equipment, including a pneumatic otoscope head and appropriately sized speculum to achieve a good air seal. When, despite proper speculum size, a seal is difficult to obtain, the head and tubing should be checked for air leaks. If none are found, application of a piece of rubber tubing to the end of the speculum (shown attached to the otoscope), or use of a softer speculum, may solve the problem. (Reproduced with permission from Zitelli and Davis, 1987.)

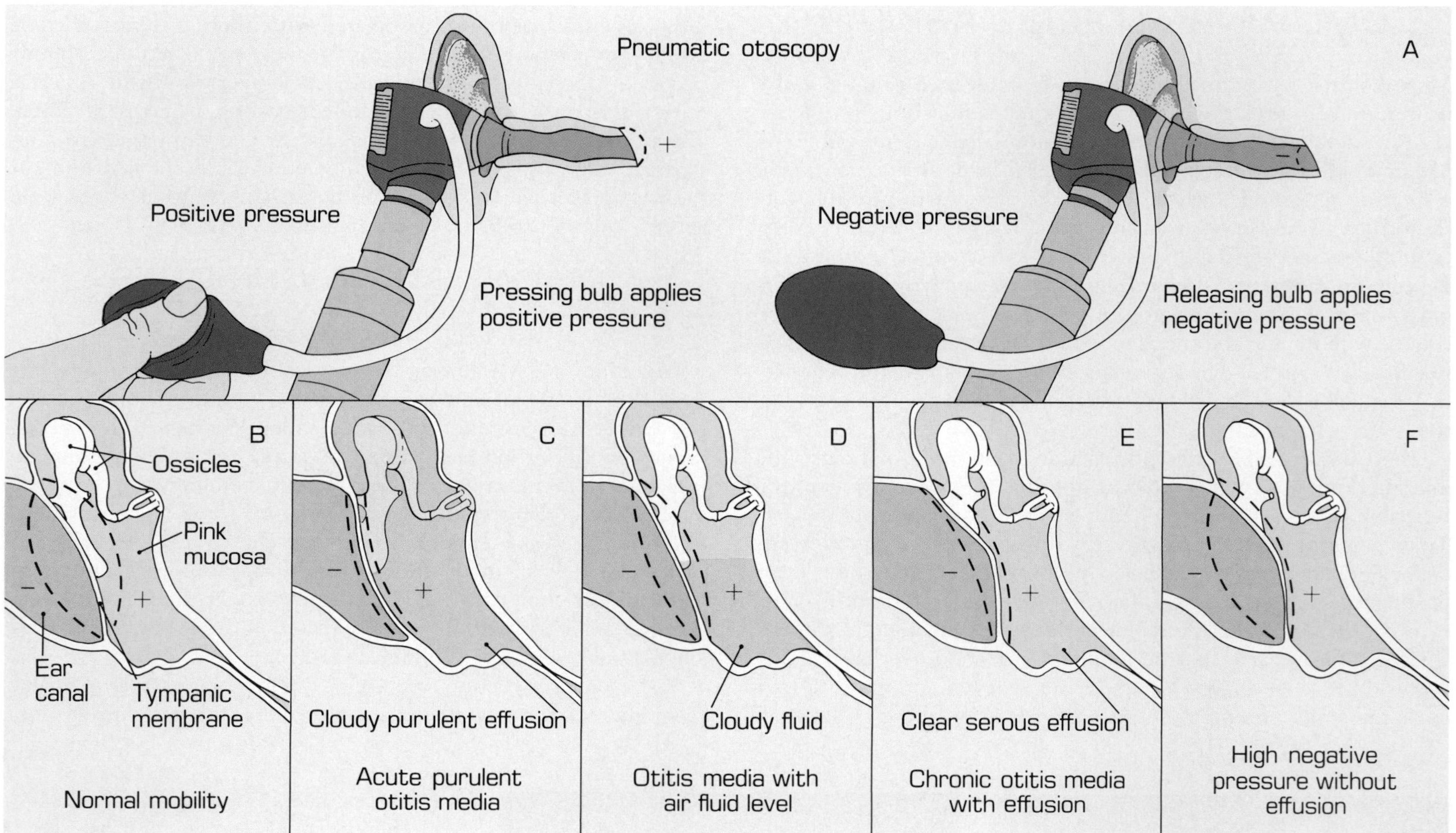

11.11 The technique and findings of pneumatic otoscopy. (A) The speculum is inserted into the ear canal to form a tight seal. The bulb is then gently and slowly squeezed and released, while the mobility of the drum is assessed. Pressing on the bulb applies positive pressure; letting up applies negative pressure. (B) With normal mobility, the drum moves inward and then back. (C) In cases of acute otitis media in which the middle ear is filled with purulent material, the drum bulges toward the examiner, and moves minimally. (D) In cases of acute otitis media with an air-fluid level, mobility may be nearly normal. In some patients, however, the drum may be retracted, indicating increased negative pressure. If this is the case, mobility on positive pressure may be reduced while the movement on negative pressure is nearly normal or only mildly decreased. This is the same pattern as that seen commonly in children with chronic serous otitis (E). In cases of high negative pressure with no effusion (F), application of positive pressure produces little or no movement. On negative pressure, the drum billows back toward the examiner. (Adapted with permission from Zitelli and Davis, 1987.)

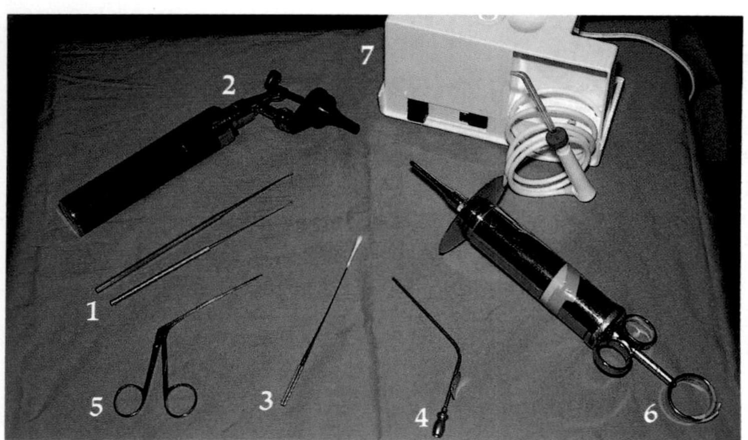

11.12 Equipment for cleaning the external auditory canal. The curette (1) is the implement most commonly used to remove cerumen. Use of a surgical otoscope head (2) makes the process considerably easier. Additional implements include: cotton wicks (3) and a suction tip (4) for removal of discharge or moist wax, alligator forceps (5) for foreign bodies, an ear syringe (6), and a motorized irrigation apparatus (7) for removing firm objects or impacted cerumen. Lavage is contraindicated when there is a possible perforation of the tympanic membrane. If the motorized apparatus is used for irrigation, it must be kept on the lowest power setting, to avoid traumatizing the eardrum.

the external ear canal to permit an adequate examination. The equipment necessary to clean the ear canal is shown in **11.12**. The normal tympanic membrane is thin, translucent, neutrally positioned, and mobile. The ossicles, particularly the malleus, are generally visible through it. Adequate assessment requires that the physician take note of the major characteristics of the tympanic membrane – its thickness, degree of translucence, position, and mobility to applied pressure. The normal tympanic membrane and landmarks are illustrated in **11.13A** and can be easily recognized in the normal eardrum shown in **11.13B**.

The bulging eardrum in **11.14** indicates the presence of excessive middle-ear fluid and documents effusion. The presence of marked erythema and hyperemia point to a clinical diagnosis of acute otitis media. Sometimes the presence of air bubbles (**11.15**) and fluid levels documents OME. The presence of a retracted eardrum suggests negative pressure and possibly atelectasis within the middle ear. **11.16** shows a retracted eardrum. Acute otitis media may, by virtue of increasing middle-ear pressure, result in acute perforation of the tympanic membrane. On presentation, the canal may be filled with pus. Careful removal of the pus with a cotton wick usually reveals an inflamed drum with

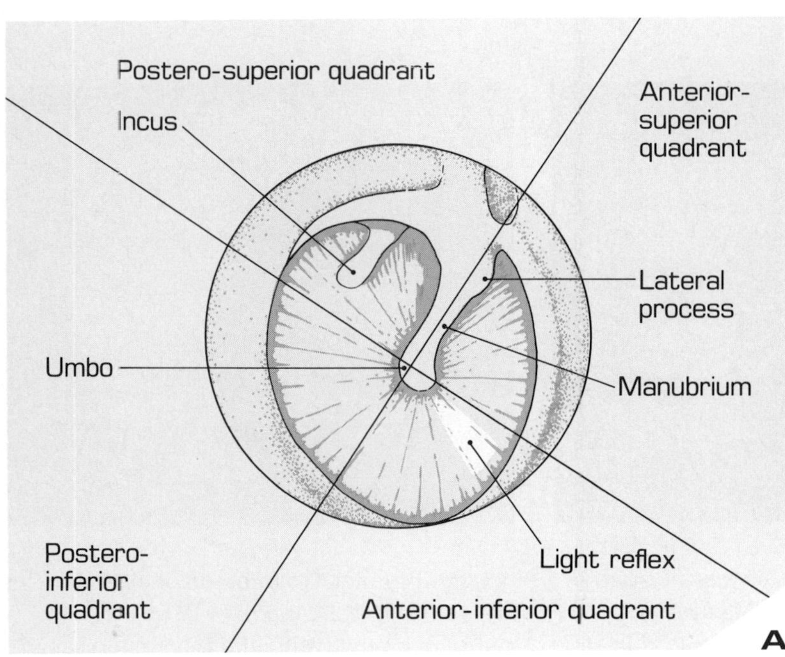

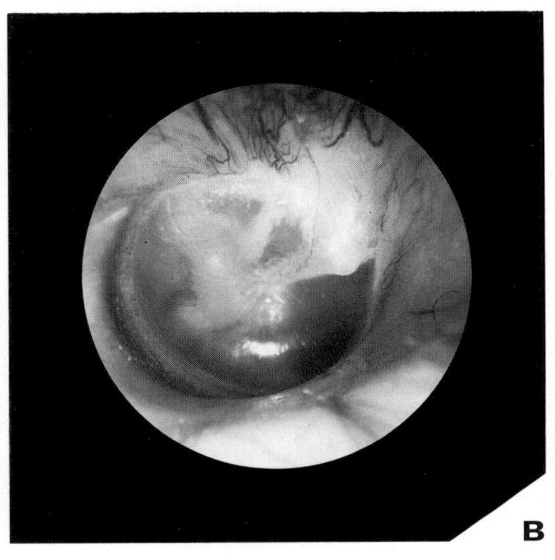

11.13 (A) The normal landmarks of the tympanic membrane. (B) Photograph of a normal tympanic membrane.

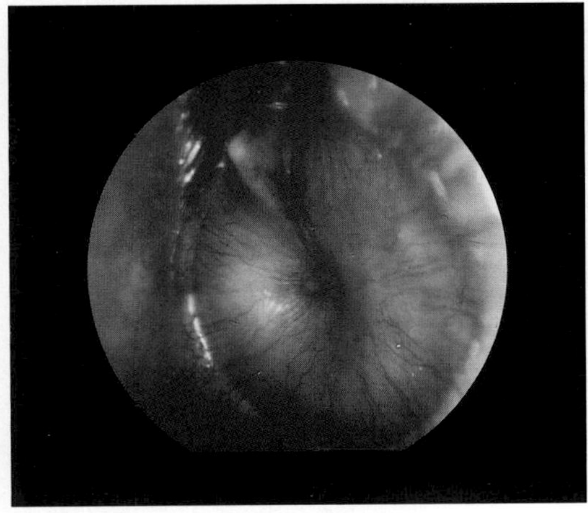

11.14 Acute otitis media. This is a typical drum seen by otoscopy, showing an erythematous, bulging tympanic membrane. The light reflex and mobility are reduced, and landmarks are partially obscured.

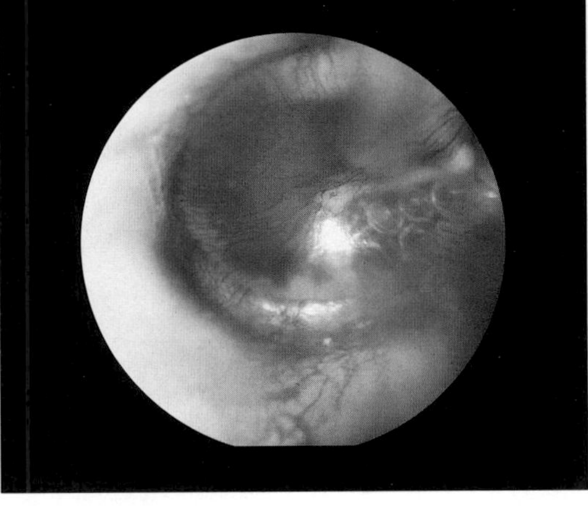

11.15 This drum, seen on otoscopy to show air bubbles, documents OME. There is a loss of normal landmarks.

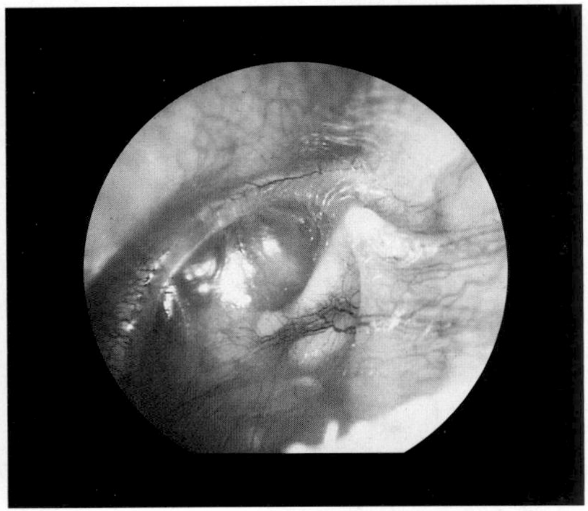

11.16 A retracted eardrum represents atelectasis with negative middle-ear pressure. This is seen in recurrent or protracted OME.

perforation (**11.17**). **11.18** shows the outcome of neglected otitis with recurrent inflammation and development of cholesteotoma.

Persistence of OME in spite of adequate therapy for more than 4–6 months and the presence of a hearing deficit are indications for a myringotomy and insertion of ventilation tubes. This facilitates hearing and reduces the frequency of recurrent otitis. **11.19** shows an eardrum with a tympanostomy tube in place.

Follow-up examinations

After initiating an appropriate course of antibiotic and analgesic therapy for the acute or chronic otitis media, follow-up physical examination is important. This is best done 3–4 weeks after diagnosis and the start of therapy, when resolution of the effusion and inflammation can be expected in over 50% of asymptomatic patients. Of course, symptomatic patients must be seen sooner to ascertain whether the selected antibiotic therapy was appropriate and that no potential complications have developed. The purpose of the re-examination is to identify those patients who are at risk for having a persistent effusion. As shown in **11.20**, 10% of patients with acute otitis, even after appropriate antibiotic therapy, still have OME 12 weeks after diagnosis. Therefore, OME may be diagnosed as an acute otitis, the residual of a treated otitis, or as an occult finding on physical examination in a patient without an apparent antecedent infection.

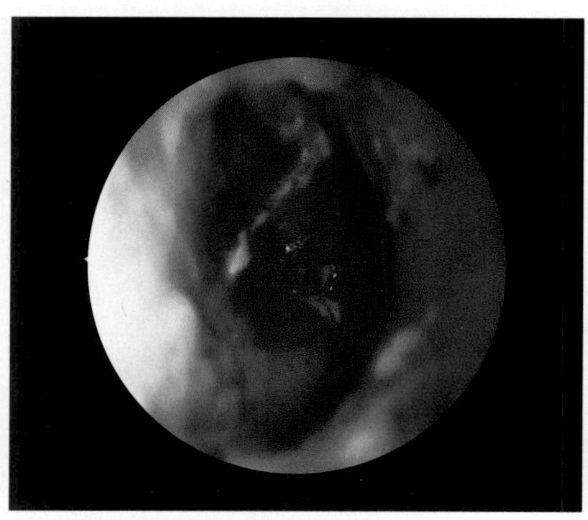

11.17 Acute otitis media with perforation. In this child, increased middle-ear pressure with acute otitis resulted in perforation of the tympanic membrane. The drum is thickened, and the perforation is seen at 3 o'clock. (Reproduced with permission from Zitelli and Davis, 1987.)

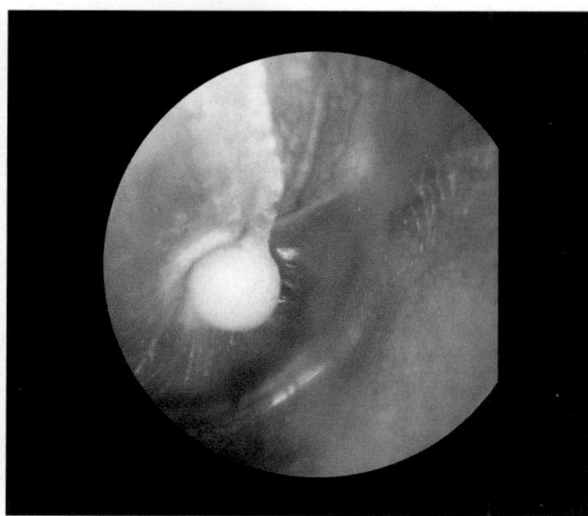

11.18 Cholesteatoma. This mass lesion, which consists of an epithelial cyst, is growing within the eardrum of this child. (Reproduced with permission from Zitelli and Davis, 1987.)

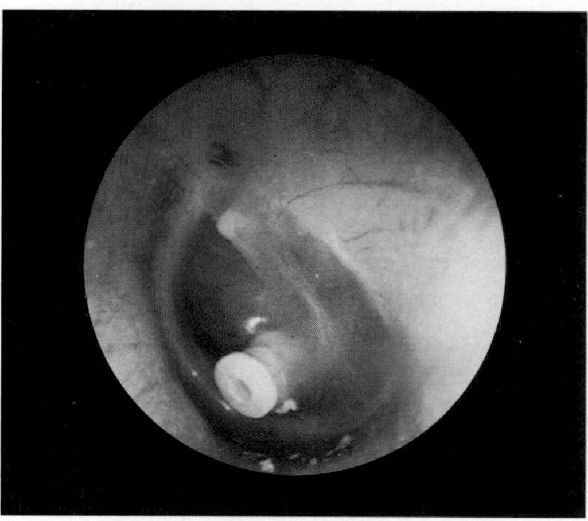

11.19 Tympanic membrane of a patient with chronic otitis media with a tympanostomy (ventilation) tube in place. The tube serves to ventilate the middle ear, improve hearing, and reduce the frequency of infection.

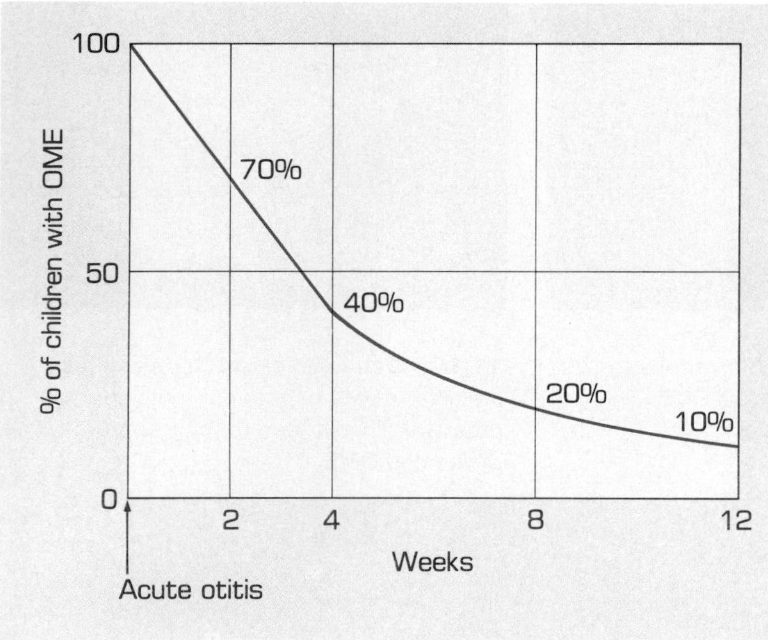

11.20 The persistence of middle-ear effusion (MEE) after an initial episode of OME treated with amoxicillin for 10 days: 70% of the children still had MEE after 2 weeks, 40% had MEE after 1 month, 20% had it after 2 months, and 10% had it after 3 months. (Modified with permission from Teele *et al.*, 1980.)

Tympanometry

The use of the tympanometer in the assessment of potential ear disease has been recognized as a valuable adjunct in the management of OME. When otoscopic findings are unclear or otoscopy difficult to perform, tympanometry can be very useful in evaluating children over 6 months of age. This instrument (**11.21**), which measures the compliance of the eardrum as well as middle-ear pressure, is also helpful in clinical practice in confirming the diagnosis of OME. Thus, many allergists have incorporated tympanometry into their office practices. **11.22** illustrates typical tympanometric findings in patients with various types of middle-ear pathologies. An audiogram is also necessary for the management of recurrent and chronic OME. The evaluation of a potential conduction hearing deficit as a complication of this disease is an important aspect of patient man-

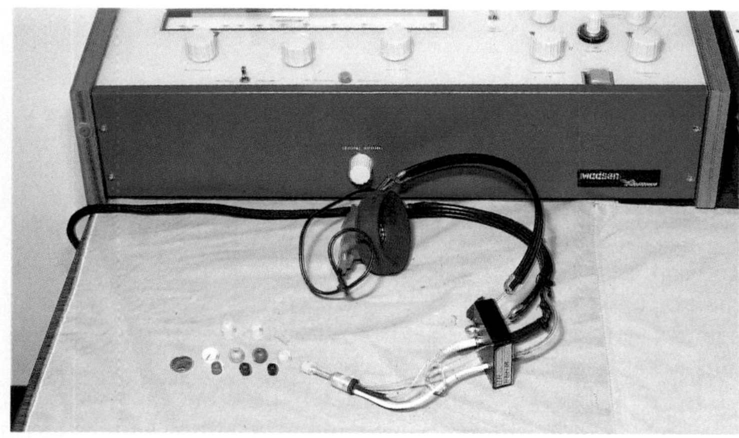

11.21 The apparatus and the variety of ear tips available for tympanometry. The tympanometer measures membrane compliance and middle-ear pressure. (Reproduced with permission from Zitelli and Davis, 1987.)

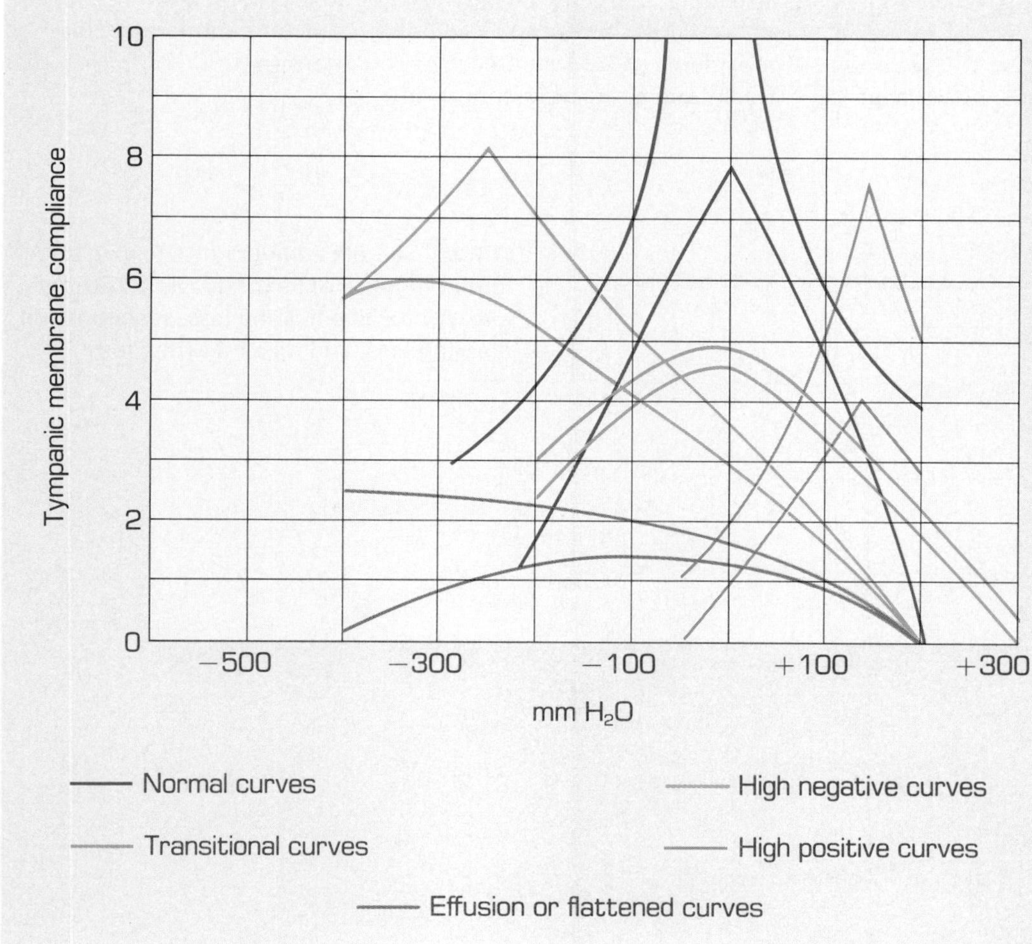

11.22 Tympanometric patterns of various conditions of the middle ear. Normal curves (red): the lower curve is typical of normal ears. The open top curve shows high compliance, but is a normal variant in young children. With these curves, there is only a 1–2% probability of MEE. Transitional curves (blue): show compliance that is intermediate between the high, normal peaks and the flattening seen with most effusions. The lower curve has a steep gradient, and a 14% probability of associated effusion. The upper, more gradual curve, because of its rounded peak, has an 82% probability of effusion. Effusion or flattened curves (purple): show decreased tympanic membrane compliance or mobility, with an 82% chance of associated effusion. Seen in patients with acute otitis, chronic otitis, or with thickened or scarred tympanic membranes. High negative curves (green): are characteristic of increased negative middle-ear pressure. Otoscopy may show retraction or movement primarily on negative pressure. The lower, more gradual curve has a 67% probability of associated effusion; the upper, peaked curve has a 29% probability. High positive curves (orange) : reflect increased positive middle-ear pressure. The lower curve has a 57% probability of effusion or ear disease and is seen commonly in early acute otitis media. The upper curve has only a 10% probability or effusion. (Adapted with permission from Zitelli and Davis, 1987.)

agement and must not be ignored. **11.23** illustrates the audiogram of a patient with a conduction hearing deficit as compared to a patient with a sensorineural hearing loss.

DIFFERENTIAL DIAGNOSIS

ALLERGY

If allergy, and specifically allergic rhinitis, is suspected from the history and confirmed by physical examination as a risk factor for the development of OME, then an allergic evaluation is suggested to confirm this suspicion. Prick skin-testing is preferred to serologic tests (RAST, FAST, ELISA, etc.) for the detection of IgE antibodies to specific allergens because of the increased sensitivity and lower cost of these tests (*see* Chapter 3). Total serum IgE levels are usually not especially helpful for the evaluation of allergic rhinitis, because only a third of these allergic individuals have elevated total serum IgE. In addition, total serum IgE does not assist in defining specific allergen sensitivity.

IMMUNE DEFICIENCY SYNDROME

The possibility of an immune deficiency syndrome should be included in the differential diagnosis if the physician decides that the child has had undue susceptibility to infections. When a child with chronic, recurrent, or persistent OME also has had recurrent sinusitis, pneumonia, or other infections in addition to the recurrent upper respiratory infections, then immunologic assessment is indicated to evaluate potential immune deficiency syndromes. The initial laboratory tests performed should include quantitation of serum IgG, IgA, and IgM, as well as a complete blood count, including a leukocyte count and differential to ascertain the absolute lymphocyte count. A delayed skin test to *Candida* can be applied to assess cell-mediated immunity. Additional laboratory tests to assess specific functional serum antibodies, serum IgG subclasses, T and B lymphocytes, as well as complement function, are discussed in detail in Chapter 17.

TREATMENT

MEDICAL

The management of OME consists of choosing the appropriate antibiotics. Amoxicillin with clavulanic acid is the antibiotic of choice for initial therapy. For recurrence, or if a beta-lactamase producing *H. influenzae* or *M. cartarrhalis* is suspect, then either amoxicillin with clavulanic acid, erythomycin with sulfa, or a cephalosporin are suggested. Trimethaprim with sulfa has been used less often. Decongestants are widely used but their efficacy has not been documented in controlled studies. If allergic rhinitis is documented in association with OME, then allergy management should include antihistamine therapy and avoidance of offending allergens. If these are not effective, then intranasal topical steroids, intranasal cromolyn, and immunotherapy may be considered. **11.24** summarizes the appropriate therapy for otitis media and associated conditions.

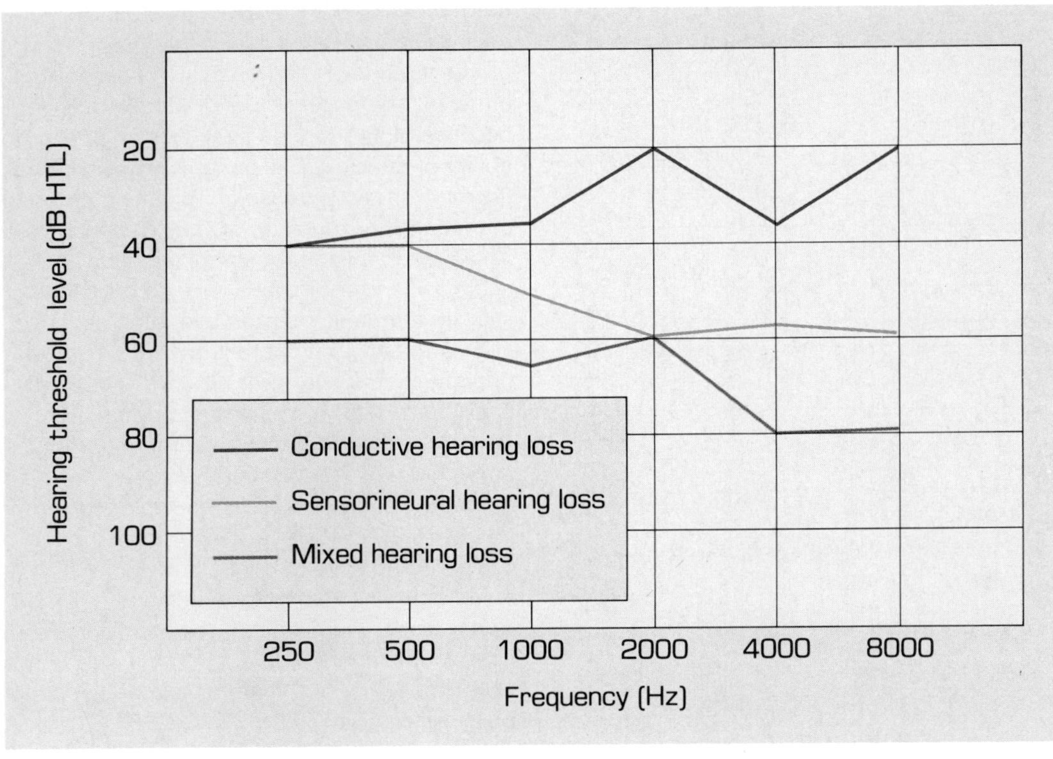

11.23 Sample audiograms showing three different types of hearing loss in the right ear: conductive hearing loss, sensorineural hearing loss, and mixed hearing loss.

SURGICAL

The surgical management of OME includes insertion of tympanostomy (ventilation) tubes to promote drainage of persistent unresolved effusions and to improve hearing (**11.19**). With recognition of the sequela of chronic OME, this surgical procedure has become the most frequently performed operation in the United States. Many physicians have questioned the increasing popularity of this surgery and have cautioned against its potential abuse. Indications for consultation with an otolaryngologist to consider insertion of tympanostomy tubes include the following:

- Appropriate medical management has not been successful in alleviating the OME.
- The OME was documented as recurrent with three or more episodes in the preceding 6 months.
- OME has persisted for more than 4–6 months.
- Persistent conductive hearing deficit was documented.

Adenoidectomy has also been recommended to relieve extrinsic eustachian tube obstruction caused by peritubular lymphoid tissue. Both of these surgical procedures appear beneficial in certain patients, but documentation of their efficacy has not yet been established in controlled, double-blind studies.

THERAPY FOR OTITIS MEDIA AND ASSOCIATED ALLERGIES

Condition	Treatment
OME	**Antibiotics** Amoxicillin Amoxicillin with clavulinic acid Erythromycin with sulfa Cephalosporin Trimethaprim with sulfa **Decongestants (efficacy unconfirmed)** Pseudoephedrine Phenylephrine
Chronic OME	**Surgery** Tympanostomy tubes Adenoidectomy **Steroids (efficacy unconfirmed)**
Allergic rhinitis	**Allergen avoidance** **Antihistamines** Chlorpheniramine Terfenadine Astemizole Loratadine **Intranasal topical steroids** Beclomethasone Fluticasone Triamcinolone Budesonide **Intranasal cromolyn** **Immunotherapy**

11.24 Therapy for otitis media and associated allergies.

REFERENCES

Bernstein JM: Recent advances in immunologic reactivity in otitis media with effusion. *J Allergy Clin Immunol*, 81:1004, 1988.

Bluestone CD, Doyle WJ: Anatomy and physiology of eustachian tube and middle ear related to otitis media. *J Allergy Clin Immunol*, 81:997, 1988.

Bluestone CD, Klein JO: *Otitis Media in Infants and Children*, W.B. Saunders, Philadelphia, 1988.

Doyle WJ, Skiner DP,Hayden F, Buchman C, Fireman P: Nasal and otological effects of experimental Influenza A virus infection. *Am Otol Rhinol Laryngol*, 103:59–69, 1994.

Fireman P. Nasal allergy: A risk factor for middle ear disease. *Ann. Allergy*, 58:395, 1987.

Fireman P. New concept of pathogenesis of otitis media with effusion. *Immunol Allergy Clinics North America*, 7:133, 1987.

Teele DW, Klein JO, Rosner BA: Epidemiology of otitis media in children. *Ann Otol Rhinol Laryngol*, 89(suppl 68):5, 1980.

Welliver RC: Allergy and middle ear effusions: fact or fiction, in Bernstein JM, Ogra PL (eds): *Immunology of the Ear*, Raven Press, New York, 1987.

Zitelli BJ, Davis HW (eds): Pediatric otolaryngology. *Atlas of Pediatric Diagnosis*, C.V. Mosby, St Louis, Chapter 20, 1987.

CHAPTER 12

Allergic Immunologic Ocular Diseases

Lee A. Wiley
Robert C. Arffa
Philip Fireman

Allergic and immunologic ocular diseases are influenced by the unique anatomy and physiology of the eye and ocular adnexa. For appropriate diagnosis and therapy, it is important for the clinician to be thoroughly familiar with the anatomy of the eye and its associated structures as illustrated in **12.1–12.3**. In this chapter, we describe how immunologic processes have been adapted to deal efficiently with the environmental antigens that continually impact on the eye, and how these processes can contribute to allergic disease. These ocular diseases are then discussed in terms of their clinical presentations, pathologies, and treatments.

NORMAL OCULAR ANATOMY

CONJUNCTIVA

Conjunctiva, the mucosa of the ocular surface, is comparable to other epithelia, such as those lining the gut and bronchi, that are exposed to the environment and subjected to a barrage of antigens and microorganisms. The conjunctiva and associated regional lymphoid tissues acquire and process antigens to produce sensitized T- and B-cells, thus providing a mechanism of immune response well-adapted to the surveillance of an exposed surface. Immunoreactive cell populations vary within the different layers and anatomical regions of conjunctiva (**12.4**). The lymphocytes of the conjunctival epithelium are mainly CD_8 cells. Langerhans cells, which function in the afferent limb as antigen-presenting cells, are most plentiful in the epibulbar and forniceal conjunctiva. These Langerhans cells participate in ocular contact allergy and corneal homograft rejection. The substantia propria of the conjunctiva is populated by a nearly equal proportion of CD_8 (cytotoxic/suppressor) and CD_4 (helper/inducer) T-cells. A smaller population of B-cells arranged in lymphoid aggregates is present in the fornices (**12.4**). Mast cells are present in the substantia propria of the conjunctiva and tissues of the eyelid, as are dendritic cells. Plasma cells are adjacent to the accessory lacrimal tissue. Lymphatics of the conjunctiva and eyelid drain laterally to the preauricular and parotid nodes and medially to the submandibular nodes.

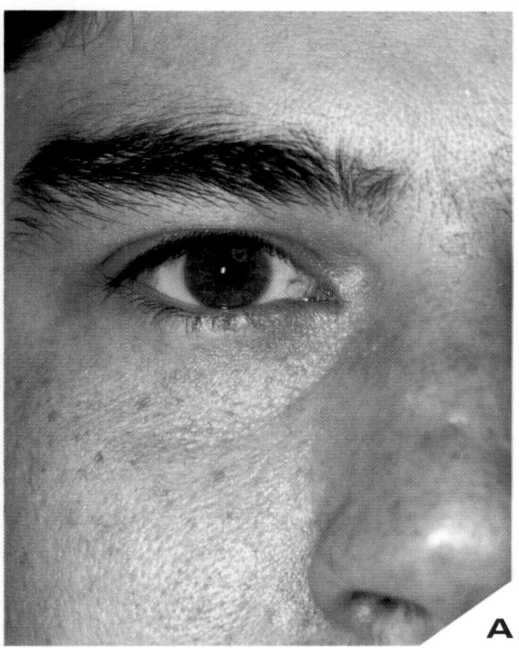

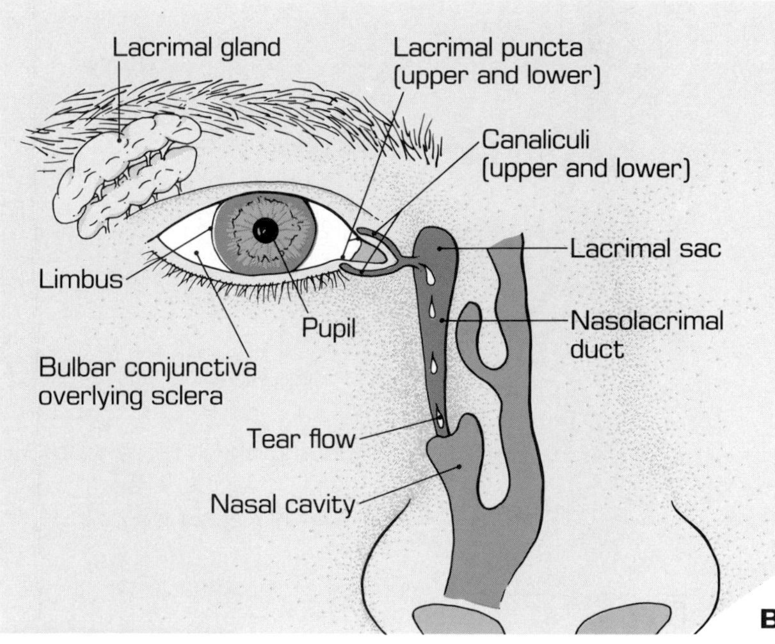

12.1 (A) The external landmarks of a normal eye. (B) Diagrammatic representation of the external landmarks of a normal eye and lacrimal system.

THE LACRIMAL GLANDS

The lacrimal glands are located in the superotemporal orbits and are responsible for production of the aqueous component of tears (*see* **12.1** and **12.5**). The tears contain secretory IgA antibodies and many other substances, such as lysozyme, that may be important to host defense.

Lymphoid aggregates composed of B-cells, macrophages, dendritic cells, and CD_4 (helper/inducer) T-cells, are active in local antigen processing which leads to the development of IgA-producing plasma cells. The aggregates associated with the intralobular ducts of the lacrimal gland have a high proportion of plasma cells, the majority producing IgA (**12.5**). This IgA is taken up by the lacrimal gland acinar cells which contribute the IgA secretory pieces that allow transport of the dimeric secretory IgA to the gland lumen. The components of the classic and alternative complement system are also present in tears. The lymphatic channels of the lacrimal gland drain to the preauricular and cervical nodes.

THE CORNEA

The cornea is the transparent and avascular major optical component of the eye (*see* **12.3**). It has no blood or lymphatic vessels, but in the non-inflamed eye Langerhans cells are found in the epithelium, with greatest density at the limbus and decreasing toward the central cornea. As in the conjunctiva, the Langerhans cells express DR antigen and present antigens to lymphoid tissue. Complement components are found throughout the corneal stroma. Immune complex-mediated disease often initially affects the peripheral cornea, presumably as a result of its proximity to the limbal vasculature. Vascularization of the cornea is accompanied by the development of lymphatic channels and both of these diminish the relative immune privilege of the cornea (*see* **12.17** and **12.18**).

THE LENS

The lens is a biconvex structure located in the posterior chamber behind the pupil. It aids in forming a focused image on the photoreceptor area, the retina (*see* **12.3**). It has been proposed that since proteins of the lens are 'sequestered' from the immune system, they might be recognized as foreign antigens. The tolerance to lens antigens may be overcome when a large amount of lens material is released in combination with trauma-induced inflammation and/or microbial contamination.

CONJUNCTIVAL AND CORNEAL ALLERGIC DISEASES

The most commonly encountered allergic ocular disorders are allergic conjunctivitis (hay fever), vernal keratoconjunctivitis, atopic keratoconjunctivitis, and giant papillary conjunctivitis. These conditions can range in severity from the minimally symptomatic allergic conjunctivitis to the visually threatening atopic keratoconjunctivitis. Although the immunopathogenesis of these diseases varies, mast cells play a significant role, since many of them are present in the substantia propria of the conjunctiva and eyelid (*see* **12.4**). Basophils are also involved in the cellular infiltrate of several allergic ocular disorders. The distinguishing clinical features of the conditions are shown in **12.6**.

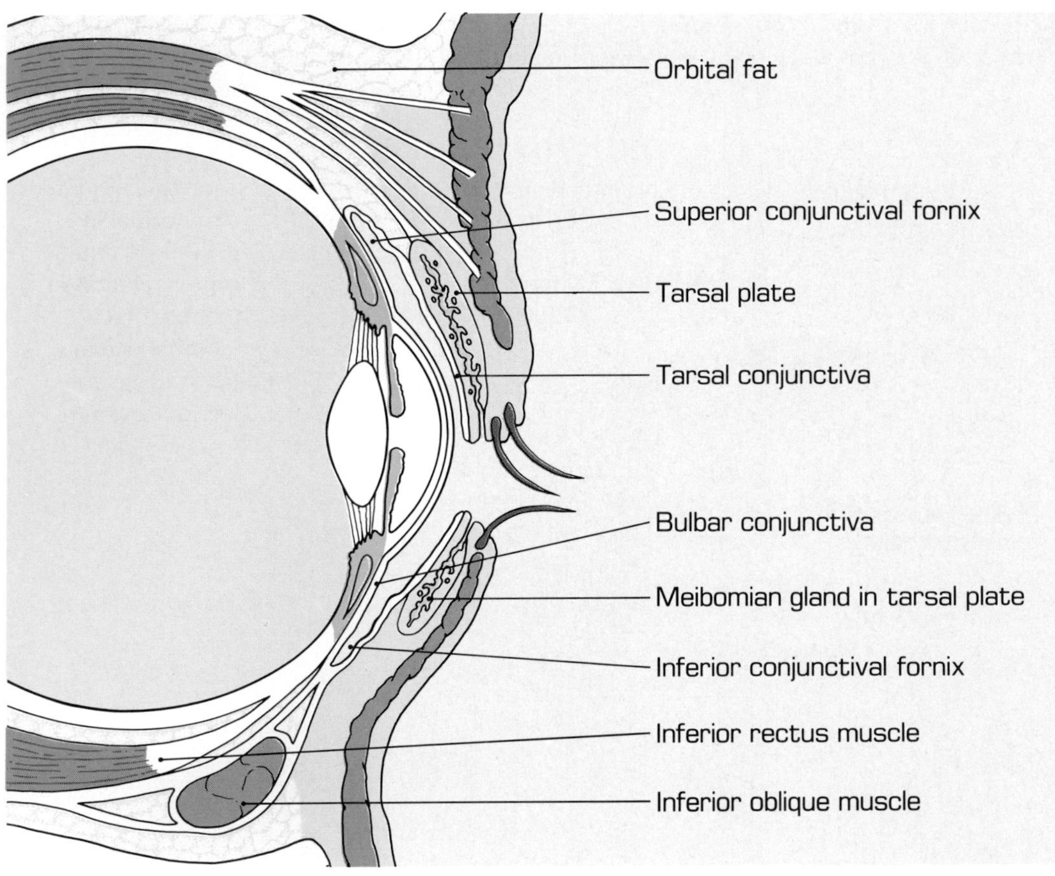

12.2 Sagittal view of the eyelids and the ocular orbit.

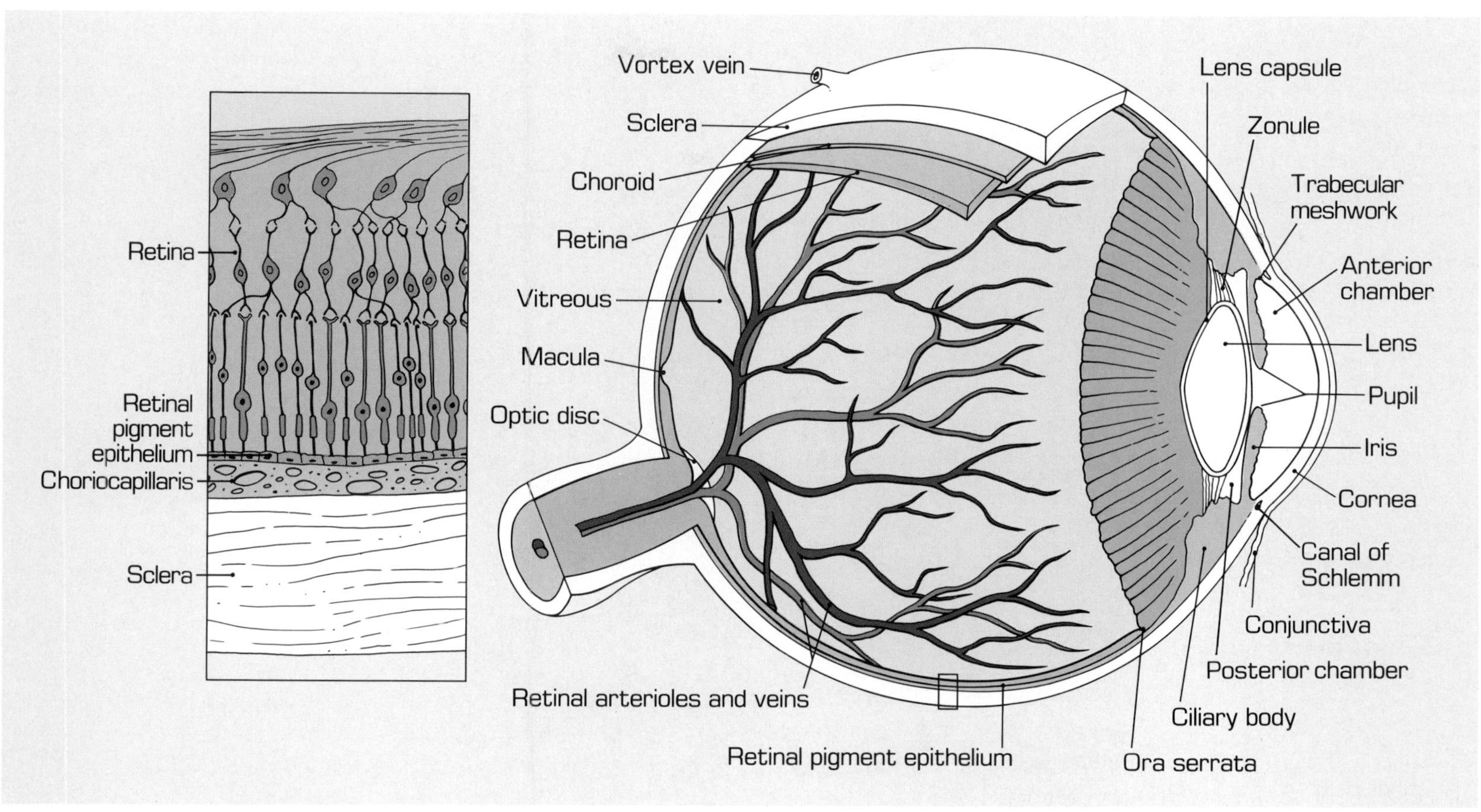

12.3 The internal structures of the eye.

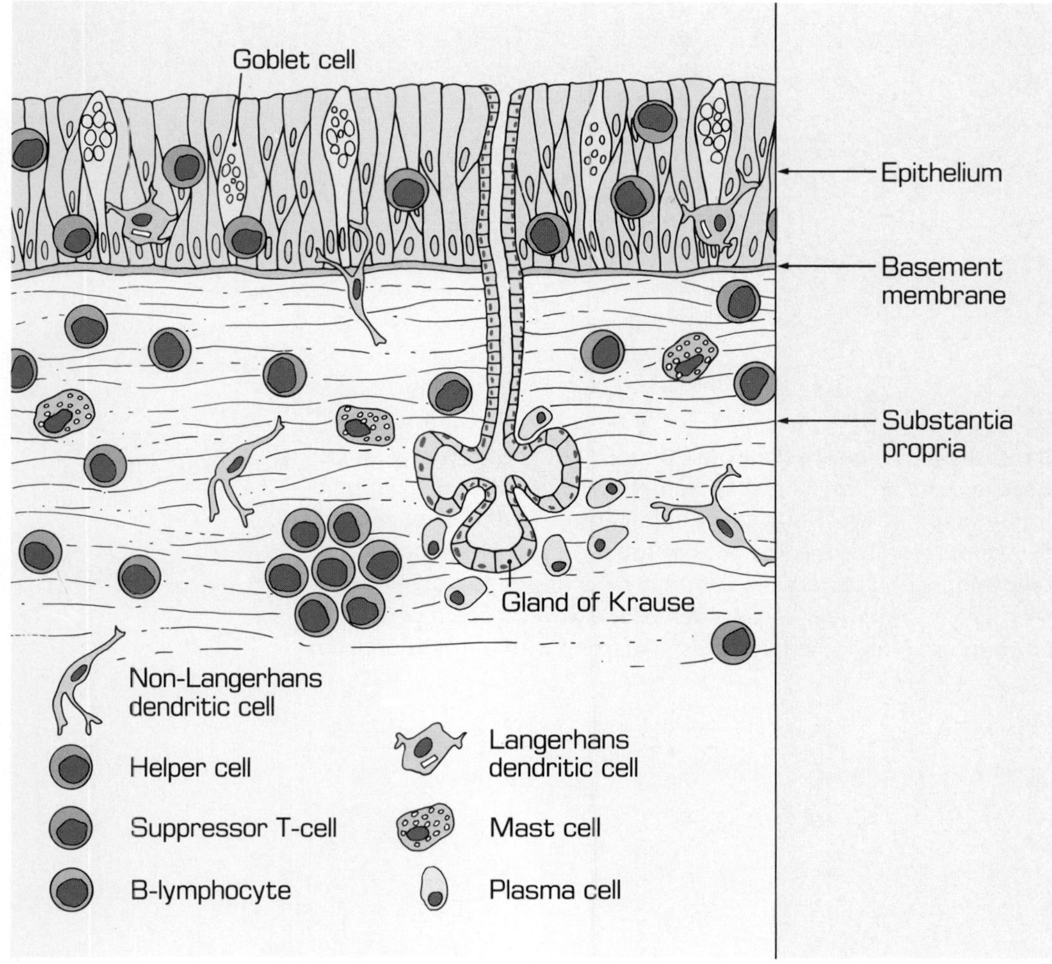

12.4 A diagram of the immunohistology of the conjunctiva. Only T-lymphocytes are present in the epithelium, with a preponderance of suppressor/cytotoxic T-cells. Dendritic Langerhans cells are also present in the epithelium. The substantia propria contains an equal proportion of helper and suppressor T-lymphocytes. Non-Langerhans dendritic cells and mast cells reside in the substantia propria as well. Aggregates of lymphoid cells, including B-lymphocytes and plasma cells, are found in association with the accessory lacrimal glands, also known as glands of Krause. (Adapted with permission from Sacks *et al.*, 1986.)

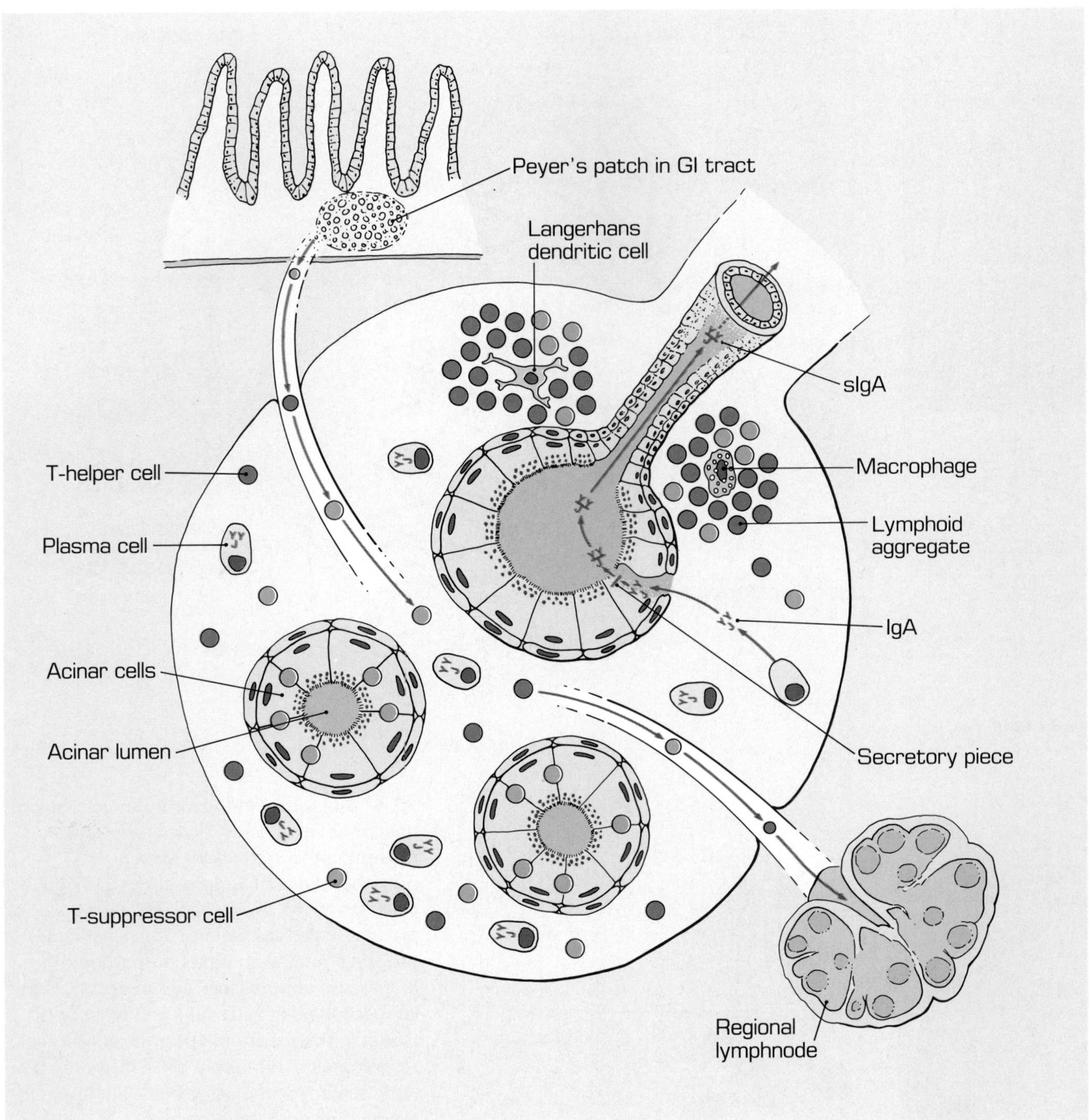

12.5 The immunologic structure of the lacrimal gland. Plasma cells are distributed throughout the lacrimal gland interstitium. They produce dimeric IgA, which diffuses into the acinar cells. A secretory piece is added, allowing transport of the immunoglobulin into the acinar lumen. Within the lacrimal gland epithelium, T-suppressor cells outnumber T-helper cells, and in the gland interstitium, T-suppressor cells remain more numerous. B-lymphocytes are found in periductular aggregates, sometimes in association with Langerhans dendritic cells or macrophages, which process and present antigens. Interaction with other mucosal lymphoid tissue, such as the Peyer's patch of the intestine, as well as regional lymph nodes, is possible through migrating lymphocytes. (Adapted with permission from Wieczorek *et al.*, 1988.)

CLINICAL CHARACTERISTICS OF ALLERGIC, VERNAL, AND ATOPIC CONJUNCTIVITIS

	Allergic conjunctivitis	Vernal conjunctivitis	Atopic conjunctivitis
Pathogenesis	Type 1 IgE-mediated hypersensitivity reaction to environmental antigen	Chronic, Type 1 IgE-mediated hypersensitivity reaction Cutaneous basophilic hypersensitivity may play a role	Chronic, Type 1 IgE-mediated hypersensitivity Cutaneous basophilic hypersensitivity and deficient cellular immunity may also play a role
Seasonal variation	Often seasonal; worsens with high pollen counts Associated with allergic rhinitis	Exacerbation in spring or summer More prevalent in warm climates	No seasonal variation
Ages affected	All ages	3–25 years; 80% of cases occur under 14 years of age	Begins in late teens; many cases remit at age 40–50
Conjunctival eye disease	Conjunctival injection and edema (chemosis)	Upper tarsal conjunctiva with giant papillae Limbal form shows gelatinous papillae at limbus	Papillary conjunctivitis of lower palpebral conjunctiva Conjunctival scarring and symblepharon may occur
Corneal complications	No corneal ulceration or scarring	Shallow vernal ulcer with vascularization	Deep corneal vascularization and corneal melting in severe cases
Conjunctival scraping	Eosinophils rarely seen	Often many eosinophils and free eosinophilic granules More than two eosinophils per high-power field is pathognomonic	Rare eosinophils and no free eosinophilic granules
Eyelids	Periorbital and eyelid edema	Swelling and ptosis of upper lids	Atopic dermatitis of lids Poor apposition of lids to globe resulting from scarring of eyelid skin

12.6 Comparison of clinical characteristics of allergic (hay fever), vernal, and atopic conjunctivitis.

ALLERGIC (HAY FEVER) CONJUNCTIVITIS

Clinical presentation

Patients with allergic conjunctivitis complain of itching, tightness, and swelling around their eyes. Affecting people of all ages, this very common condition is often associated with other atopic disorders, such as allergic rhinitis (*see* Chapter 9). It may be seasonal or perennial, depending on the provocative antigens, and there is often a family history of allergy. While there may be conjunctival edema, injection, and lid swelling, the symptoms often far exceed the objective findings (**12.7**). Although eosinophils may be present in the conjunctival substantia propria, they are seldom found in the epithelium and are not routinely detected in a conjunctival scraping. In addition to the history, skin testing or *in vitro* IgE antibody determinations are the chief methods of identifying the offending allergens (*see* Chapter 3).

Pathogenesis

The pathogenesis of allergic conjunctivitis involves a Type I hypersensitivity reaction initiated by the binding of an antigen to a specific IgE-receptor molecule on the sensitized mast cell. The specific binding of the allergen results in the generation and release of mast cell inflammatory mediators, such as histamine, leukotrienes, prostaglandins, and neutrophil and eosinophil chemotactic factors. The ocular tissues can manifest both early (15–60 minutes) and late-phase (2–6 hours) IgE-mediated allergic reactions.

Treatment

The treatment of allergic conjunctivitis consists of limiting the patient's exposure to the allergen, once it has been identified. Cool compresses applied to the orbital areas may provide some symptomatic relief. Topical antihistamines, such as the recently released levocabastine, that inhibit the H_1 receptor reduce itching and tearing. Topical vasoconstrictors reduce conjunctival injection, and many vasoconstrictor–antihistamine combinations are available. Topical cromolyn is also effective in preventing the allergic reaction. Non-steroid anti-inflammatory agents, such as ketoralek 0.5%, have been shown to reduce conjunctival inflammation and provide subjective improvement. Lodoxamide 0.1%, a topical mast-cell stabilizer, may be used four times a day during the peak allergen exposure to inhibit the release of inflammatory mediators. Low-doses should be used sparingly because they may precipitate steroid-induced glaucoma and cataracts, or they may exacerbate microbial infections. Patients with allergic rhinoconjunctivitis respond well to allergen hyposensitization.

VERNAL KERATOCONJUNCTIVITIS

Clinical presentation

Vernal keratoconjunctivitis is a bilateral, recurrent conjunctivitis that affects young people, 3–25 years of age. The term vernal refers to the seasonal (spring and summer) exacerbation of symptoms. However, there may not be a direct association between symptoms and seasonal allergens. This disorder is more prevalent in warm

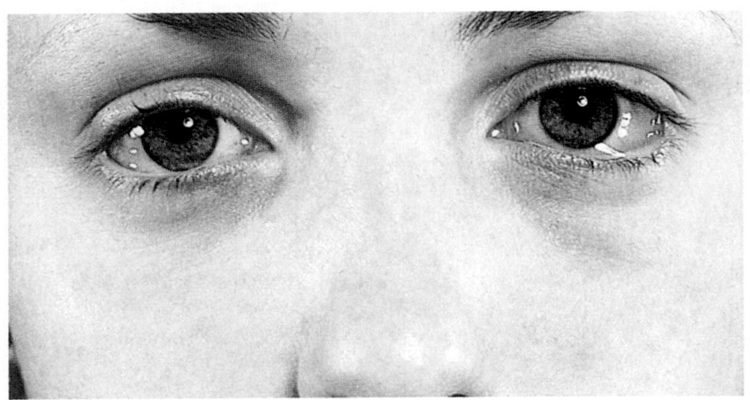

12.7 Allergic conjunctivitis with marked conjunctival edema and slight injection. This is often associated with allergic rhinitis (hay fever). (Reproduced with permission from Spalton *et al.*, 1984.)

climates and may remit in cooler climates. The symptoms of itching and photophobia may be severe, and it is fortunate that most patients become less symptomatic in their twenties. There are two forms of the disease: *palpebral* and *limbal*. The palpebral form affects the upper tarsal conjunctiva, with the appearance of large flat-topped elevations, termed giant papillae. Generally over 1 mm in diameter, these papillae can be seen easily (without magnification) on eversion of the upper lid (**12.8**). The limbal form exhibits a gelatinous papillary hypertrophy of the limbal conjunctiva (**12.9**), often with chalk-white concretions of eosinophils, called Trantas' dots. The cornea may be affected with a fine punctate epithelial cell loss or with a vernal corneal ulcer (**12.10**). Lens opacities develop in some patients. Conjunctival scraping typically reveals many eosinophils. Increased levels of serum IgE can be present, as well as specific IgE antibodies to environmental allergens. The majority of patients have a history of other atopic conditions and familial allergic disease.

Pathogenesis

Although the large number of eosinophils and degranulated mast cells in the tissue suggest an important role for Type I hypersensitivity, this mechanism cannot explain all the findings. The giant papillae contain newly synthesized collagen and massive numbers of mast cells, eosinophils, basophils, and lymphocytes. It has been suggested that a T-cell mediated, delayed hypersensitivity contributes to the disease process.

Treatment

Cold compresses and topical vasoconstrictors with antihistamines may provide relief in mild cases. Topical cromolyn sodium has also been found effective and may be combined with vasoconstrictors and antihistamines. Lodoxamide has demonstrated efficacy and may be combined with topical NSAIDs and antihistamines. Reduction of systems reduces the mechanical trauma of eye rubbing, which may contribute to the release of mast-cell mediators and the development of a vernal corneal ulcer.

For moderate disease, topical corticosteroids may help in the early phase of treatment, allowing taper to the more innocuous regimen of mast-cell stabilizers and NSAIDs. High doses (up to 1.5 g/day) of oral aspirin have been useful in some recalcitrant cases. Other topical immunodilators, such as cyclosporin, may offer other therapeutic options. Allergen immunotherapy may be employed if specific disease-associated IgE antibodies are documented. Severe cases may benefit from a brief course of systemic steroids.

ATOPIC KERATOCONJUNCTIVITIS

Clinical presentation

Atopic keratoconjunctivitis (AKC) is a chronic bilateral keratoconjunctivitis that occurs in patients with atopic dermatitis. The symptoms of itching and burning may be severe. Advanced cases often have a stringy, mucopurulent discharge. This allergic disorder is

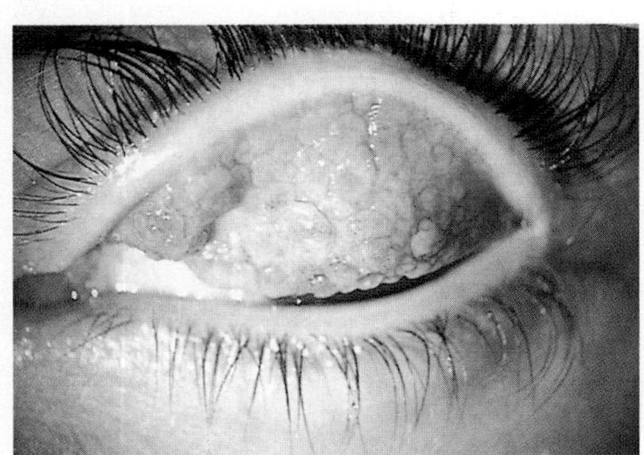

12.8 Vernal conjunctivitis, palpebral form. The giant papillary elevations are seen easily without magnification.

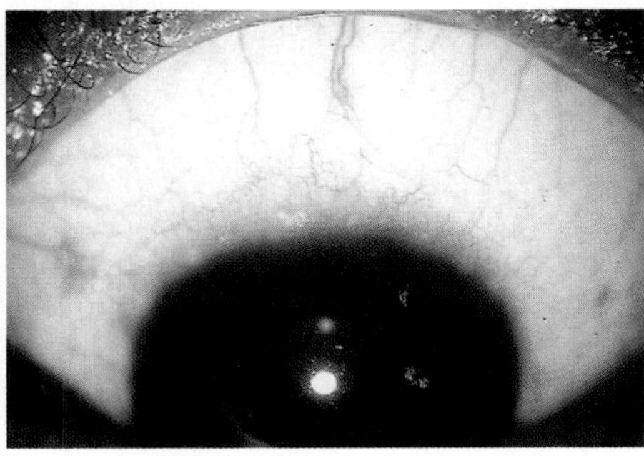

12.9 Vernal conjunctivitis, limbal form. Note the gelatinous papillary elevations of the limbal tissue.

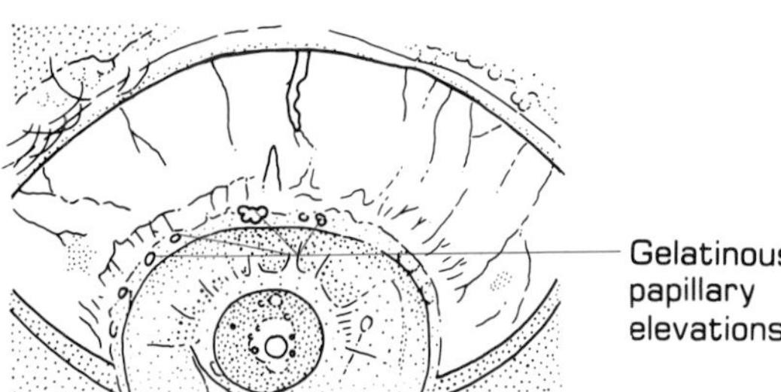

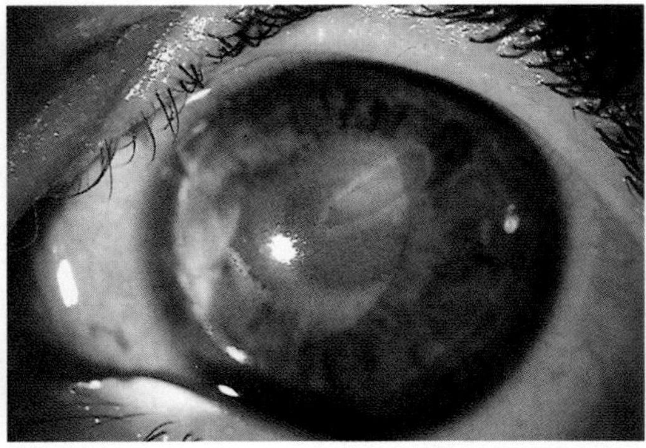

12.10 Vernal conjunctivitis with vernal corneal ulcer.

most common in men and teenage boys, tending to remit by the age of 50. The lids are thickened, indurated, and lichenified (**12.11A**), sometimes with sufficient scarring to prevent apposition of the eyelid to the globe. There is often a chronic staphylococcal infection of the eyelid margins, with lid margin hyperemia and crusty deposits on the lashes. The inferior palpebral and forniceal conjunctiva are affected by a chronic papillary conjunctivitis (**12.11B**). The limbal conjunctiva may be thickened with gelatinous elevations. Corneal changes can be severe: superficial scarring, vascularization, recurrent epithelial ulceration, and corneal perforation are vision-threatening complications (**12.11C**). Approximately 10% of patients with atopic dermatitis develop cataracts (**12.12**).

Pathogenesis

The pathogenesis of AKC may be similar to that of atopic dermatitis (*see* Chapter 15). Serum IgE, as well as allergen-specific IgE, antibodies are elevated in the majority of patients, sometimes waxing and waning with the symptoms. Mast cell counts are increased in inflamed tissues. In atopic dermatitis, surface IgE has been detected not only on mast cells and basophils, but also on macrophages and dendritic cells, suggesting another pathway by which IgE may trigger inflammation. The deficiency of suppressor T-cells in the related condition of atopic dermatitis provides further evidence of abnormal cell-mediated immunity.

Treatment

A regimen similar to the other allergic diseases, hinging on a mast-cell stabilizer and utilizing topical NSAIDs and antihistamines (levocabastine) may be employed. A special caution with topical corticosteroids must be exercised due to the propensity to corneal melting and infection. Artificial tear supplements and topical mucolytic agents may be used to relieve the symptoms associated with concurrent stringy mucopurulent discharge.

OTHER RELATED CONDITIONS

There are several other conjunctival and corneal diseases of note. *Giant papillary conjunctivitis* (**12.13**) occurs when the upper lid meets a foreign body, such as a contact lens, prosthesis, or exposed suture. The papillae, composed of collagen, are heavily infiltrated with eosinophils, basophils, and mast cells. Scrupulous cleansing to remove contact lens protein deposits, a change to a different lens design, and the use of cromolyn or topical anti-inflammatory agents may allow a patient to continue wearing lenses.

Inflamed, scaly, periocular skin, lid margin hyperemia, and conjunctival injection are characteristic of *contact dermatoconjunctivitis* (**12.14**). Scarring of the forniceal conjunctiva, punctal closure, and foreshortening of the lower eyelid skin, with poor apposition to the globe, may occur. This Type IV hypersensitivity response may

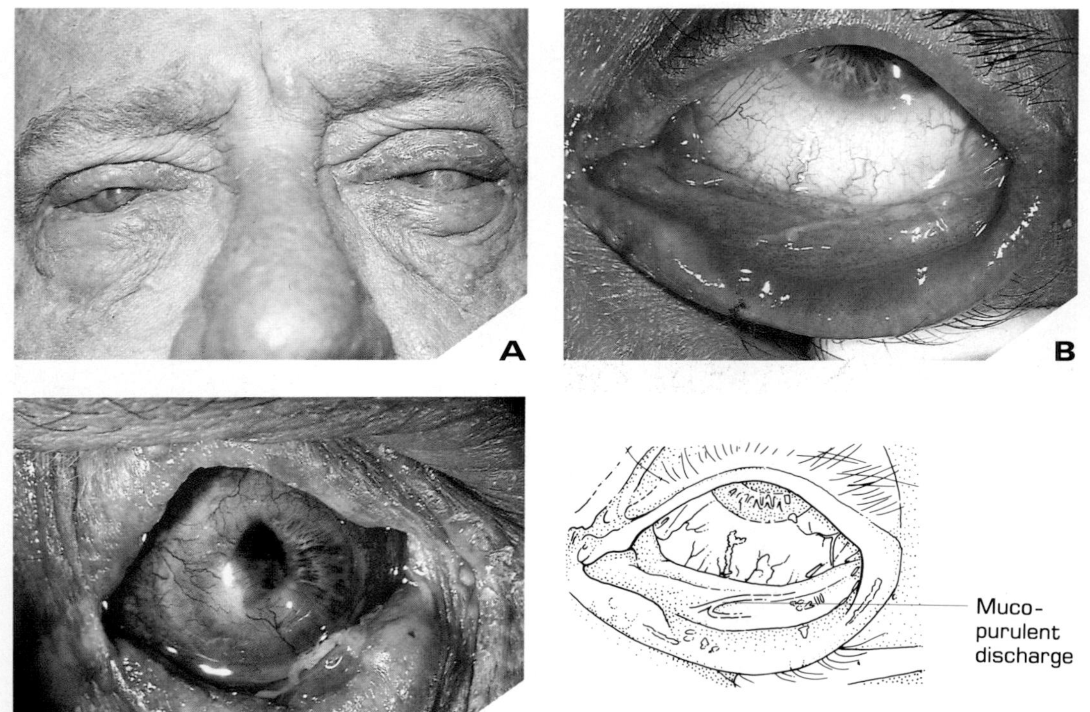

12.11 (A) Atopic keratoconjunctivitis with thickened, indurated eyelids. Note the loss of lashes. The left eye has undergone application of tissue adhesive for a corneal perforation. (B) Atopic keratoconjunctivitis with chronic papillary conjunctivitis. Note the stringy mucopurulent discharge often seen in this disorder. (C) Atopic keratoconjunctivitis with corneal scarring and vascularization.

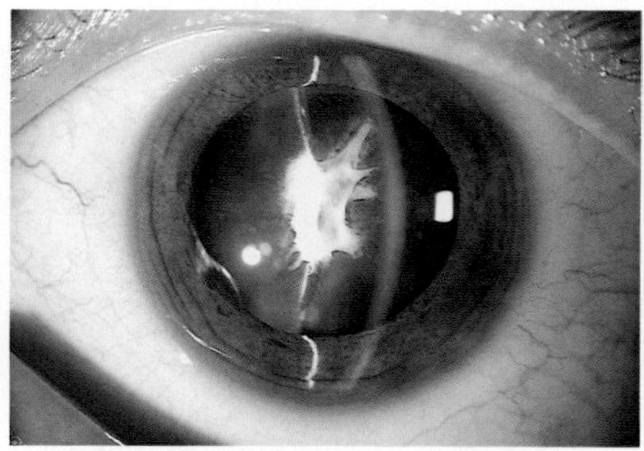

12.12 Cataract seen in patient with atopic dermatitis.

occur in reaction to topical application of many substances, including cosmetics and ophthalmic medications, such as neomycin, epinephrine, and atropine.

In *phlyctenular keratoconjunctivitis* (**12.15**), an elevated, actively inflamed corneal lesion usually ulcerates and then spontaneously resolves within several weeks, leaving a visible scar. This condition is believed to be a Type IV hypersensitivity response to microbial antigens from *Staphylococcus*, *Candida*, or tuberculosis. Lid scrubs and topical antibiotics may decrease exposure to the inciting antigen, and topical corticosteroids may speed resolution of the inflammation, limiting the scarring of the visual axis.

Catarrhal marginal infiltrates begin in the anterior corneal stroma, parallel with the limbus, and show a lucid interval of clear

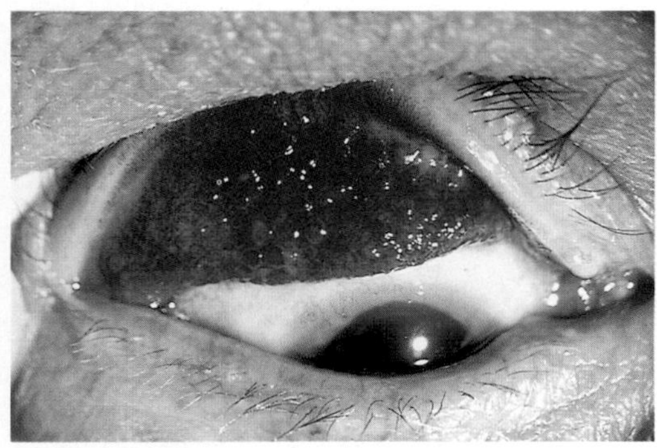

12.13 Characteristic lesions of giant papillary conjunctivitis. These hobnail-like elevations of the upper tarsal conjunctiva, evident on eversion of the upper eyelid, occur when the upper lid meets a foreign body, such as a contact lens, prosthesis, or exposed suture.

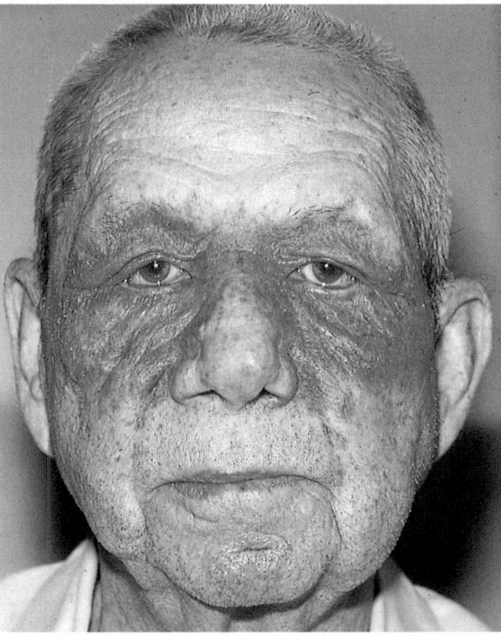

12.14 Contact dermatoconjunctivitis reaction to neomycin, with characteristic inflamed, scaly, periocular skin, lid margin hyperemia, and conjunctival injection. Scarring of the forniceal conjunctiva, punctal closure, and foreshortening of the lower eyelid skin with poor apposition to the globe may occur.

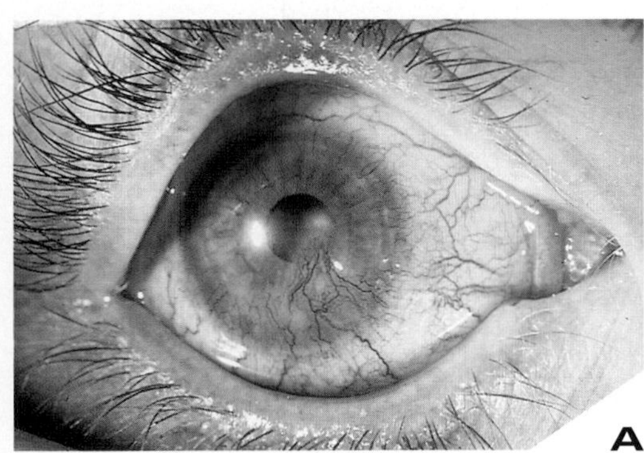

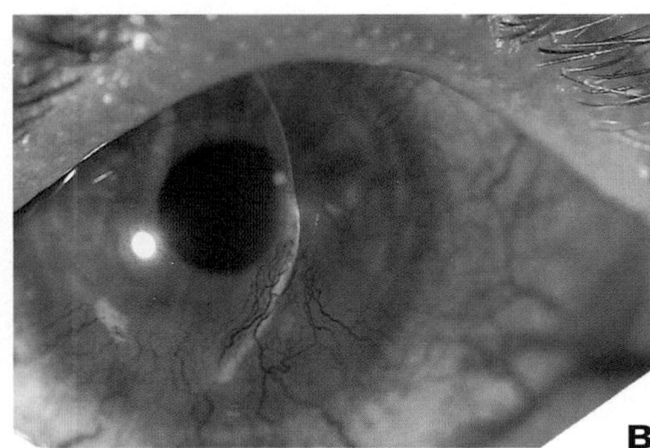

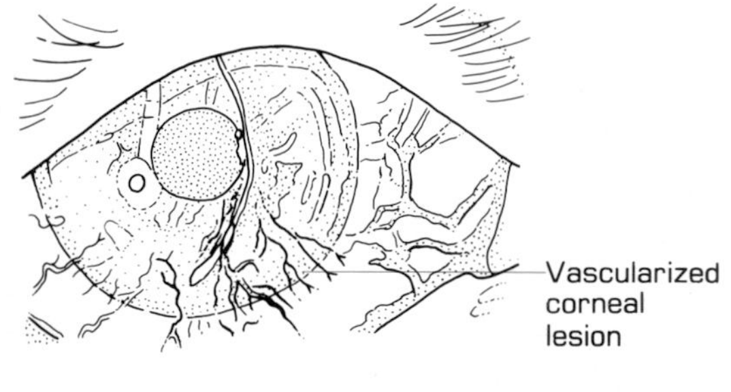

12.15 (A) The characteristic triangular, vascularized corneal scar of phlyctenular keratoconjunctivitis. (B) Closer view detailing the elevated, actively inflamed corneal lesion. This elevated area usually ulcerates and then spontaneously resolves within several weeks, leaving a visually disabling scar.

cornea (**12.16**). Often multiple, these lesions can spread circumferentially and ulcerate, mimicking an infectious corneal ulcer. This self-limited process may be due to immune complex deposition in the cornea provoked by antigens from infectious agents. The condition often responds to treatment of the associated blepharitis with lid scrubs, antibiotics, and judicious use of topical corticosteroids.

Peripheral ulcerative keratitis (**12.17**) occurs in conjunction with collagen vascular diseases, such as rheumatoid arthritis, systemic lupus erythematosus, relapsing polychondritis, progressive systemic sclerosis, Wegener's granulomatosis, and polyarteritis nodosa. It manifests as inflammation, ulceration, and thinning of the cornea and adjacent sclera. Control of the systemic disease is the most effective therapeutic approach. In a series of patients with rheumatoid arthritis and necrotizing scleritis or peripheral ulcerative keratitis, reduced mortality was observed with the use of systemic immunosuppressive medications.

Mooren's ulcer (**12.18**) is a rare, chronic, inflammatory disease of the peripheral cornea characterized by progressive thinning and loss of the anterior corneal stroma. Topical steroids, resection of the inflamed limbal conjunctiva adjacent to the ulcer, and systemic immunosuppression represent the stepwise approach most often used to treat this disease. Mooren's ulcer has recently been associated with chronic hepatitis C infections – these cases have responded to interferon alpha-2b therapy.

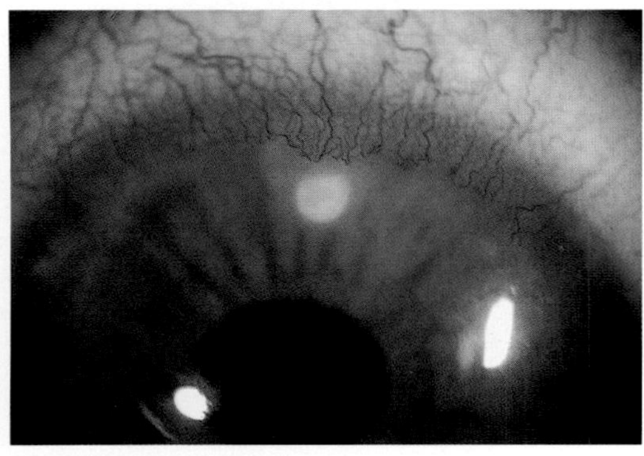

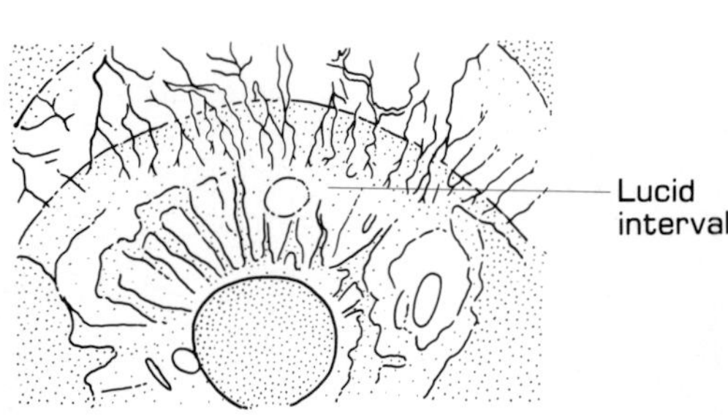

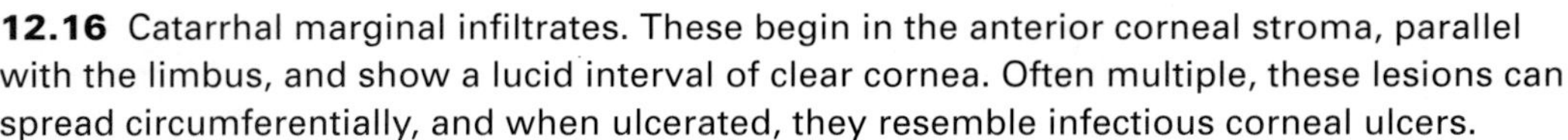

12.16 Catarrhal marginal infiltrates. These begin in the anterior corneal stroma, parallel with the limbus, and show a lucid interval of clear cornea. Often multiple, these lesions can spread circumferentially, and when ulcerated, they resemble infectious corneal ulcers.

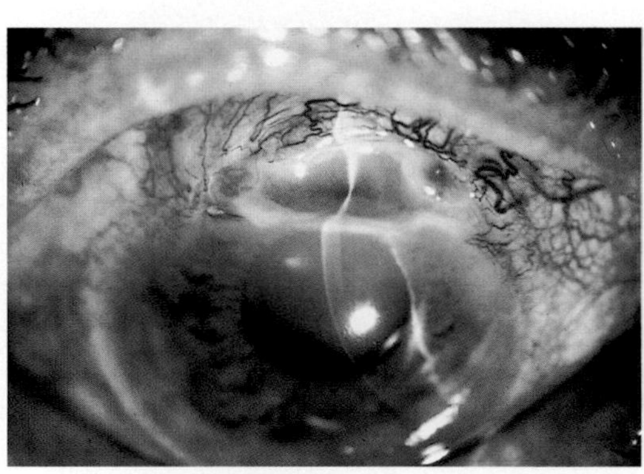

12.17 Inflammation, ulceration, and thinning of the cornea and adjacent sclera, characteristic of peripheral ulcerative keratitis. This condition occurs in conjunction with other collagen vascular diseases, including rheumatoid arthritis (as in this case), systemic lupus erythematosus, relapsing polychondritis, progressive systemic sclerosis, Wegener's granulomatosis, and polyarteritis nodosa.

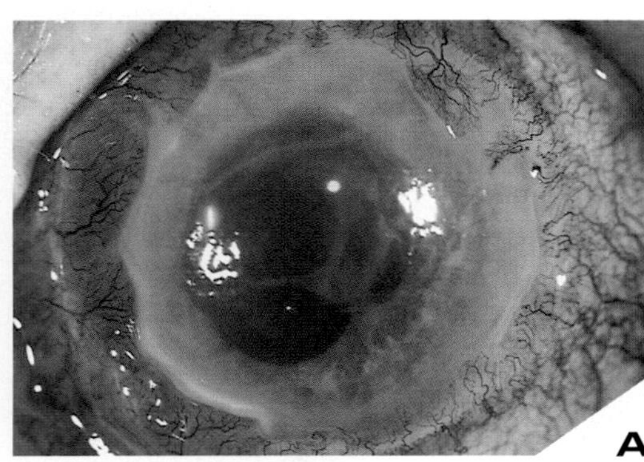

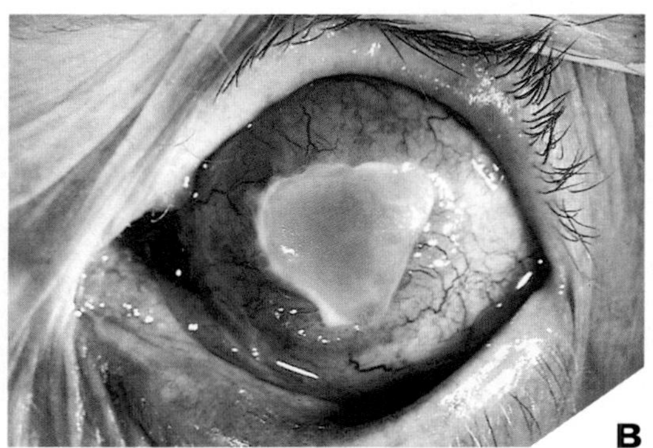

12.18 Mooren's ulcer is a rare, chronic inflammatory disease of the peripheral cornea, characterized by progressive thinning and loss of the anterior corneal stroma. Circumferential and central progression is illustrated by the appearance (A) on presentation and (B) 3 months later. The cellular infiltrate in the conjunctiva adjacent to the ulcer, and evidence of lymphocyte stimulation by corneal antigen, suggest a local autoimmune phenomenon.

SCLERAL DISEASES

The opaque wall of the globe is called the sclera (*see* **12.3**). It is avascular, composed primarily of collagen and elastic tissue. The episclera is a fibrovascular membrane that encases the sclera, provides nutrition, allows smooth movement of the globe, and, together with the muscle sheaths to which it is fused, prevents excess movement. The eye and orbit can be thought of as a modified ball-and-socket joint, the episclera being analogous to a synovial membrane. Many of the collagen vascular diseases that cause inflammation of joints may also cause scleritis or episcleritis (**12.19**).

Inflammation of these deeper structures can usually be differentiated from conjunctival inflammation by history and clinical examination. Deep eye pain occurs with scleral inflammation, but does not occur with conjunctivitis. Most important is examination of the sclera in daylight. Deep vascular inflammation appears violet, and with increased scleral thinning the dark choroid may be better observed. Since scleritis is often bilateral and recurrent, scleral thinning may be apparent in the fellow eye, or in uninflamed areas of the same eye. The involved tissue is tender – this does not occur in conjunctivitis. Blanching of the more superficial conjunctival vessels may be obtained with topical phenylephrine 10% (**12.20**), revealing persistent inflammation of the episcleral vessels.

EPISCLERITIS AND SCLERITIS

Clinical presentation

Episcleritis is often asymptomatic, but may be accompanied by a sensation of warmth or pricking in the eye. The onset is usually sudden. Episcleral vascular engorgement may occur in three patterns: sectoral, diffuse, or nodular (**12.21**). No scleral edema or necrosis is observed. The eye is rarely tender to the touch, and vision is always normal.

DISEASES ASSOCIATED WITH EPISCLERITIS AND SCLERITIS

Infectious diseases
— Herpes simplex
— Herpes zoster
— Tuberculosis

Inflammatory diseases
— Rheumatoid arthritis
— Reiter's disease
— Systemic lupus erythematosus
— Dermatomyositis
— Polyarteritis nodosa
— Ankylosing spondylitis

Metabolic diseases
— Gout
— Syphilis
— Lyme disease
— Wegener's granulomatosis
— Psoriasis
— Cranial arteritis
— Inflammatory bowel disease
— Behçet's disease
— Relapsing polychondritis

12.19 Diseases associated with episcleritis and scleritis.

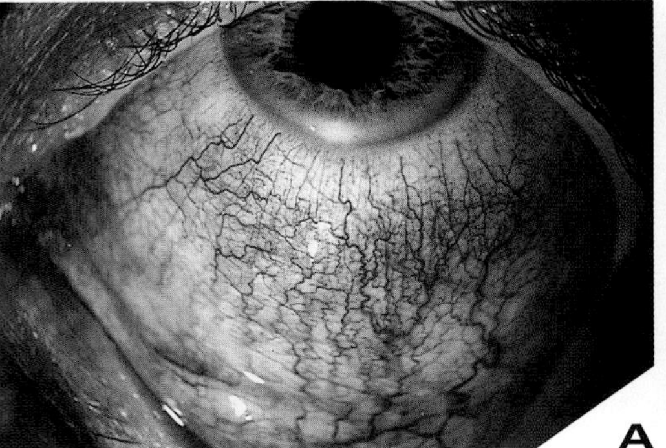

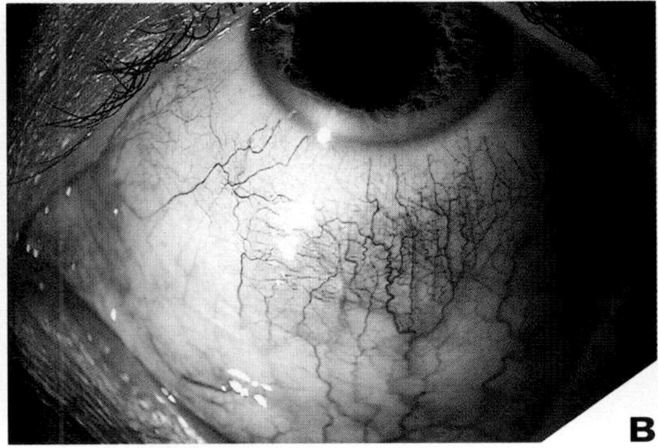

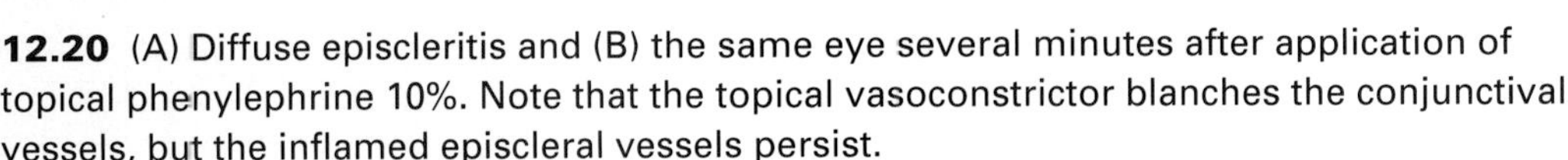
12.20 (A) Diffuse episcleritis and (B) the same eye several minutes after application of topical phenylephrine 10%. Note that the topical vasoconstrictor blanches the conjunctival vessels, but the inflamed episcleral vessels persist.

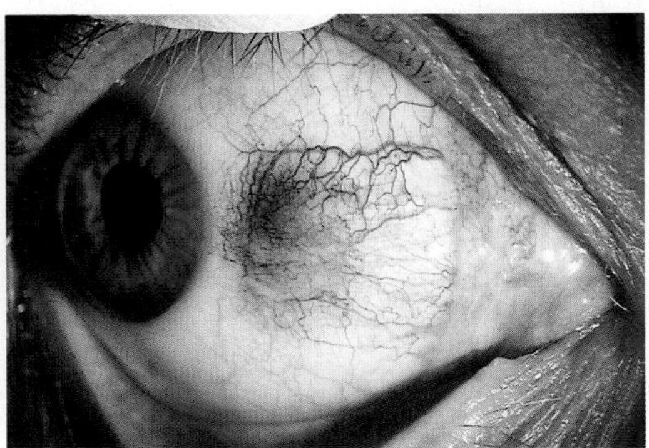

12.21 Nodular episcleritis.

In contrast, scleritis is usually gradual in onset, developing over several days. In most cases, the predominant symptom is a deep, penetrating pain, that may be severe, radiating outward to adjacent structures. Lacrimation and photophobia may occur, and visual acuity may be reduced, particularly in posterior scleritis.

Clinically, scleritis can be divided into five different types. *Nodular anterior scleritis* has one or more localized areas of scleral inflammation without necrosis. In contrast to nodular episcleritis, these nodules are tender and immovable over underlying tissue. *Diffuse anterior scleritis* is characterized by more widespread anterior scleral involvement (**12.22**). *Necrotizing anterior scleritis* with inflammation is associated with the greatest morbidity, owing to regions of vascular occlusion and loss of scleral substance (**12.23**). Attacks can lead to total destruction of the sclera, with bulging of the ocular contents or even perforation and loss of the eye.

Scleromalacia perforans cause scleral loss without signs or symptoms of inflammation and occurs almost exclusively in chronic rheumatoid arthritis patients (**12.24**). *Posterior scleritis* is not associated with anterior inflammation, and the diagnosis is frequently missed. Retinal examination may indicate exudative detachments, choroiditis and choroidal folds, or vitritis (**12.25**). A computed tomography (CT) scan of a patient with posterior scleritis is shown in **12.26**, demonstrating the increased radiodensity of the involved right sclera.

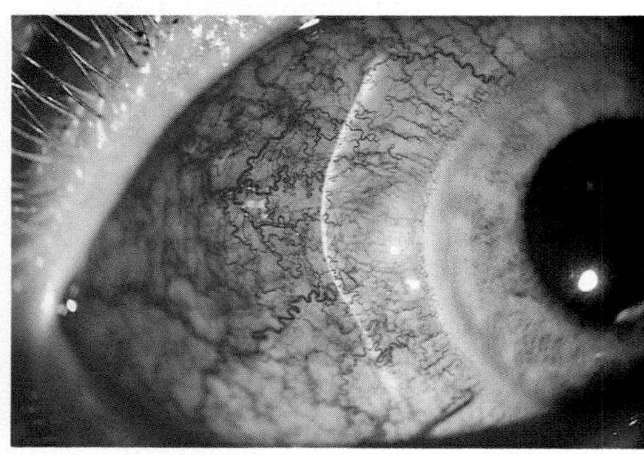

12.22 Diffuse anterior scleritis.

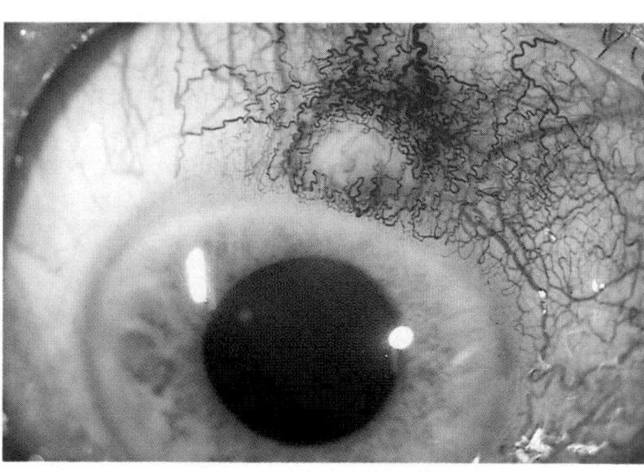

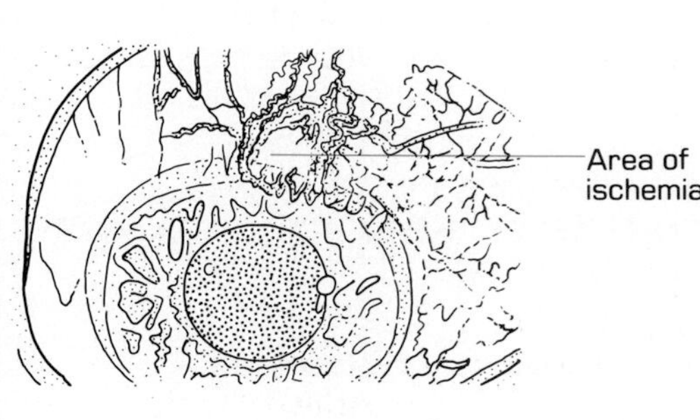

12.23 Necrotizing anterior scleritis with a nodular inflammation pattern. Note the ischemic area of the nodule.

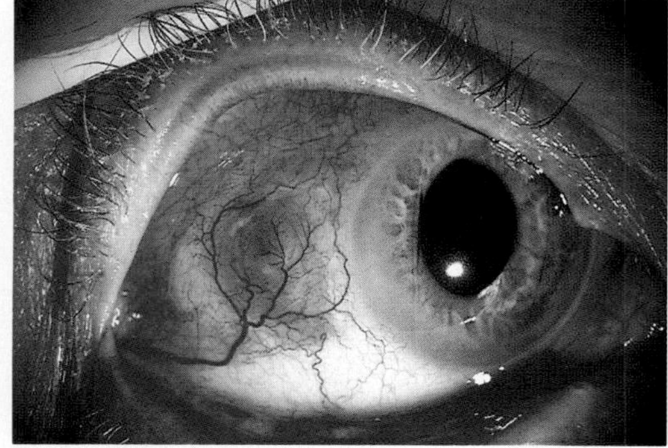

12.24 *Scleromalacia perforans* in a patient with rheumatoid arthritis.

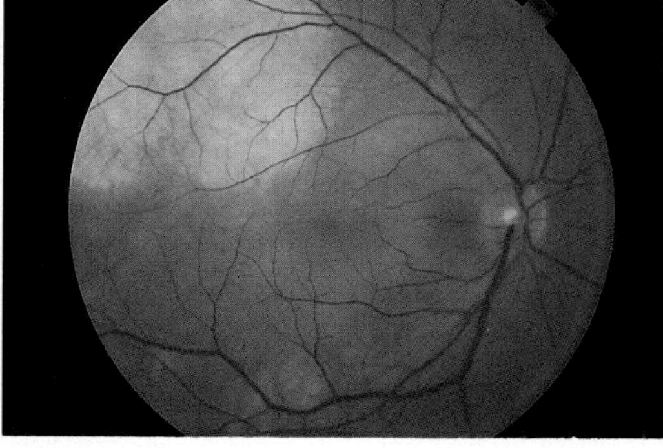

12.25 Retina of a patient with posterior scleritis. Note the areas of choroidal inflammation.

Pathogenesis

A number of diseases have been associated with scleritis and episcleritis (*see* **12.19**). Rheumatoid arthritis is the most common, but no single etiology can be identified in over 50% of patients. A lymphocytic infiltrate has been observed in episcleritis, but in scleritis, the inflammatory response is granulomatous, with fibrinoid necrosis surrounded by palisading fibroblasts, lymphocytes, plasma cells, polymorphonuclear cells, and occasional giant cells. Immune complex vasculitis is also seen, and may play a role in the scleral inflammation associated with connective tissue diseases. Scleritis in rheumatoid arthritis patients with severe articular and extra-articular disease indicates a poor prognosis; if untreated, most of these patients die within 5 years. Scleritis may indicate systemic activity in lupus erythematosus.

Treatment

Episcleritis usually resolves without treatment in 2–3 weeks, although the nodular form may last up to 2 months. If the symptoms warrant, topical steroids speed its resolution. Attacks often recur, but do not cause permanent damage or affect vision. Only very rarely does episcleritis progress to scleritis.

Topical steroids are seldom sufficient for treatment of scleritis. Systemic non-steroidal anti-inflammatory agents are often effective in non-necrotizing disease, and should be the first choice in primary episodes or mild recurrences; indomethacin, 70–100 mg/day, or tolmetin, 600–1800 mg/day, are often effective. If avascular areas are present, or in severe or unrelenting disease, systemic prednisone 80–120 mg/day is required. Sufficient treatment is given to obtain quiescence of inflammation, allowing taper to NSAIDs or immunosuppressive agents, such as methotrexate or azathioprine. Scleritis may be an important warning of the need to treat a systemic autoimmune disease.

UVEAL DISEASES

The uvea is composed of the iris, ciliary body, and choroid (*see* **12.3**). They are densely pigmented, vascular structures whose main

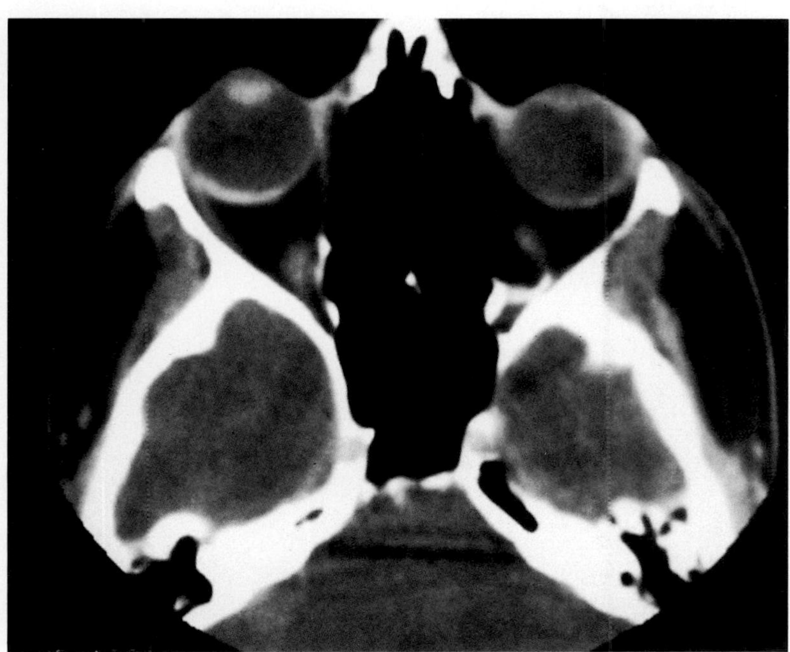

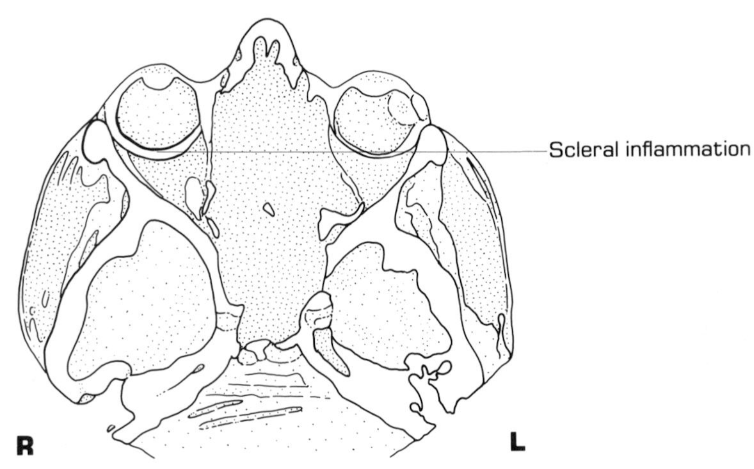

12.26 CT scan of patient with posterior scleritis. Note the area of inflammation of the right sclera.

function is to supply nutrition to the eye. In addition, the muscles of the iris and ciliary body, respectively, control the pupillary aperture and the accommodative status of the lens. Uveitis is inflammation of any portion of the uvea or retina, and can be caused by a wide variety of infectious agents and systemic diseases (**12.27**). However, in the majority of cases, no etiology can be found.

UVEITIS

Uveitis is often classified according to the primary focus of the inflammation. *Iritis* (anterior uveitis) frequently occurs in the HLA-B27-related diseases, including ankylosing spondylitis, Reiter's syndrome, and psoriatic arthritis. *Iridocyclitis* is characterized by inflammation of the iris and ciliary body. The chronic iridocyclitis seen in pauciarticular juvenile rheumatoid arthritis (JRA) (**12.28**) exemplifies the damaging sequelae of this inflammation. Ocular inflammation is most frequent in seronegative, antinuclear antibody test (ANA)-positive, pauciarticular disease, and it may cause severe damage despite apparently normal, non-inflamed sclera and conjunctiva. Regular ophthalmic evaluation of patients with JRA is important, as early diagnosis and prompt therapy with topical steroids and dilating agents appear to lessen the ocular complications (**12.29**).

DISEASES ASSOCIATED WITH ANTERIOR AND POSTERIOR UVEITIS

Anterior uveitis (iritis, iridocyclitis)

Connective tissue diseases
Ankylosing spondylitis
Reiter's syndrome
Psoriatic arthritis
Juvenile rheumatoid arthritis
HLA-B27-associated diseases

Infectious diseases
Herpes zoster
Herpes simplex
Syphilis

Other
Sarcoidosis
Glaucomatocyclitis crisis
Heterochromic iridocyclitis

Predominantly posterior uveitis (affecting choroid, retina, retinal vessels, optic nerve, vitreous)

Infectious diseases
Toxoplasmic retinochoroiditis
Herpes zoster
Herpes simplex
Cytomegalovirus
Syphilis
Candida
Tuberculosis
Presumed ocular histoplasmosis
Nematode granuloma

Other
Pars planitis
Sarcoidosis
Bird-shot chorioretinitis
Behçet's disease
Vogt–Koyanagi–Harada syndrome
Sympathetic ophthalmia

12.27 Listing of diseases associated with anterior and posterior uveitis.

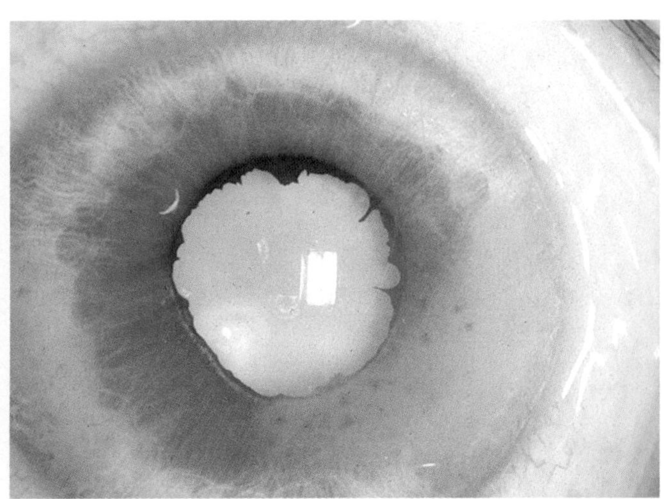

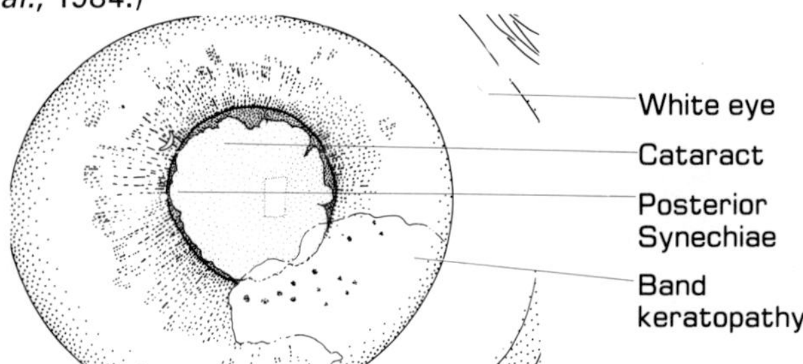

12.28 The chronic iridocyclitis of juvenile rheumatoid arthritis (JRA). This disease process can cause adhesions of the iris to the lens, cataract, calcium deposition in the cornea, and glaucoma. Severe damage may result despite apparently normal, non-inflamed sclera and conjunctiva. Early diagnosis and prompt therapy with topical steroids and dilating agents are essential to prevent or limit ocular damage. (Reproduced with permission from Spalton *et al.*, 1984.)

Intermediate uveitis manifests a more widespread inflammation of the vitreous, with many vitreous cells coalescing to form clumps and veils (**12.30**). A fibrovascular membrane and a layer of cellular debris may begin to form on the peripheral retina, a condition known as pars planitis (**12.30B**).

In *retinitis* and *choroiditis* (posterior uveitis), the major sites of inflammation are the retina and its vasculature (the choroid). Signs of inflammation may be present in the anterior chamber and vitreous. Behçet's disease commonly exhibits an occlusive retinal arteritis and periphlebitis (**12.31**). Patients with Behçet's

GUIDELINES FOR THE FREQUENCY OF OPHTHALMOLOGIC EXAMINATIONS IN CHILDREN WITH JRA[a]

JRA subtype at onset	Age of onset < 7 yr[b]		≥ 7 yr[c]
Pauciarticular			
+ANA	H[d]		M
–ANA	M		M
Polyarticular			
+ANA	H[d]		M
–ANA	M		M
Systemic	L	L	L

[a]High risk (H) indicates ophthalmologic examinations every 3–4 months. Medium risk (M) indicates ophthalmologic examinations every 6 months. Low risk (L) indicates ophthalmologic examinations every 12 months. ANA, antinuclear antibody test.

[b]All patients are considered at low risk 7 years after the onset of their arthritis, and should have yearly ophthalmologic examinations indefinitely.

[c]All patients are considered at low risk 4 years after the onset of their arthritis, and should have yearly ophthalmologic examinations indefinitely.

[d]All high risk patients are considered at medium risk 4 years after the onset of their arthritis.

12.29 Guidelines for the frequency of ophthalmologic examinations in children with juvenile rheumatoid arthritis. (Reprinted with permission from *Pediatr*, **92**:295, 1993.)

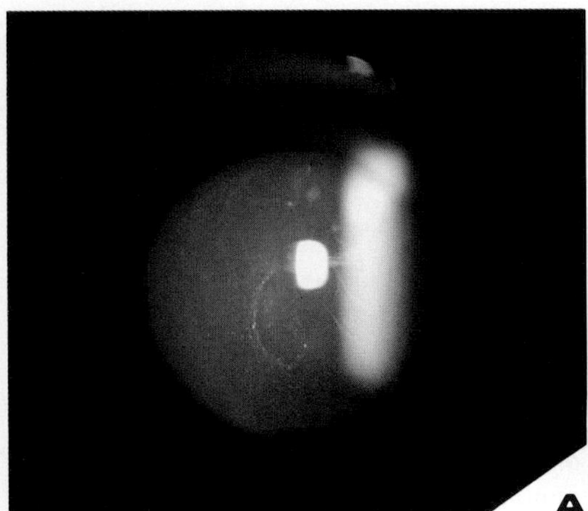

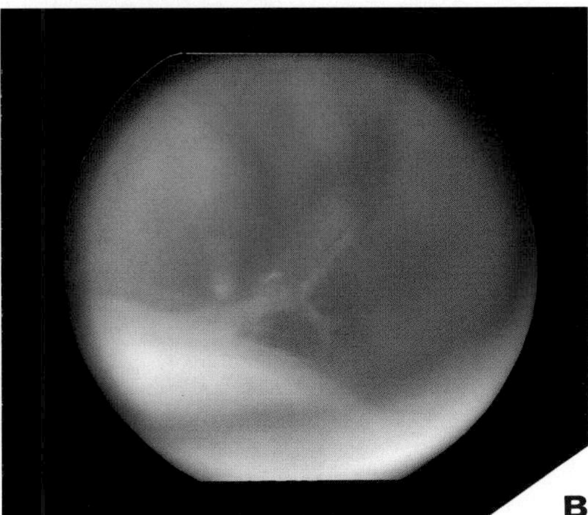

12.30 (A) Opacities of intermediate uveitis. Vitreous inflammatory debris can coalesce to form vitreous opacities, visible to the patient as dark 'floaters.' These inflammatory vitreous opacities can be seen by the examiner via retroillumination as shiny particles against the retinal red reflex. (B) By pressing on the inferior–anterior sclera near the limbus, the anterior retina (pars plana) of this patient can be brought into view. It is covered with a white inflammatory membrane extending into the vitreous. This condition may also be associated with optic nerve papillitis and macular edema.

disease frequently show aphthous ulcers of the mouth and genitalia, erythema nodosum, polyarthritis, and central nervous system disorders, in addition to the retinal abnormality. There is a strong association between this disease and HLA-B51. Short-term therapy with corticosteroids is helpful, but long-term systemic immunosuppression with cyclosporin seems more effective.

Vogt–Koyanagi–Harada syndrome (**12.32**) and *sympathetic ophthalmia* (**12.33**) primarily involve the choroid. The former, a diffuse granulomatous uveitis, involves the choroidal vessels and overlying pigmented epithelium, as well as the retina. Patients with this syndrome often show a loss of pigmentation of the eyelashes (poliosis) along with vitiligo and alopecia. The central nervous system manifestations of Vogt–Koyanagi–Harada include deafness, tinnitis, and seizures. Systemic corticosteroids, given topically and via periocular injection, are the proper modalities for this disease.

Sympathetic ophthalmia is characterized by the presence of Dalens–Fuchs nodules – collections of inflammatory cells beneath the retinal pigmented epithelium, which arise bilaterally, following the injury of one of the eyes. Through an unknown mechanism, the penetration of one eye provokes the formation of these nodules in the fellow (sympathizing) eye. The process can begin anywhere from 10 days to decades after surgical or traumatic ocular penetration. If, however, the injured eye is removed prior to the onset of inflammation in the fellow eye, sympathetic ophthalmia does not occur.

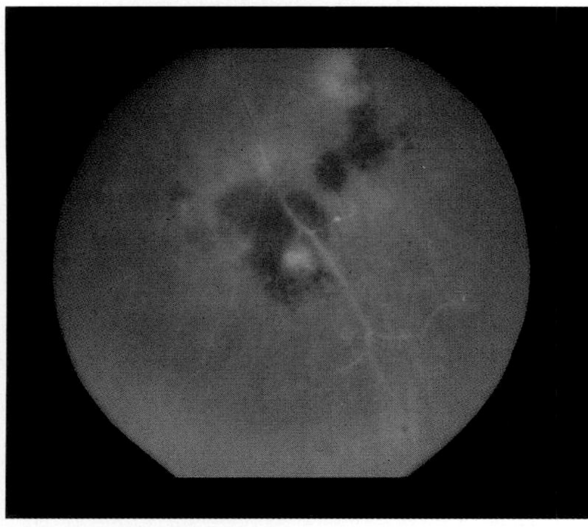

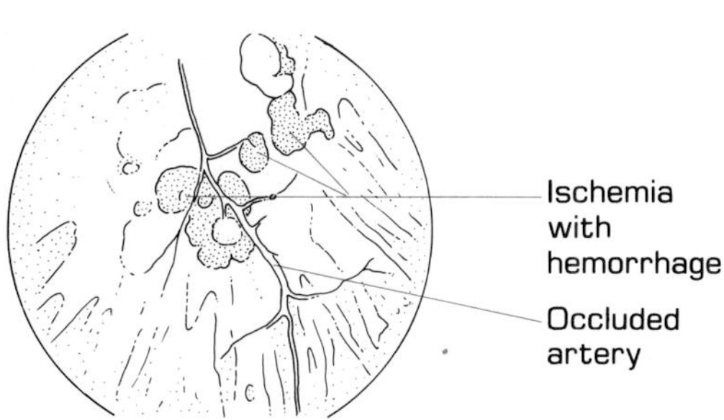

12.31 Occlusive retinal vasculitis in Behçet's disease. Note the occluded, whitened artery. Distal to the vascular occlusion is an area of retinal ischemia with hemorrhage.

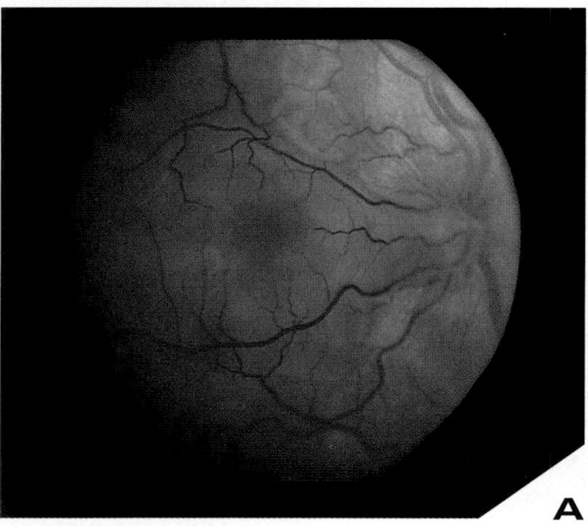

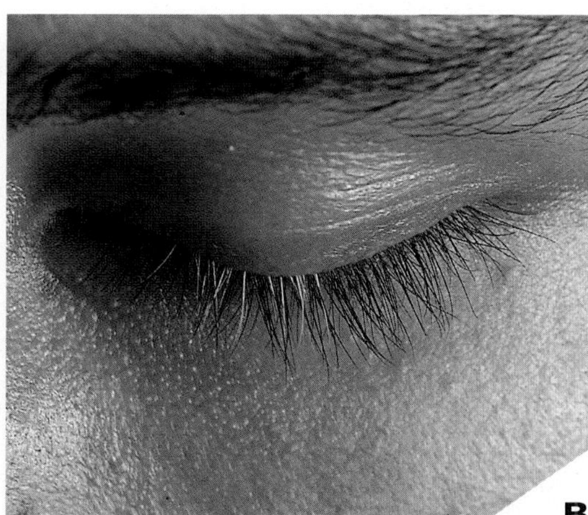

12.32 (A) The diffuse exudative choroiditis of Vogt–Koyanagi–Harada syndrome. This chronic, diffuse, granulomatous uveitis involves the choroidal vessels, the overlying pigmented epithelium, and the retina. (B) Loss of pigmentation of the eyelashes (poliosis) is often seen, along with vitiligo and alopecia.

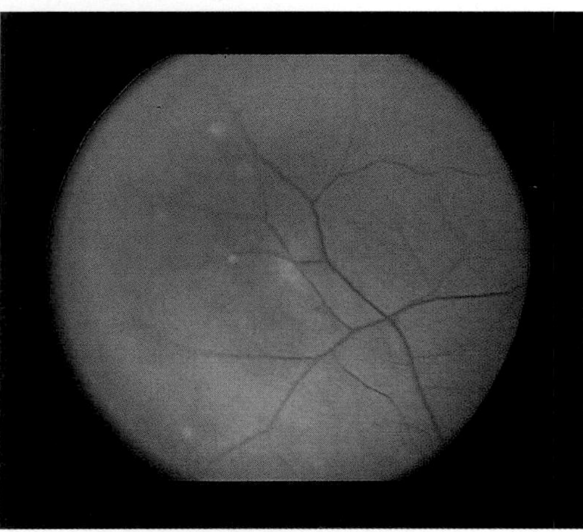

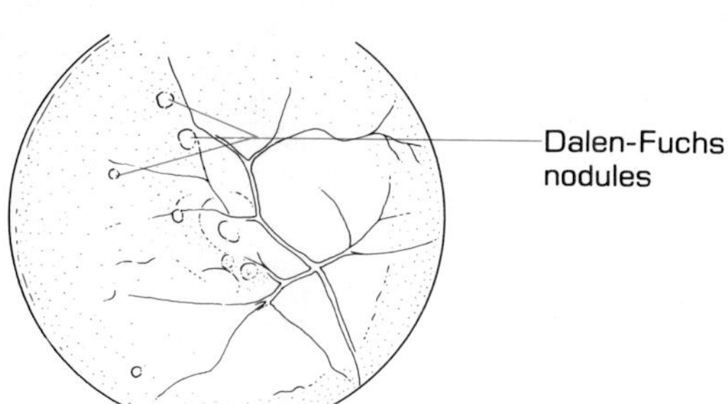

12.33 The yellowish lesions shown here are Dalen–Fuchs nodules – collections of inflammatory cells beneath the retinal pigmented epithelium. They are characteristic of sympathetic ophthalmia. This condition is a bilateral chronic panuveitis that follows penetrating injury of one eye. The mechanism by which penetration of one of the eyes provokes this response in the sympathetic eye is, as yet, unknown.

Clinical manifestations

A patient with acute iritis usually experiences sudden onset of redness, photophobia, tearing, pain, and decreased vision. This can be difficult to differentiate from conjunctivitis without biomicroscopic (slit lamp) examination, but the pain and light sensitivity are more marked in iritis. The conjunctiva is injected, especially surrounding the cornea (**12.34**). The pupil may be smaller in the inflamed eye. Inflammatory precipitates, called keratitic precipitates (**12.35**), may form on the back of the cornea. Inflammatory nodules can develop on the iris or at the pupillary margin (Koeppe nodules) (**12.36**), and adhesions may form between the iris and the cornea or the lens (see **12.28**).

Inflammatory cells may be observed in the vitreous and may coalesce to form opacities visible to the patient as 'floaters' (see **12.30A**). Vasculitis is characterized by exudation, sheathing of vessels, hemorrhage, and vascular closure (**12.37**) The retina may become edematous from the leaking vessels, resulting in decreased vision. Inflammatory exudate in the retina and choroid appears white or yellow.

Leakage from inflamed choroidal vessels often results in the collection of fluid beneath the retina, causing a serous detachment. In eyes with hazy media, examination by an ophthalmologist skilled in the use of the indirect ophthalmoscope is necessary to assess the full extent of the diseases.

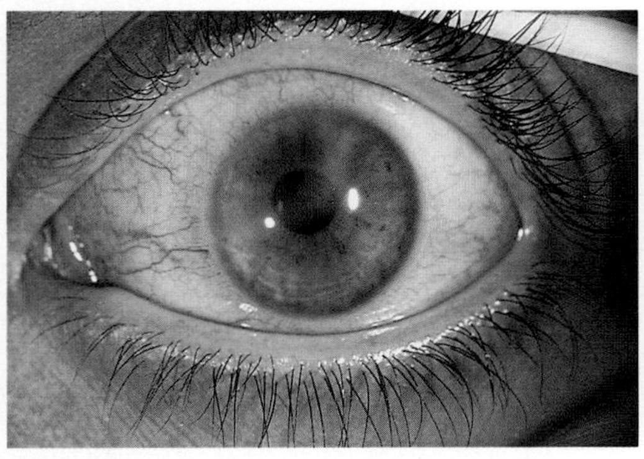

12.34 Iritis with circumlimbal flush. Note the ring of perilimbal injection so characteristic of iritis.

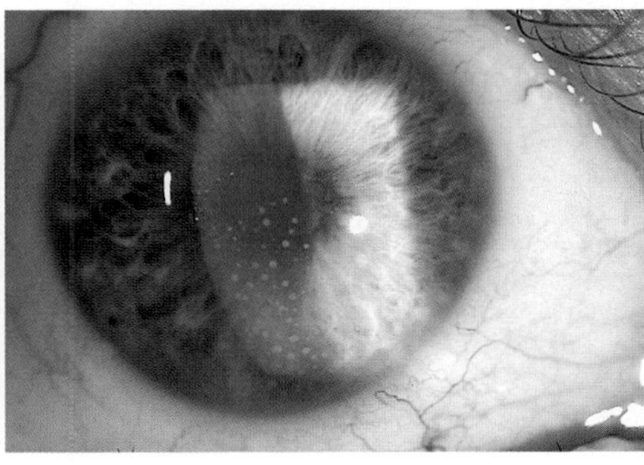

12.35 Inflammatory (keratitic) precipitates seen on the posterior surface of the cornea.

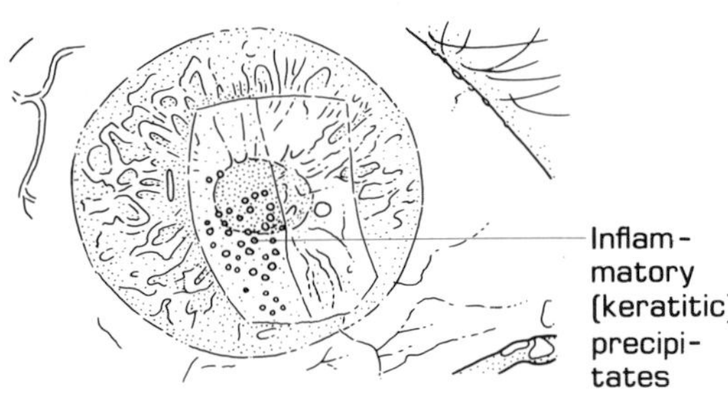

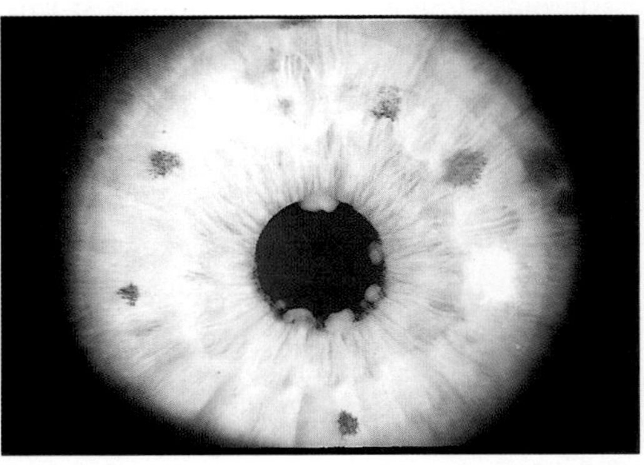

12.36 Uveitis with iris nodules (Koeppe nodules).

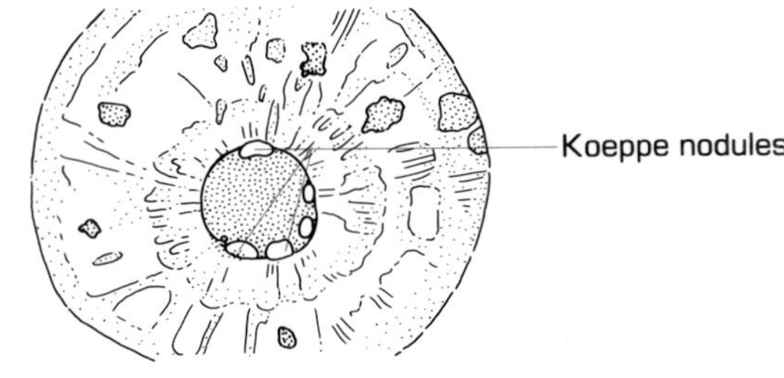

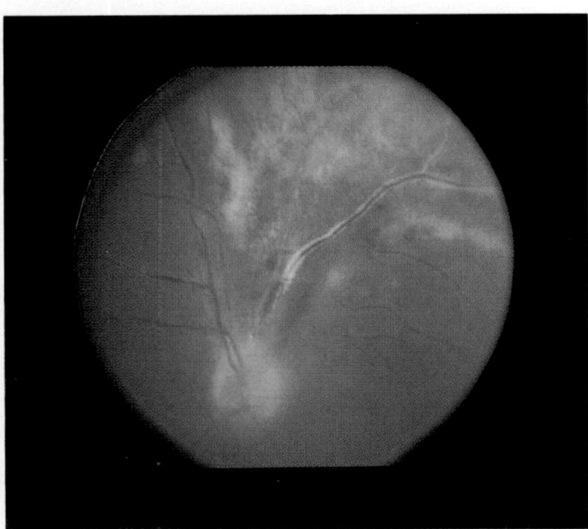

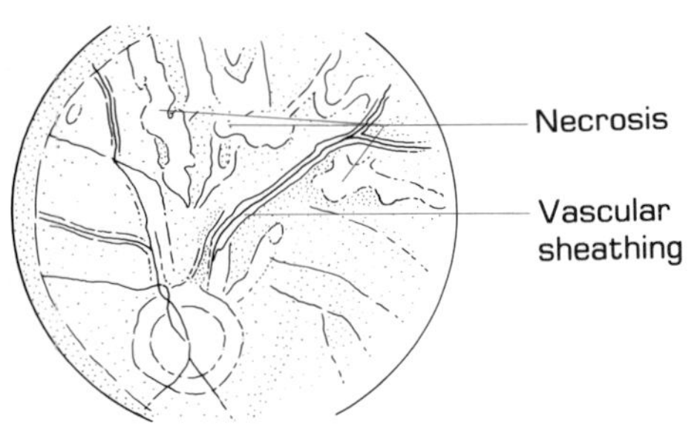

12.37 Vascular sheathing, edema, necrosis, and hemorrhage of the retina. These findings are characteristic of cytomegalovirus (CMV) retinitis.

Treatment

Therapy is best approached by the identification and treatment of any underlying systemic condition. Often, however, this is not possible, and non-specific treatment of uveitis is usually initiated with a topical corticosteroid, such as prednisolone acetate 1%, and pupillary dilatation/cycloplegia with atropine or scopolamine. More severe inflammation may require oral non-steroidal anti-inflammatory agents (indomethacin) or corticosteroids. Periocular corticosteroids injections may control inflammation, while minimizing the side effects. In recalcitrant cases or in steroid intolerant patients, cyclophosphamide or cyclosporin may be successful.

Topical therapy is not sufficient for inflammation of the posterior uvea, the retina, and the choroid. Systemic or periocular corticosteroid administration is required. If this is not successful, other immunosuppressive agents may be used.

ACKNOWLEDGEMENT

The authors acknowledge the excellent photographic assistance of Diane Curtin and Joseph Warnicki.

REFERENCES

Abelson MB, Schaefer K: Conjunctivitis of allergic origin – immunologic mechanisms and current approaches to therapy. *Surv Ophthalmol*, 38, Suppl., 1993.

Allansmith MR, Ross RN: Ocular allergy and mast cell stabilizers. *Surv Ophthalmol*, 34(4):229–244, 1986.

Foster, CS, Forstot SL, Wilson LA: Mortality rate in rheumatoid arthritis patients developing necrotizing scleritis or peripheral ulcerative keratitis: effects of systemic immunosuppression. *Ophthalmology*, 9:1253–1263, 1984.

Dinning WJ: Therapy-selected topics, in Kraus-Mackiw E, O'Connor GR (eds): *Uveitis: Pathophysiology and Therapy,* Thieme, New York, pp 211–219, 1986.

Nussenblatt RB, Palestine AG: *Uveitis: Fundamental and Clinical Practice,* Year Book, Chicago, 1989.

Sacks EH, Wieczorek R, Jakobiec FA, Knowles DM: Lymphocyte subpopulations in the normal human conjunctiva: a monoclonal antibody study. *Ophthalmology*, 93(10):1276–1283, 1986.

Smolen G, O'Connor GR (eds): *Ocular Immunology,* 2nd edn, Little, Brown and Co., 1986.

Spalton DJ, Hitchings RA, Hunter PA: *Atlas of Clinical Ophthalmology*, Gower, London, pp 5.2, 10.9, 1984.

Watson P: Diseases of the sclera and episclera, in Duane TD (ed.): *Clinical Ophthalmology,* Harper and Row, Philadelphia, 1987.

Wieczorek R, Jakobiec FA, Sacks EH, Knowles DM: Immunoarchitecture of the normal human lacrimal gland: relevancy for understanding pathologic conditions. *Ophthalmology*, 95(1):100–109, 1988.

CHAPTER 13

Food Hypersensitivity

S. Allan Bock

The study of food hypersensitivity has been fraught with much unnecessary confusion and misdiagnosis. This chapter presents a practical approach to the investigation of food hypersensitivity which is applicable to nearly any patient encountered in clinical allergy practice. This discussion contains clinical information on our current understanding of the mechanisms, presentation, diagnosis, treatment, and natural history of these reactions.

PATHOGENESIS

Adverse reactions to foods are known to occur by one of several mechanisms:

- Carbohydrate intolerance, especially lactase deficiency, which is surely the most common cause of adverse reactions to food.
- Toxic reactions due to natural constituents of food, compounds added during processing, or contaminants acquired during storage.
- Symptoms due to strongly held beliefs about the effects of food.
- Hypersensitivity (allergic) reactions due to immune mechanisms, which are the main focus of this chapter.

It is also likely that there exist biochemically mediated reactions which have not yet been discovered (**13.1**). New information about allergic and/or inflammatory mechanisms is accumulating and is helping our understanding of the mechanism of food allergy and directions for future treatment. Particularly exciting is the growing understanding of the role of cytokines and adhesion molecules in the pathogenesis of atopic dermatitis.

Every symptom known to man has, at one time or another, been blamed on food. The list of foods incriminated is endless. However, most confirmed reactions to foods have elicited only gastrointestinal, cutaneous, and respiratory symptoms (**13.2**). Isolated respiratory symptoms due to a food hypersensitivity reaction are unusual, and behavioral symptoms as the *sole* manifestations of adverse reactions to foods are difficult to reproduce. The former continues to be an area of active investigation (Bock, 1992; James *et al.*, 1994).

Gastrointestinal symptoms reproduced during double-blind, placebo-controlled food challenge (DBPCFC) have included nausea, vomiting, diarrhea, and abdominal pain. Cutaneous reactions have included urticaria, angioedema (**13.3 and 13.4**), atopic dermatitis (**13.5**), and non-specific erythematous rashes. Respiratory

DIFFERENTIAL DIAGNOSIS OF ADVERSE FOOD REACTIONS
1. Deficiency of interstitial enzymes (disaccharidase deficiency)
2. Toxins in food (natural or added)
3. Psychological reactions (strongly held beliefs)
4. Hypersensitivity/allergy
5. Biochemical reactions not yet defined

13.1 Differential diagnosis of food allergy. The table lists the five general categories into which nearly all adverse food reactions fall.

and ocular manifestations have included sneezing, rhinorrhea, ocular and pharyngeal pruritus, wheezing, cough, and laryngospasm. Occasionally, a devastating combination of the above is accompanied by hypotension or other symptoms and results in anaphylaxis. The mechanisms by which these symptoms are elicited are outlined in **13.6**.

SYMPTOMS ASSOCIATED WITH FOOD HYPERSENSITIVITY

Confirmed during objective challenge

Gastrointestinal	Skin	Respiratory	Ocular	Other
Abdominal pain	Urticaria	Rhinorrhea	Pruritus	Anaphylaxis (hypotension)
Nausea	Eczema	Sneezing	Lacrimation	Migraine headache
Vomiting	Angioedema	Coughing	Edema	Arthritis (1 case)
Diarrhea	Erythema	Wheezing	Injection	
'Colic'		Laryngospasm		
		Pruritus		

Not yet confirmed during objective challenge

Hyperactivity due to sugar
Headache (not migraine)
Collagen vascular disease
Otitis media
Ménière's disease
Urinary problems including eneuresis
'Tension fatigue syndrome'
Learning disorders
Acne

13.2 Symptoms associated with food hypersensitivity grouped according to the organ systems affected. Many commonly reported symptoms, including headaches, acne, otitis media, and eneuresis, have yet to be confirmed by objective challenge. Behavioral symptoms, including irritability and mood changes, have been found in association with many of the symptoms listed. However, behavioral symptoms as the sole manifestation of an adverse food reaction have rarely been reproduced during objective food challenge.

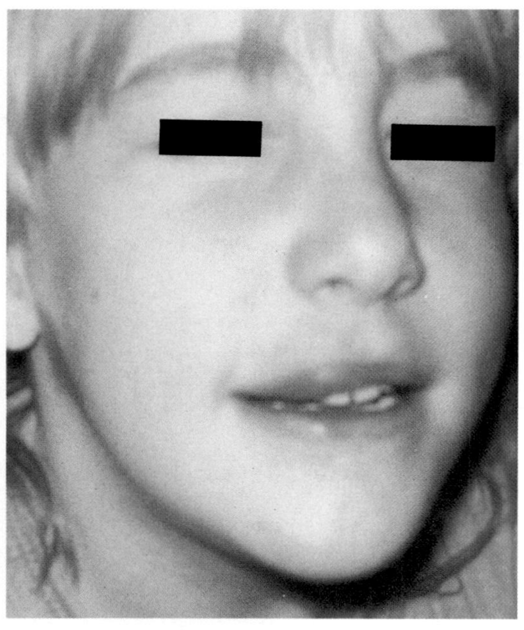

13.3 Angioedema of the lip. This reaction occurred in a child following ingestion of fish during an objective food challenge.

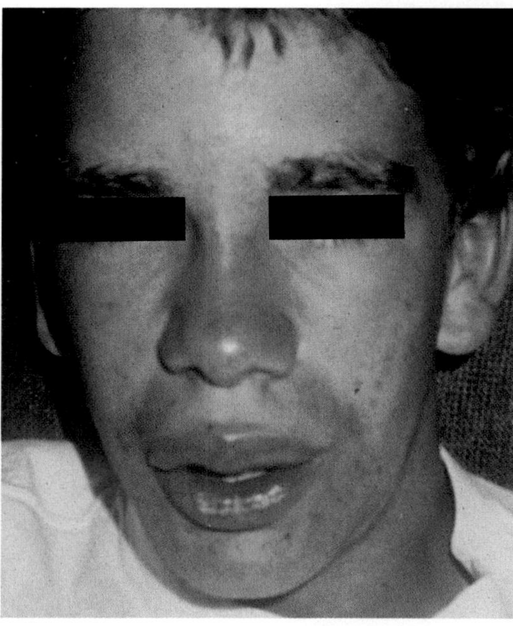

13.4 Appearance of patient following challenge with cottonseed protein. (Photo courtesy of Dr F.M. (Dan) Atkins, Denver, Colorado.)

NATURAL HISTORY

The natural history of adverse food reactions has two components: the development and subsequent loss of food hypersensitivity. Observations concerning the development of food hypersensitivity and other atopic symptoms in children have been made during studies which attempted to prevent the development of atopic disease in infancy (Zeiger *et al.*, 1992). These observations are discussed later in this chapter.

Almost all the data concerning the ongoing natural history of allergy symptoms due to food have been obtained in children. However, a thorough study has shown that adult patterns are similar to those seen in children (Pastorello *et al.*, 1989). Younger children with confirmed hypersensitivities to milk, soy, and egg seem to be the ones most likely to lose the problem as they grow (Bock, 1982). This has even been found true in nine youngsters with histories of anaphylaxis to specific food proteins (Bock, 1985). At the present time, longitudinal investigation of those nine children has revealed that none of them any longer shows life-threatening reactions to foods that were initially identified as producing anaphylaxis. The longer a reaction continues to occur, or the older a child is at the time that the DBPCFC confirms a hypersensitivity, the less likely it is that the reactions will disappear. Children with peanut hypersensitivity appear to be very unlikely to lose their reactivity, especially if the problem persists for a few years (Bock and Atkins, 1989).

There is a great deal of discussion in the allergy literature about cross reactions among food families. However, it is a disservice to patients to presume that there is cross reactivity among foods, even within the same food family (Bernhisel-Broadbent and Sampson, 1989). These botanical relationships do not necessarily have clinical relevance. Each food stands alone, and cross reactivity among foods even in the same 'family' must be *proven*, not assumed. Several recent studies have shown a lack of cross reactivity among foods in the same botanical family. In fact, there seems to be more 'cross reactivity' between birch pollen and certain fruits and

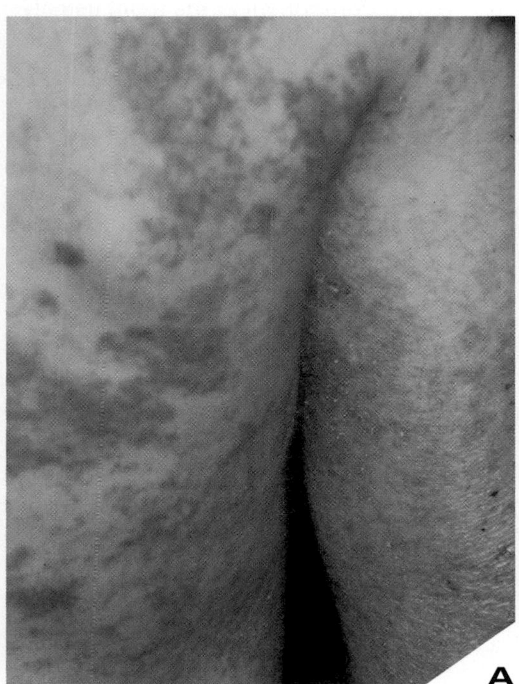

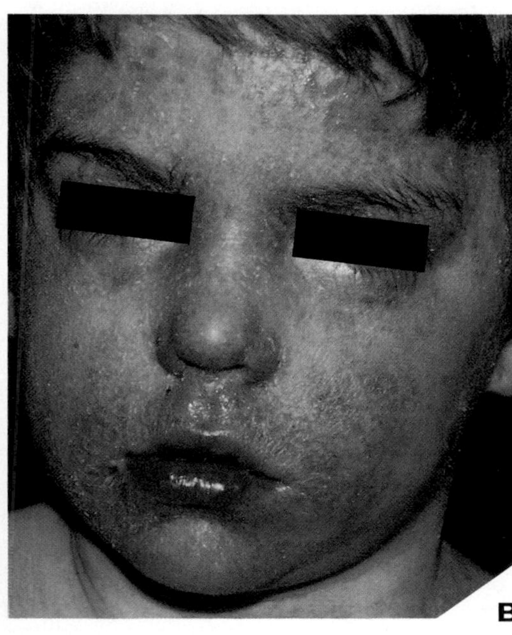

13.5 Exacerbation of atopic dermatitis on (A) the arms and (B) the face of a young boy following food challenge. (Photo courtesy of Dr Hugh A. Sampson, Johns Hopkins University School of Medicine.)

between ragweed and melons, than between different legumes. Therefore, each food under suspicion must be evaluated individually. An important point to remember is that patients with specific food-protein hypersensitivity can tolerate the purified oils of these proteins. For example, patients with reactions to peanuts, even if severe, can tolerate pure peanut oil because the pure oil lacks peanut protein. This has also been shown to be true for soy and sunflower seed oils. However, if these oils have been used to cook foods to which an individual is hypersensitive, then exposure to the 'contaminated' oil may elicit symptoms. It is also important to be aware that even after food hypersensitivity has been 'outgrown,' and the patient tolerates the food when it is ingested, sensitization as detected by the presence of IgE antibody on skin testing may persist.

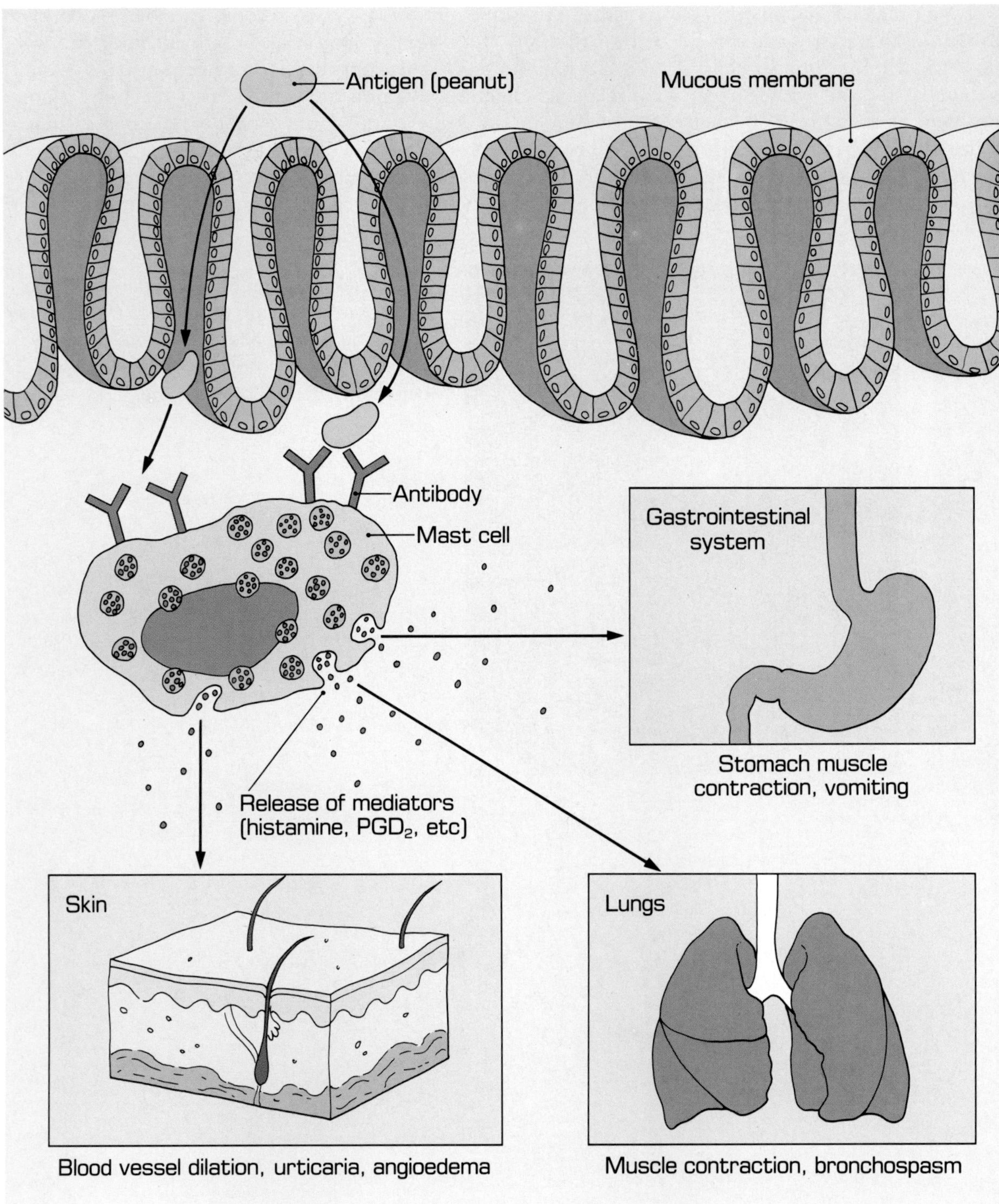

13.6 Schematic representation of the immunologic events underlying the clinically recognizable symptoms of food hypersensitivity. These processes are set in motion when a hypersensitive individual is exposed to an antigenic food. The antigenic component of the food, usually a protein, binds to immunoglobulins on the surfaces of mast cells. This triggers the degranulation of the mast cells and the release of a wide range of inflammatory mediators, resulting in the end-organ changes characteristic of allergy.

AN APPROACH TO PATIENTS COMPLAINING OF ADVERSE REACTIONS TO FOOD

13.7 presents a step-wise approach to the patient complaining of symptoms which might be due to food ingestion. Following acquisition of the history and consideration of the differential diagnosis, the clinician must design a double-blind, placebo-controlled food challenge to test whether administration of the food in question reproduces the history described by the patient. Appropriate laboratory tests may be undertaken either to provide further information about the diagnosis or to suggest a likely mechanism. Once the history has been confirmed, the clinician can design a plan of management.

TAKING THE HISTORY

13.8 lists the important facts which must be elicited in order to reproduce the history as described by the patient. Usually, in medicine, a physician acquires a patient's history to make the diagnosis; but because of the confusion and misinformation surrounding adverse reactions to foods, the purpose of the history in this context is to establish a symptom pattern which the allergist then attempts to confirm or refute through the blind food-challenge. Therefore, certain facts must be recorded, such as a detailed description of symptoms, timing from ingestion of the food to onset of symptoms, the quantity of food required to produce symptoms, and the frequency with which the reaction has been noted in the past.

AN APPROACH TO THE DIAGNOSIS OF FOOD HYPERSENSITIVITY

1. Acquire a thorough history which can be used to design a challenge
2. Consider the differential diagnosis
3. Perform double-blind, placebo-controlled food challenges (DBPCFC)
4. Perform appropriate laboratory tests
5. Design a plan of management

13.7 A step-wise approach to the diagnosis of food hypersensitivity.

POINTS TO CONSIDER WHEN TAKING THE HISTORY

1. Description of the symptoms
2. Time between ingestion of food and onset of symptoms
3. Most recent occurrence
4. Number of times reaction has been noted
5. Minimum quantity of food required to elicit symptoms

13.8 Key points for consideration when taking the history of a patient complaining of food allergy. The function of the history in this clinical context is to provide a profile of symptoms which are to be either confirmed or refuted through direct, blind challenge.

13.9 and **13.10** present algorithms which can be very helpful to physicians in determining for themselves, and also in explaining to the patient, how the evaluation will proceed. **13.9** presents the procedure to be followed when a specific food is suspected. This is the simpler situation, since the specific food or foods can be tested by eliminating them from the diet. If the symptoms persist following elimination of the food, it is not likely that the food in question is causing the reaction. If the symptoms do disappear during the period in which the food is eliminated, and reoccur when the food is replaced in the diet, then a DBPCFC should be arranged.

13.10 covers the more complicated situation in which the patient does not have a specific suspicion about which food or foods may be causing an adverse reaction. An elimination diet (**13.11**) is used to determine whether or not the symptoms remit. Symptoms which persist after 7–14 days on a strict elimination diet (which may even include use of an elemental diet) are not likely to be related to ingested substances. Prolonged elimination diets, beyond 2 weeks, rarely produce additional benefit and may be nutritionally harmful. On the other hand, symptoms which disappear on elimination diets may then be explored in accord with the

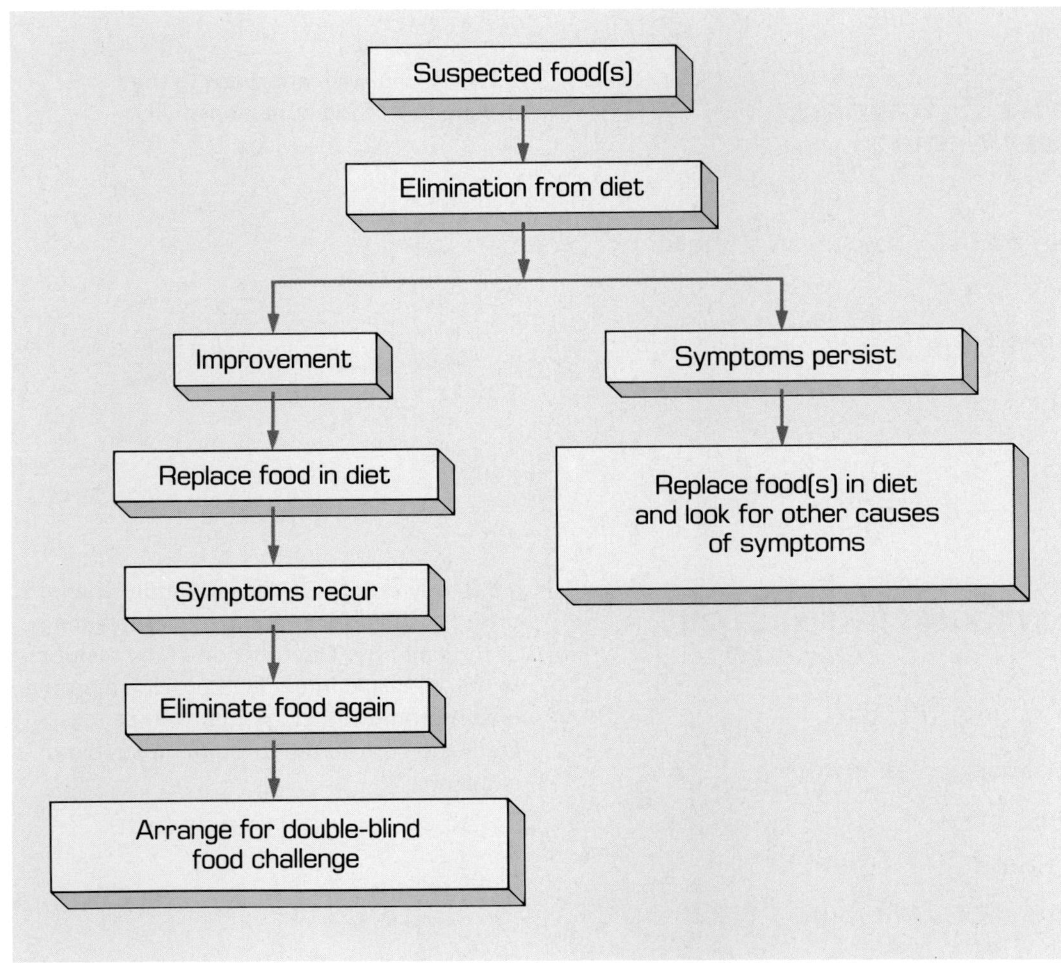

13.9 Schematic representation of the steps involved in the evaluation of possible food hypersensitivity when a specific food is suspected. This is the simplest situation; the suspected food can simply be eliminated from the diet. If symptoms persist, it is unlikely that this food is the cause. If symptoms resolve, the food should be tested by DBPCFC. (Adapted with permission from Bock, 1988.)

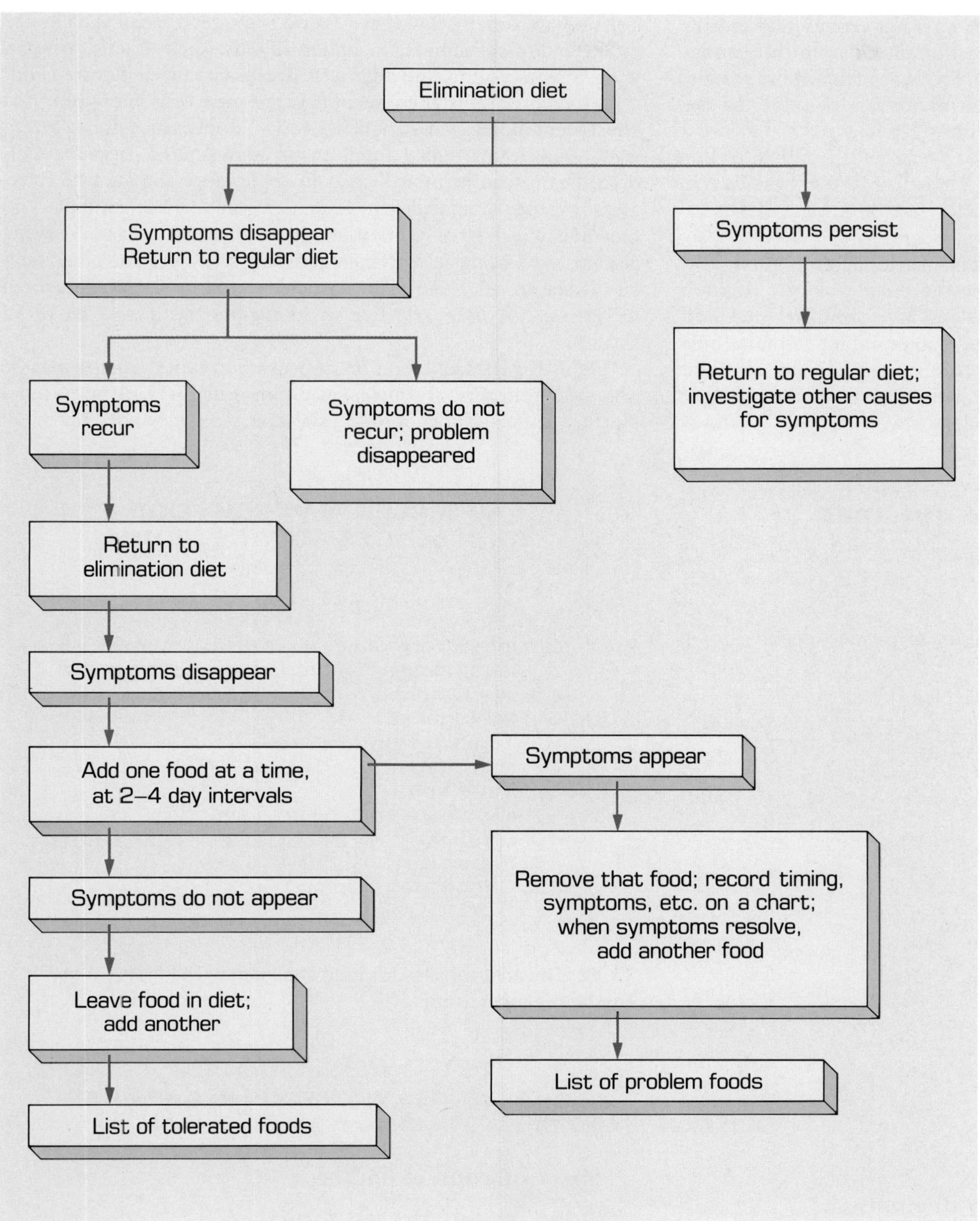

13.10 Algorithm for evaluation of possible food hypersensitivity in cases in which no specific food is suspected. These situations are more complicated, and require the use of an elimination diet. Symptoms persisting beyond 14 days of an elimination diet are not likely to be due to ingested food. (Adapted with permission from Bock, 1988.)

algorithm as outlined. Elimination diets are not very useful for cases in which the symptoms are occasional or sporadic. In these situations, symptom diaries may pin-point food suspicions more readily. As a general rule, however, food diaries are rarely useful and are tedious for both doctor and patient.

THE DOUBLE-BLIND, PLACEBO-CONTROLLED FOOD CHALLENGE

13.12 lists the vehicles in which challenge foods may be hidden. Certainly, capsule challenges are the most desirable for research purposes, since they are the most likely to hide completely the food from the patient's detection. In young babies, infant formulas hide or mask most foods being tested. In this context, it is not the child from whom the food is being hidden, but rather the parent or other caregiver. Iced, vanilla-flavored elemental formulas, such as Tolerex® (Vivonex), have been found to be very useful vehicles for hiding many substances, including liquids, such as oils, vinegar, wine, flavors, colors, and additives. Because it may be flavored with a dark-colored substance, such as grape juice or grape syrup, it is effective in hiding many challenge foods. Apple sauce is also a very useful vehicle for hiding foods to be administered to young children. Grains can be mixed easily in apple sauce and are well tolerated by most young children. Chocolate pudding is a good place to hide nuts which have been ground in a coffee grinder and are being administered using an incremental dosing schedule. The other vehicles listed are each useful in particular situations. Grape-flavored ice cream has been effective in hiding the distinctive flavor of shrimp.

Foods for encapsulation or suspension in other vehicles may be obtained from several sources, as outlined in **13.13**. A mortar and pestle, a coffee grinder, a food processor, a simple scale, and small

SAMPLE ELIMINATION DIET

Food permitted

Rice in any form (rice cakes and rice cereal especially helpful)

Pineapple, Apricots, Cranberries, Peaches, Pears, Apples — also canned fruit and juices of these

Lamb
Chicken

Asparagus
Beets
Carrots
Lettuce
Sweet potatoes

White vinegar
Olive oil
Honey
Cane or beet sugar
Salt
Safflower oil

Avoid all foods not on this list

13.11 Sample elimination diet. This diet is not nutritionally complete, and should only be used for short periods of time (less than 14 days) and when there is a clear clinical indication for it. Elimination diets are of little value when the patient's symptoms are occasional or sporadic.

VEHICLES IN WHICH FOOD CHALLENGES MAY BE HIDDEN

1. Capsules
2. Infant formulas
3. Iced, vanilla-flavored elemental formulas
4. Apple sauce
5. Milkshakes
6. Tapioca–fruit mixtures
7. Hamburger
8. Tuna fish
9. Ice cream with heavy flavoring
10. Lentil soup
11. Popsicles
12. Chocolate pudding

13.12 Effective vehicles for food challenges. The first four are among the most useful.

CHALLENGES WITH FOOD IN CAPSULES

No. 1 opaque capsules

Dried or dehydrated foods

Nuts: powdered, using mortar and pestle or coffee grinder
Grains: used as purchased.
Freeze-dried meats: available from camping or sporting goods stores
Dried or freeze-dried fruits and vegetables: available from camping or sporting goods stores

13.13 Preparation of food for challenge via capsules or suspension.

containers are useful adjunctive equipment. Nuts, cereal grains, and non-fat, powdered, dry milk are readily available in most supermarkets, and the popularity of camping in the United States has resulted in the widespread availability of freeze-dried meat, fruit, and vegetables. If it seems cumbersome to place these foods in capsules, they may be suspended in one of the other vehicles described. **13.14** presents the weight of foods in individual capsules as used at Johns Hopkins University School of Medicine.

SINGLE CHALLENGES

The administration of food challenges can be reduced to a fairly reproducible sequence of steps. **13.15** outlines a protocol which may be undertaken quite readily without making patients particularly ill. A challenge should be designed on the basis of the patient's specific history. It is practical to start with one-half the amount of challenge food expected to produce symptoms. Incremental increases approximately doubling the previous amount are given at intervals slightly longer than expected to produce symptoms.

These steps are fairly straightforward in patients who have histories of prompt onset of symptoms, which is the situation in most cases that allergists are asked to evaluate. However, there are many patients in whom delayed reactions need exploration. If the allergist is properly prepared, these situations are only slightly more problematic. For example, in cases in which the patient reports symptoms only after eating a certain food once a day for three or four days, it is perfectly acceptable to have the patient come to the physician's office in the morning, ingest the challenge, and then resume normal activity. The patient should be instructed to call the allergist when symptoms begin. These patients rarely complain of severe or life-threatening symptoms, and thus the risk in these situations is negligible.

MULTIPLE CHALLENGES

A slightly more cumbersome set of circumstances arises when multiple challenges over multiple days are required to elicit symptoms. In these cases, it may be necessary to allow the patient to take the

SAMPLE WEIGHT EQUIVALENT FOR FOOD CHALLENGE

Food	Wet weight (g)	Dry weight (g)	Weight/capsule (g)
Egg	2.36	0.59	0.59
Milk	6 (ml)	0.61	0.61
Peanut	1.83	0.44	0.44
Wheat	0.90	0.90	0.90
Soy	2.83	0.68	0.68
Corn	8.25	0.66	0.66
Beef	4.10	0.57	0.57
Shrimp	3.28	0.59	0.59

13.14 Dry and wet weight equivalents of common foods. This table provides measurements of dried food weights in individual capsules as used in food challenges at the Johns Hopkins University School of Medicine. (Reproduced with permission from Bock, *et al.*, 1988, p. 993.)

ADMINISTRATION OF FOOD CHALLENGE

1. Design challenge to reproduce history with respect to quantity and timing, without making the subject too uncomfortable.
2. Start with approximately one-half the amount expected to produce any symptoms.
3. Give incrementally increasing amounts (about double), at intervals slightly longer than those expected to produce symptoms.
4. If multiple challenges over multiple days are required to elicit symptoms, give the necessary amount two or three times per day.
5. It may be necessary to 'cross' the placebo and active food up to three times when attempting to elicit subjective symptoms that occur hours after challenge.
6. Have patient or observer maintain a symptom record.
7. When the double-blind challenge is negative after 8–10 g of dried food or the equivalent, the food must be placed openly in the diet, preferably under observation, and consumed in the usual and customary portions. Preparation should be in the usual manner. This will confirm the fact that there is no reaction.

13.15 Steps in the administration of an uncomplicated, placebo-controlled food challenge. This sequence of steps works in nearly all contexts. It is essential to begin with a sufficiently small amount of the suspected food, to avoid a severe adverse reaction.

capsules home so that they may be self-administered 2–3 times per day. Self-administration should be allowed only for patients who can be relied upon not to attempt to discern the contents of the capsules. It is crucial in each of these situations that a placebo be used. The best placebos for use in capsules are either dextrose, which is readily available, or another food which is not on the patient's list of suspicions. Particularly for subjective symptoms, it may be necessary to cross over the active and the placebo challenge three times each. In other words, the placebo and the suspect food are given alternately on three occasions, in a varying sequence. The placebo could be given twice consecutively and then the suspect food and placebo alternated.

Throughout the challenge period, the observer or patient should maintain a symptom record. A crucial step in the process occurs when the blind challenge is negative up to approximately 8–10 g of food in either solid (dried) or liquid form. The food *must* be placed openly in the diet, preferably under observation, and consumed in the usual and customary portions. This allows the clinician to eliminate many of the questions which are often raised about matters such as the digestion, preparation, and combination of foods.

13.16 briefly summarizes the results of double-blind, placebo-controlled food challenges in 630 children with histories of adverse reactions to foods. As may be seen clearly from the data, the histories are confirmed less than 40% of the time. However, a substantial number of children in this series of selected patients were found to have food hypersensitivity. This ongoing study has also shown that:

- When food hypersensitivity is confirmed, it is frequently to fewer foods than were suspected in any individual patient.
- The list of foods for which confirmation has been obtained does not include some of the most notorious 'food villains,' specifically chocolate (and only one reaction to corn).

Although not shown in **13.16**, this study has investigated numerous and varied histories of delayed reactions which have not been reproduced during double-blind food challenges in children over 3 years of age. In children under 3 years, delayed onset reactions have been confined to gastrointestinal symptoms, and in one youngster to an unusual but reproducible skin rash. The gastrointestinal problems were protein enteropathies. The nature of the skin rash was not determined since no biopsy was permitted. These findings have been confirmed in a number of studies at other institutions.

LABORATORY TESTING FOR FOOD HYPERSENSITIVITY

Despite efforts by many investigators all over the globe to find a laboratory procedure which would render food challenges unnecessary, no acceptable, highly reliable test has yet been found. Immune mechanisms are best documented by detection of IgE via skin or *in vitro* tests in association with objectively confirmed symptoms during double-blind, placebo-controlled food challenges (Bock *et al.*, 1988). Gastroenteropathies, especially due to cow's milk, soy, and gluten proteins, are suspected but not proven examples of non-IgE immune-mediated reactions. The involvement of IgG and its subclasses in the production of adverse reactions to food has been the subject of speculation, but has not been proven. Measurements of IgG immunoglobulin subclasses and immune complexes should currently be regarded as experimental and not for the regular clinical evaluation of patients. Skin testing for the confirmation of IgE to food protein, though not diagnostic in and of itself, still seems to be the most reliable method available (Bock and Sampson, 1994).

At the present time, the best reason for doing skin tests is to select those patients with histories suggestive of IgE-mediated food

RESULTS OF DOUBLE-BLIND, PLACEBO-CONTROLLED FOOD CHALLENGES IN CHILDREN

Patients undergoing DBPCFC	630
Patients with positive DBPCFC	235 (37%)
Number of food challenges – DBPCFC	1419
Number of positive DBPCFC	313 (22%)

Foods:				
	Egg	85	Chicken	2
	Peanut	74	Turkey	1
	Milk	69	Banana	1
	Nuts	32	Rye	1
	Soy	17	Squash	1
	Fish	10	Hot dog	1
	Wheat	7	Crab	1
	Pea	5	Corn	1
	Shrimp	3		

TOTAL: 313

Egg, Milk, Peanut, Wheat, Soy = 252 or 81% of total

13.16 Summary of the results of double-blind, placebo-controlled food challenges (DBPCFC) in 630 children suspected of being hypersensitive to one or more of the foods listed. The study showed that just under 40% of the reported symptoms were confirmable through challenge. Eggs, peanuts, and milk were the most commonly confirmed allergenic foods.

hypersensitivity in whom blinded food challenges should be undertaken. In patients with histories of fairly immediate onset of symptoms, negative skin tests most likely indicate that no reaction will occur when the food is ingested. These tests may, however, have low positive predictability, since they may detect asymptomatic hypersensitivity. Radioallergosorbent testing (RAST) gives information very similar to skin testing, but in most clinical settings it is substantially more expensive and, therefore, hard to justify in the current medical–economic climate. Many other tests have been proposed for diagnosing food hypersensitivity, but currently none of these have been proved sufficiently efficacious to justify introduction into clinical practice.

CHRONIC DIARRHEA AND FOOD HYPERSENSITIVITY

One problem for which allergists are consulted, but for which there are no good laboratory tests, is chronic diarrhea. Many children with chronic diarrhea, and an equal number of adults with chronic bowel disease, find their way to allergists' offices to be evaluated for possible food allergy. Generally, these patients have not received satisfactory assistance in their efforts to find an explanation for their bowel problems. **13.17** presents an extreme example of what can happen when a foreign protein damages the small intestine. The mechanism by which this damage occurs is not known. Although there is substantial evidence that the immune system is intimately involved with the process, it may not be responsible for the pathophysiology. This small bowel biopsy specimen was taken from a 9-month-old infant who had recurrent bouts of diarrhea, which had initially been blamed on infection. Following hospitalization and treatment with intravenous fluids and antibiotics, the youngster was fed a cow's milk formula. Shortly thereafter, he was found to be very pale and listless, with a decreased blood pressure. Several hours later, a profuse watery diarrhea ensued, suggesting the movement of a great deal of fluid into the intestine. Less than 24 hours later, the biopsy was obtained, showing a grossly flattened jejunal mucosa. This is an extreme example of protein enteropathy. Cow milk and soy protein enteropathies appear to be transient and almost invariably resolve by the third birthday. Gluten sensitive enteropathy (celiac disease) appears to be a life-long illness and should be followed through childhood and adulthood by a specialist in gastrointestinal diseases (Bock and Sampson, 1994).

Allergic gastroenteropathy and eosinophilic esophagitis and gastroenteritis have been increasingly reported in the past few years. The exact pathophysiology and molecular mechanisms remain to be elucidated and the symptom constellations can be quite varied. However, there is increasing evidence that immune mechanisms are involved and that food proteins may initiate the pathophysiologic events.

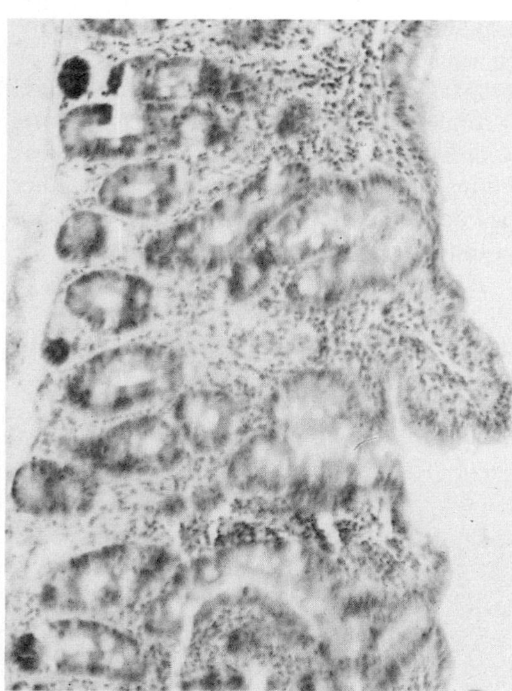

13.17 Small bowel biopsy section from a 9-month-old boy suffering recurrent, profuse diarrhea due to cow's milk enteropathy. Although the mechanism responsible for the flattening of the jejunal mucosa and other histopathologic changes is not known, there is strong evidence suggesting immune system involvement.

MANAGEMENT OF PATIENTS WITH PROVEN FOOD HYPERSENSITIVITY

A general protocol for the management of patients with food hypersensitivities is outlined in **13.18**. At the present time there is no acceptable preventive medication for proven food hypersensitivity. Avoidance, with regular rechallenge, is the preferred mode of management. This is because the natural history of food hypersensitivity, especially in children, strongly supports the claim that many patients outgrow their symptomatic food reactions. Injection therapy for life-threatening food hypersensitivities, which are often as severe as reactions to insect venom, would seem desirable, but as yet no one has determined a safe protocol by which to accomplish this goal. Thus, for the time being, avoidance and rechallenge over time, as described in **13.19**, is the optimal mode of management. Depending upon the severity of the initial and subsequent reactions, the culprit food should be regularly re-introduced at varying intervals until it is clear that the food problem is either going to be outgrown or may never be outgrown, as can occur with peanut hypersensitivity. Although patients with probable food-induced anaphylaxis do require attention from allergists, the methods described in this chapter are not suitable for their ongoing care and should not be applied as described. The general topic of anaphylaxis is covered in Chapter 4.

13.20 presents some considerations regarding the feeding of atopically predisposed infants. This is an area in which our knowledge is in a rapid state of flux: there is an accumulating body of information which appears quite regularly in the allergy literature. The reader is referred to one of several excellent reviews on this subject and also to the multiple studies which have appeared (Zeiger *et al.*, 1992). Studies suggest that the use of elimination diets may only delay the onset of adverse reactions to foods or of atopic dermatitis. Very few studies have demonstrated a decrease in the frequency of rhinitis or asthma in the groups with dietary intervention from birth. Research in this area is ongoing and it may be hoped that one day primary prevention will become a reality. In the meantime rapid diagnosis and prompt intervention with secondary prevention by identification and elimination of offending foods is the best approach. (Avoidance of cigarette smoke, dust mites, and viral infection in infancy may offer better hope for the prevention of asthma and rhinitis in atopically predisposed children.)

ANAPHYLAXIS TO FOOD

Although anaphylaxis is covered elsewhere (*see* Chapter 4), a few points specific to food-induced anaphylaxis are appropriate. As already mentioned, food-induced anaphylaxis can occur in very young children. When the food responsible for the reaction is egg or milk, the problem may remit to the extent that the food no longer causes life-threatening symptoms (Bock, 1985). When peanuts, tree nuts, and shellfish are responsible for producing anaphylaxis it may be a life-long condition. Ongoing studies in multiple centers suggest that children rarely 'outgrow' anaphylactic symptoms to those foods. In addition to foods commonly reported to produce anaphylaxis, spices have increasingly been incriminated. Examples include coriander and cumin seed (Bock, 1993).

The diagnosis of food-induced anaphylaxis can usually be confirmed by obtaining a careful and thorough history and by careful skin testing so that challenges are not necessary. However, in some situations when the responsible food cannot be easily identified and there are several possible culprits, then careful challenges under controlled conditions may be required. Additionally, there may be confounding factors such as exercise prior to eating.

In most situations symptoms occur immediately and if treated appropriately they remit totally. However, there have been reports of symptoms recurring several hours after the initial treatment was administered. These reactions have been termed 'biphasic'. Whether they are truly biphasic may depend upon the effectiveness of the initial treatment in the elimination of the reaction, rather than just the

MANAGEMENT OF PATIENTS WITH PROVEN FOOD HYPERSENSITIVITY

1. Avoidance (with regular rechallenge).
2. Corticosteroids may be important in a few, rare conditions (e.g., eosinophilic gastroenteritis, secretory diarrhea).
3. Avoid use of medications such as cromolyn or antihistamines; they have not been proven efficacious in well-controlled studies.
4. Injection therapy for food hypersensitivity should not be done, except under experimental protocols.

13.18 Management guidelines for proven food hypersensitivity.

suppression of it. Further research is required to unravel this observation (Sampson *et. al.*, 1992).

Education is the most important part of the prevention of food-induced anaphylaxis. Teaching patients to be very wary about what they eat and to be aware of the potential contamination of food substances which should be safe is very important. Educational information is available from the FOOD ALLERGY NETWORK (4744 Holly St., Fairfax, VA 22030, USA). All persons with food-induced anaphylaxis should carry emergency epinephrine which can be self-administered.

Exciting advances have occurred in our ability to diagnose and understand food hypersensitivity during the past 20 years. Let us hope that the next 20 years will lead to further understanding of the basic mechanisms and to treatments which will rapidly reverse the problem.

LONGITUDINAL CHALLENGES[a]

1. In patients with DBPCFC-proven food hypersensitivity, repeat the challenge 1–3 months after the initial positive challenge.
2. If the results of the rechallenge are positive, repeat the challenge in 1–6 months, depending on the severity of the reaction.
3. If the results are positive for the third time, repeat the challenge at 6–12 month intervals, until the reaction either disappears or shows signs of long-lasting remission.

[a]These recommendations do not apply to patients with a history of food-induced anaphylaxis.

13.19 Protocol for administration of regular, repeated challenges during follow-up.

FEEDING THE ATOPICALLY PREDISPOSED INFANT

1. Allow a normal prenatal maternal diet.
2. Encourage breast feeding for at least 6 months, with Nutramigen as the only supplement.
3. Advise the nursing mother to avoid eggs, peanuts, and possibly fish. Avoidance of dairy products may be considered.
4. Delay introduction of solid food as follows:
   6–12 months: vegetables, rice, meat, fruit
   12–18 months: cow's milk, wheat, corn, citrus, soy
   24 months: egg
   36 months: peanuts, fish

13.20 Considerations regarding the feeding of atopically predisposed infants. Although these recommendations are in a state of flux, changing with new clinical discoveries, they remain a reasonable approach to the care and management of these young patients.

REFERENCES

Bernhisel-Broadbent J, Sampson HA: Cross-allergenicity in the legume botanical family in children with food hypersensitivity. *J Allergy Clin Immunol*, **83**:435–440, 1989.

Bock SA: The natural history of food sensitivity. *J Allergy Clin Immunol*, **69**:173–177, 1982.

Bock SA: The natural history of severe reactions to foods in young children. *J Pediatr*, **107**:676–680, 1985.

Bock SA: *Food Allergy: A Primer for People*, Vantage, New York, 1988.

Bock SA, Atkins FM: The natural history of peanut allergy. *J Allergy Clin Immunol*, **83**:900–904, 1989.

Bock SA, Lee W-Y, Remigio L, Holst A, May CD: Appraisal of skin tests with food extracts for the diagnosis of food hypersensitivity. *Clin Allergy*, **8**:559–564, 1978.

Bock SA, Sampson HA, Atkins FM, Zeiger RS, Lehrer S, Sachs M, Bush RK, Metcalfe DD: Double-blind, placebo-controlled food challenge (DBPCFC) as an office procedure: a manual. *J Allergy Clin Immunol*, **82**: 986–997, 1988.

Bock SA: Respiratory reactions induced by food challenges in children with pulmonary disease. *Pediatric Allergy Immunol*, **3**:188–192, 1992.

Bock SA: Anaphylaxis to coriander: A sleuthing story. *J. Allergy Clin Immunol*, **91**:1232–1233, 1993.

Bock SA, Sampson HA: Food allergy in infancy. *Pediatr Clin of N Am*, Oct. 1994 (in press).

James JM, Bernhisel-Broadbent J, Sampson HA: Respiratory reactions provoked by double-blind food challenges in children. *Am J Respir Crit Care Med*, **149**:59–64, 1994.

Pastorello EA, Stocchi L, Pravettoni V, Bigi A, Schilke ML, Incorvaia C, Zanussi C: Role of the elimination diet in adults with food allergy. *J Allergy Clin Immunol*, 84:475–483, 1989.

Sampson HA, Albergo R: Comparison of results of skin tests, RAST, and double-blind, placebo-controlled food challenges in children with atopic dermatitis. *J Allergy Clin Immunol*, **74**:26–33, 1984.

Sampson HA, Mendelson L, Rosen JP. Fatal and near-fatal anaphylactic reactions to food in children and adolescents. *N Engl J Med*, **327**:380–384, 1992.

Zeiger RS, Heller S, Mellon MH, Halsey JF, Hamburger RN, Sampson HA: Genetic and environmental factors affecting the development of atopy through age 4 in children of atopic parents: a prospective randomized study of food allergen avoidance. *Pediatr Allergy Immunol*, **3**:110–127, 1992.

CHAPTER 14

Allergic Contact Dermatitis

Raymond G. Slavin

Allergic contact dermatitis, or dermatitis venenata, is a skin condition commonly seen by primary care physicians. Since new, potentially sensitizing chemicals are continually being brought into use, the flow of patients with this condition can only be expected to continue. Contact dermatitis is the most common occupational disease and, as such, it is of tremendous importance to both the individual and society (*see* Chapter 6). The diagnosis of allergic contact dermatitis, and especially the discovery of its cause in a given case, requires all of the patience, thoroughness, and acumen that the physician can offer. However, in recent years, the extraordinary success of corticosteroids in treating allergic contact dermatitis may have dulled the interest and perhaps lessened the clinician's desire to take the time necessary to discover the offending agent through history, physical examination, and diagnostic patch testing. The fact that fatalities and serious systemic complications of allergic contact dermatitis are rare may have also contributed to a diminished interest.

From the viewpoint of the patient with allergic contact dermatitis, this cavalier lack of concern is quite unjustified. The disease causes great discomfort and is frequently disabling. The chronic nature of the condition may provoke depression, and many patients must endure frequent hospitalization in addition to the limitations imposed on their pursuit of employment or recreation. Few patients are more grateful to their physicians than those for whom allergic contact dermatitis has been diagnosed, the inciting agent identified, and a plan for avoidance proposed.

CLINICAL FEATURES

GENERAL PROFILE

Allergic contact dermatitis (**14.1**) may appear at any age, but is most common in the middle aged and elderly. It is equally common

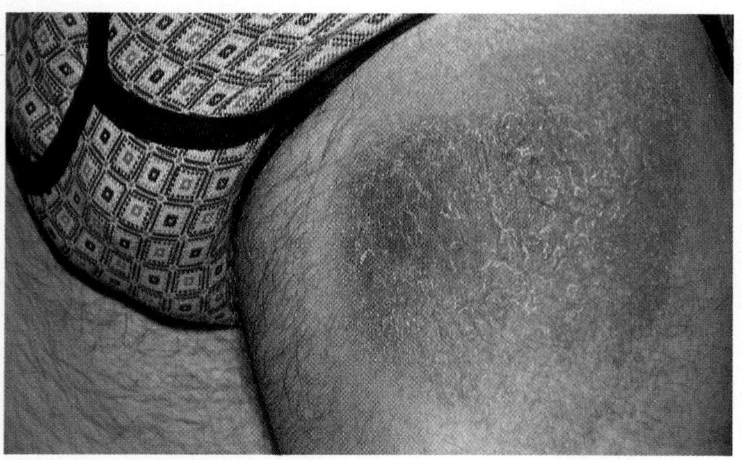

14.1 Contact dermatitis reaction to phosphorus sesquisulphide. The patient had been carrying a match-box in his pocket. The offending agent was found in the striker on the side of the match-box. This serves to illustrate an important point: clothing or other material in between the skin and the allergen does not necessarily prevent contact dermatitis. (Reproduced with permission from duVivier, 1986.)

in the general and atopic populations, and a history of concomitant or family allergy is of no help. Little is known about the prevalence of contact allergy in the general population. Sensitivity to nickel (**14.2A** and **14.2B**) is approximately 6% in general, with a striking prevalence in women, of the order of 10% versus 1% in men.

The interval between exposure to the causative agent and the arising or clinical manifestations is usually 12–48 hours. The incubation period (i.e., the time between initial exposure to the agent and the development of skin sensitivity) may be as short as two or three days in the case of a strong sensitizer, such as poison ivy (**14.3**), or as long as several years for a weak sensitizer, such as chromate. If a sufficient amount of allergen from the sensitizing exposure remains to react with the sensitized skin when the incubation period has elapsed, a spontaneous flare-up may occur at the site of sensitization. Once sensitivity is established, it generally persists for many years.

PHYSICAL EXAMINATION

The clinical appearance of allergic contact dermatitis depends upon the stage at which the patient presents. In the acute stage, erythema, papules, and vesicles predominate, usually accompanied by edema and, occasionally, bullae (**14.4**). Edema may be profound in areas of loose tissue, such as the eyelids and genitalia. Acute allergic con-

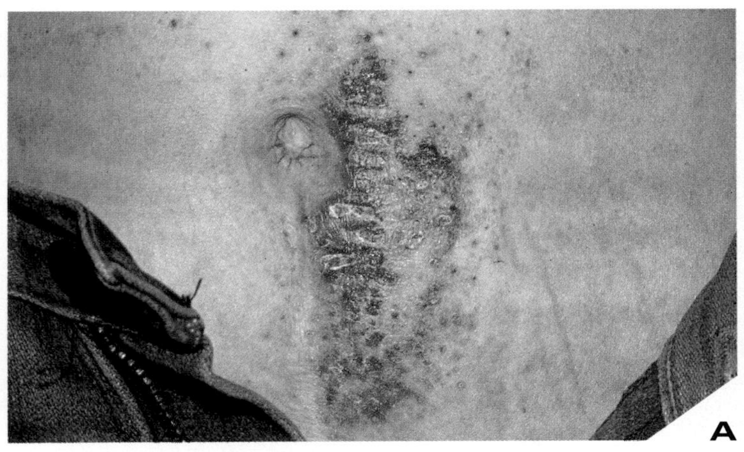

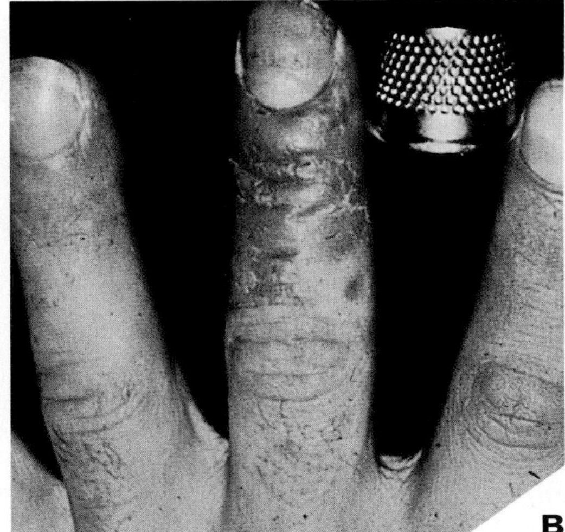

14.2 Nickel sensitivity. (A) Dermatitis from contact with the zipper and stud of jeans. (B) Dermatitis from nickel in sewing thimble. Patients with nickel sensitivities should avoid contact with this metal. (A: Reproduced with permission from duVivier, 1986; B: Courtesy of Medcom, Inc.)

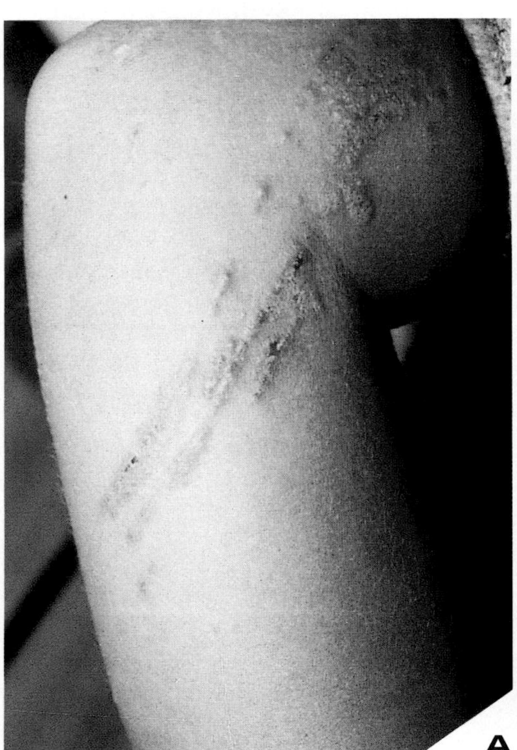

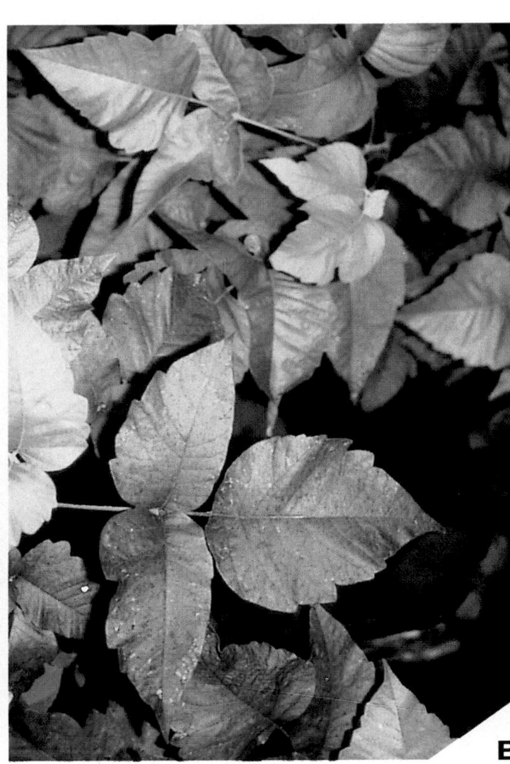

14.3 Poison ivy dermatitis. (A) Pruritic vesicles, often arranged in linear streaks, are typical of poison ivy dermatitis, the most common form of contact dermatitis in the US. (B) The poison ivy plant is characterized by shiny, deep-green leaflets ordered in patterns of three. (Reproduced with permission from Mallory and Zitelli, 198.)

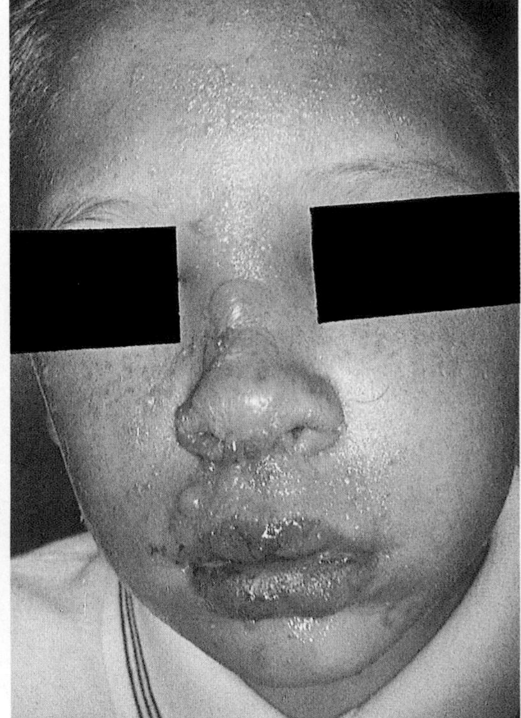

14.4 Acute stage of allergic contact dermatitis. Note the presence of vesicles and bullae typical of the condition. (Courtesy of Medcom, Inc.)

tact dermatitis of the face may result in a marked degree of periorbital swelling that resembles angioedema (**14.5**).

In the subacute phase, vesicles are less pronounced and there is evidence of crusting, scaling, and the beginning of lichenification. In the chronic stage, few papulovesicular lesions are evident, and thickening, lichenification, and scaliness predominate (**14.6**).

Skin areas vary in their susceptibility to sensitization by contact allergens. The eyelids, neck, and genitalia are among the most easily sensitized areas. The palms, the soles, and the scalp are more resistant, since the skin is characteristically thicker. Pressure, friction, and perspiration seem to promote the process of sensitization, and a tissue that is already irritated, inflamed, or infected has heightened susceptibility. A good clinical example is afforded by the common occurrence of contact dermatitis in sites of stasis dermatitis that have been treated with anti-bacterial or anti-fungal creams or ointments (**14.7**).

More often than not, the location of the dermatitis is the place at which the patient's skin surface made direct contact with the allergen (**14.8–14.11**). However, the relationship between the dermatitis and the direct contact allergen may not always be so obvious, and

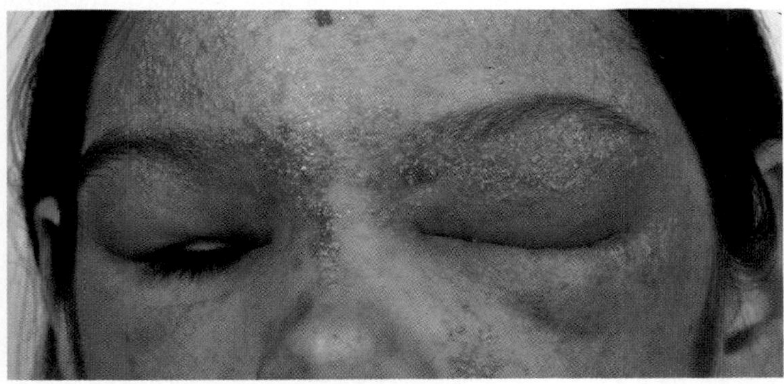

14.5 Periorbital contact dermatitis. In some cases, acute reactions occurring around the eyes may produce a marked degree of periorbital swelling that resembles angioedema. In this case, the reaction occurred after application of mepyramine maleate to the eyelid. (Reproduced with permission from duVivier, 1986.)

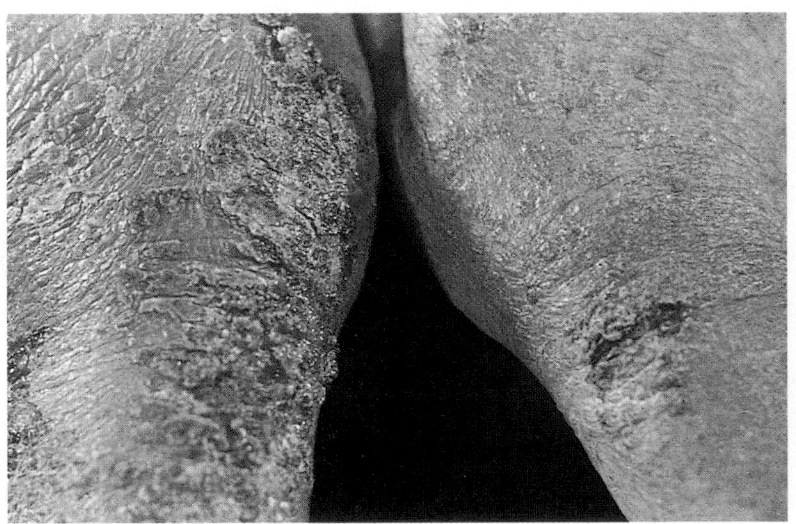

14.6 Chronic stage of allergic contact dermatitis. This stage is typified by scaliness, fissuring, and lichenification of the reactive area(s). (Courtesy of Medcom, Inc.)

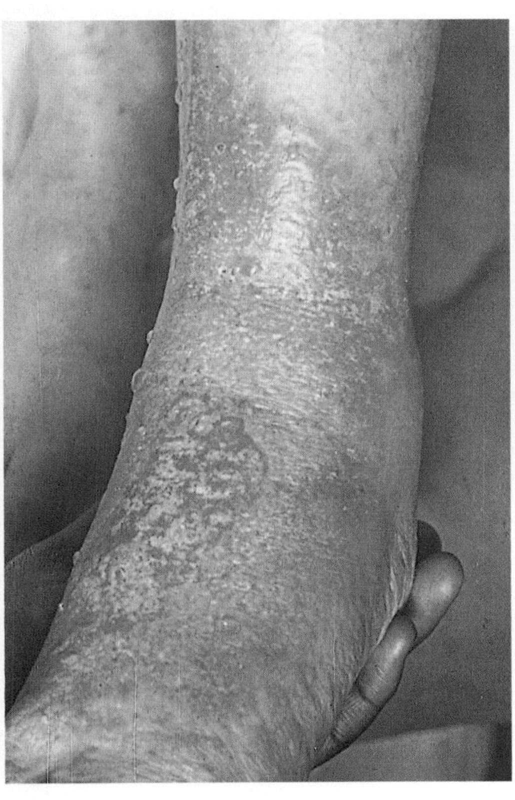

14.7 Allergic contact dermatitis due to application of an ointment to an area of stasis dermatitis.

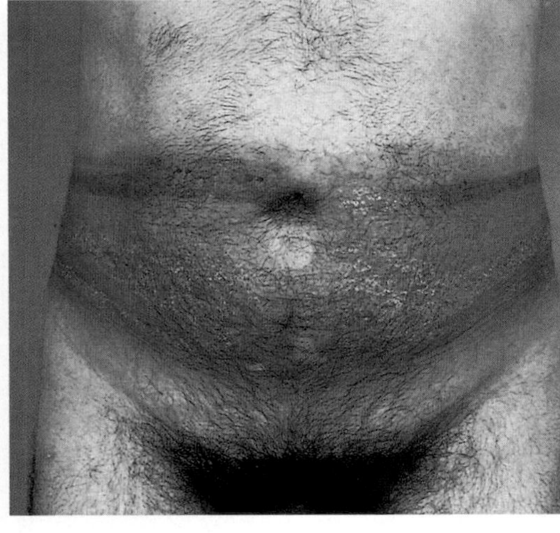

14.8 Contact dermatitis due to formaldehyde in the elastic band of the patient's underwear. (Courtesy of Medcom, Inc.)

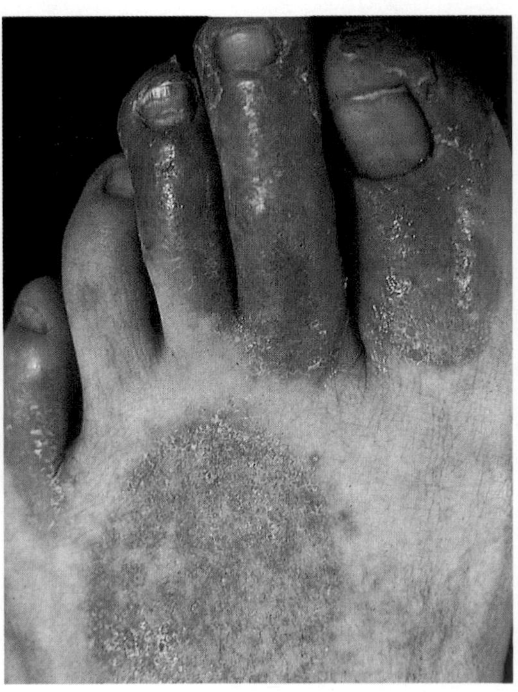

14.9 Dermatitis on the foot, arising as a result of contact with potassium dichromate. This chemical is used in the process of tanning leather for shoes. (Courtesy of Medcom, Inc.)

the ability to associate certain areas of involvement with particular types of exposure is extremely helpful (**14.11**).

IMMUNOLOGIC MECHANISMS IN CONTACT DERMATITIS

AFFERENT PHASE

Allergic contact dermatitis represents the cutaneous analogue of delayed, or cell-mediated, hypersensitivity. The inductive, or afferent limb, of the disorder begins when the skin comes into contact, intentionally or otherwise, with a hapten (**14.12**). A low molecular-weight organic or non-organic substance which is non-immunogenic in and of itself, a hapten combines with a protein carrier to form an immunogenic complex, such that the specificity of the subsequent immune response is directed at both the hapten and the carrier.

Strong evidence indicates that Langerhans cells are crucially important in the induction of contact sensitivity. These dendritic epidermal cells cannot be seen on light microscopy of routine histologic skin sections, but they can be identified easily by means of special stains (**14.13**). They possess Ia antigens, receptors for complement and for the Fc portion of IgG, and appear to contain surface proteins that act as carriers for contact allergens. Each Langerhans cell has up to 12 dendrites with terminal podia forming a reticuloepithelial trap for contact antigens (haptens). The cell ingests the antigen by pinocytosis, partially degrades it, then brings to its surface peptides that bind to the Ia antigen (**14.14**). The antigen processed by the Langerhans cells is then presented to T-helper cells either in the skin or in the paracortical area of the draining lymph node (see **14.12**). It takes approximately 18–24 hours from

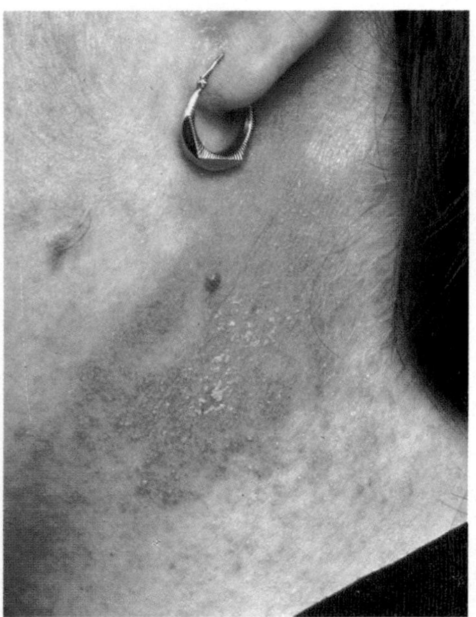

14.10 Reaction to perfume. The dermatitis is found at the sites of application, particularly on the sides of the neck. (Reproduced with permission from duVivier, 1986.)

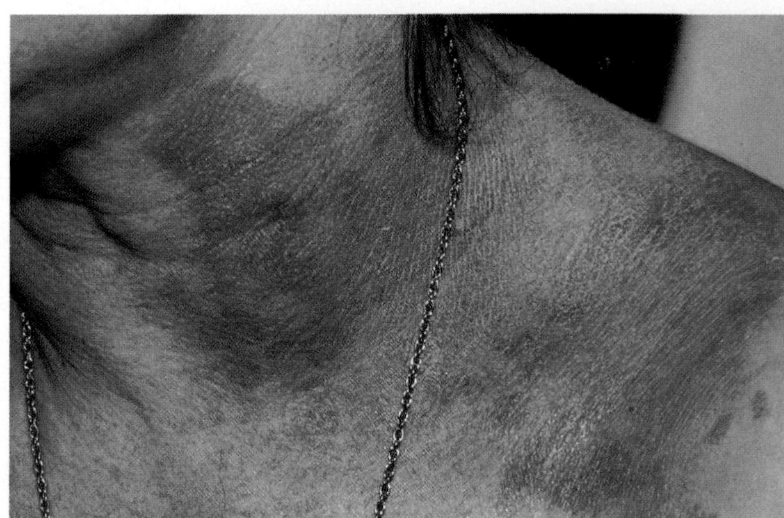

14.11 Contact dermatitis on the neck and shoulders provoked by contact with nail polish. In this case, the reaction did not occur on the nails or the hands, but on the skin surfaces which the patient touched while her nails were still wet. (Reproduced with permission from duVivier, 1986.)

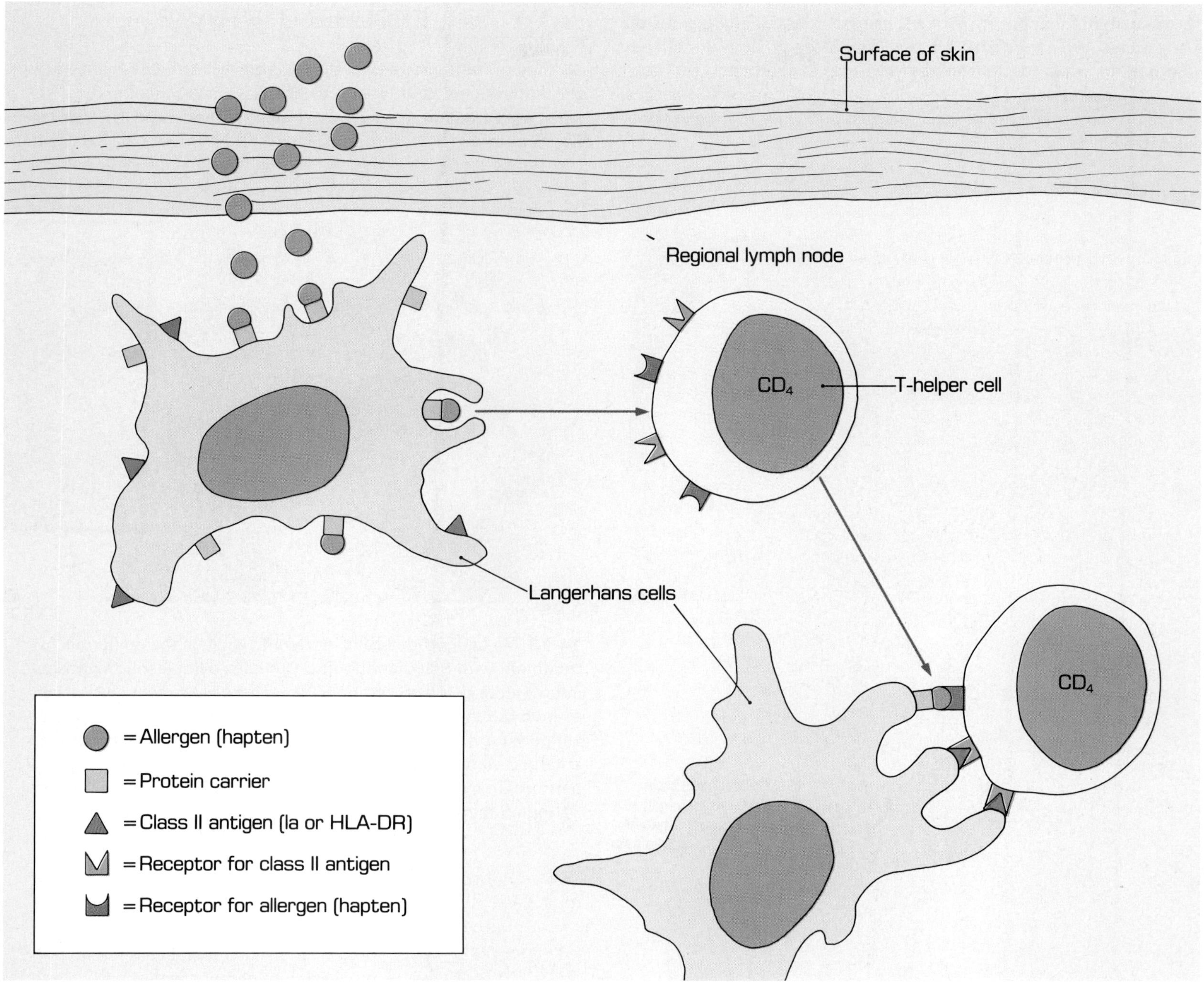

14.12 The inductive or afferent phase of allergic contact dermatitis. The process begins when the skin comes into contact with a hapten – a low molecular weight substance that is not, in and of itself, immunogenic. The hapten combines with protein carriers on the surface of the epidermal Langerhans cells, thus forming immunogenic complexes. These cells, which collectively form an epithelial trap for contact antigens (haptens), ingest the hapten–protein complexes, degrade them, and bring peptides to their surfaces. The antigens so processed are then presented to the cutaneous T-helper cells.

the time of initial application of a sensitizing dose of allergen for the Langerhans cells to arrive in the lymph node. For an allergic response to proceed, the antigen-bearing Langerhans cells must contact CD_4+ T-cells (T-helper cells) that have, on their surfaces, specific receptors for the contact allergen and class II antigen (Ia or HLA-DR).

EFFERENT PHASE

As they present antigens to the receptor-bearing CD_4 lymphocytes, the Langerhans cells produce and release interleukin-1 (IL-1), a substance thought to activate T-cell synthesis and the release of interleukin-2 (IL-2) and interferon-γ (IFN-γ) (**14.15**). Recent data

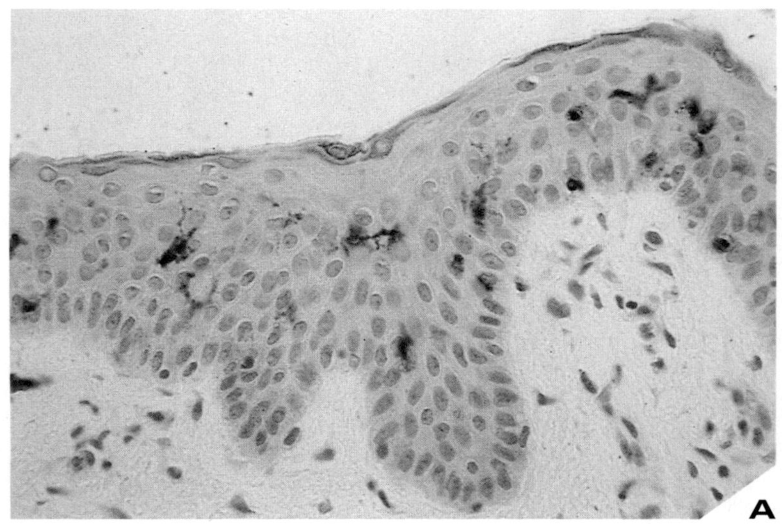

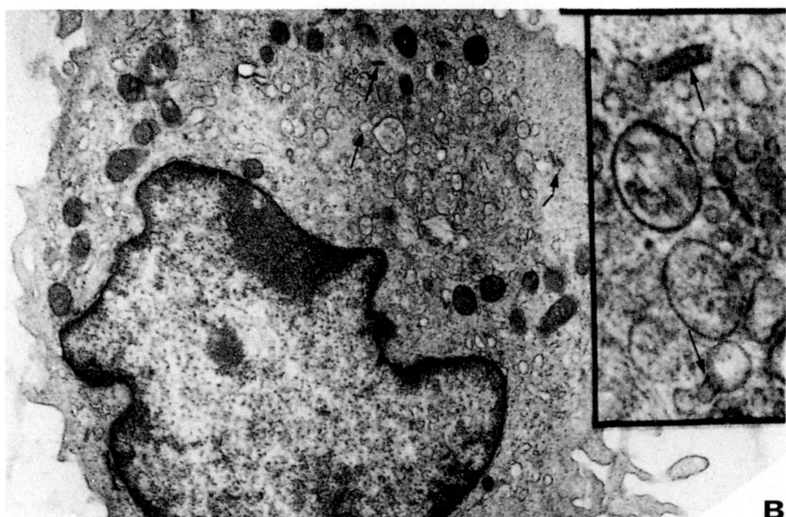

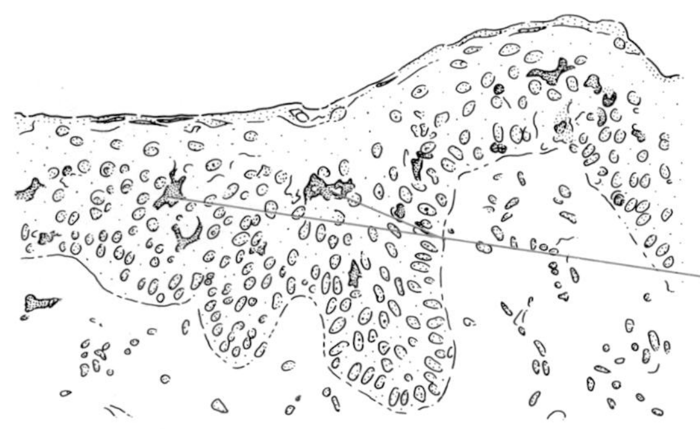

14.13 (A) Langerhans cells rendered visible in the epidermis by treatment with S-100 antibodies. Complex cytoplasmic extensions interdigitate between keratinocytes. These cells must be specially stained to be seen on light microscopy. (B) Electron micrograph of a Langerhans cell in a dermal lymphatic vessel. The inset shows an enlarged view of the cell's granules. (A: Reproduced with permission from True, 1990; B: Reproduced with permission from Dr. Inga Silberberg-Sinakin.)

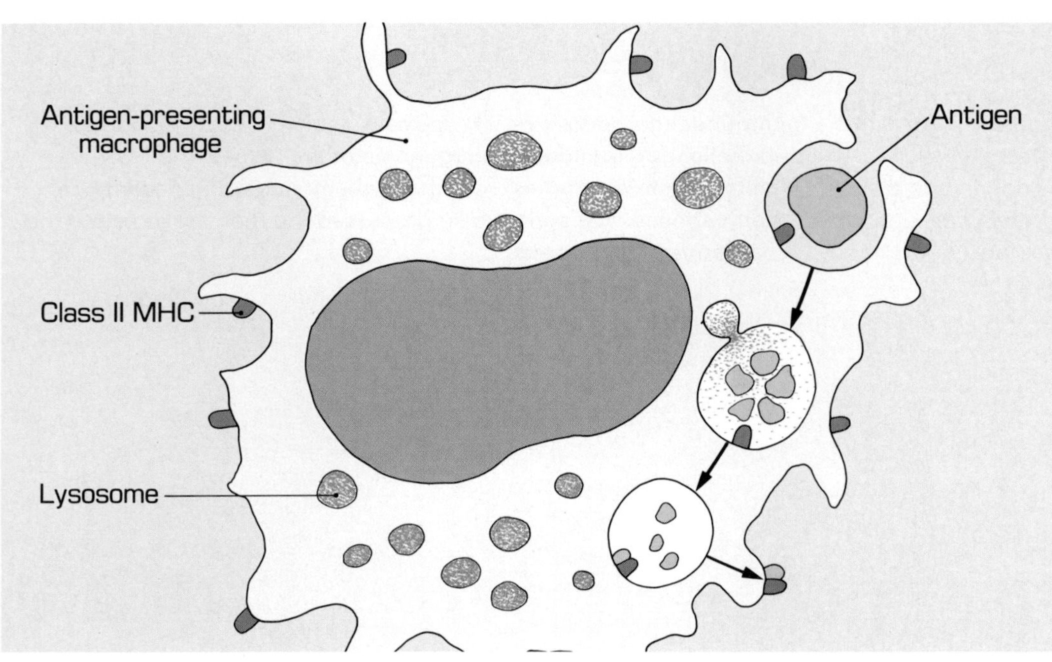

14.14 Schematic representation of the processing of haptens within the Langerhans cell. The antigen is taken in and broken down into its component peptides. Certain of these determinants are then expressed on the cell surfaces in association with a major histocompatibility complex. Once on the surfaces of the Langerhans cells, they are presented to the CD_4 cells.

suggest that IL-1 may also increase antigen-presenting cell function and up-regulate Ia expression on the Langerhans cells themselves. IL-2 acts non-specifically to stimulate T-cells with and without specific antigen receptors, causing them to proliferate and secrete IFN-γ. IFN-γ, or immune interferon, activates cytotoxic T-cells, natural killer (NK) cells, and macrophages that cause the epidermal spongiosis (intercellular edema) and dermal infiltrate that are the histologic hallmarks of allergic contact hypersensitivity (**14.16**).

The specifically sensitized CD_4 helper T-cells localize the response to the site of challenge via production of IL-2 and IFN-γ. They also provide the immunologic memory that accounts for the more intense and rapid response to contact allergens upon -

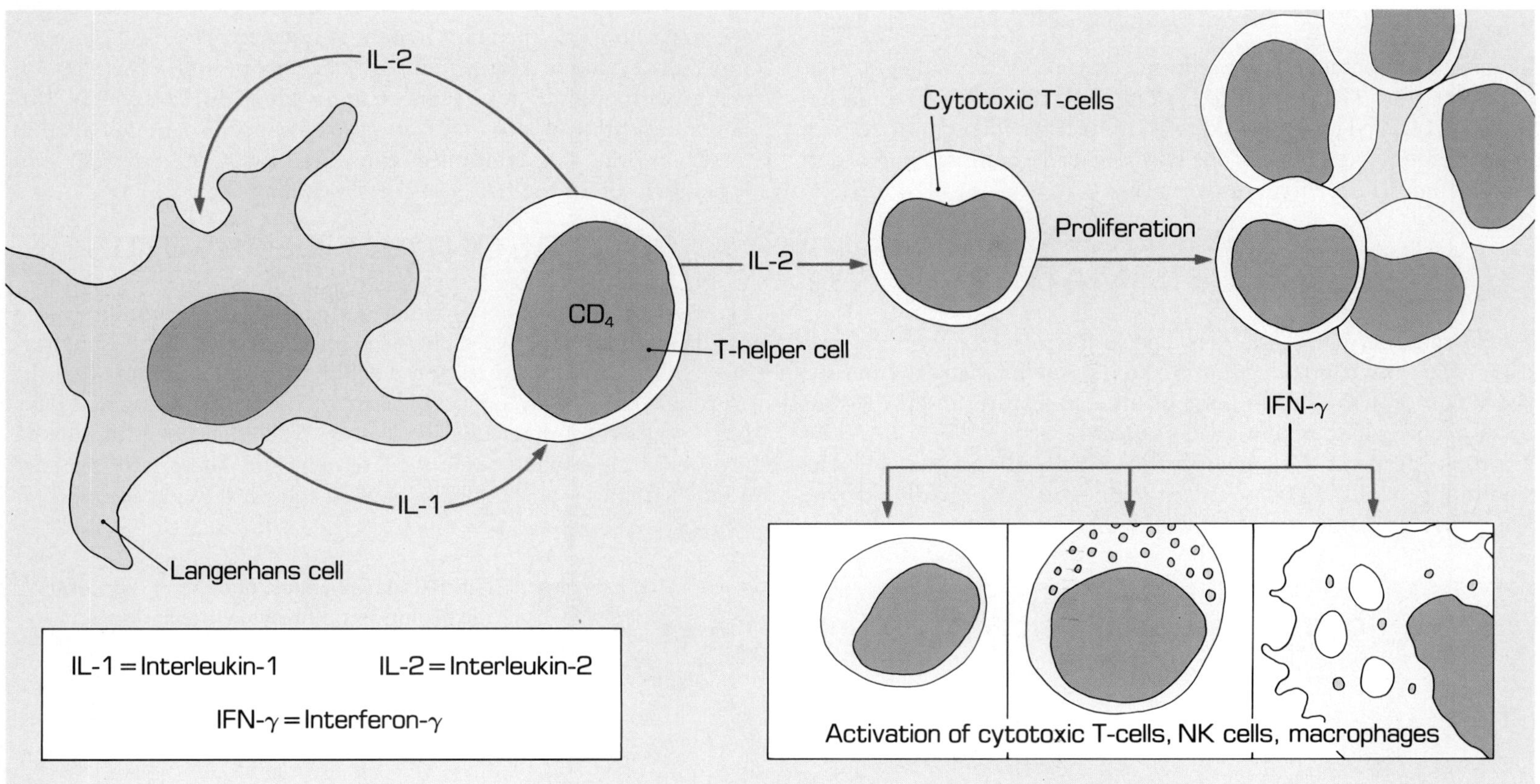

14.15 The efferent phase of allergic contact dermatitis. As they present the processed antigens to the CD_4 cells, the Langerhans cells also release interleukin-1 (IL-1). This cytokine triggers the T-cell synthesis of IL-2, which non-specifically activates other T-cells, and of interferon IFN-γ, which activates the cytotoxic T-cells, natural killer (NK) cells, and macrophages. These changes culminate in the epidermal spongiosis and dermal cellular infiltration that are characteristic of allergic contact dermatitis. In this way, the specifically sensitized CD_4 cells are responsible for the localization of the immune response.

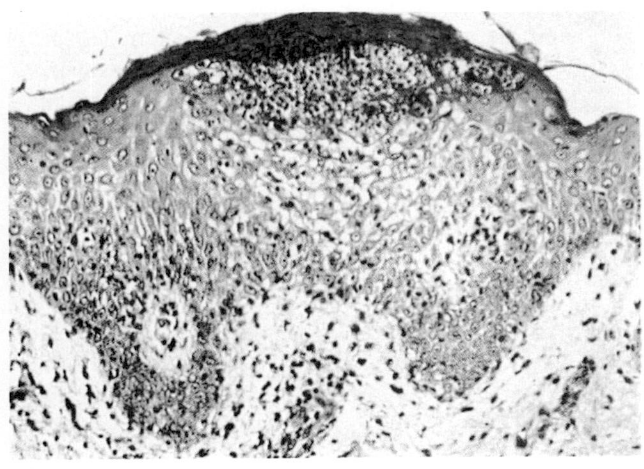

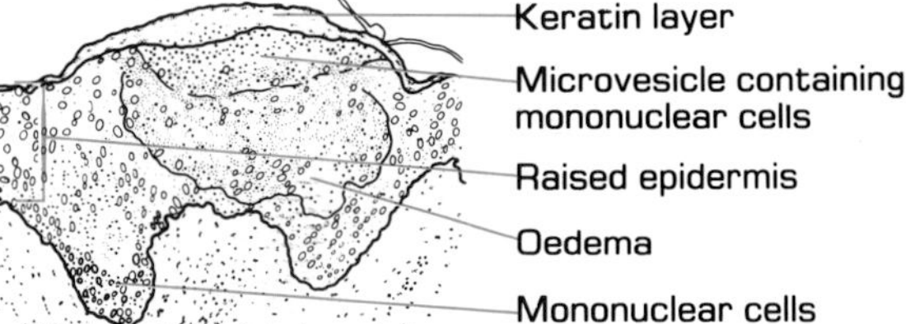

14.16 Histology of contact dermatitis. This section depicts the histologic changes typical of contact hypersensitivity. Mononuclear cells have infiltrated the epidermis, pushing it outward. The epidermal layer also contains microvesicles, and shows evidence of marked edema. The dermal layer is infiltrated by large numbers of leukocytes. hematoxylin and eosin stain, × 130. (Reproduced with permission from Roitt, 1985.)

re-exposure. Since T-cells are more numerous, owing to intense proliferation following the primary exposure, there is an increased likelihood that, on re-exposure to the antigen, the Langerhans cells encounter the specifically sensitized T-cells within the skin *before* they can migrate to the draining lymph node.

DIFFERENTIAL DIAGNOSIS

A number of contact skin conditions exist other than allergic contact dermatitis. These are listed, along with their proposed mechanisms, in **14.17**. The skin conditions most frequently confused with allergic contact dermatitis are seborrheic dermatitis, atopic dermatitis, and primary irritant dermatitis.

SEBORRHEIC AND ATOPIC DERMATITIS

In seborrheic dermatitis, there is a general tendency toward oiliness of the skin, and a predilection of the lesions for the scalp and the nasolabial folds. Pruritus is not a prominent feature, and the lesions tend to be irregular, with a greasy coating.

Atopic dermatitis is covered thoroughly in Chapter 15. The condition generally has its onset in infancy or early childhood. The skin is dry; also, although pruritus is a prominent feature, it appears before the lesions and not after them, as is the case with allergic contact dermatitis.

PRIMARY IRRITANT DERMATITIS

The dermatitis caused by a primary irritant is a simple chemical or physical insult to the skin. For example, the condition commonly called 'dish-pan hands' is caused by household detergents. Prior sensitization to the primary irritant is not necessary, and the reaction can develop in a large number of normal persons. The eruption begins with mild dryness, redness, and scaling. **14.18A** and **14.18B** illustrate a primary irritant reaction to entrapped soaps and alkalies under a ring. On continued exposure, fissuring, crusting, and lichenification of the backs of the hands may occur (**14.19**).

PHOTOCONTACT DERMATITIS

Photosensitivity, or photocontact dermatitis, is an eruption caused by the interaction between chemical and ultraviolet light. The diagnosis of any photosensitization reaction is based on finding that the eruption occurs only on those parts of the individual which have been exposed to ultraviolet irradiation. The sensitizer is usually an ingested drug – sulfa compounds, tetracycline, and griseofulvin are good examples – or a topically applied substance, such as a coal tar extract.

CATEGORIES OF CONTACT DERMATITIS

Type	Mechanism
Primary irritant	Non-immunologic
Photoirritant or phototoxic	Non-immunologic; requires ultraviolet light exposure
Allergic contact	Immunologic; delayed hypersensitivity
Photoallergic contact	Immunologic; requires ultraviolet light exposure
Contact urticaria	Non-immunologic, immunologic (IgE-mediated), and combination mechanisms

14.17 Classification of contact dermatitis according to pathogenic mechanisms.

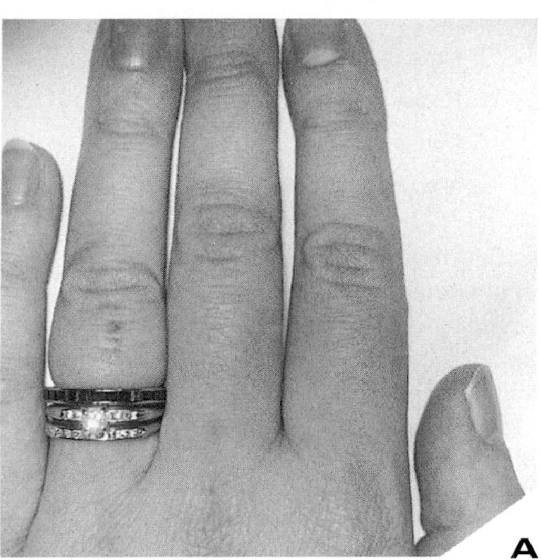

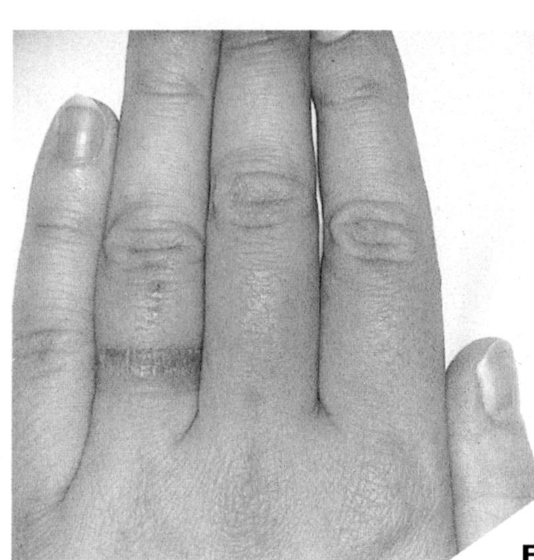

14.18 (A) Primary irritant reaction caused by the accumulation of soaps and alkalies underneath the patient's ring. (B) Removal of the ring reveals the severity of the reaction. (Courtesy of Medcom, Inc.)

Phototoxicity

Photoreactions can take two forms: in the first, the phototoxic reaction, cell damage can occur on the first exposure to sunlight. No sensitization period is required and the mechanism is non-immunologic. As in primary irritant reactions, the severity of the symptoms is dose-related. The clinical appearance of the phototoxic reaction is usually that of an exaggerated sunburn reaction (**14.20**).

Contact photoallergic dermatitis

The second form of photoreaction is a true contact photoallergic dermatitis. The patient makes contact with a photosensitizing substance and then has a delayed hypersensitivity reaction induced by ultraviolet light of an appropriate wavelength. An incubation period is required, so there is no reaction on first exposure. In this form of reaction, the sensitizing allergen undergoes a chemical alteration on exposure to the ultraviolet components of sunlight. The concentration of drug necessary for a reaction is usually low, and the clinical appearance of the reaction is largely eczematous, in contrast to the intense erythema and inflammatory response of phototoxic reactions (**14.21**).

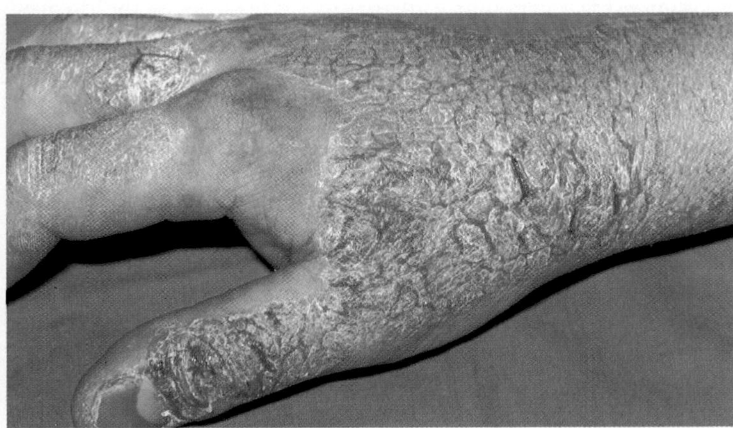

14.19 Primary irritant dermatitis of the backs of the hands. This patient, a garage mechanic, was in constant contact with irritant substances. Reactions like this are common in individuals whose occupations require their hands to be repeatedly immersed in water and/or allergenic chemicals. When it occurs in the context of household chores, it is referred to as 'dish-pan hands.' (Reproduced with permission from duVivier, 1986.)

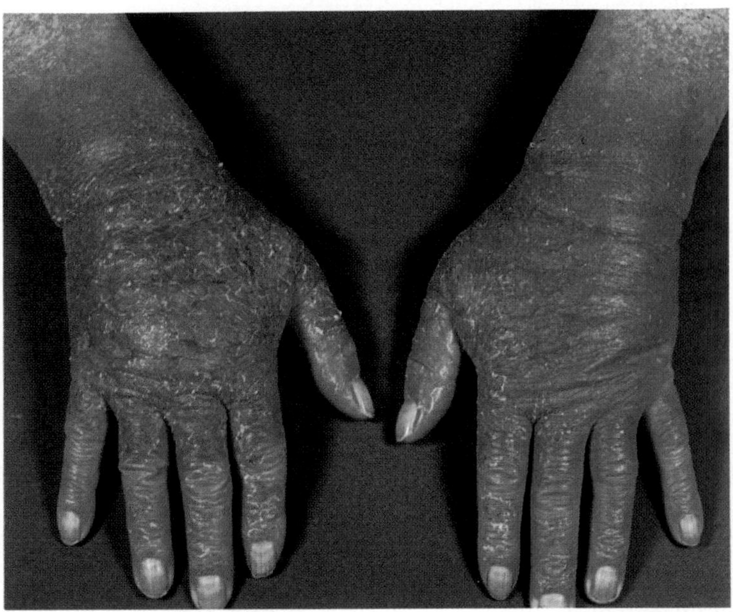

14.20 Phototoxic contact dermatitis. Erythema and edema arose secondary to the ingestion of a thiazide diuretic drug and subsequent exposure to sunlight. (Reproduced with permission from duVivier, 1986.)

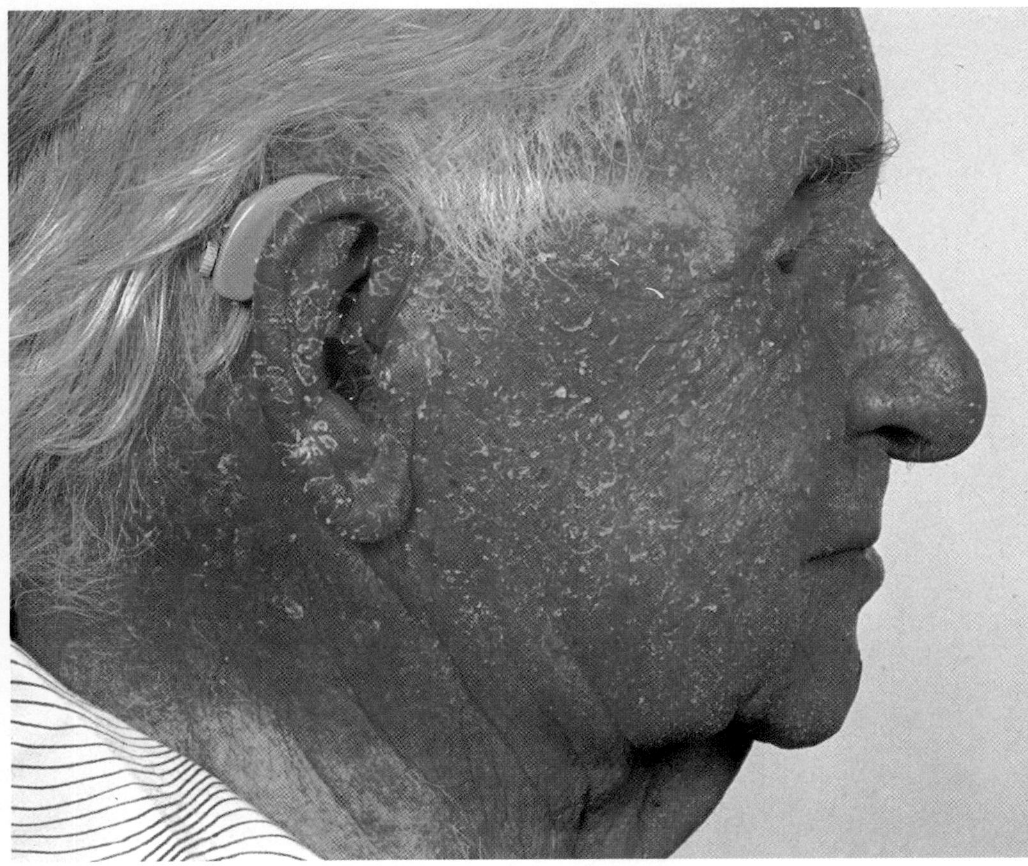

14.21 Photoallergic contact dermatitis. This reaction, a true allergic dermatitis, is distinguished from phototoxic dermatitis by the scaly, eczematous appearance of the skin. Phototoxic reactions are usually intensely erythematous, rather than eczematous, but the distinction is not always clear. Some drugs are capable of causing both phototoxic and photoallergic reactions. (Reproduced with permission from duVivier, 1986.)

CONTACT URTICARIA

A final form of contact dermatitis is contact urticaria (*see* Chapter 16). This is an immediate wheal-and-flare response generated by a wide variety of contactants. There are three categories of contact urticaria based on the mechanism of action. The first is non-immunologic and affects nearly all individuals. It occurs as a result of the direct release of mediators from mast cells triggered by substances from stinging arthropods or plants, like the nettle. The second is allergic, and probably represents a Type I hypersensitivity reaction due to foods, such as fish and eggs, or medications, such as penicillin. The third category arises from an unknown mechanism and appears to combine features of both the allergic and non-allergic types. A common cause is ammonium persulfate, an oxidizing agent in hair bleach.

DIAGNOSIS

PATCH TESTING

The most-nearly definitive diagnostic test for contact dermatitis is patch testing, which can be thought of as creating the disease in miniature. The idea is to apply the suspected allergen to the skin with the intention of producing a small area of allergic contact dermatitis (**14.22**). The test generally takes 48–96 hours, although a reaction may appear after 24 hours in markedly sensitive patients. When the patch is removed, the area is inspected for the gross appearance of a localized dermatitis resembling the patient's primary lesions. One must remember, however, that a positive finding is not absolute proof that the test substance is the cause of the dermatitis. A positive skin test simply indicates sensitivity; it may reflect a previous, unrelated episode of dermatitis or it may be without clinical relevance at all. The positive patch test must always be correlated with the patient's history and physical appearance.

Choosing test substances

Choosing the appropriate substances for patch testing is important. Frequently, the history and physical examination reveal the cause of the dermatitis, and the patch test serves only as corroboration (**14.23**). On other occasions, the history and location of the dermatitis suggest a particular category of exposure; in these cases, patch testing should be tailored to the particular category. These include the patient's occupation, hobbies, household articles, clothing, cosmetics, plant exposures, and topical medications. In some instances, there may be little or no suggestion of the offending agent, in which case application of a standard group of substances known to be common causes of allergic contact dermatitis is indicated. The contents of a standard screening tray are listed in **14.24**. **14.25** lists some common skin sensitizers and their most frequent forms or sources of exposure.

Precautions

Several precautions must be observed in patch testing. The test material itself may sensitize the patient and, accordingly, patch tests, especially repeated tests, should not be done unnecessarily. One must also avoid provoking non-specific inflammation. In other words, the test material must be dilute enough so that it would not

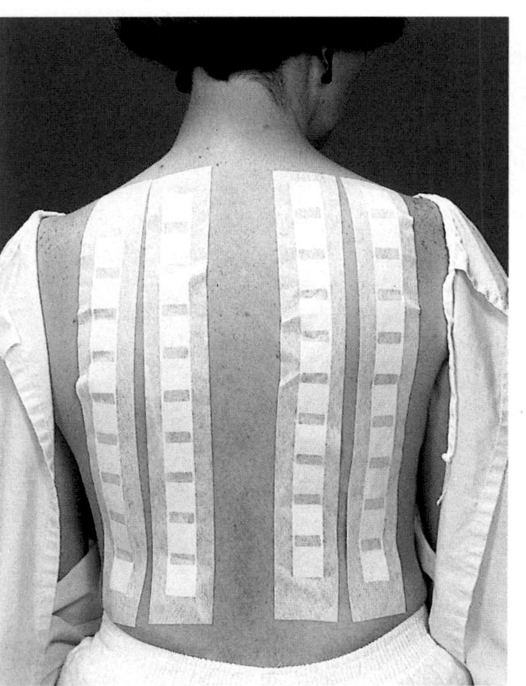

14.22 Placement of a diagnostic patch-test series on the back of a patient complaining of symptoms possibly indicative of contact allergy.

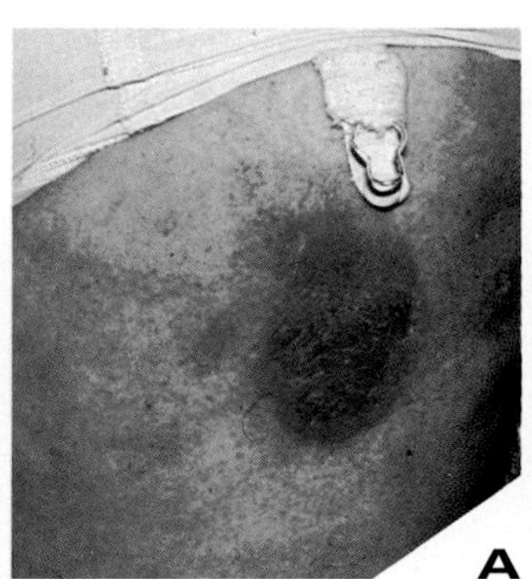

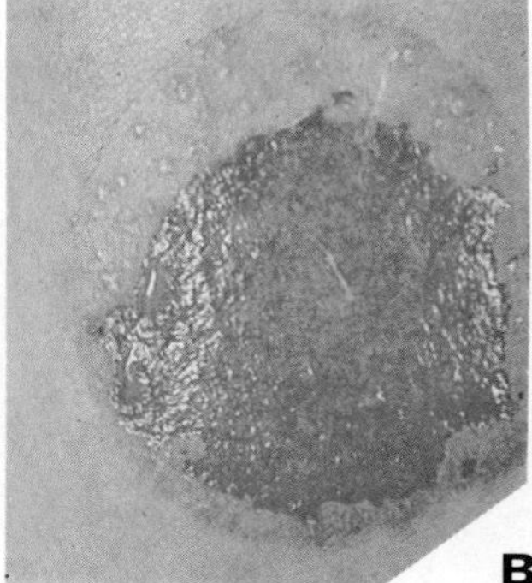

14.23 Comparison between the actual, clinically observed contact dermatitis, and the dermatitic response to patch testing. (A) This eczematous lesion was provoked by sensitivity to certain components of the rubber of the patient's undergarment. (B) The suspected allergen was patch-tested, and produced a similar eczematous lesion within 72 hours, confirming the allergenicity of the substance. (Reproduced with permission from Roitt, 1985.)

ALLERGENS AVAILABLE IN STANDARD SCREENING PATCH TEST KIT

Benzocaine, 5%

Mercaptobenzothiazole, 1%

Colophony, 20%

ρ-Phenylenediamine, 1%

Imidazolidinyl urea (Germall 115), 2%

Cinnamic aldehyde, 1%

Lanolin alcohol (wool wax alcohols), 30%

Carba mix, 3%

Neomycin sulfate, 20%

Thiuram mix, 1%

Formaldehyde (contains methanol), 1%

Ethylenediamine dihydrochloride, 1%

Epoxy resin, 1%

Quaternium 15, 2%

ρ-*tert*-Butylphenol formaldehyde resin, 1%

Mercapto mix, 1%

Black rubber p -phenylenediamine mix (PPD), 0.6%

Potassium dichromate, 0.25%

Balsam of Peru, 25%

Nickel sulfate (anhydrous), 2.5%

14.24 Listing of allergens available in a standard screening patch testing kit. (Reproduced with permission from Slavin and Ducomb, 1989.)

COMMON SKIN SENSITIZERS IN ALLERGIC CONTACT DERMATITIS

Agent	Source
Ethylenediamine hydrochloride	Antifungal cream Aminophylline Hydroxyzine Antihistamines
ρ-Phenylenediamine	Hair dye Fur dye Black, blue, or brown clothing
Thiuram	Rubber compounds (vulcanization accelerator) Fungicides Wood preservatives
Formalin, formaldehyde	Cosmetics Insecticides Apparel (drip-dry, wrinkle-resistant, water-repellent)
Potassium dichromate	Leather (chrome tanned) Yellow paints
Paraben	Cosmetics Pharmaceuticals
Epoxy resin	Adhesives
Sodium hypochlorite	Bleach Cleansing agents
Carba mix	Rubber Lawn and garden fungicides
Imidazolidinyl urea	Cosmetics (preservatives)
Mercaptobenzothiazole	Rubber compounds (accelerator) Anticorrosion agents
ρ-β-Naphthylamine	Rubber compounds (antioxidant)
ρ-*tert*-Butylphenol	Rubber compounds Plastics Adhesives
Mercury	Topical ointments Disinfectants
Nickel	Coins Jewelry Buckles Clasps Door handles
Copper	Coins Alloys Insecticides Fungicides

14.25 Listing of common skin sensitizers and the sources or vehicles in which they are most often found. (Reproduced with permission from Slavin and Ducomb, 1989.)

have a primary irritant effect in a substantial number of normal controls. This precaution is especially important when the test substance has not been obtained as a standard patch-test material.

Patch testing should not be performed in the presence of an acute or widespread contact dermatitis. False-positive reactions may be obtained because of increased skin reactivity. A positive test reaction involving the offending agents may cause the dermatitis to flare. Patients should be carefully instructed at the time the patches are applied to remove any patch that causes severe irritation. If such a patch is left in place for the full 48 hours, the area may actually slough.

Standardized systems

A number of standardized patch-testing systems have been developed. Both North American and international contact dermatitis research groups have recently adopted the AL-test as the standardized method for epicutaneous testing. This device employs a cellulose antigen-bearing disk attached to a polyethylene-coated aluminum paper backing (**14.26**). An alternative is the Finn Chamber, which consists of a shallow aluminum cup holding the test material, affixed to the skin with tape (**14.27**). Its major advantage is that reaction sites are smaller than with the AL-test and more patches can be applied. The thin-layer, rapid-use epicutaneous (TRUE) test

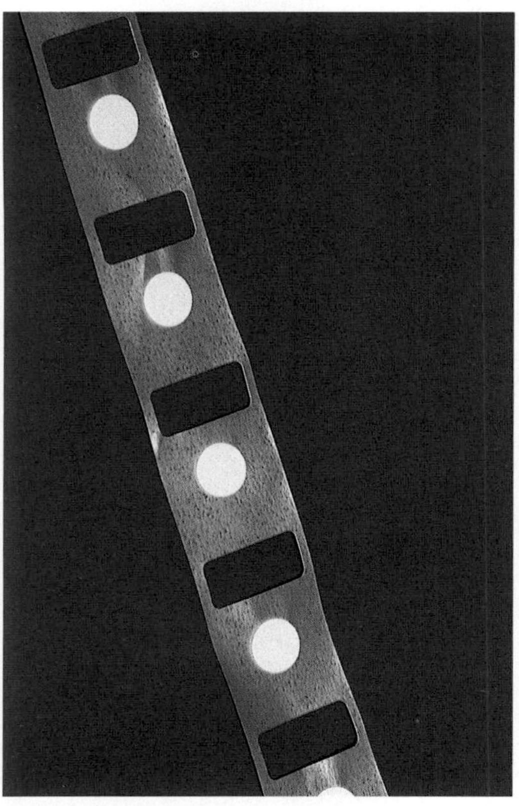

14.26 Close-up view of the AL-test system. (Courtesy of Hollister–Stier Laboratories.)

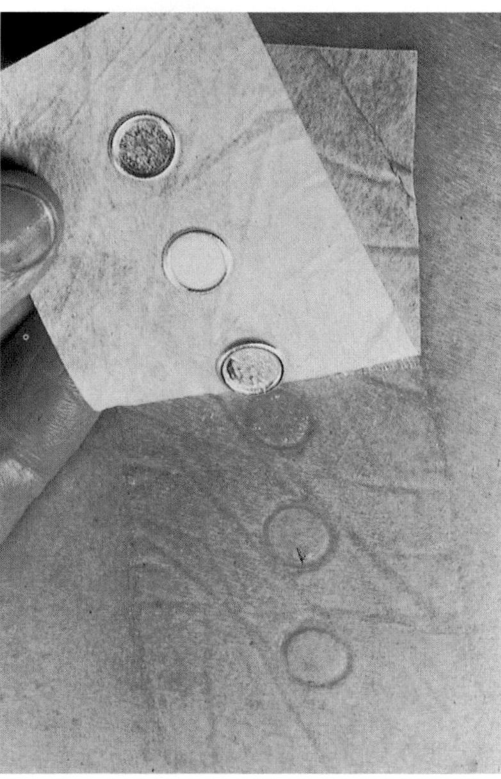

14.27 Close-up view of the Finn chamber testing system. (Courtesy of Hermal Pharmaceutical Laboratories.)

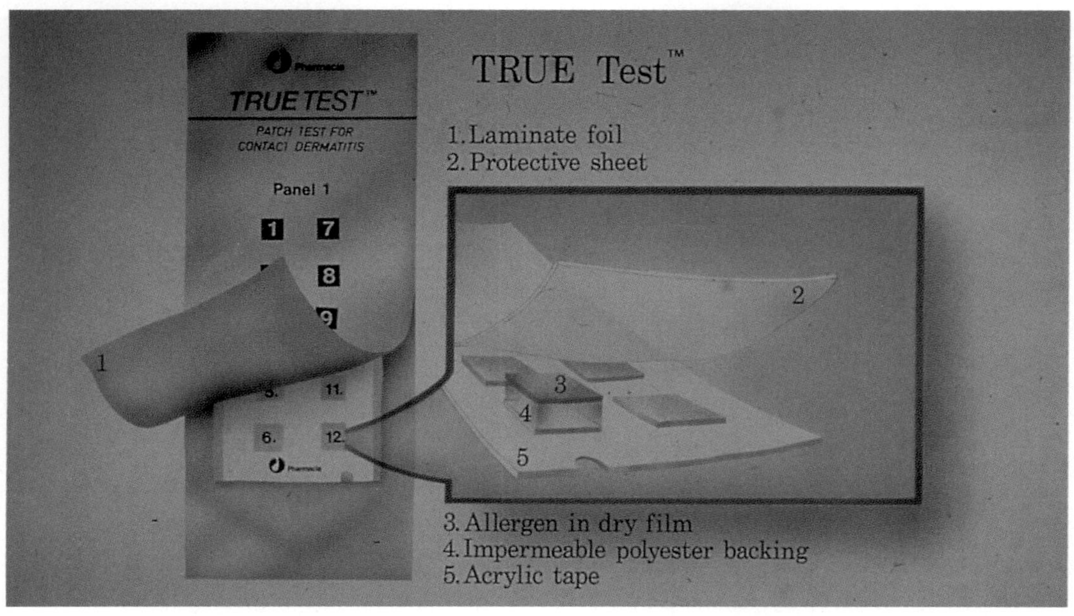

14.28 Components of the TRUE test. (Allergen Patch Test TRUE Test™ has been licensed for distribution in the United States by Glaxo Dermatology.)

is a standardized, ready-to-apply patch test system made of polyester covered with a film of allergens incorporated into a hydrophilic polymer. The patches are mounted on non-woven cellulose tape with acrylic adhesive, covered with siliconized plastic, and packed in an airtight and light impermeable envelope (**14.28**). When the test strip is affixed to the skin (**14.29**), perspiration hydrates the film and transforms it into a gel, releasing the allergen.

MANAGEMENT OF ALLERGIC CONTACT DERMATITIS

TREATMENT OF MILD REACTIONS

General management strategies are outlined in **14.30**. For limited, localized allergic contact dermatitis, cool tap-water compresses and a topical corticosteroid are the preferred modalities. Hydrocortisone is the only corticosteroid that should be applied to the face. The compresses minimize oozing, are very economical, and are easy for patients to make from a soft, smooth cotton cloth, such as a diaper or tea towel. Further, the compresses facilitate the absorption of a topical steroid, and enhance its anti-inflammatory property. The steroids should be in the form of a cream, not an occlusive ointment.

TREATMENT OF ACUTE REACTIONS

For extensive or edematous acute reactions, systemic corticosteroids are warranted. A large initial dosage of prednisone, of the order of 40–60 mg per day for an adult patient, should be given with a slow taper over a period of 2 weeks. The slow taper prevents rebound flare and minimizes side effects.

PREVENTION

In terms of prophylaxis, it is important to avoid the offending antigen as much as possible. In this light, it should be emphasized once again that the determination of exactly what substances provoke the reaction is vital, if the patient is to practice proper environmental control. The use of protective clothing is beneficial, as are newly available barrier creams, such as Ivy Shield (Interpro, PO Box 1823, Haverhill, MA 01831).

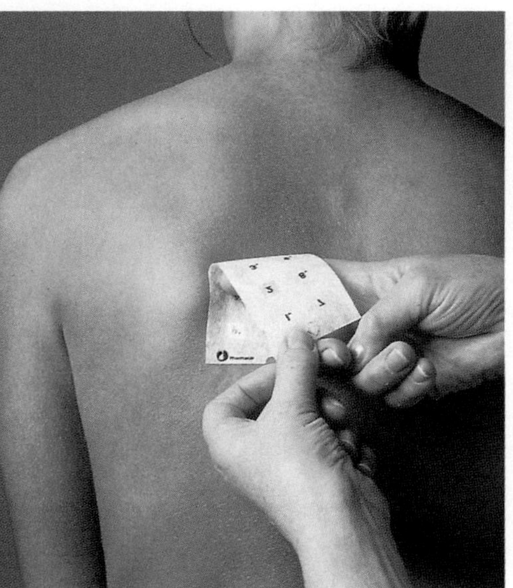

14.29 TRUE test strip being fixed to the skin. (Allergen Patch Test TRUE Test™ has been licensed for distribution in the United States by Glaxo Dermatology.)

MANAGEMENT OF ALLERGIC CONTACT DERMATITIS

Limited, localized reaction
Cool tap-water compresses
Topical corticosteroid cream

Extensive, acute reaction
Oral prednisone: 40–60 mg per day initially (adult); slow taper over 2 weeks

Prophylaxis
Antigen avoidance
Protective clothing
Barrier creams

14.30 Protocol for the management of allergic contact dermatitis.

REFERENCES

DuVivier A: *Atlas of Clinical Dermatology*, Gower, London, 1986.
Mallory SB, Zitelli JA: Pediatric dermatology, in Zitelli BK, Davis HW (eds): *Atlas of Pediatric Physical Diagnosis*, Gower, New York, pp 8.1–8.27, 1987.
Roitt IM, Brostoff J, Male DK: *Immunology*, Gower, London, 1985.
Slavin RG, Ducomb DF: Allergic contact dermatitis. *Hosp Pract*, **24**;41A, 39–51, 1989.
True LD: *Atlas of Diagnostic Immunohistopathology*, Gower, New York, 1990.

CHAPTER 15

Atopic Dermatitis

Philip Fireman

Atopic dermatitis, described by some clinicians as infantile eczema, is a chronically recurrent, genetically influenced skin disorder of early infancy, childhood, and young adulthood. Although it was initially described in the nineteenth century, it was not until 1935 that Hill and Sulzberger first characterized the clinical entity. The term atopy, derived from the Greek word which means 'strange thing', was introduced in 1923 by Coca and Cooke to describe a cohort of patients with asthma and allergic rhinitis who demonstrated immediate wheal-and-flare reactions upon skin testing with a variety of environmental allergens. The sera of these patients contained skin sensitizing antibodies that were subsequently characterized as IgE immunoglobulins. It was later recognized that these atopic individuals also frequently manifested the itchy, eczematous dermatitis which was labeled atopic dermatitis.

The physical distribution of the skin eruption varies with age, as shown in **15.1.** During infancy, the rash can occur over all of the body surface except the diaper area (**15.1A**). It tends to be worse on the cheeks and the extremities, especially the flexural areas. During childhood (**15.1B**), the skin eruptions tend to localize in the flexures, such as the antecubital and popliteal fossae, on the neck, and on the ankles. The flexural eruption can persist through childhood to adulthood, when foot and hand involvement becomes common (**15.1C**).

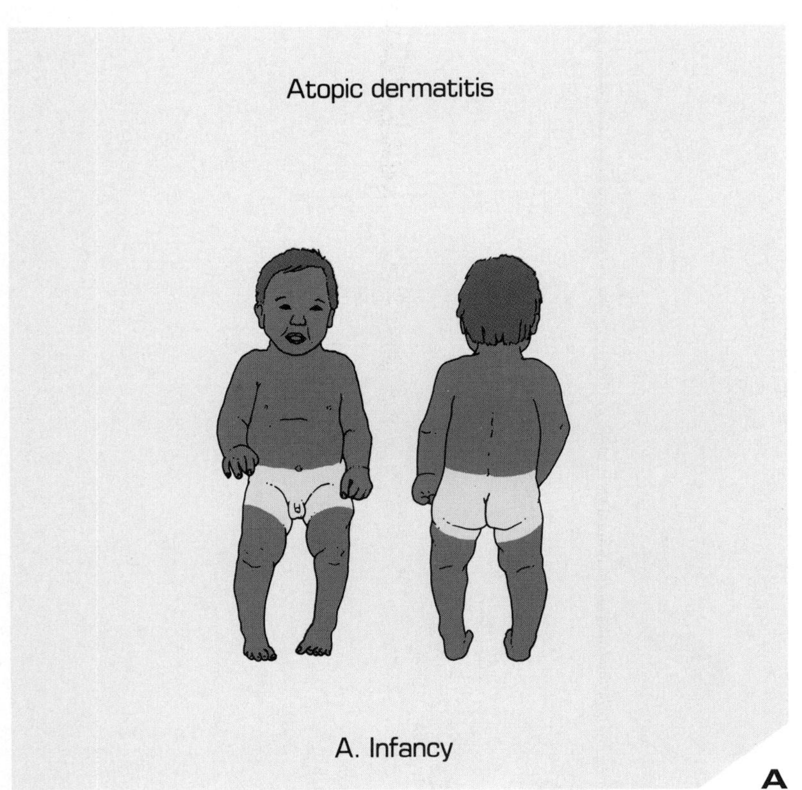

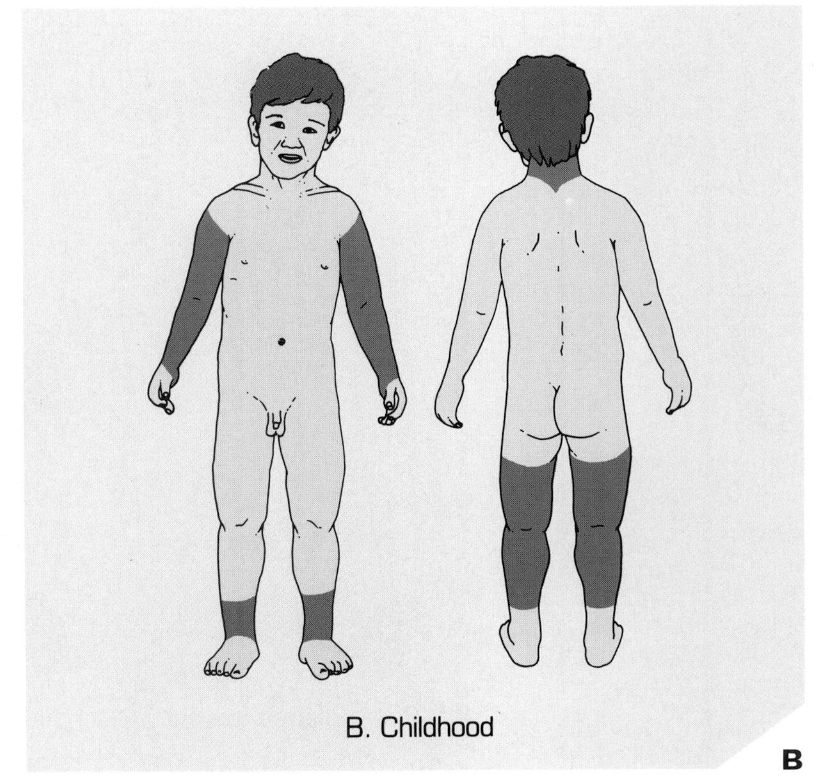

15.1 Characteristic distribution of lesions of atopic dermatitis in infancy, childhood, and adulthood. (A) In infancy, widespread lesions may be generalized, sparing only the diaper area. The head and neck, as well as the flexural and extensor surfaces of the distal extremities, are often severely involved. (B) In older childhood, lesions tend to involve the flexural surfaces of the upper and lower extremities, as well as the neck. With severe flares of disease activity, the rash may become more generalized.

EPIDEMIOLOGY

Although data are not precise, recent surveys reveal that atopic dermatitis is rather common, with an incidence of 7 per 1000 individuals in the United States. The prevalence is highest among children, affecting 3–5% of all children between 6 months and 10 years of age. Although the onset of atopic dermatitis in the first months of life has only rarely been reported, nearly 60% of patients can be expected to have an initial outbreak by their first birthday. Another one-third present between 1–5 years' old. Onset of disease in late adulthood is unusual and should alert the clinician to the possibility of other diagnoses.

In families with a history of allergic rhinitis or asthma, nearly one-third of the children can be expected to develop skin lesions of atopic dermatitis. Inversely, in patients with atopic dermatitis, one-third can be expected to have a personal history of allergic rhinitis or asthma, with two-thirds showing a family history of these disorders. Half of those manifesting the dermatologic condition in infancy or childhood ultimately go on to develop allergic respiratory symptoms later in life. Atopic dermatitis does not appear to be linked to the histocompatibility locus antigen (HLA), as has been described in allergic rhinitis. Rather, it seems to be inherited as an autosomal trait with multi-factorial recessive influences.

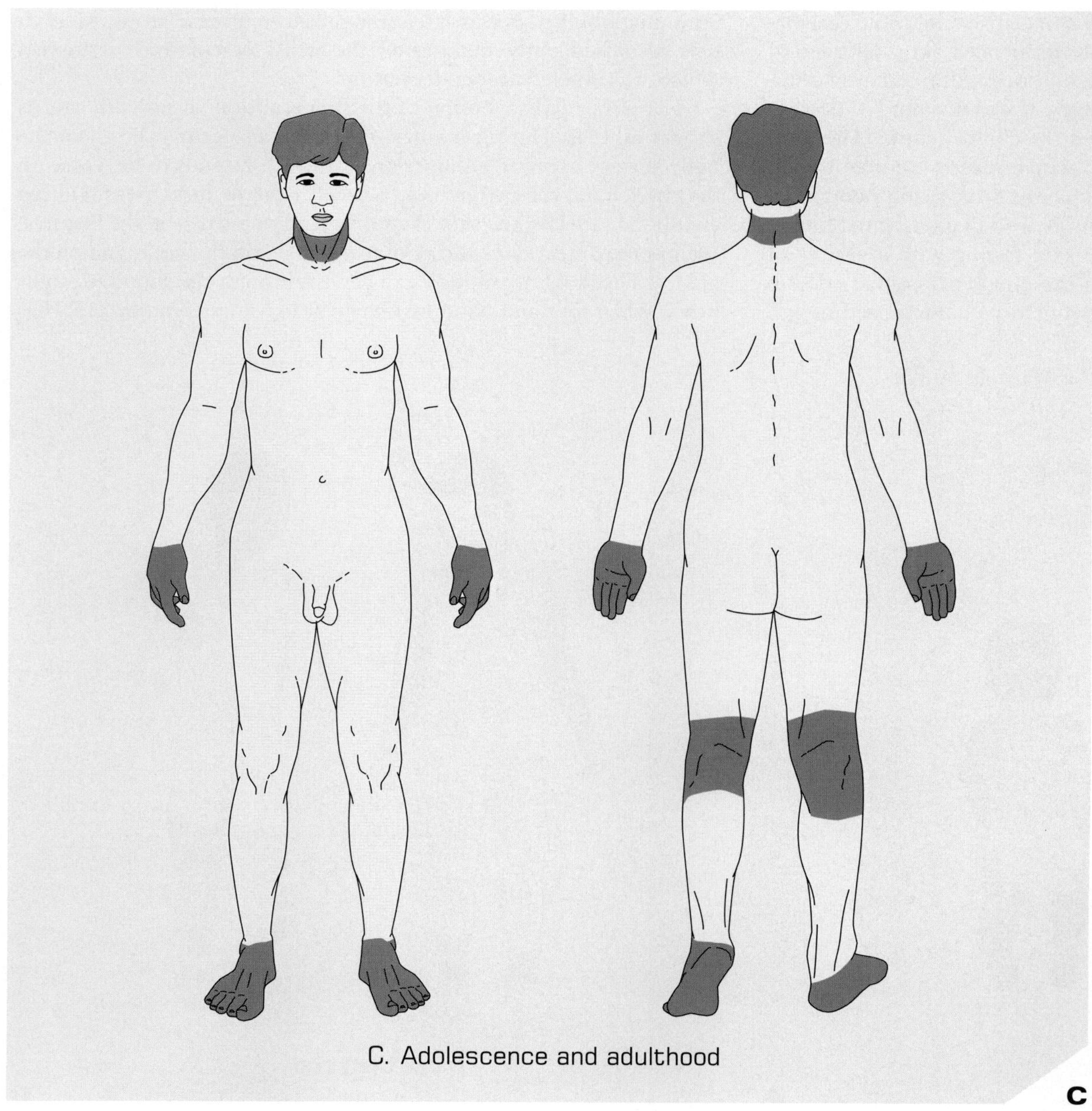

C

15.1 cont. (C) In adults, the lesions are usually restricted to the flexural creases. However, in some patients, involvement of the neck, as well as of the palms and soles, may become particularly prominent.

PATHOGENESIS

Although the precise etiology and pathogenesis of atopic dermatitis are unknown, an immunologic basis, and particularly an allergic mechanism, has been suggested, owing to its frequent association with other atopic and immunologic disorders (**15.2**). A number of factors have been shown to trigger IgE-mediated wheal-and-flare reactions in patients with atopic dermatitis. However, the connection between positive immediate skin reactions and cutaneous disease activity has not been established.

Since the discovery, in 1966, of the IgE class of immunoglobulins and, later, the relationship of IgE antibodies to allergic rhinitis and asthma, several correlations between IgE and atopic dermatitis have been shown. In patients with atopic dermatitis, serum IgE levels are increased three- to four-fold and, occasionally, by as much as ten times the normal value. Levels tend to be highest in patients with concomitant allergic respiratory disease. In many patients, the degree of IgE elevation corresponds to the level of disease activity. Serum levels of IgE may decrease in patients whose skin remains in remission for a year or longer. However, in a small subset of patients with typical atopic dermatitis, IgE serum levels remain normal even during exacerbation of the skin disease.

Up to 80% of patients may also have defects in cell-mediated immunity as manifested clinically by increased susceptibility to viral and fungal infections. Decreased responses in delayed hypersensitivity skin tests to candidal, streptococcal, and trichophyton antigens are common (**15.3**). At some time during the course of disease, patients may demonstrate a relative inability to be sensitized to contact antigens, such as dinitrochlorobenzene. *In vitro* responses of lymphocytes to phytohemagglutinin and concanavalin A may also be reduced. Use of monoclonal antibody markers have permitted the demonstration of decreased numbers of circulating T-cells and a relative increase in the number of T(CD_8) helper cells in some patients with atopic dermatitis. Leukocyte chemotaxis may also be suppressed by increased serum IgE and histamine. Unfortunately, these findings are inconsistent from patient to patient, and may vary even in the same patient over the course of clinical disease.

Histamine has been proposed by many investigators as the primary chemical mediator released in the various pharmacologic and immunologic reactions of atopic dermatitis. It is well-known for its ability, upon intradermal injection, to produce cutaneous pruritus, which is a characteristic finding in atopic dermatitis. Other mediators of inflammation, including prostaglandins, kinins, and neuropeptides, may also be implicated. A number of precipitating factors, including foods, environmental allergens (animal dander, pollen, molds), and bacterial infection, may trigger atopic dermatitis through reactions with specific IgE antibodies or other mechanisms which promote the generation and release

DISEASES ASSOCIATED WITH ATOPIC DERMATITIS

Allergic diseases
Allergic rhinitis
Asthma
Food allergy

Immunodeficiency diseases
Wiskott–Aldrich syndrome
Ataxia telangiectasia
Hyper-IgE syndrome

15.2 Allergic and immunodeficiency diseases associated with atopic dermatitis.

IMMUNOLOGIC ABNORMALITIES ASSOCIATED WITH ATOPIC DERMATITIS

Humoral immunity
Increased immediate hypersensitivity to environmental antigens
Increased serum IgE levels

Cell-mediated immunity
Decreased delayed hypersensitivity skin tests
Decreased T-cells and function
Decreased T-cell proliferation to PHA, Con A
Decreased suppressor–cytotoxic T(CD_8) cells

Leukocyte function
Increased cutaneous viral disease
Decreased leukocyte chemotaxis

15.3 Abnormalities of humoral immunity, cell-mediated immunity, and leukocyte function associated with atopic dermatitis.

of histamine or other inflammatory mediators into cutaneous tissues (**15.4**). A decreased itch threshold promotes excessive rubbing and excoriation which, in concert with the provoked inflammation, results in acute and frequent chronic eczematoid dermatitis.

CLINICAL PRESENTATION

The term eczema, which means 'boil over', is used by many clinicians when referring to infantile atopic dermatitis. However, most dermatologists use the word eczema as a morphologic term to characterize an acute dermatitis which displays erythema, scaling, vesicles, and crusts (**15.5A**). Dermatitis is a general term which incorporates all the clinical findings of an acute inflammation of the skin, as well as chronic inflammatory skin disease. The chronic changes typical of atopic dermatitis include scaling, pigmentary changes, and lichenification, a thickening of the skin with accentuation of normal skin markings (**15.5B**). Although these acute and chronic manifestations are characteristic of atopic dermatitis, they are also seen in a number of other skin disorders.

The distribution and morphology of skin lesions in atopic dermatitis are often diagnostic, and the clinical findings show a characteristic pattern of evolution. In infancy, lesions tend to be widespread, involving the trunk, scalp, face, and flexor, as well

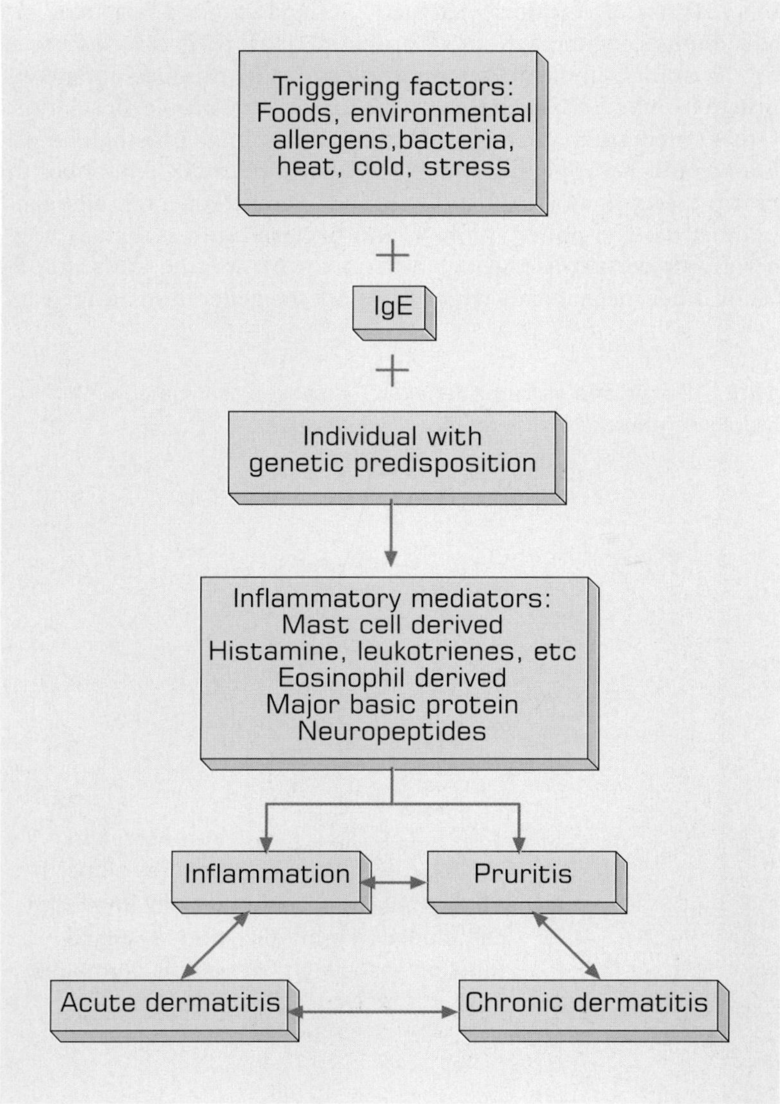

Triggering factors:
Foods, environmental
allergens, bacteria,
heat, cold, stress
+
IgE
+
Individual with
genetic predisposition
Inflammatory mediators:
Mast cell derived
Histamine, leukotrienes, etc
Eosinophil derived
Major basic protein
Neuropeptides
Inflammation
Pruritis
Acute dermatitis
Chronic dermatitis

15.4 Schematic representation of the processes by which external factors, including foods, bacteria, and environmental allergens, trigger the release of cutaneous inflammatory factors, resulting in pruritus and inflammation of the skin of susceptible individuals. Secondary manipulation of the skin (i.e., rubbing and excoriation due to a decreased itch threshold) produces many of the symptoms of acute and chronic dermatitis. Dermatitic changes in the skin result in further pruritus, thus potentiating an escalating cycle of increasing clinical findings, particularly during flare periods.

as extensor surfaces of the extremities (**15.6**). The diaper area is invariably spared, probably because it is protected from drying and from secondary manipulation by the patient. Exposed sites, including the face, scalp, hands, and feet, may present with acute vesicles, crusts, and erythema. The infant is often irritable, sleeps poorly, and scratches or rubs the affected areas incessantly. Growth and development, however, are usually normal.

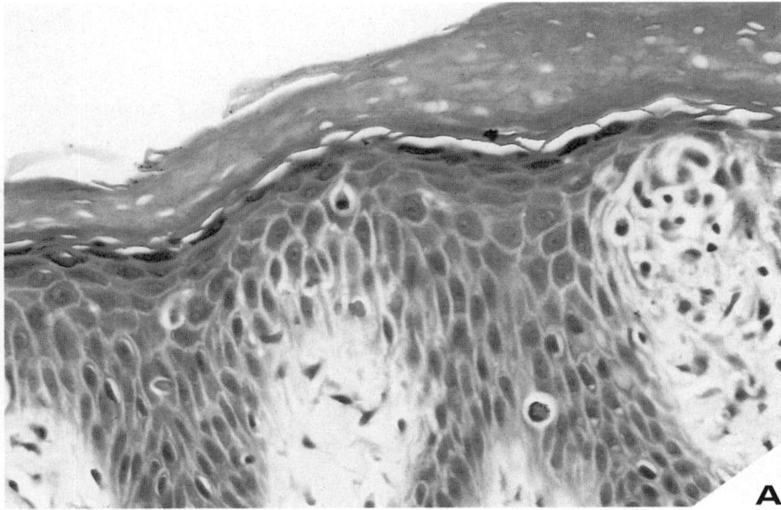

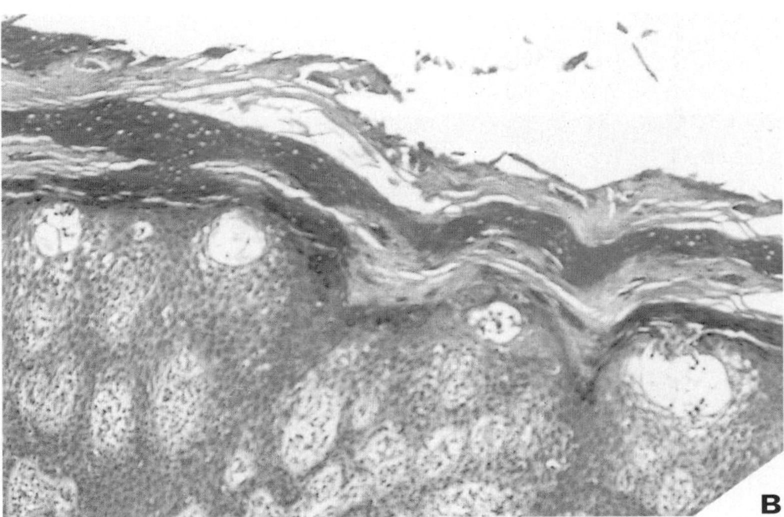

15.5 Histologic differences between acute and chronic dermatitis. (A) Acute dermatitis is characterized by erythema, vesicles, exudates, and crusts. Histologic findings include acanthosis (thickening of the epidermis), spongiosis (intercellular edema), and vesicle formation. (B) Chronic dermatitis is characterized by scaling, pigmentary changes, and lichenification. Histologic findings include marked acanthosis, mild spongiosis, and chronic (lymphohistiocytic) dermal inflammation.

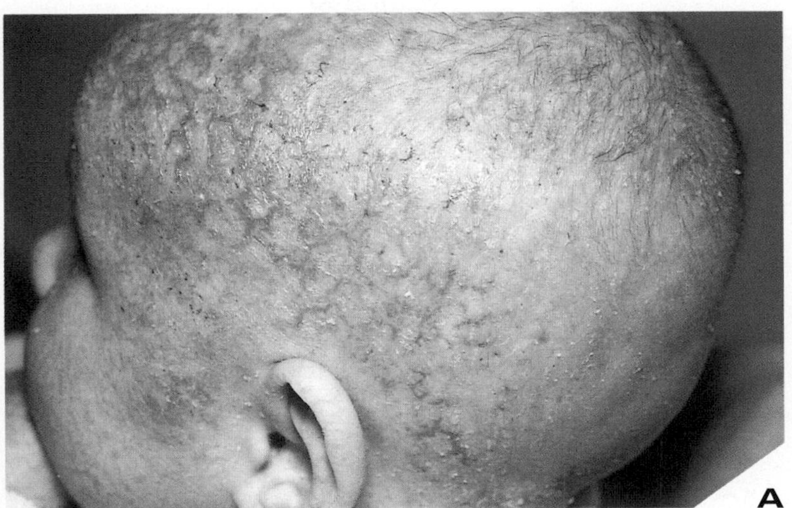

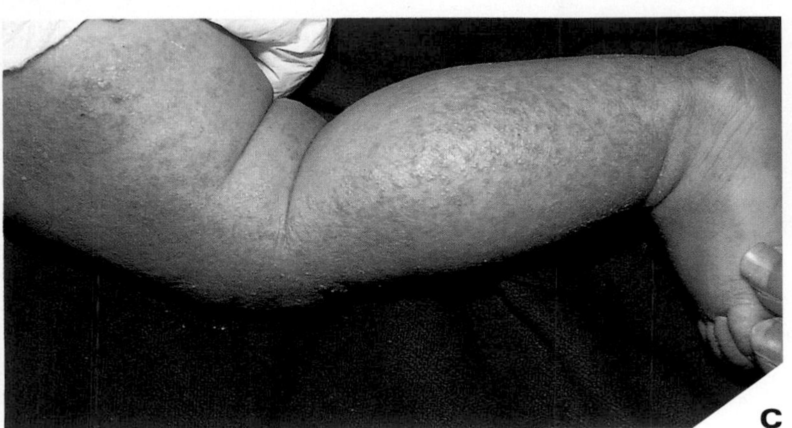

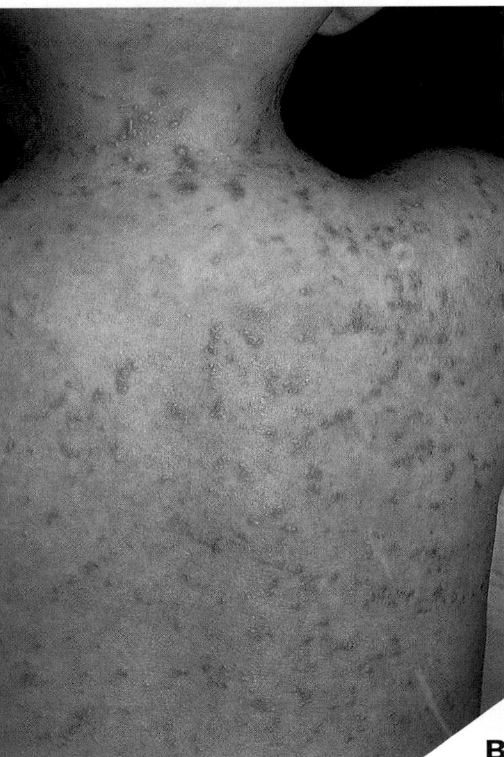

15.6 Atopic dermatitis of infancy, with involvement of (A) the face and scalp, (B) the trunk, and (C) the extremities. Erythema, scaling, and crusting are not restricted to the flexures alone; usually the diaper area is the only portion of the skin surface that is spared.

Although some school-age children present with disseminated skin lesions, in most cases the dermatitis is restricted to the flexural surfaces (15.7). The commonly involved areas include the antecubital and popliteal fossae, with extension above and below these sites. The anterior flexural surfaces of the ankles, neck, and face are also commonly affected. Lichenification, as well as hypo- and hyperpigmentation, may be marked.

While 50% of patients experience spontaneous resolution of the dermatitis at puberty, and the other half markedly improve, a small subset of patients manifest the disease well into adult life. In adolescents and adults, the skin rash tends to be localized to the flexural creases, and chronic hand dermatitis may represent the only manifestation of atopic dermatitis. However, in some patients, widespread disease persists or flares intermittently (15.8).

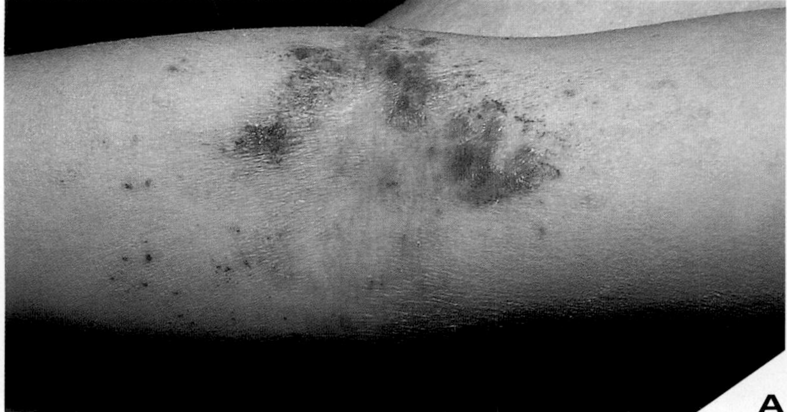

A

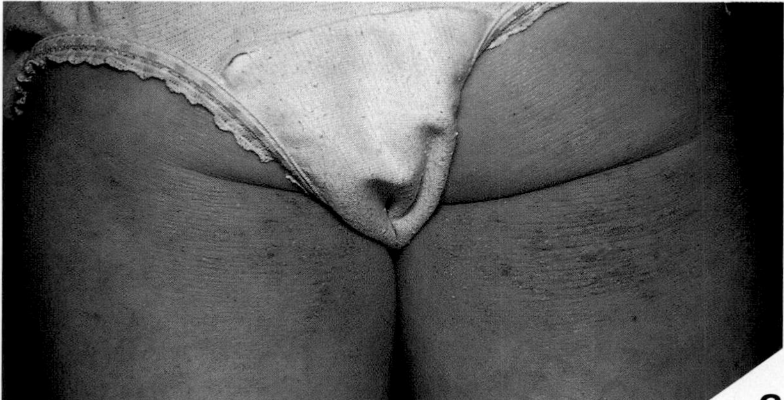

C

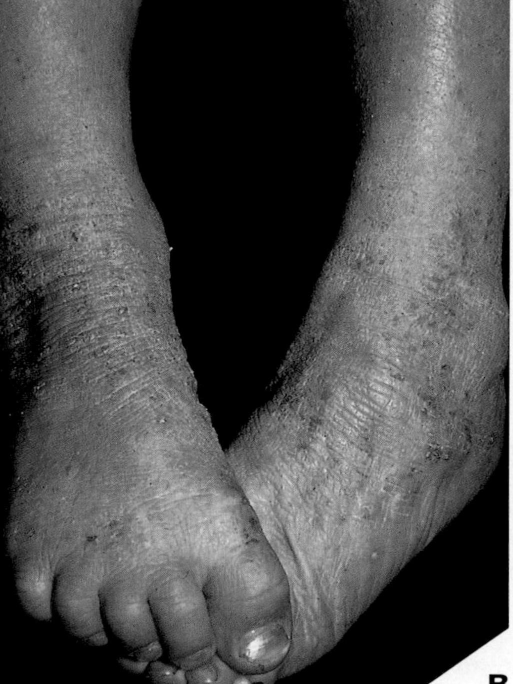

B

15.7 Atopic dermatitis of childhood, with lesions on (A) the arm, (B) the legs, and (C) the creases of the buttocks. In childhood, dermatitis involves the flexural surfaces of the upper and lower extremities. The neck, ankles, wrists, and posterior thighs may be severely affected.

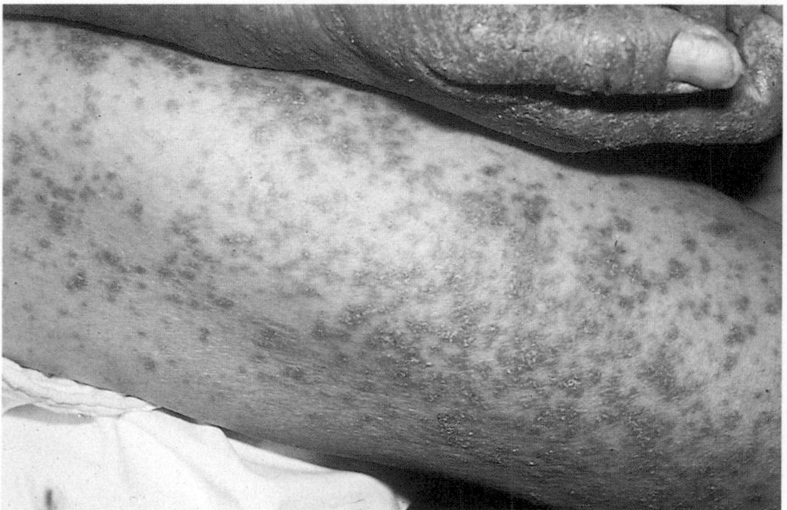

15.8 Hand dermatitis. Chronic hand dermatitis, with persistent scaling and lichenification, may be the only manifestation of atopic dermatitis in older children and adults. However, severe, widespread, and acute dermatitis may erupt occasionally, as in this 50-year-old man.

ASSOCIATED CLINICAL FINDINGS

NUMMULAR ECZEMATOUS DERMATITIS

Although this disorder is distinct from atopic dermatitis, clinicians frequently use the term to describe the discrete, coin-shaped erythematous patches seen on many patients with atopic disease (**15.9**). Lesions typically appear as tiny papules and vesicles, which form confluent patches on the arms and legs. Nummular lesions may be extremely pruritic and are difficult to treat, particularly during the winter months when the incidence seem to reach its peak.

PRURIGO NODULARIS

While chronic rubbing results in lichenification and scratching in linear excoriations, individuals who pick and gouge at their itchy, irritated skin tend to produce markedly thickened papules known as prurigo nodules (**15.10**). Although prurigo nodularis is not specific to atopic dermatitis, many patients with these nodules also have an atopic diathesis, manifesting allergic rhinitis, asthma, or food allergy. Frequently, there are other stigmata of atopic dermatitis as well. These lesions tend to be localized to the extremities, although widespread cutaneous involvement is observed in some cases.

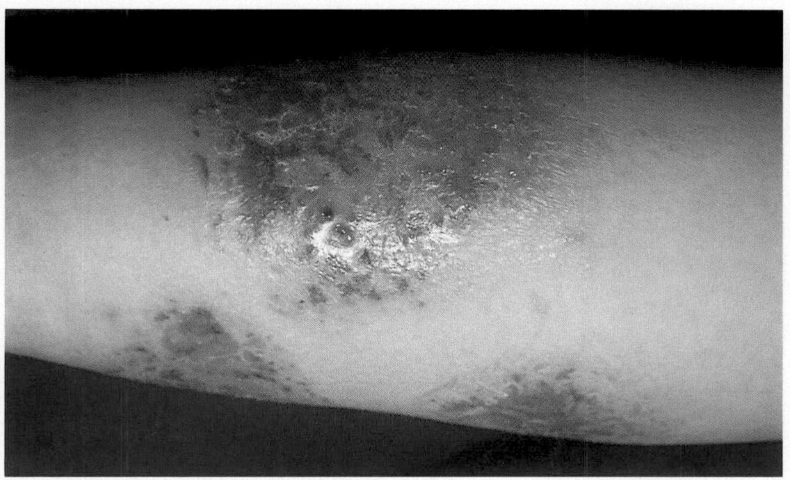

15.9 Nummular eczema. Acute, vesicular, and crusted coin-shaped patches erupt on the extremities of individuals with this disease. The term 'nummular eczema' is also used to describe chronic, circular patches on the extremities and trunks of atopic patients.

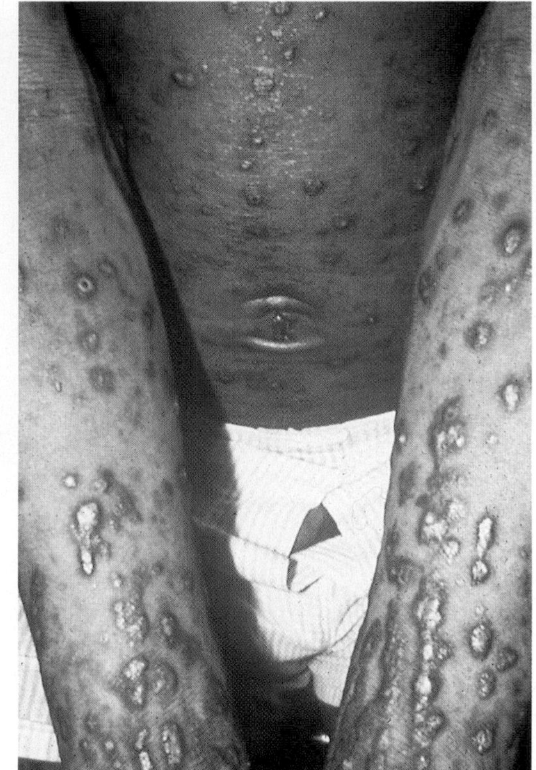

15.10 Prurigo nodularis. Widespread, lichenified nodules involve the trunk and extremities of an adolescent with severe atopic dermatitis. Lesions may be particularly resistant to treatment.

FOLLICULAR ECZEMA

Although a small number of patients with atopic dermatitis initially present with a predominance of follicular papules, virtually all atopics develop these 2–4 mm follicular lesions at some time during their clinical course (**15.11**). Lesions are usually widespread on the trunk, but with careful observation they can also be found on the extremities, particularly during early flares of disease activity. In patients with chronic disease, discrete papules may be obscured by excoriations and lichenification, particularly in the flexural creases.

ICHTHYOSIS VULGARIS

Hyperlinear palms and soles typical of autosomal dominant congenital ichthyosis vulgaris are common findings in patients with atopic dermatitis (**15.12**). Retained polygonal scales are usually evident on the distal lower extremities, but they may also show a generalized distribution on occasion. Keratosis pilaris, characterized by horny follicular papules, may also be noted on the upper arms, medial thigh, and cheeks. This results from localized perifollicular retention of scales. The etiologic connection between congenital ichthyosis and keratosis is unknown.

INFRAORBITAL FOLDS

Often referred to as Dennie's lines or Morgan folds, extra infraorbital folds have been suggested as being indicative of atopy (**15.13**). In many patients, they represent current or past local inflammation produced by persistent scratching and rubbing of these tissues. Although not specific for atopic dermatitis, it may be a useful finding when seen in association with other diagnostic physical signs.

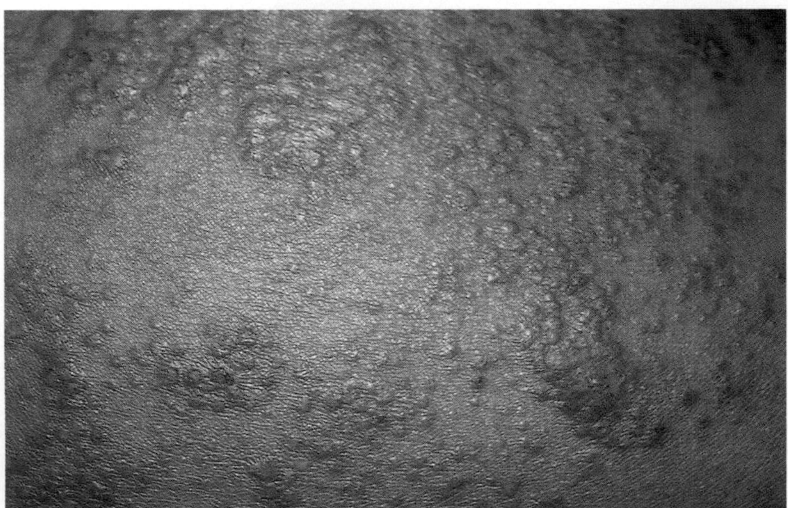

15.11 Follicular eczema. In certain cases, follicular papules may be the only manifestation of atopic dermatitis. These lesions occur in most atopics at some time during the course of their disease, as in this adolescent with follicular eczema on his back.

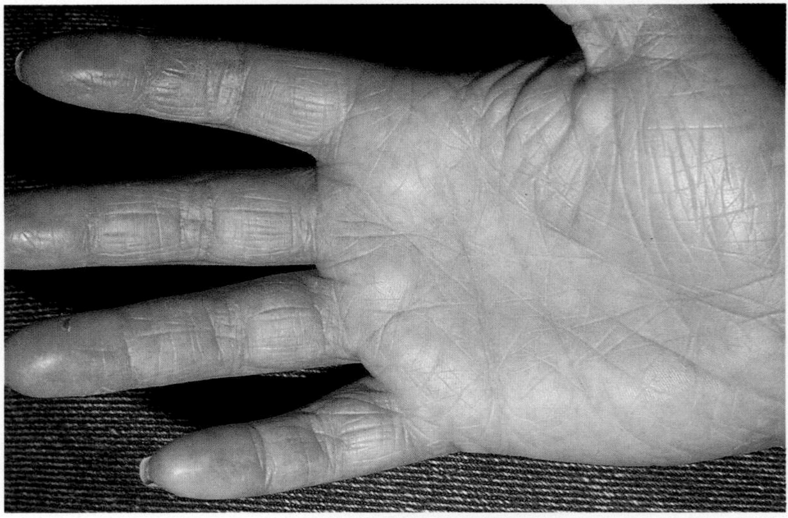

15.12 Ichthyosis vulgaris. Hyperlinearity of the palms and soles was marked in this woman with atopic dermatitis and ichthyosis vulgaris. She had two children with mild atopic dermatitis, showing similar manifestations on the palms and soles, and thick scaling on the anterior surfaces of their lower legs.

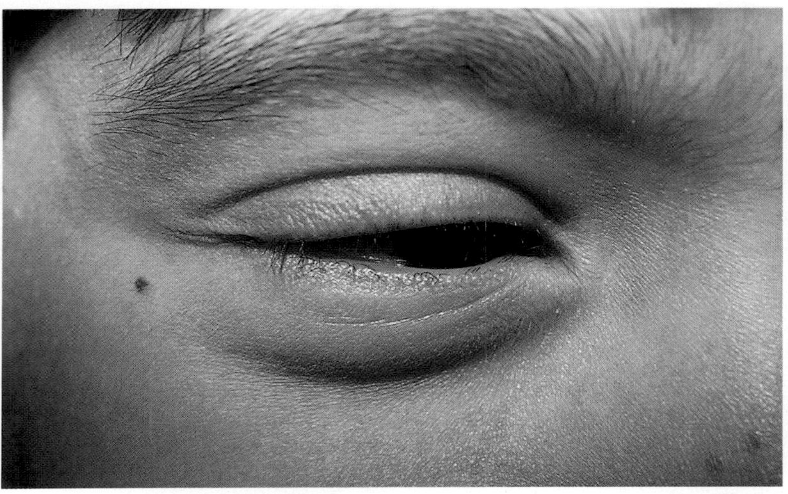

15.13 Edema of the infraorbital folds. Eyelid edema and lichenification due to chronic rubbing resulted in the development of an extraorbital fold. Although not specific to atopic dermatitis, this feature should suggest such a diagnosis when seen in association with other, more pathognomonic findings.

PIGMENTARY CHANGES

Post-inflammatory hyperpigmentation and hypopigmentation occur commonly in atopics, especially in the setting of chronic disease (**15.14A** and **15.14B**). Although pigmentary changes may be quite prominent, this is not always the case; subtle and poorly demarcated areas of hypopigmentation in atopics are referred to as pityriasis alba (**15.15**). Changes are most marked in darkly pigmented individuals or in lighter skinned patients following tanning in the sun. The extremities and face are the most commonly involved areas of the body. Although some post-inflammatory pigmentary changes persist indefinitely, fading of hyperpigmented patches and repigmentation of lightened areas usually occur during prolonged remissions. The pigmentary changes tend to be exacerbated during the flare periods of atopic dermatitis.

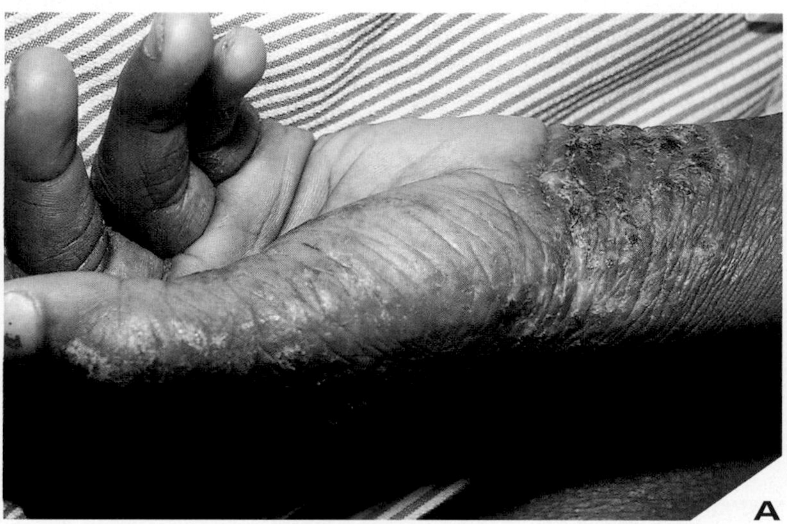

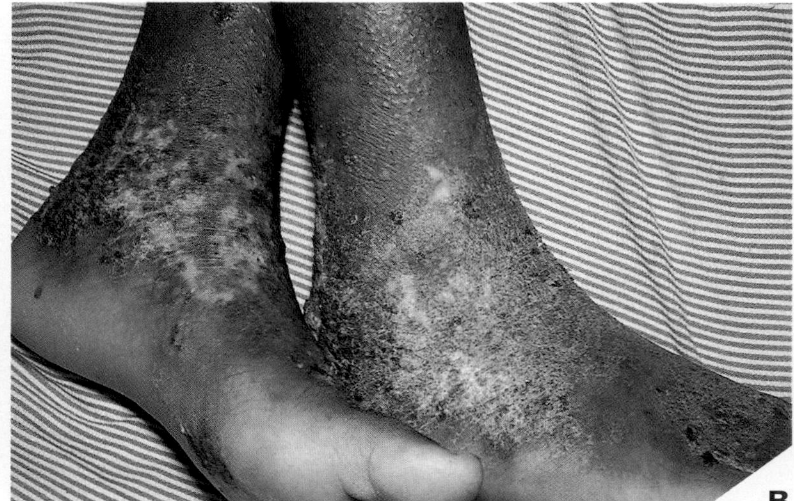

15.14 Post-inflammatory pigmentary changes of atopic dermatitis. Changes in pigmentation are marked on (A) the hands and (B) the feet of this 9-year-old girl with severe, chronic atopic dermatitis. In this child, the pigmentary changes are associated with lichenification and crust formation.

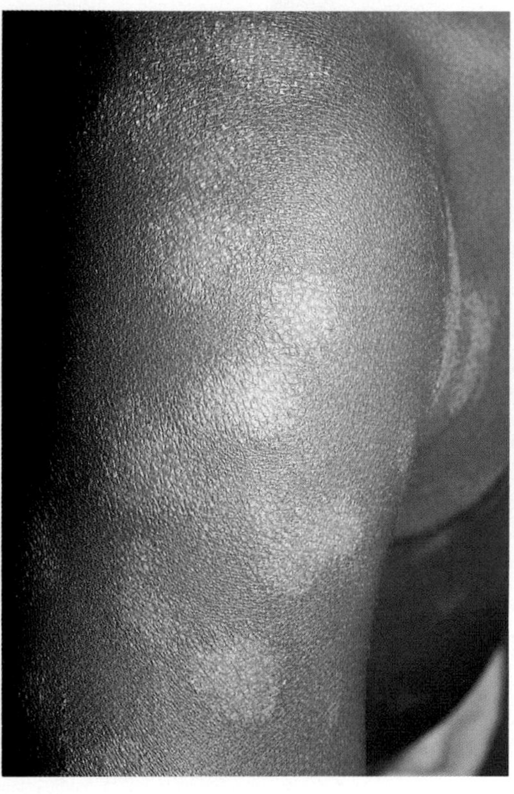

15.15 Pityriasis alba. In some atopics, subtle inflammation may result in poorly demarcated areas of hypopigmentation known as pityriasis alba. Lesions are most prominent in darkly pigmented individuals.

HAND DERMATITIS

Involvement of the hands is common at all ages, and may be the only manifestation of disease in adolescents and adults. The reactions are commonly triggered by contact irritants. Clinical findings include dry, scaly patches on the palms, and frequent fissuring of the palms and fingers. Dyshidrosis, or formation of deep-seated inflammatory vesicles on the palms and along the sides of the fingers, may produce intense pruritus. Involvement of the paronychial skin may result in separation of the nail from the underlying nail bed (onycholysis), as well as in yellowing and pitting of the nail plate (**15.16**).

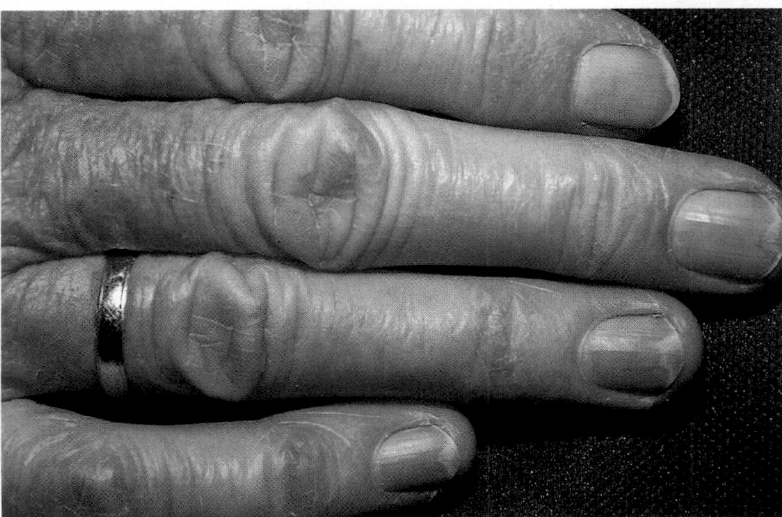

15.16 Nail dystrophy. Nail changes, including onycholysis and pitting, may occur when chronic dermatitis affects the fingertips, as in this 45-year-old woman.

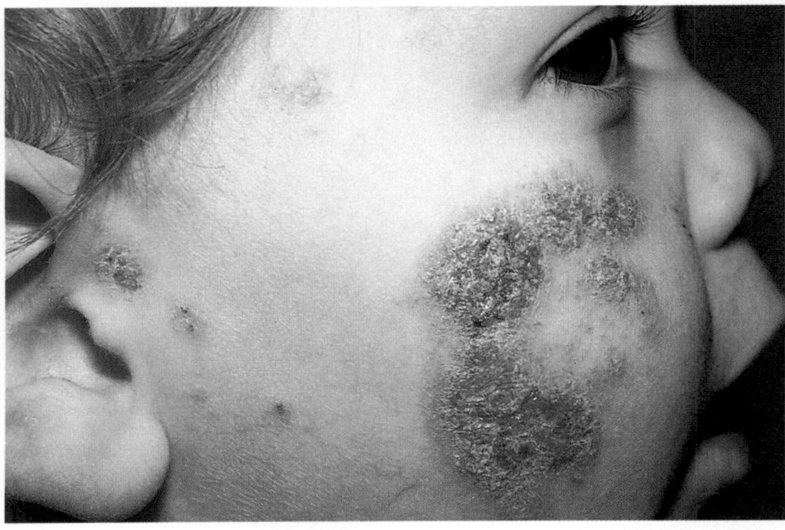

15.17 Impetigo. Honey-coloured crusts on an erythematous base are typical of secondary impetigo in a child with severe eczema. Group A beta-hemolytic *Streptococci* were cultured from the facial crusts.

COMPLICATIONS

Secondary bacterial infection is the most frequent complication of atopic dermatitis. Since it may also trigger an acute exacerbation of clinical disease, early recognition and treatment are mandatory. Crusted, exudative patches should suggest a diagnosis of secondary infection (**15.17**). Although Group A beta-hemolytic *Streptococci* are frequently found in these areas, many investigators have proposed a predominant role for *Staphylococcus aureus*. In contrast to normal individuals, many atopic dermatitis patients show *S. aureus* on the skin even during periods of clinical remission. During flares, cultures from uninvolved skin are frequently positive for this pathogen. Acute onset of bullous lesions should particularly suggest a diagnosis of staphylococcal impetigo. Certain strains of *S. aureus* produce a soluble exotoxin, which may result in a widespread sunburn-like erythema, and denudation and crusting of the skin, referred to as staphylococcal scalded-skin syndrome (SSSS) (**15.18**). This reaction should be considered in any patient, particularly an infant or toddler, who presents with an erythroderma of acute onset. Although defects of cellular immunity are not found consistently among patients with atopic dermatitis, many show evidence of serious or persistent infection with viral or fungal organisms.

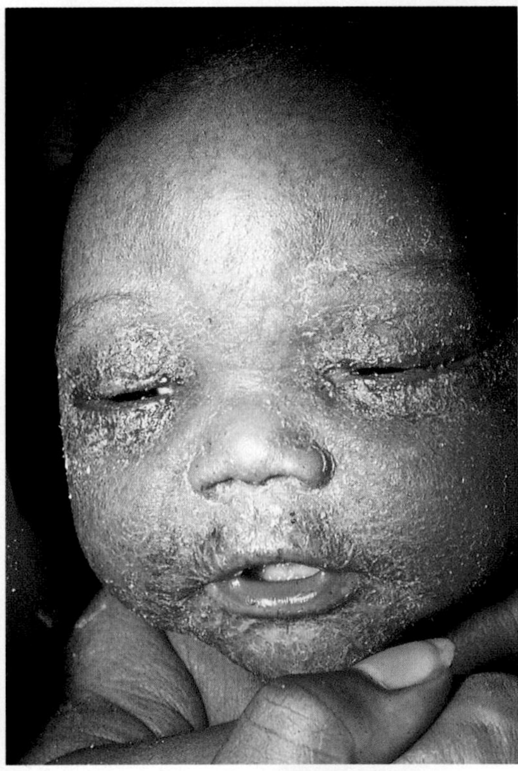

15.18 Staphylococcal scalded-skin syndrome (SSSS). The condition is evident in this infant with generalized red skin, weeping, and crusting around the eyes and mouth. *Staphylococcus aureus* was cultured from the facial crusts.

Herpes simplex may produce devastating cutaneous and, on rare occasions, disseminated visceral disease in patients with atopic dermatitis. The acute development of vesicles or denuded areas, which typically begin in areas of previous dermatitis but can spread to uninvolved areas, should suggest the diagnosis of eczema herpeticum or primary cutaneous *H. simplex* (**15.19A**). Tzanck smears (**15.19B**) and viral cultures confirm the clinical diagnosis, and systemic anti-viral therapy with acyclovir should be started immediately.

A number of other organisms, including the virus that causes molluscum contagiosum (**15.20**), and dermatophytes such as *Trichophyton rubrum*, may produce chronic, recalcitrant infections in atopic patients.

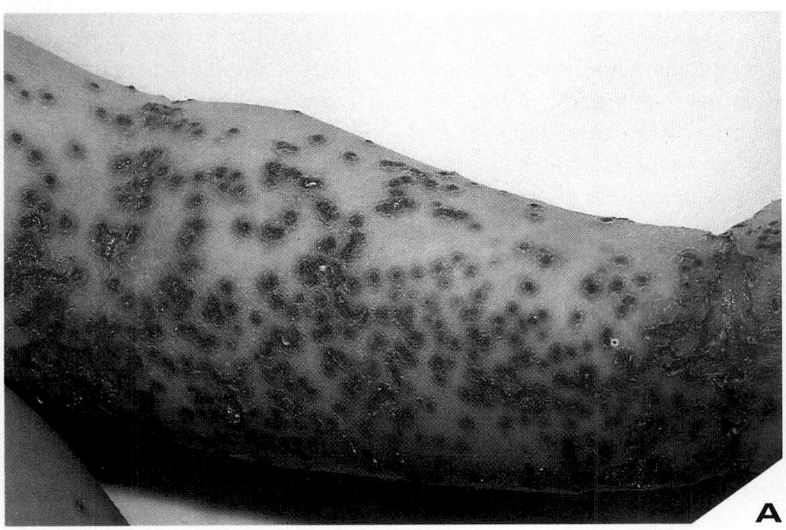

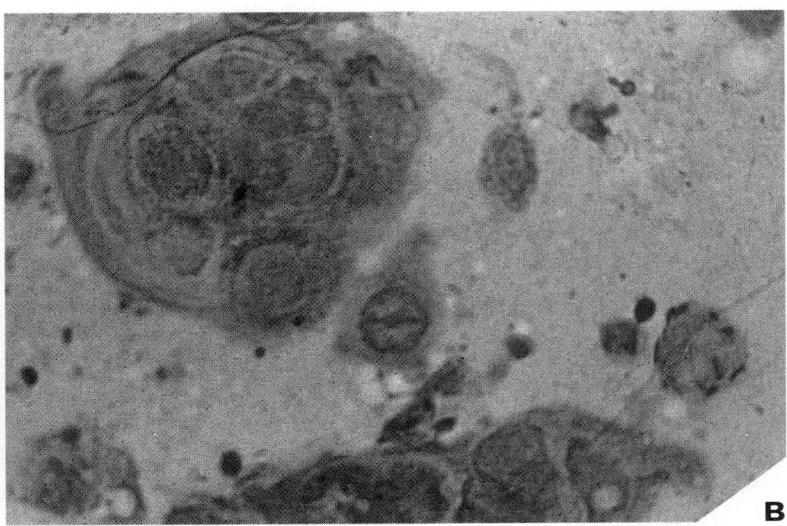

15.19 *Herpes simplex.* (A) Eczema herpeticum, the primary cutaneous manifestation of *H. simplex* in an atopic, spread rapidly over the trunk and extremities of this 10-month-old girl. (B) A Tzanck smear from an intact vesicle demonstrated multinucleated giant cells typical of *H.*. The giant cell is surrounded by acantholytic epidermal cells. This finding is specific for blisters caused by *H. simplex* and *Varicella zoster* infections. However, these two blistering viral eruptions can only be differentiated from one another by viral culture.

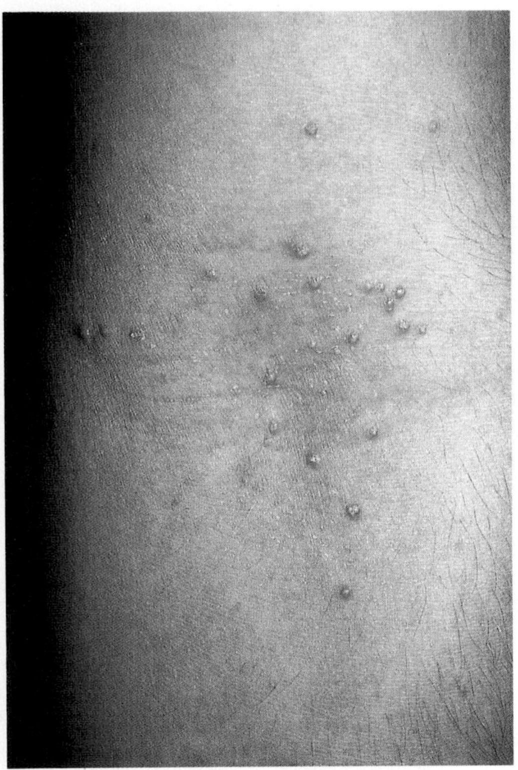

15.20 Mulloscum contagiosum. Typical umbilicated papules of molluscum contagiosum are seen on the arm of a young atopic. The virus producing these lesions may be recalcitrant to treatment in individuals with atopic dermatitis.

DIAGNOSIS

Many atopic patients show immediate hypersensitivity to multiple environmental allergens, and allergy testing is indicated in the evaluation of any patient with persistent atopic dermatitis. Evidence for this hypersensitivity includes elevated serum levels of IgE, as well as positive skin tests or serum IgE antibodies directed toward a wide variety of allergen types, including foods, pollens, and molds (*see* Chapter 3). However, some patients with atopic dermatitis have normal levels of IgE, and neither skin tests nor serum RAST tests have been found to correspond consistently with known potentiators of disease activity in individual patients.

DIFFERENTIAL DIAGNOSIS

Atopic dermatitis is a clinical diagnosis – characteristic cutaneous findings in a patient with a family history of atopy should suggest the disorder. To aid in diagnosis, several investigators have proposed a number of primary and secondary criteria (**15.21**).

A number of conditions may mimic the clinical findings of atopic dermatitis. In infancy, seborrheic dermatitis typically begins with an angry, scaly dermatitis in the inguinal creases. Lesions may spread to the entire diaper area, axillae, neck, and flexures of the arms and legs (**15.22**). The eruption is typically associated with a scaly scalp dermatitis (cradle cap) and retroauricular maceration. Unlike atopic dermatitis, onset of lesions is frequent during the first month of life, and there is little or no pruritus. Moreover, the diaper area is usually spared in atopic dermatitis. Some infants may demonstrate manifestations of both atopic and seborrheic dermatitis and observation over several months may be required to differentiate these disorders.

An irritant or allergic contact dermatitis must also be differentiated from atopic dermatitis (*see* Chapter 14). In infants, contact eruptions are often restricted to the diaper area (**15.23**). In older

DIAGNOSTIC CRITERIA FOR ATOPIC DERMATITIS

Major criteria (all required for diagnosis)	Common findings (at least two)	Associated findings (at least four)
Pruritus Typical morphology and distribution of rash	Personal or family history of atopy Immediate skin test reactivity White dermographism Anterior subcapsular cataracts	Ichthyosis, xerosis, hyperlinear palms Pityriasis alba Keratosis pilaris Facial pallor, infraorbital darkening Dennie–Morgan folds Keratoconus Hand dermatitis Repeated cutaneous infections

15.21 Diagnostic criteria for atopic dermatitis. This disease is likely when a patient shows both of the major criteria, plus at least two of the common or at least four of the associated findings. (Adapted with permission from Hanifin and Lobitz, 1977.)

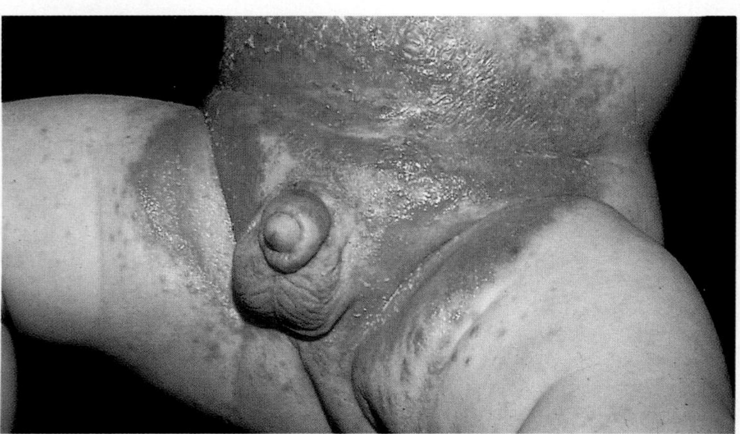

15.22 Seborrheic dermatitis. Red, greasy, scaling patches began in the inguinal creases and spread to involve much of the diaper area in this infant. The rash may become more widespread, with general involvement of the skin creases, as well as the face, scalp, trunk, and extremities. (Reproduced with permission from Mallory and Zitelli, 1987.)

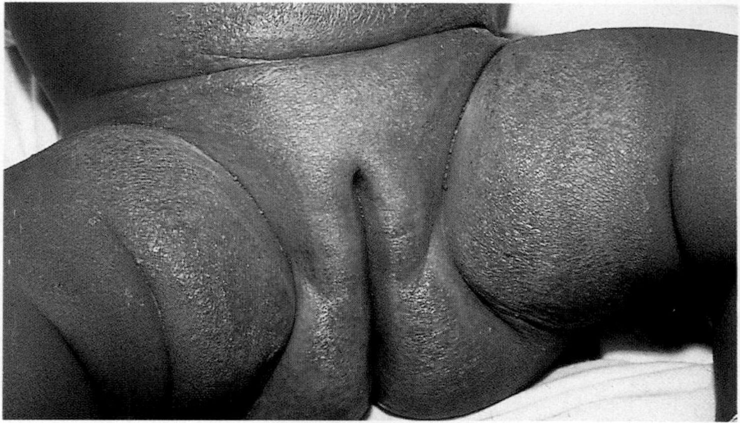

15.23 Irritant dermatitis. Irritant contact dermatitis in infants tends to involve the convex surfaces while sparing the creases, as in this child with red, scaly, diaper dermatitis. (Reproduced with permission from Mallory and Zitelli, 1987.)

children and adults, contact dermatitis typically develops in unusual, asymmetric patterns. Irritants and allergens, however, may exacerbate an underlying atopic rash, and occasional widespread contact eruptions may obscure the differentiation.

Acrally distributed dermatitic eruptions, such as papular acrodermatitis [Gianotti–Crosti syndrome (**15.24A**)] and acrodermatitis enteropathica (**15.24B**) may thwart the clinician. Fortunately, papular acrodermatitis, which is triggered by a number of viral infections, is self-limited and asymptomatic. Acrodermatitis from zinc deficiency may be differentiated by associated symptoms, including hair loss, diarrhea, and irritability. In time, the eruption of acrodermatitis enteropathica may also produce persistent, erosive patches around the mouth, groin, and anal area – manifestations which are unusual in atopic dermatitis.

Psoriasis is a common, pruritic, papulosquamous eruption which may mimic atopic dermatitis, particularly before the psoriatic plaques become fully established. Psoriasis tends to involve the extensor surfaces of the extremities, sacrum, umbilicus, and scalp, and nail pitting is typical. Although lesions may be extremely localized (**15.25A**), widespread plaques (**15.25B**) may also appear.

Scabies may produce a difficult diagnostic dilemma. The eruption tends to appear first in the finger webs, wrists, arm pits, breast, umbilicus, genitals, ankles, and feet (**15.26**). In infants the scalp, palms, and soles may also be involved. The presence of linear burrows in these areas may be diagnostic. However, after several weeks to months of clinical disease, many patients develop a widespread eczematous eruption and lichenification or excoriation may obliterate the primary lesions. Scabies should be considered in any patient with acute onset of severe itching, worse at night, particularly if there is no antecedent history of atopic dermatitis or if the onset of disease is in adolescence or adulthood. A careful history of rash and pruritus in close contacts should also be elicited.

Recently, atopic dermatitis eruptions have been identified in several immunodeficiency syndromes, including Wiskott–Aldrich, ataxia telangectasia, X-linked agammaglobulinemia, and hyper-IgE syndromes (*see* Chapter 17, **17.13**).

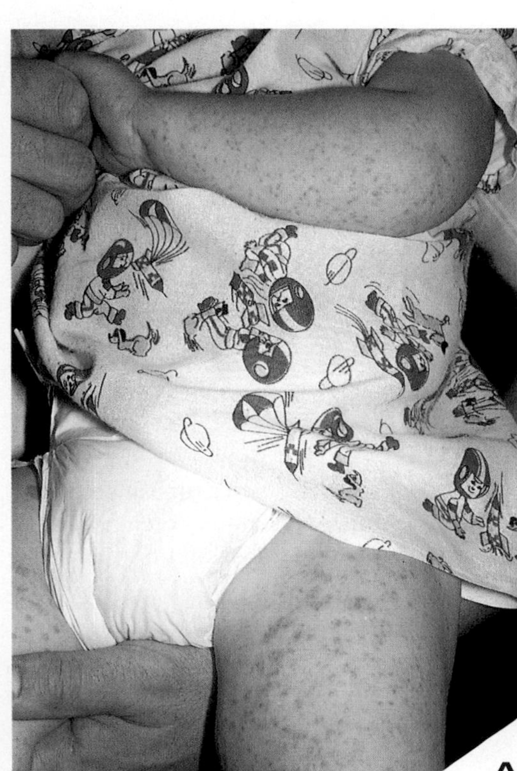

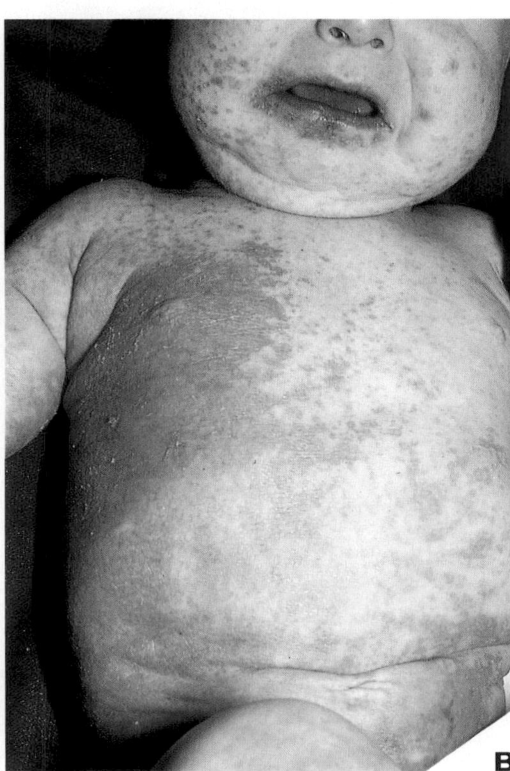

15.24 (A) Papular acrodermatitis. The asymptomatic, edematous, red papules which erupted on the arms and face of this 18-month-old boy were associated with mild upper-respiratory symptoms. The rash resolved in 6 weeks. (B) Acrodermatitis enteropathica. Red, scaly, and erosive patches developed on the hands, feet, face, flanks, and diaper area of this 8 month-old boy, in association with diarrhea, hair loss, and poor growth. All symptoms promptly disappeared with zinc supplementation.

TREATMENT

Therapeutic measures should be individualized depending on the morphology of the skin lesions, distribution of the lesions, and age of the patient. Infants, for instance, may benefit from aggressive efforts directed toward protection of their skin from environmental irritants and excoriating fingers. Loose-fitting cotton clothing with long sleeves and foot coverings may be optional.

Although bathing and the use of soaps was once thought to exacerbate atopic dermatitis, increasing evidence contradicts this view. Daily baths in the summer and on alternating days in the winter, followed by liberal application of lubricants help to cleanse and hydrate the skin. Emollients should be tailored to the patient to increase compliance. In general, greasy, occlusive preparations are safest and most effective. However, some patients may prefer less occlusive agents (**15.27**). Mild soaps may help to reduce bacterial colonization and the risk of secondary infection. Their use should be restricted to areas such as the groin, axilla, and umbilicus where bacteria are most likely to thrive. Ultraviolet light therapy may also be helpful, but should be supervized by a dermatologist or specialist familiar with its application.

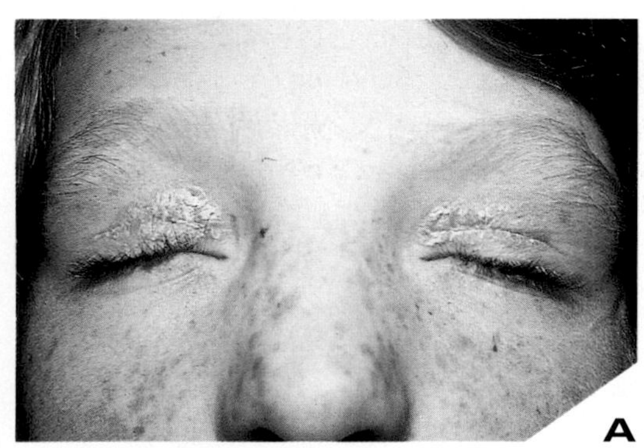

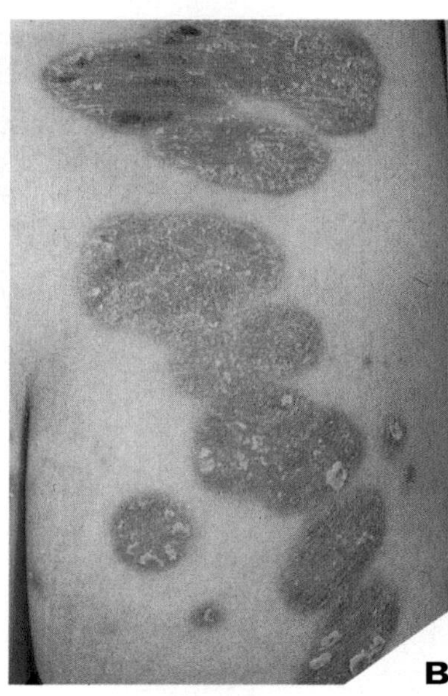

15.25 Psoriasis. (A) Localized psoriatic plaques, such as the eyelid lesions of this 9-year-old boy, may resemble contact dermatitis. (B) Erythematous plaques topped by a silver scale are typical of psoriasis. (B: Reproduced with permission from Mallory and Zitelli.)

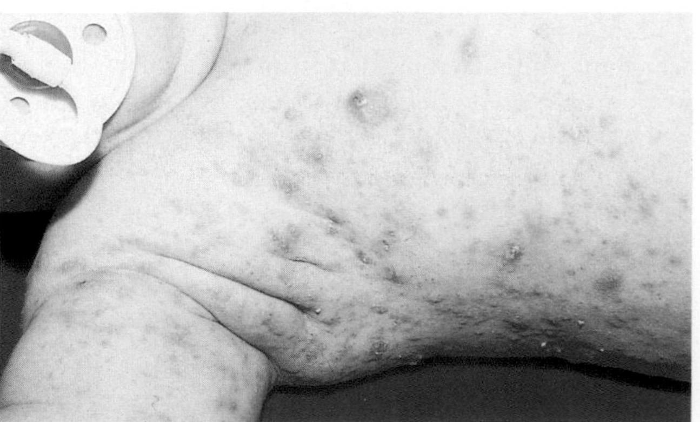

15.26 Scabies. Pruritic, erythematoid papules and vesicles cover the arm and trunk of this infant. The widespread distribution of the lesions, and the associated pruritus and dermatitis, may suggest atopic dermatitis to the unsuspecting clinician. (Reproduced with permission from Mallory and Zitelli, 1987.)

RELATIVE GREASINESS OF COMMON SKIN LUBRICANTS

Lubricant	
Petrolatum	More greasy ↑
Aquaphor® ointment base	
Mineral oil	
Eucerin® cream	
Acid mantle® cream	
Keri® lotion	
Lubriderm® lotion	
Complex 15® phospholipid moisturizing cream and lotion	—
Cetaphil® lotion	
Carmol® 10% lotion	
LactiCare® lotion	
Moisturel® skin lubricant–moisturizer	
Neutraderm® lotion	
Shepard's® skin cream	↓ Less greasy

15.27 Scale of the relative greasiness of many commonly prescribed skin lubricants. (Reproduced with permission from Cohen, 1985.)

STEROIDS

Low- and medium-potency topical steroids are particularly useful during periods of increased disease activity. Twice-daily applications should be restricted to the worst areas of atopic dermatitis, and should be tapered as soon as possible. Practitioners should select a few preparations in the low- and medium-potency categories and explore the availability and cost of these medications in their community (**15.28**). Medium potency agents are useful in open, unoccluded areas, whereas low potency preparations are safer for areas of thin or occluded skin, such as the face, neck, axillae, and groin. High-potency steroids are useful only when intense disease activity is limited to small areas of involvement, such as the hand or foot. Even in this setting, quantities used should be carefully monitored. High potency steroid creams should not be applied to the face. In some patients with self-limited seasonal disease, there may be a place for short courses of systemic corticosteroids.

POTENCY OF TOPICAL STEROID PREPARATIONS

Group	Generic name	Trade name US	Trade name UK	
1	Clobetasol propionate	Temovate® cream 0.05%	Dermovate® cream 0.05%	High potency
	Betamethasone dipropionate	Diprolene® cream 0.05%	—	↑
2	Amcinonide	Cyclocort® ointment 0.1%	—	
	Betamethasone dipropionate	Diprosone® ointment 0.05%	Diprosone® ointment 0.05%	
	Diflorasone diacetate	Florone® ointment 0.05%	—	
	Halcinonide	Halog® cream 0.1%	—	
	Fluocinonide	Lidex® cream 0.05%	Metosyn® cream 0.05%	
	Fluocinonide	Lidex® ointment 0.05%	Metosyn® ointment 0.05%	
	Diflorasone diacetate	Maxiflor® ointment 0.05%	—	
	Desoximethasone	Topicort® cream 0.25%	Steidex® cream 0.25%	
3	Betamethasone dipropionate	Diprosone® cream 0.05%	Diprosone® cream 0.05%	
	Betamethasone benzoate	Benisone® gel 0.025%	—	
	Betamethasone valerate	Valisone® ointment 0.1%	Betnovate® ointment 0.1%	
4	Triamcinolone acetonide	Aristocort® ointment 0.1%	Adcortyl® ointment 0.1%	
	Flurandrenolide	Cordran® ointment 0.05%	—	
	Triamcinolone acetonide	Kenalog® ointment 0.1%	—	
	Fluocinolone acetonide	Synalar® cream 0.025%	Synalar® cream 0.025%	
5	Triamcinolone acetonide	Aristocort® cream 0.1%	Adcortyl® cream 0.1%	
	Flurandrenolide	Cordran® SP cream 0.05%	—	
	Fluocinolone acetonide	Fluonid® cream 0.01%	—	
	Triamcinolone acetonide	Kenalog® cream 0.1%	Ledercort® cream 0.1%	
	Fluocinolone acetonide	Synalar® cream 0.01%	—	
	Betamethasone valerate	Vasilone® cream 0.1%	Betnovate® cream 0.1%	
	Hydrocortisone valerate	Westcort® cream 0.2%	—	
6	Hydrocortisone 1%, urea 10%	Alphaderm® cream 1%	Alphaderm® cream 1%	
	Flumethasone pivalate	Locorten® cream 0.03%	—	
	Desonide	Tridesilon® cream 0.05%	—	
7	Hydrocortisone 1%	Hytone® cream 1%	Hydrocortisyl® cream 1%	
	Hydrocortisone 1%	Hytone® ointment 1%	Hydrocortisyl® ointment 1%	
	Dexamethasone	Hexadrol® cream 0.04%	—	
	Methylprednisolone acetate	Medrol® ointment 0.25%	—	
	Prednisolone	Meti-Derm® cream 0.5%	—	↓
8	Hydrocortisone 0.5%	Cortaid® cream	Efcortelan® cream	Low potency

15.28 Potency ratings for the available topical steroids. (Modified from Cohen, 1985.)

ANTIHISTAMINES

Where eczema is severe, antihistamines may help to relieve pruritus. It has been suggested that the classic first-generation antihistamines are beneficial because of their sedative effect. Consequently, antihistamines such as diphenhydramine (Benadryl®) may be better tolerated if administered at bedtime. The newer, second generation, non-sedating antihistamines, such as astemizole, ceterizine, loratidine, and terfenadine, are also effective in many patients (*see* Chapter 9, Allergic Rhinitis, for a discussion of antihistamine therapy). Although they may be taken throughout the day, tachyphylaxis to a given antihistamine may develop after prolonged therapy, and it may be necessary to change the class of antihistamine prescribed.

ANTIBIOTICS

Secondary bacterial infections are frequently associated with exacerbation, and may cause an acute flare of atopic dermatitis. This complication should initiate prompt intervention. Oral antibiotics, such as erythromycin or, alternatively, cephalosporins and semisynthetic penicillins, are indicated when infection is evident. If the infection is widespread, parenteral antibiotics may be necessary. Localized patches of infection may be managed with topical antibiotics, such as bacitracin and mupirocin. Appropriate cultures should be obtained in severe or disseminated infections prior to the initiation of antibiotic therapy.

During acute flares with vesicle and crust formation, applications of warm water compresses three times a day for 15–20 minutes, topical lubricants, such as Eucerin®, and oral antibiotics should result in rapid improvement of impetiginized areas. In chronic disease, liberal use of emollients, judicious use of low- and medium-potency topical steroids twice daily, antihistamines, and avoidance of environmental irritants and allergens may bring symptomatic relief.

While it is important to try to control the itch, a child with atopic dermatitis should not be placed in physical restraints, and the older patient should not be burdened by psychosocial constraints. Most patients with chronic atopic dermatitis are troubled by the effect of the rash on their physical appearance. Therefore, emotional support and psychological counseling may be helpful adjuncts in the care of these patients.

REFERENCES

Cohen BA: Common dermatoses of childhood. *American Family Physician*, **32**(4): 186–203, 1985.

Hanifin JM: Basic and clinical aspects of atopic dermatitis: a review. *Ann Allergy*, **52**:368–375, 1984.

Hanifin JM: Atopic dermatitis. *J Am Acad Dermatol*, **6**:1–13, 1982

Hanifin JM, Lobitz WC: New concepts of atopic dermatitis. *Arch Dermatol*, **113**:663, 1977.

Krafchik B: Eczematous dermatitis, in Schachner LA, Hansen RC: *Pediatric Dermatology*, Churchill-Livingstone, pp 695–724, 1988.

Leung D, Rhodes R, Geha RS: Atopic dermatitis, in Fitzpatrick TB, Eisen ZA, Wolff K, Freedburg IM, Austen KF (eds): *Dermatology in General Medicine*, McGraw-Hill, New York, pp 1385–1408, 1987.

Mallory SB, Zitelli BJ: Pediatric dermatology, in Zitelli BJ, Davis HW (eds): *Atlas of Pediatric Physical Diagnosis*, Gower, London, pp 8.1–8.27, 1987.

Sampson HA: Pathogenesis of eczema. *Clin Exp Allergy*, **20**:459–467, 1990.

CHAPTER 16

Urticaria and Angioedema

Michael D. Tharp
Macy I. Levine
Philip Fireman

INTRODUCTION

Urticaria, commonly called hives, is characterized by pale or erythematous localized swellings of the skin, without surface scaling, which vary in size and shape. Sometimes surrounded by a red halo, these lesions can coalesce, and are always associated with itching. Angioedema, also known as giant urticaria, is manifested by a more generalized swelling of the skin, due to deep dermal and subcutaneous edema. Thus, these lesions have poorly defined borders and often retain normal skin color. Angioedema commonly affects the eyelids, lips, tongue, genitalia, hands, feet, and, rarely, the larynx, gastrointestinal tract, or urinary bladder.

Urticaria and angioedema are very common conditions in the general population, occurring in up to 20–25% of all people at some time during their lives. In one study of a large number of patients, 49% had both conditions, 40% had urticaria alone, and 11% had angioedema alone. These conditions may be classified as acute, which includes symptoms lasting up to 6 weeks, and chronic, which includes the presence of hives or angioedema occurring on most days for longer than 6 weeks. They are discussed together because, in general, they have similar causes and treatment.

Frequently, patients with urticaria or angioedema seek the attention of a physician who specializes in the treatment of allergic or skin diseases. Clinicians must be aware that some primary skin disorders and systemic diseases with cutaneous manifestations may mimic these lesions, and a portion of this chapter is dedicated to the differential diagnosis of these conditions.

EPIDEMIOLOGY

Urticaria and angioedema may arise in all age groups. Acute disease appears to be more common in young adults and children, at times arising from the triggering of cutaneous mast cells through antigen-specific IgE antibodies. The chronic form of urticaria or angioedema occurs much more frequently in adults, particularly in middle-aged females. Available data on the natural history of these cutaneous reactions among large groups of patients indicate that a majority of individuals with urticaria alone are free of lesions after one year, although a few continue to experience their eruption for a number of years. Similarly, approximately one-half of patients with acquired angioedema alone continue to experience the disorder for more than one year. A personal or family history of atopy may be more common in patients with acute urticaria, but this association does not appear to be a factor in patients with chronic urticaria or angioedema.

CLINICAL PRESENTATION

Because they are so common, the lesions of urticaria are often correctly diagnosed by the patient. Classically, this cutaneous eruption appears as round-to-oval, white or erythematous wheals (**16.1**). Surrounding erythema may or may not be present. Lesion size ranges from a few millimeters to several centimeters in diameter (**16.2**). Less commonly, urticarial lesions may assume annular, arcuate, or serpiginous configurations (**16.3**).

The clinical expression of urticarial lesions results primarily from upper dermal inflammation and edema. This appears clinically as:

- Normal skin surface markings (absence of scaling).
- Normal pigmentation.
- Erythema, which is indicative of vasodilatation.

Urticarial lesions are usually pruritic, and generally last less than 24 hours. In contrast to urticaria, angioedema reactions occur deep in the dermis and may involve subcutaneous tissue (**16.4A** and **16.4B**). These lesions appear as large, slightly erythematous areas with normal epidermal surface markings and poorly defined borders. Often these subcutaneous swellings are asymptomatic, but may be slightly painful. Typically, lesions of angioedema are asymmetrical.

ETIOLOGY

Numerous agents have been implicated in the provocation of urticaria or angioedema, and these include: medications, foreign sera, foods, food additives, infections, insect bites and stings, contactants, inhalants, and physical agents (e.g., heat, cold, pressure, vibration, water, light). Recently, a subset of patients with chronic urticaria have been demonstrated to have circulating antibodies to IgE receptors and IgE on the mast cell surface. It is believed that these antibodies are directly responsible for their urticaria. Emotional stress also may exacerbate these reactions. In addition, urticarial reaction patterns have been associated with certain genetic disorders, pregnancy, connective tissue diseases, and neoplasm (**16.5**).

While the origin of acute urticaria can sometimes be detected, an etiologic agent or precipitating cause is often difficult to establish in chronic disease. The association of urticaria with underlying systemic diseases is relatively uncommon, although this cutaneous reaction pattern has been linked to some disorders (**16.6**).

As is true for urticarial reactions, a definitive cause is usually not determined for many of the patients with chronic angioedema. However, hereditary angioedema must be considered in any patient with recurrent lesions, and this disorder is discussed later.

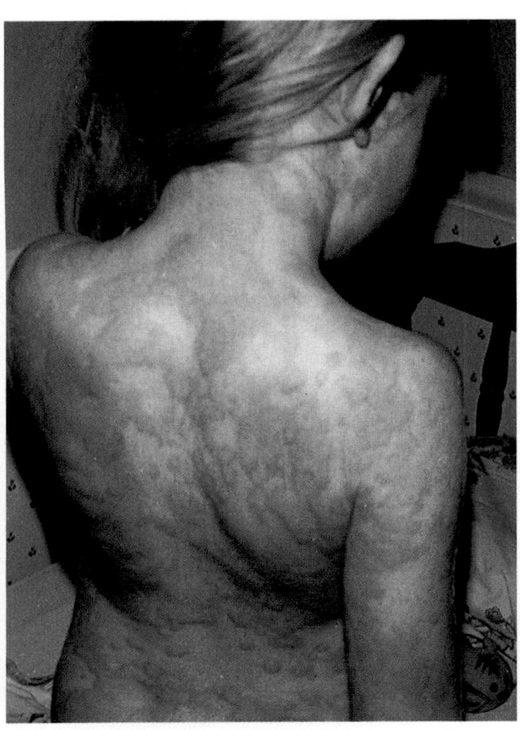

16.1 Urticarial lesions of various sizes ranging from 1 mm to several centimetres in diameter. Individual erythematous lesions may coalesce, as shown in this photograph.

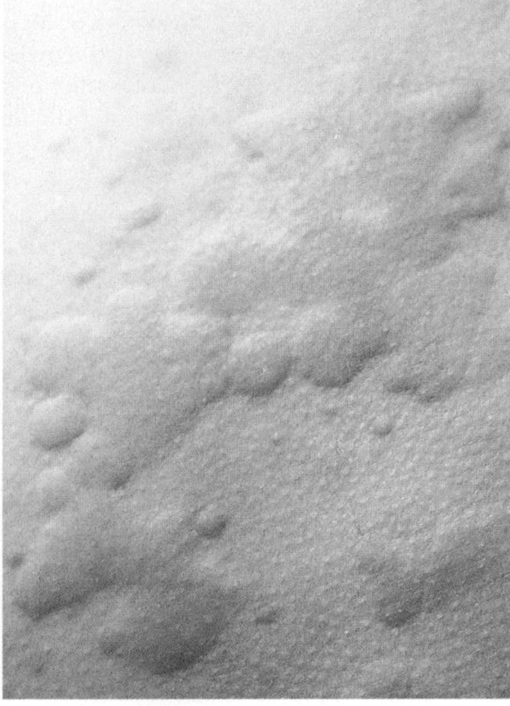

16.2 A close-up photograph of typical urticarial lesions, which may show considerable size variation.

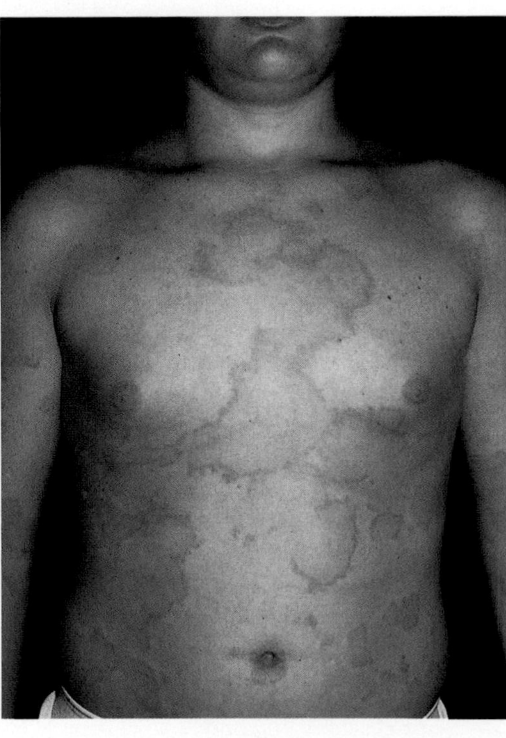

16.3 Chronic urticaria patient with annular lesions on the upper and mid-thorax, and arcuate lesions in the abdominal area. A typical serpiginous lesions is seen in the right upper abdominal quadrant.

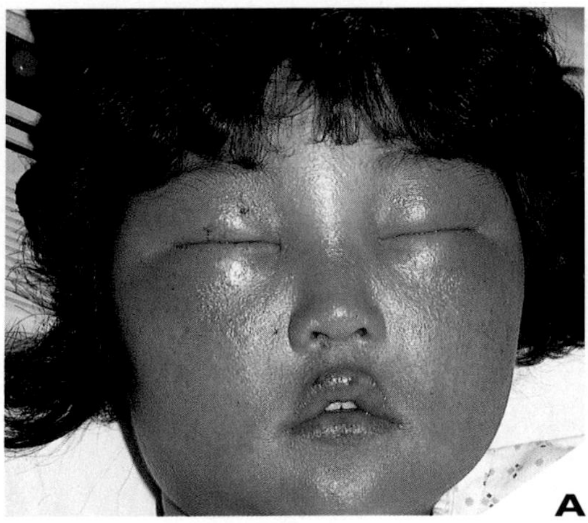

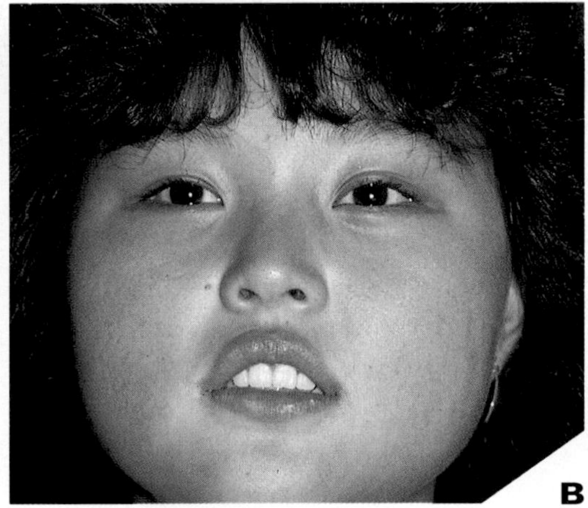

16.4 (A) Angioedema involving the periorbital areas bilaterally due to recurrent allergen exposure. (B) The patient's normal facial appearance following resolution of the reaction.

PATHOLOGY

HISTOLOGIC CHANGES

Classically, cutaneous biopsies of urticarial lesions have revealed surprisingly few histopathologic alterations. Dilatation and engorgement of superficial vessels and lymphatics in association with dermal edema is a prominent feature, and a sparse to moderate perivascular mononuclear infiltrate with few eosinophils is also typically seen (**16.7A**). However, a greater spectrum of histopathologic changes may be observed in lesional skin. Skin biopsy specimens may demonstrate a dense perivascular infiltrate consisting of mononuclear cells, neutrophils, and eosinophils, with no evidence of leukocytoclasis or endothelial cell damage (**16.7B**). Some of the urticaria patients with this histologic pattern have demonstrable circulating antibodies to IgE and IgE receptors on the mast cell surface. Rarely, a true vasculitis can be observed in lesional skin specimens, which is characterized by a neutrophil-rich, perivascular infiltrate associated with leukocytoclasis and fibrin-like deposition around dermal vessels (**16.7C**). Direct immunofluorescence studies demonstrate the presence of immunoglobulins, C_3, and/or fibrin, suggesting the presence of immune complex disease (**16.7D**). While the histopathologic alterations in lesions of angioedema have not been as extensively investigated, vasodilation and edema associated with a mixed cellular infiltrate appear to be common features. In contrast to the superficial dermal changes of urticaria, these alterations are observed primarily in the deep dermis and subcutaneous tissue.

PATHOGENESIS

Numerous clinical and pharmacologic studies suggest a primary role for the tissue mast cell in the expression of urticaria and/or angioedema. Mast-cell stimulation may result from a number of different immune and non-immune-mediated mechanisms, which are listed in **16.8**. One or a combination of these factors may be important in triggering an urticarial reaction. The early vascular changes observed in these cutaneous eruptions can be readily attributed to the release of the preformed mediator, histamine, but may also involve the elaboration of mast cell-derived prostaglandin D_2 (PGD_2) and leukotrienes (LTs). The tissue mast cells may also release several different chemotactic factors [histamine, neutrophil chemotactic factor (NCF), eosinophil chemotactic factors of anaphylaxis (ECF-A), and possibly leukotriene B_4 (LTB_4)] that result in the influx of inflammatory cells to the primary site of mast-cell activation. It is likely that the infiltration of activated leukocytes into the area leads to the release of additional cell-derived inflammatory mediators, resulting in local tissue injury and possibly provoking a second wave of tissue mast-cell activation.

Although, theoretically, this series of events could explain in total the pathogenesis of urticaria and/or angioedema, evidence suggests that the local release of neuropeptides from sensory nerve endings may play a role in the expression of these cutaneous eruptions, especially in patients with chronic disease. A number of different neuropeptides, including substance P (SP), vasoactive intestinal polypeptide (VIP), calcitonin gene-related peptide (CGRP), and neuropeptide Y (NPY), have been identified by immunocytochemical methods in sensory nerves in the dermis. When released in human skin, these substances induce a wheal-and-flare reaction. A model for potential interaction of sensory nerves with dermal mast cells is illustrated in **16.9**. When cutaneous sensory nerves are activated by some stimulus, both orthrodromic (forward) and antidromic (retrograde) action potentials may be generated. These retrograde impulses may subsequently lead to the release of one or more neuropeptides in the dermis.

Taken together, it can be postulated that skin mast-cell mediator release leads to vasodilatation, plasma extravasation, inflammatory-cell chemotaxis, and sensory-nerve stimulation. The subsequent

POTENTIAL CAUSES OF URTICARIAL REACTIONS

1. Foods
2. Medications
3. Sera
4. Infections
5. Insect bites and stings
6. Contactants and inhalants
7. Antibodies to IgE and IgE receptor
8. Physical agents (heat, cold, pressure, vibration, water, and light)
9. Psychological factors (stress)
10. Exercise

16.5 Potential causes of urtical reactions.

SYSTEMIC DISEASES ASSOCIATED WITH URTICARIAL ERUPTIONS

1. Systemic lupus erythematosus
2. Serum sickness, cryoglobulinemia
3. Juvenile rheumatoid arthritis (JRA)
4. Hyperthyroidism, hypothyroidism
5. Neoplasms
6. Mastocytosis

16.6 Systemic diseases associated with urticarial eruptions.

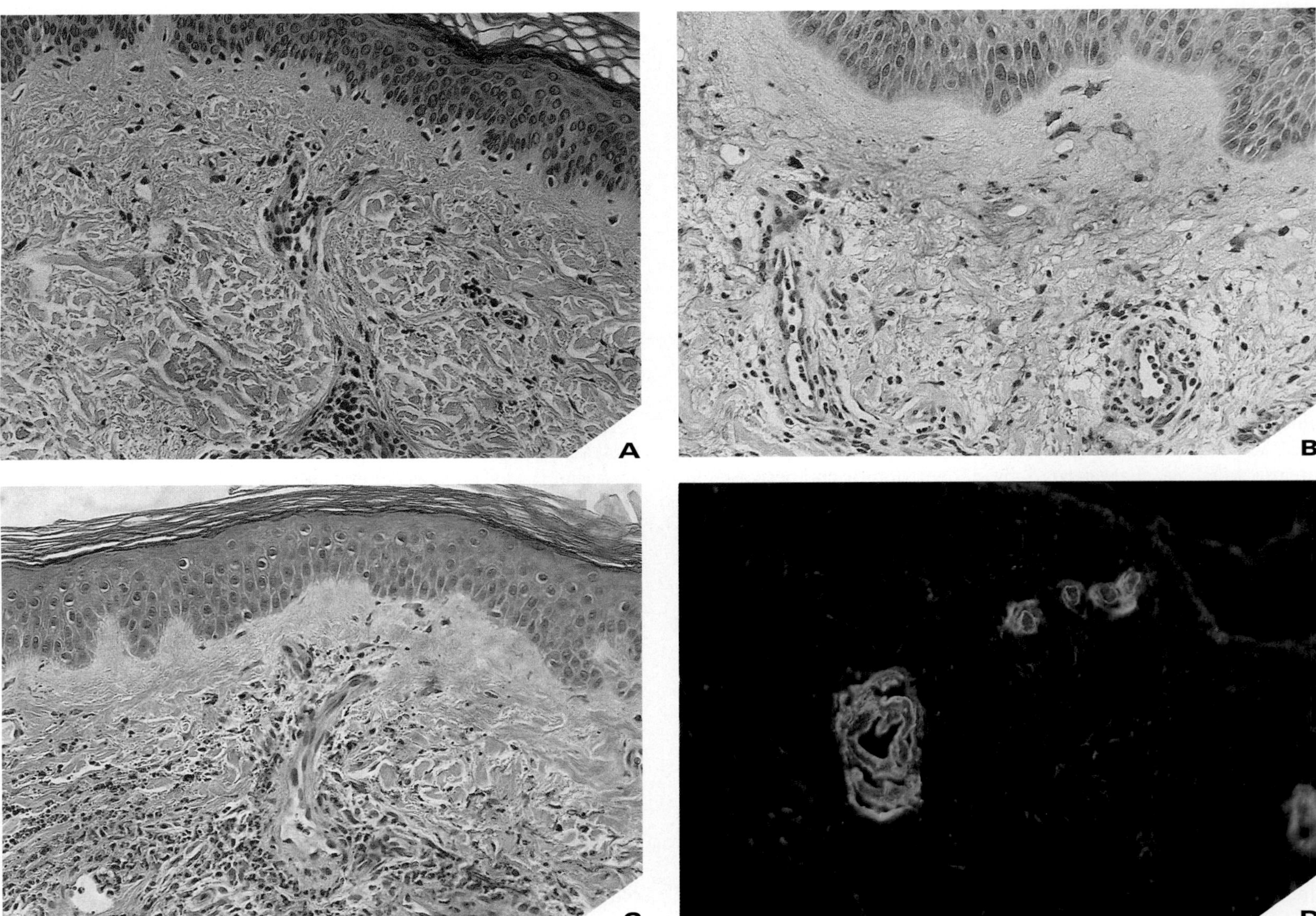

16.7 Photomicrographs of the spectrum of histologic changes in patients with urticarial lesions. (A) Typical urticaria with dermal edema and a sparse perivascular, mononuclear cell infiltrate. (B) Less commonly, one sees the accumulation of dermal plasma cells and the infiltration of neutrophils around vessels, without evidence of vasculitis in the lesional skin of some patients with urticaria. (C) Urticarial vasculitis: intense perivascular neutrophil accumulation, with damage to neutrophils (cytoclasis) and endothelial cells, are characteristic histologic features. (D) Immunofluorescent staining documents the presence of complement (C_3) and immunoglobulin (IgG, IgM) deposition around vessels in early lesions of urticarial vasculitis. This histology has been described by Jones *et al,* 1983.

POTENTIAL MECHANISMS OF MAST-CELL ACTIVATION IN CLINICAL URTICARIA

Immunologic mechanisms

Antigen reaction with specific mast-cell membrane IgE antibody

Complement anaphylatoxin (C_{3a} and C_{5a}) stimulation of specific mast-cell-associated receptors

Eosinophil-derived major basic protein activation of mast cells

Leukocyte-derived histamine releasing factor(s), stimulation of mast cells

Antibodies to IgE and IgE receptors

Non-immunologic factors that stimulate mast cells

Neuropeptides (substance P, calcitonin gene-related peptide, vasoactive intestinal polypeptide, neurokinin Y)

Hormones (gastrin, estrogen, ACTH)

Medications (aspirin, non-steroidal anti-inflammatory agents, codeine, curare, succinylcholine, polymyxin B, thiamine)

Physical stimuli (heat, cold, pressure, light)

Venoms

Radiocontrast media

16.8 Mast cell stimuli.

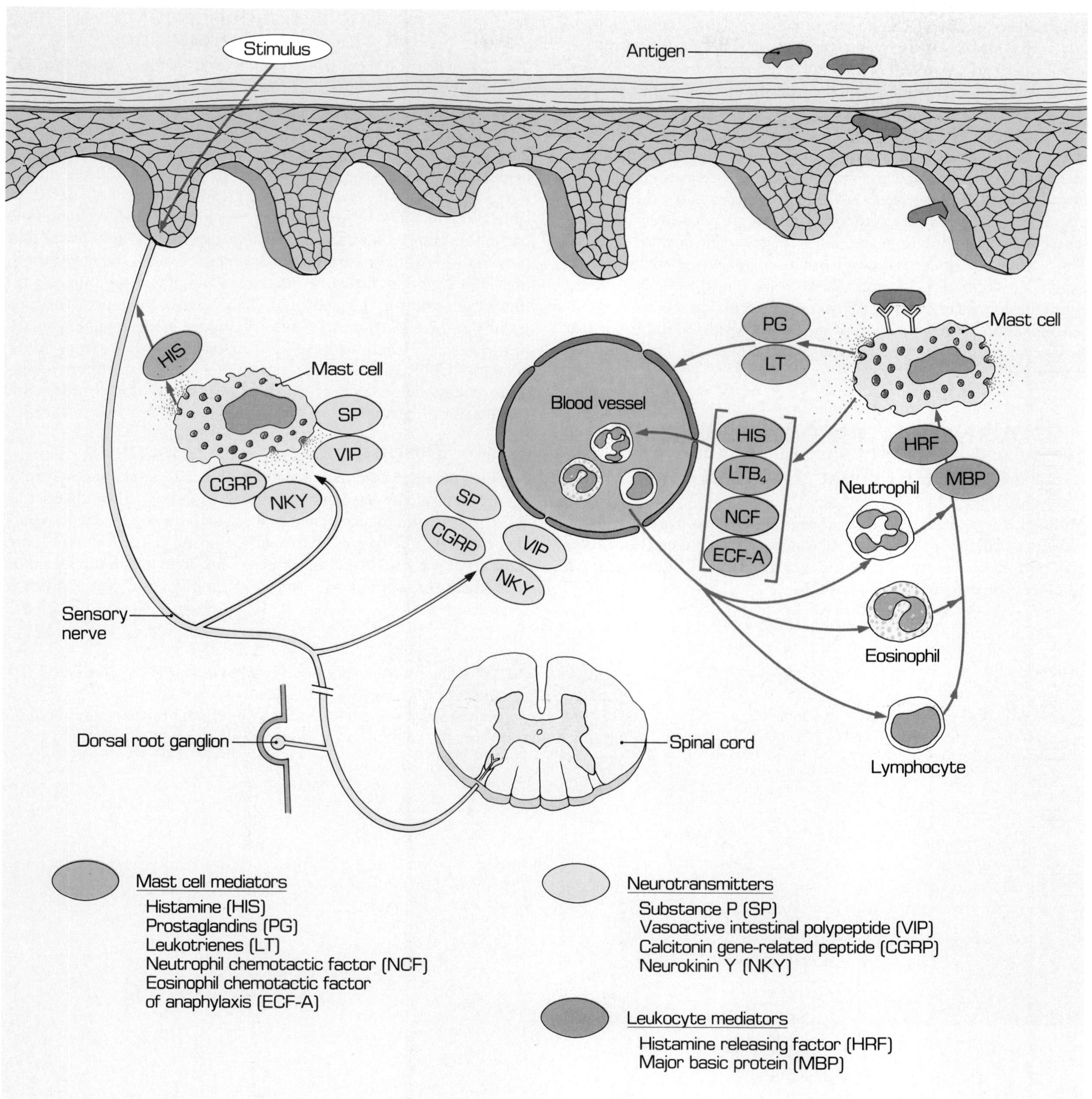

16.9 Pathogenesis of chronic urticaria. Mast cell stimulation and mediator release may be initiated through antigen cross-linking of surface-bound IgE antibodies or by histamine-releasing factors (HRFs) elaborated from leukocytes which have been activated by foreign proteins or other immune stimuli. Mast cell-derived histamine (His), prostaglandin D_2 (PGD_2), and leukotrienes (LTs) all have direct dilating effects on blood vessels, thus provoking dermal edema. These mediators also show chemotactic properties which attract leukocytes into tissues. Mast cell-derived neutrophilic and eosinophilic chemotactic factors (NCF and ECF-A, respectively) also encourage local leukocyte infiltration. Histamine, PGD_2, and possible leukocyte-derived mediators are capable of stimulating sensory nerves in the skin. While orthrodromic neuroimpulses would be expected to transmit signals to the central nervous system via the spinal cord, antidromic or retrograde neurotransmission is also theoretically possible, and these impulses may lead to the release of neuropeptides in the skin. Neuropeptides such as substance P (SP), calcitonin gene-related peptide (CGRP), vasoactive intestinal polypeptide (VIP) and neurokinin Y (NKY) are capable of causing additional vasodilation and possibly mast cell degranulation.

generation of antidromic and sensory nerve potentials could, in turn, lead to the local release of neuropeptides, which also induce vasodilatation and edema formation by their direct effects on endothelial cells, as well as cause additional mast-cell stimulation. Ultimately, the number and type of infiltrating leukocytes may dictate the severity and duration of the inflammatory reaction. Because leukocytes are known to stimulate mast-cell-mediator release, it is conceivable that these cells may perpetuate the initial reaction. Furthermore, the elaboration of leukocyte-derived lysosomal enzymes and other inflammatory mediators in the local environment may lead to additional sensory-nerve stimulation and subsequent neuropeptide release. Thus, from our understanding to date, it appears that the clinical expression of urticaria or angioedema results from a combination of pathophysiologic events. To varying degrees, this may include mast-cell activation, the elaboration of mediators, the local release of sensory-nerve peptide, and the infiltration of different groups of inflammatory cells.

DIAGNOSIS AND EVALUATION

DIFFERENTIAL DIAGNOSIS

Although the lesions of urticaria and angioedema are often easily recognized, there are instances in which other cutaneous disorders may mimic these eruptions. In these cases, careful consideration of all diagnostic possibilities is essential.

Pruritic urticarial papules and plaques of pregnancy

The term pruritic urticarial papules and plaques of pregnancy (PUPPP) refers to an intense pruritic eruption that is occasionally observed in pregnant women. Characteristically, patients with this disorder develop erythematous, urticarial plaques and papules during the last trimester of pregnancy (**16.10**). Classically, these lesions begin centrally over the abdomen and extend to involve the thighs, buttocks, and distal extremities. The facial area is usually spared. In some patients only the lower extremities are involved. Although the pathophysiologic mechanism for this disorder is unknown, skin biopsies of lesional tissue show histologic changes similar to those observed in other urticarial reactions and, therefore, suggest an important role for the mast cell. The maternal cutaneous lesions usually resolve shortly after delivery and no associated abnormalities or adverse reactions have been reported in infants from mothers with PUPPP. Patients who develop PUPPP with their initial pregnancy are not necessarily at risk for recurrence of this disorder with subsequent pregnancies.

Idiopathic urticarial vasculitis

Another disorder that may present with urticaria-like lesions is the syndrome called idiopathic urticarial vasculitis. This disorder is more prevalent in women than in men, and is associated with recurrent urticaria-like lesions. The hands, elbows, ankles, and knees are most frequently involved, and the patient often experiences pain or tenderness of cutaneous lesions in conjunction with pruritus

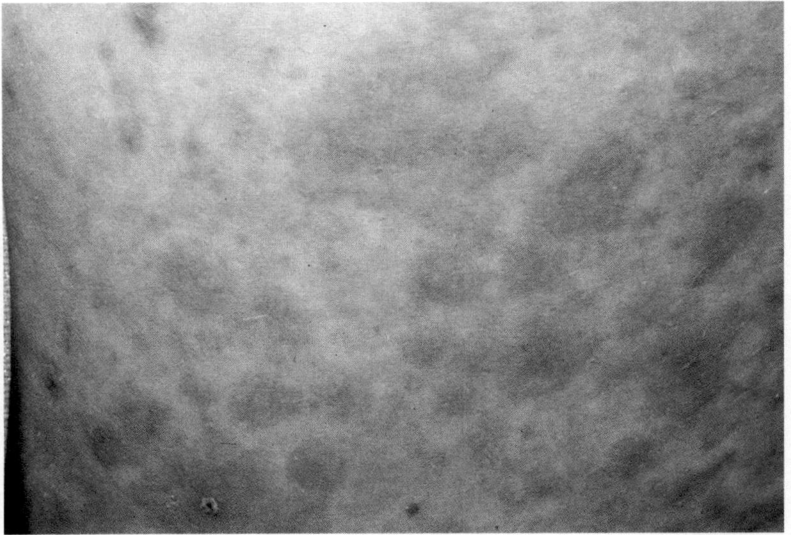

16.10 Urticaria-like eruption of pruritic urticarial papules and plaques of pregnancy (PUPPP). Characteristically, these erythematous lesions begin on the abdomen of patients during the last trimester of pregnancy, and may extend to the proximal extremities.

(**16.11A** and **16.11B**). Joint pain and stiffness are also common and usually parallel skin-disease activity. Gastrointestinal (GI) symptoms, including abdominal pain, nausea, vomiting, and diarrhea, have been temporarily associated with skin and joint involvement. Other symptoms encountered less frequently in patients with urticarial vasculitis include recurrent headaches, eye pain, and chest pain.

In addition to arthritis, other clinical signs of systemic involvement in these patients include generalized lymphadenopathy, bronchospasm, uveitis, episcleritis, and, more rarely, neurologic findings, such as pseudotumor cerebri, meningitis, and mononeuritis.

The diagnosis of idiopathic urticarial vasculitis is established by the histological changes in the skin biopsy. In the majority of patients, the hallmarks of necrotizing vasculitis are evident in cutaneous lesions and indicative of immune-complex-mediated disease. Direct immunofluorescence (DIF) studies of lesional skin from some, but not all, patients with this syndrome show complement and/or immunoglobulins within dermal vessels and/or along the dermo-epidermal junction (*see* **16.7D**). Approximately 50–60% of patients with urticarial vasculitis have detectable hypocomplementemia, most having depressed levels of the early classical pathway components (C_2 and C_4). In addition, low molecular weight (7S) Clq precipitins have been reported in the sera of some urticarial vasculitis patients. Presumably, urticaria-like lesions develop as a result of immune-complex deposition in the skin leading to complement activation and the formation of the anaphylatoxins C_{3a} and C_{5a}. These activated complement components in turn stimulate mast cells to release histamine and other mediators. A few patients with this disorder develop renal disease, ranging in severity from a focal necrotizing glomerulonephritis to a diffuse proliferative process. More recent reports also indicate that some patients with urticarial vasculitis may have an accelerated course of chronic obstructive pulmonary disease (COPD). Additional tests (antinuclear antibodies, antibodies to double-stranded DNA, cryoglobulins, circulating rheumatoid factors, false-positive VDRL, hepatitis B surface antigen) that are frequently employed for the diagnosis of connective tissue diseases or immune-complex-mediated disorders are usually either negative or of low titer in patients with urticarial vasculitis, limiting their diagnostic value in this context.

Systemic lupus erythematosus and other disorders

Urticarial lesions have been reported to occur in the rare patient with systemic lupus erythematosus (SLE). In some cases, these lesions have the typical histologic changes of urticaria, while in others there is evidence of leukocytoclastic vasculitis. Some patients with essential mixed cryoglobulinemia may also present initially with urticaria-like lesions following cold exposure. However, the presence of palpable purpuric lesions (vasculitis), Raynaud's phenomenon, and cutaneous ulcerations helps to distinguish these patients from those with uncomplicated chronic urticaria. Most patients with serum sickness develop an urticarial reaction pattern early in the course of disease. Histologically, these lesions may demonstrate typical changes of urticaria or may show

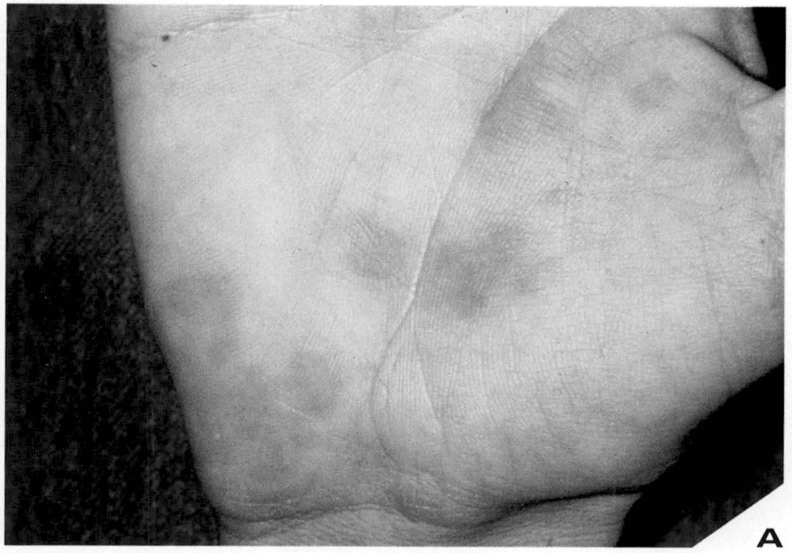

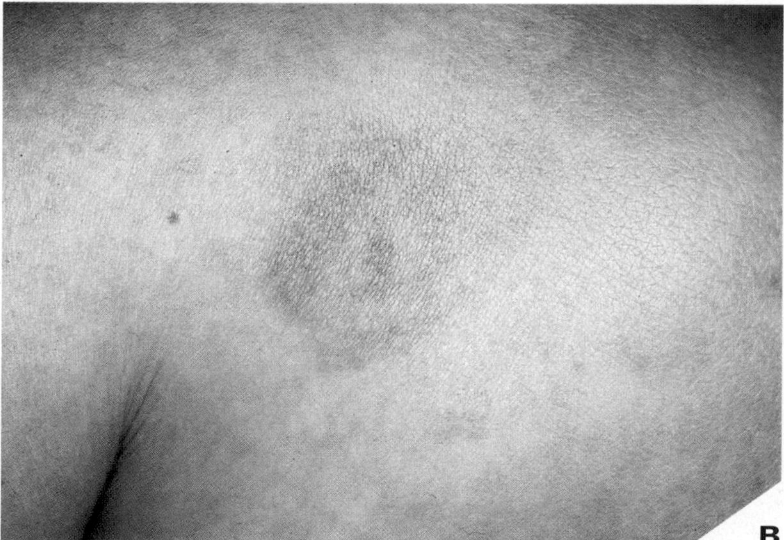

16.11 Lesions of urticarial vasculitis. (A) Palmar involvement frequently occurs in these patients and this may mimic the lesions of erythema multiforme. (B) Evidence of purpura may be seen in resolving urticarial vasculitis lesions.

more significant inflammation in the form of vasculitis. Urticarial-like papules and plaques have also been reported in children with juvenile rheumatoid arthritis, but, unlike common hives, these lesions are characteristically non-pruritic. Lesions of acute and chronic urticaria have also been reported in patients with hypothyroidism, hyperthyroidism, and occult lymphomas. Patients with mastocytosis may have dermatographism or a spontaneous urticaria-like eruption in foci of cutaneous mast-cell infiltrates (**16.12**). Recurrent episodes of urticaria and angioedema have also been described in adolescents with the rare hereditary disorder originally described by Muckle and Wells. These children experience recurrent urticarial eruptions accompanied by chills and malaise. Progressive nerve deafness and amyloidosis of the kidney develop after a variable period of time.

Hereditary angioedema

In patients with recurrent angioedema (**16.13**), several disorders should be considered in the differential diagnosis. These include hereditary angioedema (HAE), acquired deficiency of the inhibitor of C_1 esterase, and angioedema–eosinophilia syndrome. Hereditary angioedema is an autosomal disorder characterized by episodic, non-pruritic, and painless subcutaneous swellings lasting for several hours to days. The lesions are often triggered by local trauma or emotional stress, and are usually asymmetrical. Unlike acquired angioedema, an urticarial reaction pattern is rarely present in patients with this disorder. Also, a history of recurrent nausea, vomiting, and abdominal colicky pain is common in this patient population; it results from localized intestinal edema.

The onset of HAE usually begins in childhood or young adulthood. There is often a positive history of other family members with similar complaints. It is important to differentiate HAE from other causes of angioedema, because patients with this disorder may be at greater risk for laryngeal edema leading to sudden death. The underlying mechanism for HAE is a genetically determined partial deficiency of an alpha$_2$-glycoprotein, termed C_1 esterase inhibitor (C_1 INH). This serum protein normally inactivates the first component of complement. The absence of C_1 INH results in excessive consumption of the complement component, C_4. Thus, patients with HAE have chronically depressed serum levels of C_4, and during acute attacks both C_4 and C_2 levels are depressed. In approximately 85% of the patients, C_1 INH levels are low, while in the remaining 15% the protein is present in normal amounts. In this latter group, the inhibitory activity of C_1 INH is abnormal; thus, a functional C_1 INH assay is necessary to correctly identify this subset of HAE.

The underlying mechanisms for hereditary angioedema appear to involve both the activation of the complement and plasma-kinin-forming pathways. In the absence of C_1 INH activity, the stimulation of the complement cascade proceeds essentially uninhibited following minor stimuli. Generation of the anaphylatoxins, C_{3a} and C_{5a} under such circumstances would be expected to provoke mast-cell and basophil-mediator release. C_1 INH also inhibits kallikrein, Hageman factor fragments, and plasmin. Following tissue trauma, kallikrein is readily generated from high molecular prekallikrein in a patient with HAE, and as a result of inadequate C_1 INH activity, it stimulates kininogen leading to the generation of bradykinin, a

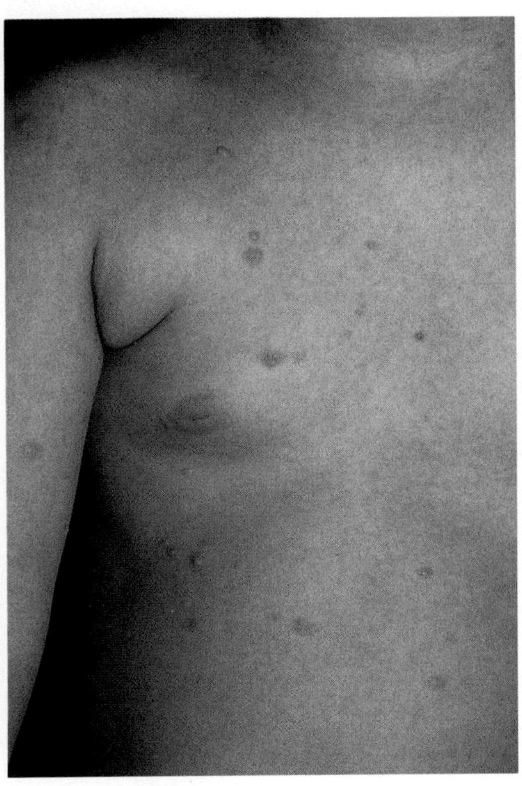

16.12 Urticarial reaction in lesions of mastocytosis. The stroking of mastocytosis skin lesions results in an urticarial response (Darier's sign). These yellow-tan papules are commonly described as urticaria pigmentosa.

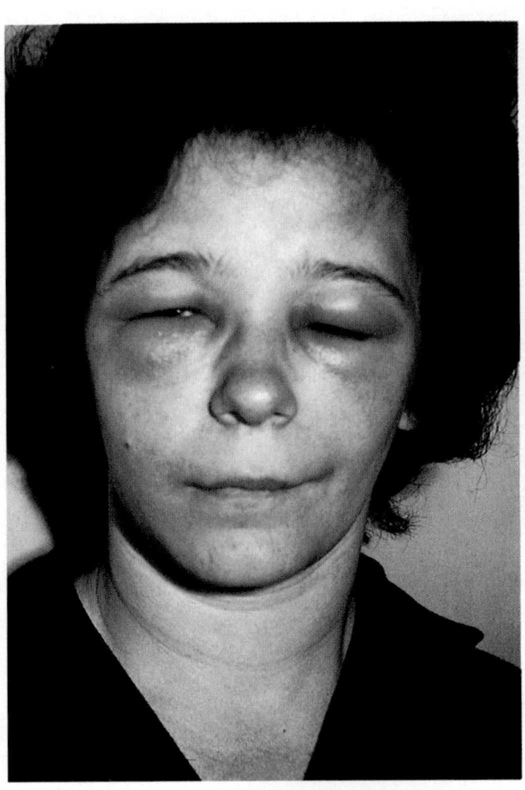

16.13 Hereditary angioedema. In this condition, the swellings frequently involve the face, including the oropharynx. The edema is typically non-erythematous and non-pruritic. These lesions can be extensive, involving the deep dermal and subcutaneous tissues.

potent vasoactive polypeptide (**16.14**). Subcutaneous injections of either the first component of complement (C_1) or kallikrein result in angioedematous lesions in patients with HAE, suggesting a role for other complement factors and the plasma-kinin-forming pathway. Both HAE variations respond to stanazolol or danazol therapy.

Acquired C_1 INH deficiency

Certain neoplastic disorders, including lymphomas and multiple myeloma, as well as pulmonary and colon carcinomas, have occasionally been associated with a clinical syndrome similar to HAE. However, unlike those with HAE, these patients often have urticarial lesions accompanying the angioedema. Referred to as acquired deficiency of serum C_1 INH, this disorder can be detected through its association with a decrease of C_4 and C_2 levels. In contrast to HAE patients, however, levels of C_1 are also depressed in this population.

Angioedema–eosinophilia syndrome

Recently, a most unusual disorder characterized by recurrent episodes of angioedema and urticaria in association with fever, prominent weight gain, and peripheral blood eosinophilia was described. Characteristically, these patients develop angioedema which persists for up to 7–10 days, and is associated with a 7–9 kg (15–20 pound) weight gain. The most striking laboratory abnormality is a marked increase in peripheral blood eosinophils (ranging from 2,760–95,0404 mm^3). Cutaneous biopsies from lesional tissue demonstrate dermal edema and perivascular lymphocytic infiltrates with scattered eosinophils. Despite few demonstrable tissue eosinophils, immunofluorescence staining for eosinophil-granule-derived major basic protein (MBP) has been uniformly positive in each skin biopsy specimen. Extensive study of each case for an underlying parasitic infection and/or antigen stimulus has been negative. The prognosis for these patients appears good in that they

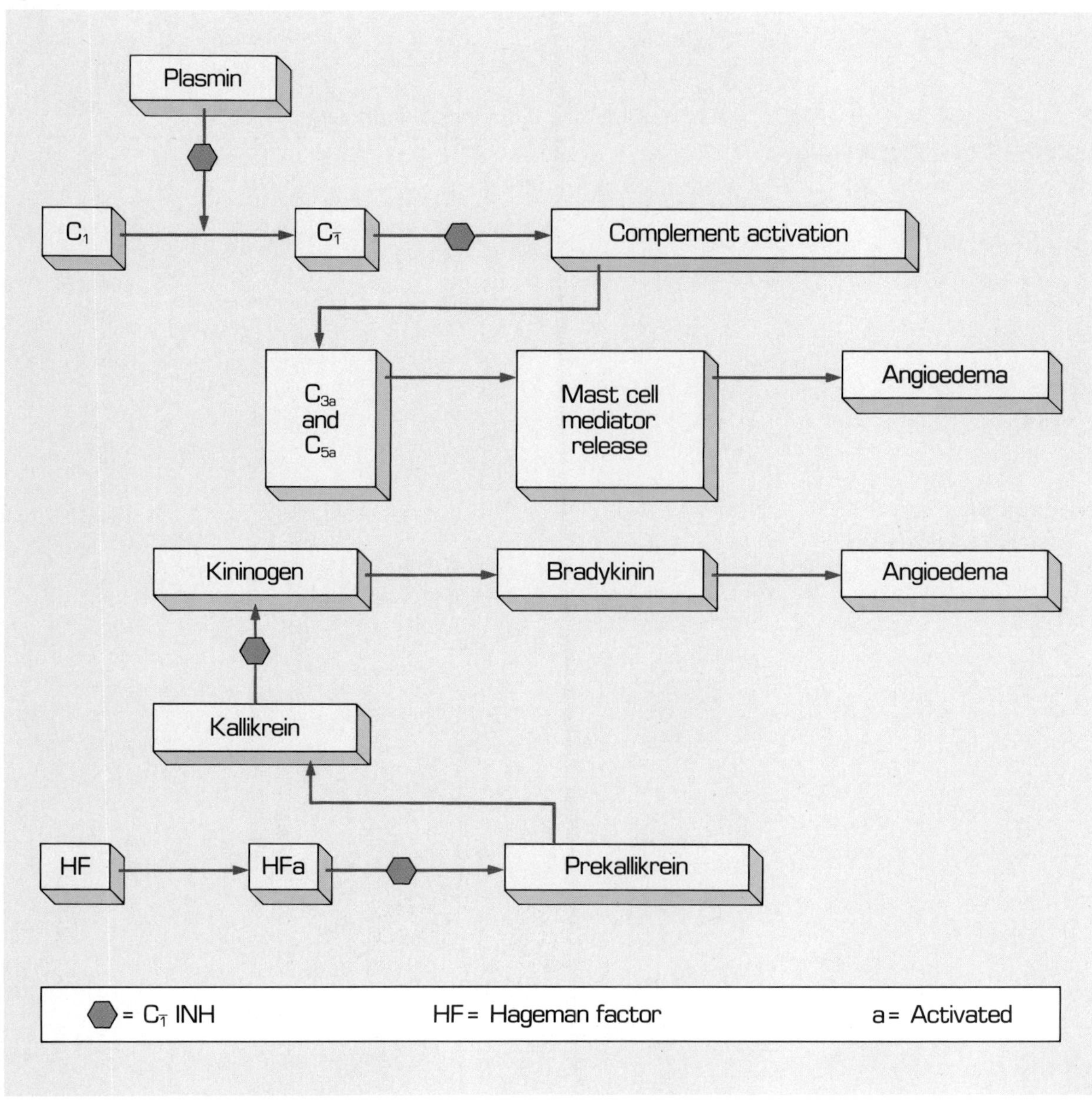

16.14 Pathogenesis of hereditary angioedema. Deficiency in C_1 esterase inhibitor (C_1–INH) leads to uninhibited complement activation and anaphylatoxin (C_{3a}, C_{5a}) formation which, in turn, stimulates mast cell mediator release. In addition, Hageman Factor (HF) activation also proceeds in the absence of C_1–INH activity, which may result in the formation of the vasodilating agent bradykinin.

respond to systemic corticosteroid therapy. Two subjects have had this disorder for at least ten years without significant disseminated disease or complications.

Other cutaneous disorders

Several other well-defined cutaneous diseases also should be considered in the differential diagnosis of urticaria or angioedema (**16.15**). The annular and arcuate morphology of some urticarial lesions must be distinguished from a group of disorders termed the figurative erythemas. This group includes erythema annulare centrifugum (**16.16A**), erythema chronicum migrans, and erythema marginatum. In contrast to urticaria, usually these eruptions are non-pruritic. Erythema annulare centrifugum, which most closely resembles an urticarial reaction pattern, can be identified by a characteristic scaling ring that trails its advancing red border. Individual lesions of erythema multiforme may also assume an urticarial morphology. However, the more typical target-like lesions are usually also present (**16.16B**).

Early in their course, some of the primary blistering disorders may appear urticarial. In particular, the autoimmune blistering diseases, dermatitis herpetiformis (**16.16C**) and bullous pemphigoid may present as pruritic papules. Similarly, *Herpes simplex* and *Herpes zoster* may begin as pruritic, slightly painful urticarial lesions, and in some instances the full clinical expression of grouped vesicles may not occur (**16.16D**). Lesion arrangement (grouped) and a focal anatomical distribution, however, provide important clinical characteristics for differentiating herpetic lesions from typical lesions of urticaria (**16.16E**). Similarly, patients with mastocytosis frequently develop urticarial wheals at the sites of focal cutaneous mast-cell infiltrates. However, close examination of the skin usually reveals the typical macular (telangiectasis macularis eruption perstans), papular (urticaria pigmentosa) (**16.12**), or nodular (mastocytoma) lesions due to dermal mast-cell infiltration. There are several disorders that may mimic lesions of angioedema. These include panniculitis, localized cellulitis, thrombophlebitis, lymphangitis, and cheilitis granulomatosa (**16.17**).

DIFFERENTIAL DIAGNOSIS OF URTICARIA

1. Urticaria of pregnancy (PUPPP)
2. Urticarial vasculitis
3. Figurative erythemas
4. Erythema multiforme
5. Dermatitis herpetiformis
6. Bullous pemphigoid
7. Herpes simplex, Herpes zoster
8. Mastocytosis

16.15 Differential diagnosis of urticaria.

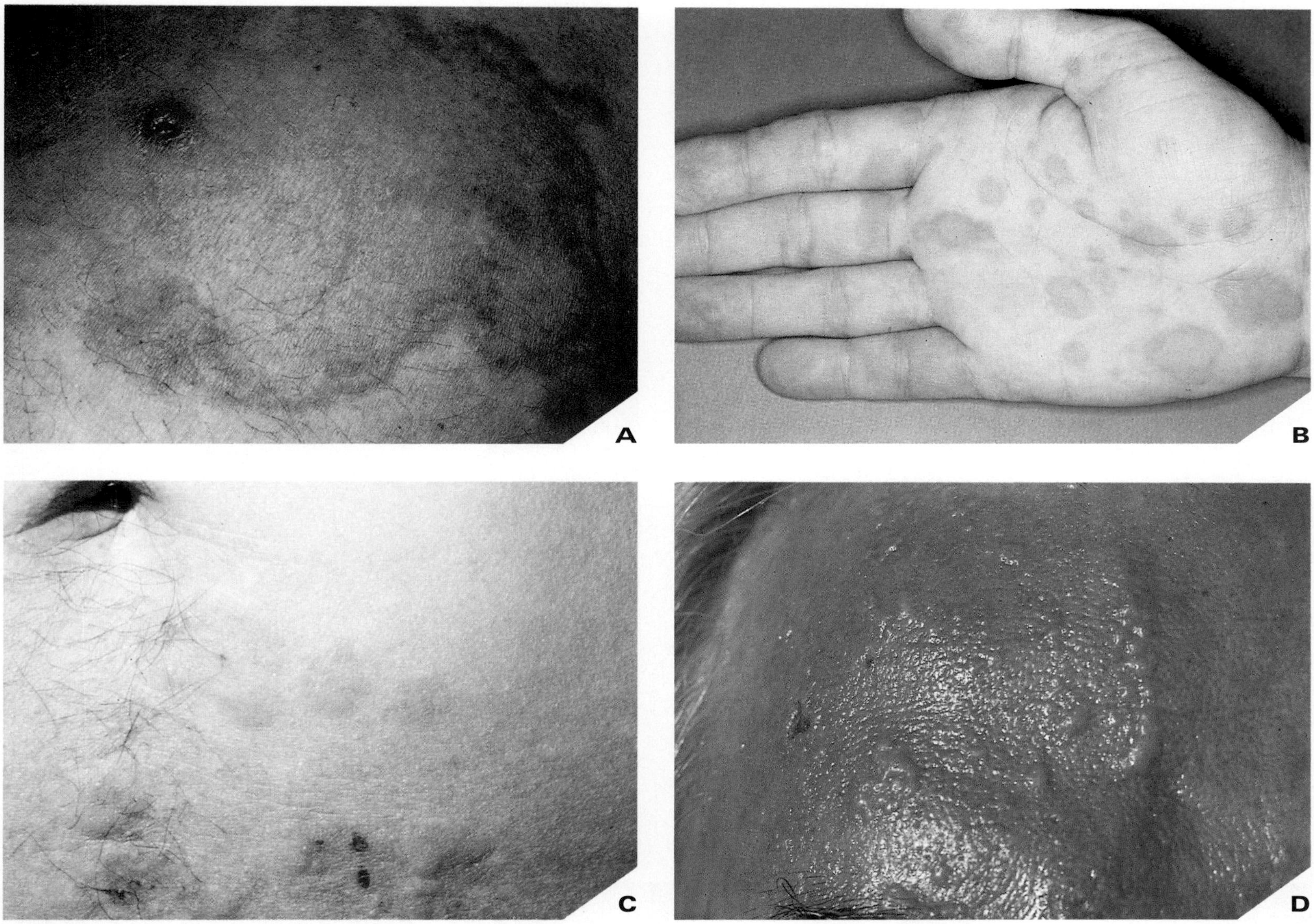

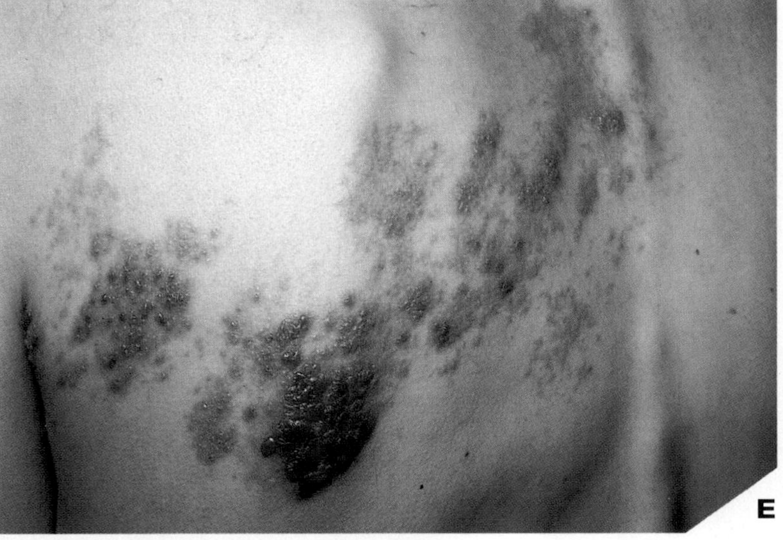

16.16 Cutaneous disorders which may appear as urticaria. (A) Erythema annulare centrifugum. (B) Erythema multiforme involving the palm. Both of these belong to the group of disorders known as the figurative erythemas. (C) Dermatitis herpetiformis. An urticaria-like eruption may be seen in early lesions of this blistering disease. (D) Edematous plaques, which may appear urticarial, in *Herpes zoster*. (E) More typically grouped lesions of *H. zoster*.

PATIENT EVALUATION

Once the clinical diagnosis of urticaria or angioedema has been established and other conditions have been excluded, careful attention to both the morphology and the anatomical distribution of lesions may provide insight into potential etiologic factors. Small, 1.0–3.0 mm, wheals with large surrounding areas of erythema suggest a diagnosis of cholinergic urticaria (**16.18**). Focal, urticarial lesions with geometric shapes (linear, angular, straight-edged) indicate the presence of external influences, as may be seen in pressure urticaria or dermatographism (**16.19A**). Similarly, urticarial lesions localized to exposed areas suggest the possibility of solar (**16.19B**) or cold-induced reactions (**16.19C**). In patients with distal extremity involvement alone, the diagnosis of papular urticaria or urticarial vasculitis should be considered (**16.11**), while small urticarial papules with a follicular-like arrangement suggest the possibility of aquagenic urticaria.

In general, when the history and physical examination fail to uncover potential etiologic factors, a skin biopsy is warranted in cases of chronic urticaria. Extensive laboratory studies, such as a complete blood count, erythrocyte sedimentation rate (ESR), urinalysis, serum chemical analyses, allergy testing, as well as sinus and dental radiographs, on the other hand, have not been very useful. **16.20** outlines a clinical algorithm for the diagnosis and management of unresponsive chronic urticaria or angioedema.

DIFFERENTIAL DIAGNOSIS OF ANGIOEDEMA

1. Hereditary angioedema (HAE)
2. Acquired C1 inhibitor deficiency
3. Angioedema–eosinophilia syndrome
4. Panniculitis, cellulitis
5. Thrombophlebitis, lymphangitis
6. Cheilitis granulomatosa

16.17 Differential diagnosis of angioedema.

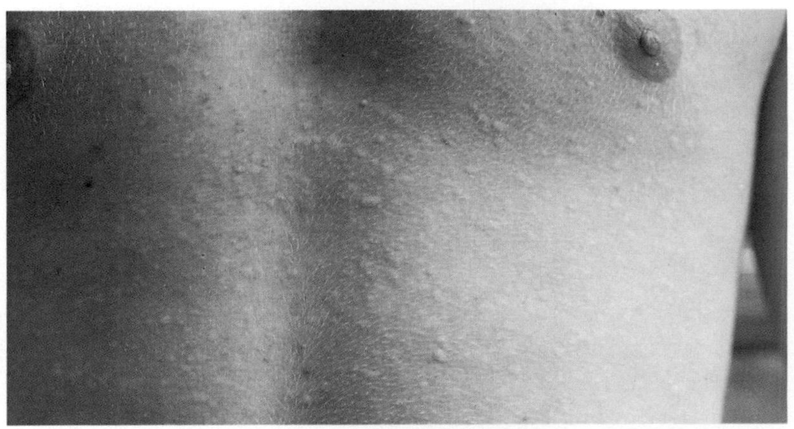

16.18 Typical lesions of cholinergic urticaria. Papules 1–3 mm in diameter, with surrounding erythema are commonly seen especially after exercise or increased body temperature.

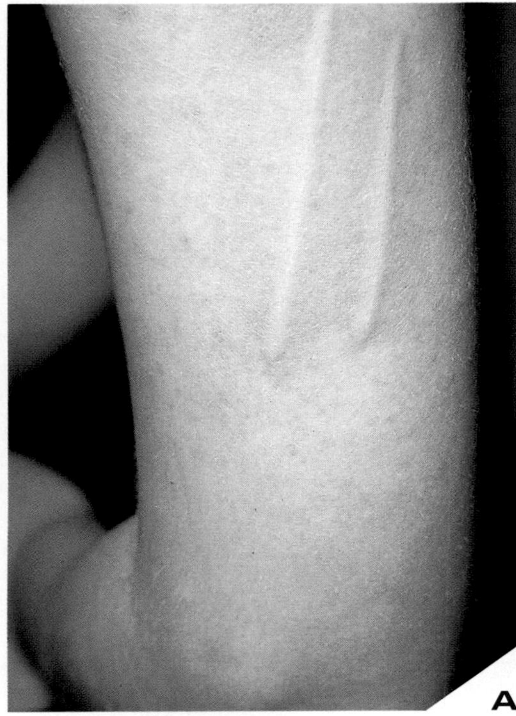

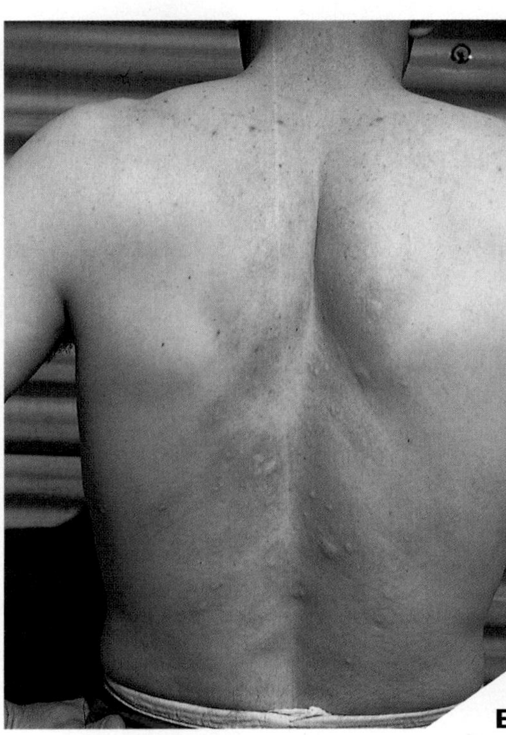

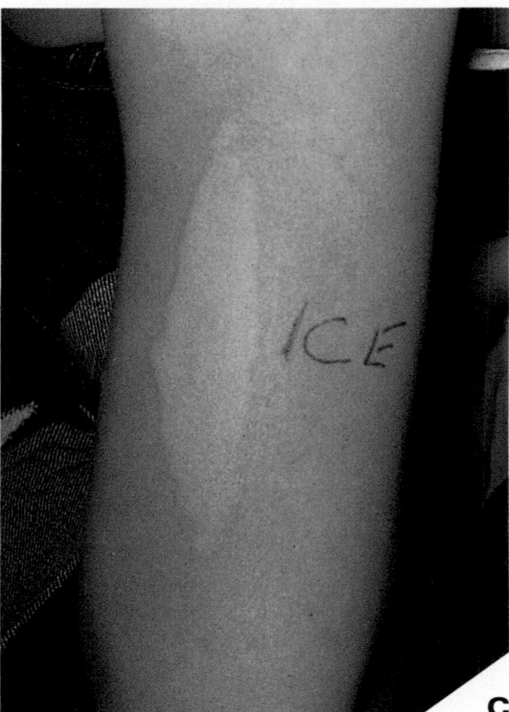

16.19 Physical urticarias. (A) Pressure urticaria. This photograph demonstrated a typical response 20 minutes after applying pressure by firmly stroking the skin with a tongue depressor. (B) Solar urticaria. This photograph was taken after 30 minutes of unprotected sunlight exposure. (C) Cold urticaria. An urticarial response minutes after removal of ice applied to the skin for five minutes.

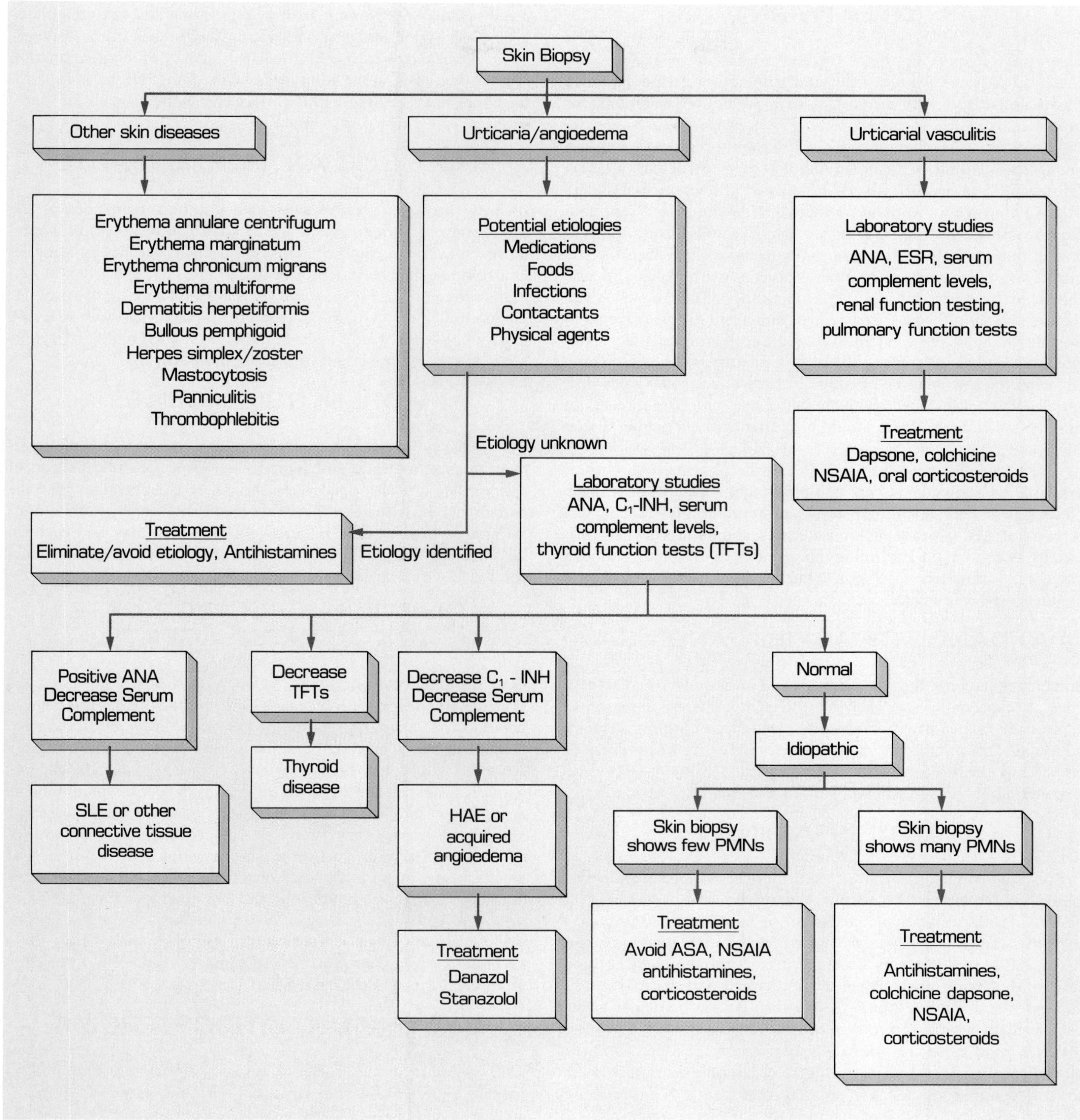

16.20 Algorithm for the diagnosis and treatment of chronic urticaria and angioedema.

TREATMENT

The most effective approach to the treatment of urticaria or angioedema is the identification and elimination of the causative agents. In patients with medication or food-induced eruptions, for example, avoidance of these substances is curative. In cases of physical urticaria, an explanation of the disease process and its initiating factors permits patients to modify their particular lifestyle. Those with cold urticaria should be warned of the potential danger of swimming in cool water and should never swim alone. Commonsense measures, such as wearing warm socks and gloves, and protecting one's face from the cold air, can markedly reduce the frequency of symptomatic episodes. Patients with solar urticaria should be instructed on the use of combined UVB and UVA sun screens and should be advised against direct sun exposure. In addition, a gradual increase in exposure to natural or artificial light may effectively induce tolerance to light in patients with solar urticaria. Chloroquine also may be effective in controlling some solar urticaria patients. Obviously, patients who have underlying infections or other systemic disorders should be treated with modalities directed specifically at these diseases.

Unfortunately, in more than 75% of the patients with chronic urticaria or angioedema, no etiologic factors can be identified. Nevertheless, because of the pruritus and undesirable cosmetic features associated with these skin eruptions, some form of therapy is usually necessary. In the following sections, a rational, although empirical, approach to the treatment of chronic urticaria or angioedema is presented.

AVOIDANCE OF ASPIRIN AND NSAIA

Some patients with chronic urticaria and angioedema may experience an exacerbation of their clinical symptoms on ingestion of aspirin and related drugs. Therefore, avoidance of aspirin and nonsteroidal anti-inflammatory agents (NSAIA) is recommended empirically. In those cases in which aspirin sensitivity is evident, patients should also avoid exposure to azo dyes and benzoates.

ANTIHISTAMINES

Because the cutaneous mast cell and its released mediators play a central role in urticarial reactions, therapy directed at blocking the effects of mast-cell-derived histamine is warranted. Histamine-1 receptor antagonists have proven to be effective in controlling many, but not all, patients with urticaria. Although most H_1 antihistamines have similar properties, individual patients may note a superior therapeutic response to one class or one particular agent, such as hydroxyzine. Cyproheptadine has been reported to be more effective than other H_1 antagonists in controlling patients with cholinergic urticaria. In some instances, a combination of two different H_1 antihistamines may prove to be superior to either alone. In this latter case, it is recommended that agents representing two different classes of H_1 antagonists be employed for maximal therapeutic benefit. The newer non-sedating antihistamines, terfenadine, astemizole, loratadine, and cetirizine appear to be as effective as other H_1 antagonists in controlling lesions of chronic urticaria. The long-acting effect of astemizole given once daily seems to be more appropriate in the management of many chronic urticaria patients. Because histamine mediates its effects through both H_1 and H_2 receptors, H_2 antagonists, such as cimetidine and ranitidine have been used in combination with H_1 antihistamines in the management of chronic urticaria. Although the efficacy of this combination remains in question, the addition of an H_2 antagonist to an H_1 antihistamine may be worthwhile in selected patients who are unresponsive to H_1 treatment alone.

TRICYCLIC ANTIDEPRESSANTS

If chronic urticaria is unresponsive to H_1 antihistamine therapy, the use of tricyclic antidepressant agents known to be potent H_1 antagonists, may be considered. Doxepin, a heterocyclic variation of amitriptyline, has been demonstrated *in vitro* to be nearly 800-fold more active at the H_1 receptor site on a molar basis than the H_1 antagonist diphenhydramine. Recently, doxepin has been reported in a double-blind study to be superior to hydroxyzine and cyproheptadine in the treatment of cold-induced urticaria.

ADRENERGIC AGENTS

The use of subcutaneous epinephrine may be helpful for the treatment of acute urticaria and angioedema. Since the clinical effects of this medication last only a few hours, it is imperative that the patient also be treated with another medication, such as an H_1 antihistamine. Oral terbutaline and ephedrine also may be beneficial for the control of urticaria and angioedema in some patients, when combined with antihistamine therapy.

DISODIUM CROMOGLYCATE AND RELATED AGENTS

Oral disodium cromoglycate may be effective in controlling the pruritus and whealing in patients with mastocytosis. However, its benefit for urticaria patients has not been substantiated. Doxantrazole, a cromoglycate-like agent which is more rapidly absorbed orally, has been shown to reduce whealing in patients with cold-induced urticaria. Ketotifen, a benzocycloheptathiophene derivative with both mast-cell stabilizing qualities and H_1 receptor antagonist activity, has been reported to control symptoms of patients with physical urticaria, chronic idiopathic urticaria, and mastocytosis. Oxatomide is a diphenylmethyl piperazine derivative of a substituted benzimidazole and has pharmacologic activities similar to ketotifen. This agent also has proven efficacious in controlling chronic urticarial reactions. Although these latter three agents are available in Europe and Canada, they are not presently approved for use in the United States.

SYSTEMIC CORTICOSTEROIDS

The use of systemic corticosteroids is sometimes indicated in patients experiencing acute urticarial reactions, especially if associated with extensive angioedema or anaphylaxis. Corticosteroids may also be effective in controlling severe exacerbations in patients with idiopathic chronic urticaria. However, they are to be avoided on a *long-term* basis in the management of patients with chronic urticaria. An exception to this statement pertains to the treatment of patients with urticarial vasculitis or the angioedema–eosinophilia syndrome, who may require daily or alternate-day systemic steroid therapy.

OTHER TREATMENTS

The calcium channel blocker, nifedipine, has been reported effective in the treatment of chronic urticaria when combined with H_1 antihistamines. Colchicine, dapsone, or sulfasalazine in conjunction with antihistamines may be helpful for the management of chronic urticaria patients who demonstrate numerous neutrophils and eosinophils without vasculitis in their skin biopsies. Some of these patients have demonstrable circulating antibodies to mast-cell IgE receptors and IgE. A subset of these patients may be poorly responsive to this combination therapy and require treatment with plasmapheresis or cyclosporin A to control their symptoms.

SUMMARY

Urticaria and angioedema represent cutaneous reaction patterns for which multiple etiologic factors have been identified. Initial evaluation of patients with urticaria or angioedema should focus on a thorough history and physical examination. When the cutaneous diagnosis is in question, a skin biopsy should be performed. Additional diagnostic testing is dictated by the information gained from the initial patient examination. Treatment of urticaria and angioedema is directed toward eliminating the etiologic agents, when possible. In instances where such factors cannot be identified or eliminated, empirical therapy should include the avoidance of aspirin and related drugs and the use of H_1 (and possibly H_2) antagonists. Initially, oral corticosteroids may be necessary to control patient symptoms. As our understanding of the forces responsible for the expression of urticaria or angioedema improve, more effective approaches to treatment should emerge.

REFERENCES

Champion RH, Roberts SDB, Carpenter RG, *et al.*: Urticaria and angioedema. A review of 554 patients. *Br J Dermatol*, **81**:588–597, 1969.

Gelfand JA. Acquired C1-esterase inhibitory deficiency and angioedema: A review. *Medicine*; **58**:321–328, 1979.

Jones RR, Bhogal B, Dash A, *et al.*: Urticaria and vasculitis: A continuum of histological and immunopathological changes. *Br J Dermatol*, **108**:695–703, 1983.

Hide M, Francis DM, Grattan CE, *et al.*: Autoantibodies against the high affinity IgE receptor as a cause of histamine release in chronic urticaria. *N Engl J Med*, **328**:1599–1604, 1993.

Kennard CD, Ellis CN: Pharmologic therapy for urticaria. *J Am Acad Dermatol*, **25**:176–187, 1991.

CHAPTER 17

Immunodeficiency Diseases

Philip Fireman

Immunodeficiency diseases range from severe, life-threatening disorders to mild or even asymptomatic conditions. On occasion they need to be considered in the differential diagnosis of allergic diseases. In these conditions, one or more abnormalities of the immune system impair the host's defense mechanisms and result in an increase in susceptibility to infections. Immunodeficiency should be suspected in any patient who has frequent or recurrent infections. Immunodeficiency diseases, however, are relatively uncommon and many other illnesses may predispose a patient to repeated infections.

17.1 lists and groups these varied conditions according to the mechanisms by which they predispose a patient to repeated infection. If the immune system is intact, some of the listed illnesses, such as dysfunctional cilia syndrome, may actually manifest hypergammaglobulinemia as an increased immune response to repeated infections. With persistent or recurrent respiratory symptoms, allergy may also be suspected. A thorough patient history and physical examination identifies many of these illnesses, and a correct diagnosis can be confirmed by the appropriate laboratory tests. If the clinician has considered and excluded these other, more common clinical syndromes, it is then reasonable to suspect a defect or deficiency of the patient's immune mechanism.

As outlined in **17.1**, immunodeficiency may be either primary or secondary. Primary immunodeficiencies are divided into four major categories, depending on the portion of the host defense system that is affected. As shown in **17.2**, these primary immune defects include

ILLNESSES WHICH INCREASE SUSCEPTIBILITY TO INFECTION – SELECTED EXAMPLES

1. **Primary immunodeficiency**
   X-linked hypogammaglobulinemia, severe combined immunodeficiency disease (SCID), DiGeorge syndrome
2. **Secondary immunodeficiency**
   Acquired immunodeficiency syndrome (AIDS), lymphoma, malnutrition, immunosuppression therapy
3. **Mucosal–skin barrier disorders**
   Dysfunctional cilia syndrome, eczema, burns,sinus tract disorders
4. **Obstructive disorders**
   Cystic fibrosis, asthma, eustachian tube obstruction
5. **Circulatory disorders**
   Sickle cell disease, diabetes, congenital heart disease
6. **Foreign bodies**
   Venous and urinary catheters, aspirated objects, artificial heart valves
7. **Unusual microbiologic factors**
   Antibiotic overgrowth, contaminated respiratory equipment, infectious contact

17.1 Conditions that increase host susceptibility to infection, with selected examples.

deficiencies of antibodies (B-lymphocytes), cell-mediated immunity (T-lymphocytes), phagocytic cells, and complement systems. Secondary immunodeficiencies occur in previously normal individuals who, as a result of some intercurrent illness or exposure, manifest compromised or defective immune responses. The most severe and devastating of these is acquired immunodeficiency syndrome (AIDS). While AIDS is, to date, irreversible, other secondary immune defects are reversible if the underlying condition or illness is corrected. The secondary immunodeficiencies are outlined in **17.3**, and are considerably more common than primary immunodeficiencies.

EPIDEMIOLOGY

The true prevalence of immunodeficiency is unknown. Good data are difficult to obtain since physicians are not required to report these diagnoses. In addition, as new immunologic technologies are being developed, additional diseases are being diagnosed. It is estimated that one case of immunodeficiency occurs in every 10,000 individuals. The genetically determined primary deficiencies are rare. In the United States, it is estimated that X-linked agammaglobulinemia occurs with a frequency of 1:50,000 and severe combined immunodeficiency disease (SCID) with an approximate frequency of 1:200,000 live births. Many primary immunodeficiencies are hereditary and congenital. Consequently, most of these illnesses are recognized in childhood, with individuals under 20 years of age comprising about 80% of the cases. During childhood there is a 5:1 male:female sex predominance for these disorders. This is reversed in adults, with a slight (1:1.4) predominance in females. As better methods of managing and treating these syndromes are developed, it is anticipated that many of these patients will survive into adulthood.

Among the immunodeficiency syndromes, B-cell or antibody defects are most common. In fact, isolated IgA deficiency may have an incidence of one per 500 individuals, If IgA deficiency is excluded,

CLASSIFICATION OF PRIMARY IMMUNODEFICIENCIES

1. **Antibody (B-lymphocyte) deficiency**
2. **Cell-mediated (T-lymphocyte) deficiency**
   T-cell deficiency alone
   With B-cell deficiency
3. **Phagocytic deficiency**
4. **Complement deficiency**

17.2 The four major categories of primary immunodeficiency.

SECONDARY IMMUNODEFICIENCIES, ASSOCIATED FACTORS, AND EXAMPLES

1. **Infectious diseases**
   AIDS, cytomegalovirus (CMV), infectious mononucleosis [Epstein-Barr (EB) virus], congenital rubella, measles
2. **Therapeutic agents (medications)**
   Steroids, radiation, immunosuppressive agents (cancer), anti-lymphocyte (T-cell) serum
3. **Neoplastic and hematologic diseases**
   Lymphoma (Hodgkin's disease), leukemia, myeloma, neutropenia, aplastic anemia, sickle cell disease
4. **Metabolic diseases**
   Protein-loss enteropathy, nephrotic syndrome, diabetes, malnutrition
5. **Trauma and surgery**
   Burns, splenectomy, anesthesia
6. **Miscellaneous**
   Lupus erythematosus, chronic hepatitis, Down's syndrome

17.3 Secondary immunodeficiencies, their associated factors, and selected examples.

B-cell defects make up about 50% of the immunodeficiency syndromes (**17.4**). T-cell deficiencies make up about 30%, with 10% of these conditions being isolated T-cell defects and 20% being combined T- and B-cell defects. Therefore, a defect of B-cell function is present in over 70% of all primary immune defects. Various defects of neutrophil and phagocyte function comprise about 20%, with complement abnormalities being the least common (under 1%).

DEVELOPMENT OF THE IMMUNE SYSTEM

Cellular (T-cell) and humoral (B-cell) immunity develops from pluripotent hematopoietic stem cells (**17.5**). These same bone marrow stem cells are also the source of polymorphonuclear leukocytes, macrophages, and monocytes, which also participate in host defense. In response to signals from the host's internal environment, these stem cells generate large numbers of lymphocytes that mature into T- and B-lymphocytes that become capable of antigen responsiveness. The thymus-dependent T-lymphocytes become responsible for cell-mediated immune responses directed against common pathogens, such as viruses and fungi. Patients with T-cell defects have severe infections with organisms that usually cause mild or limited infections. T-lymphocytes are also important in the expression of tumor cytotoxicity and homograft rejection. T-lymphocytes collaborate in immunoregulation of B-cell function via subpopulations of T-helper (CD_4) and T-suppressor (CD_8) lymphocytes. Isolated T-cell deficiencies are very rare.

Also derived from bone-marrow stem cells, the B-lymphocytes are precursors of plasma cells. Plasma cells synthesize the immunoglobulins that have functional capacity for antigen recognition, and are defined as antibodies. A lack of one or more of the immunoglobulin isotypes (IgG, IgA, IgM) constitutes humoral or serum antibody immunodeficiency, which may or may not be accompanied by decreased peripheral blood B-cells. A few patients with normal numbers of B-cells and plasma cells, as well as normal

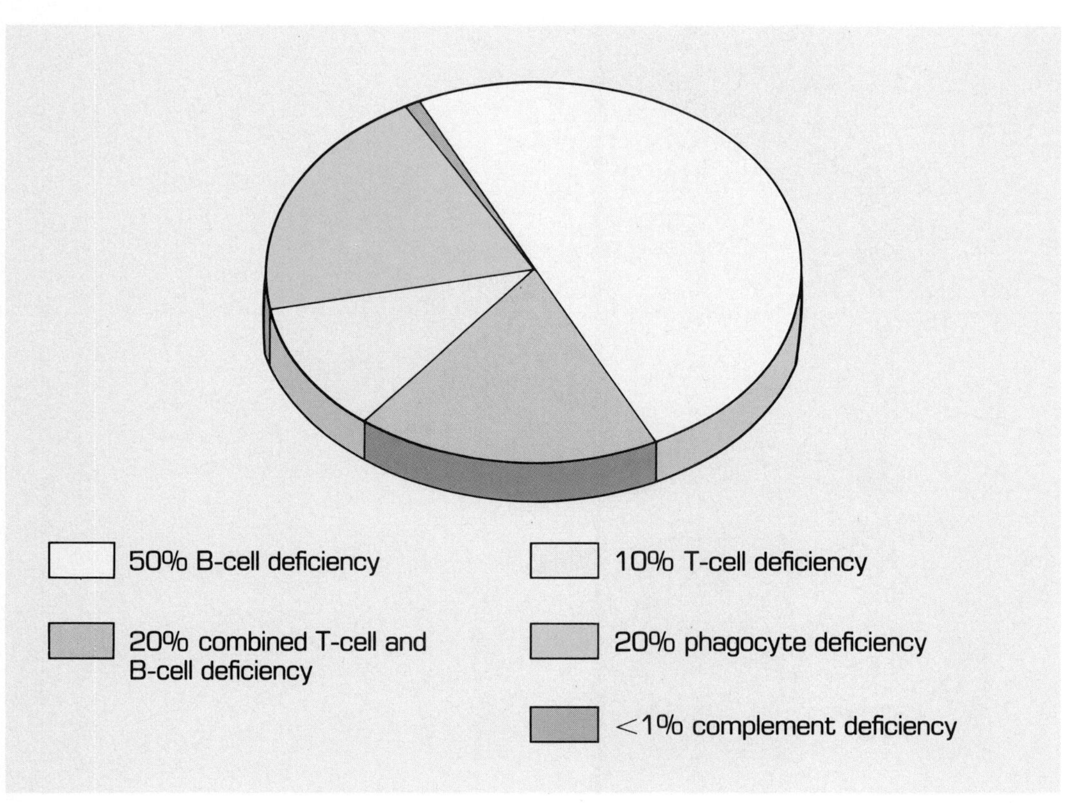

17.4 The relative distribution of the primary immunodeficiency syndromes.

serum immunoglobulin levels, are, nonetheless, immunodeficient because they lack functional antibodies. The primary combined immunodeficiencies result from abnormalities in expression of both T- and B-cells (**17.6**). Cellular antibody (T-cell) immunodeficiencies (**17.7**) or humoral antibody (B-cell) immunodeficiencies (**17.8**) arise from abnormalities in the development of T- or B-lymphocytes, respectively.

In the developing fetus, T-cells begin to appear between the eighth and tenth weeks of gestation, and are promptly accompanied by the presence of B-cells (**17.9**). Appreciable immunoglobulin syn-

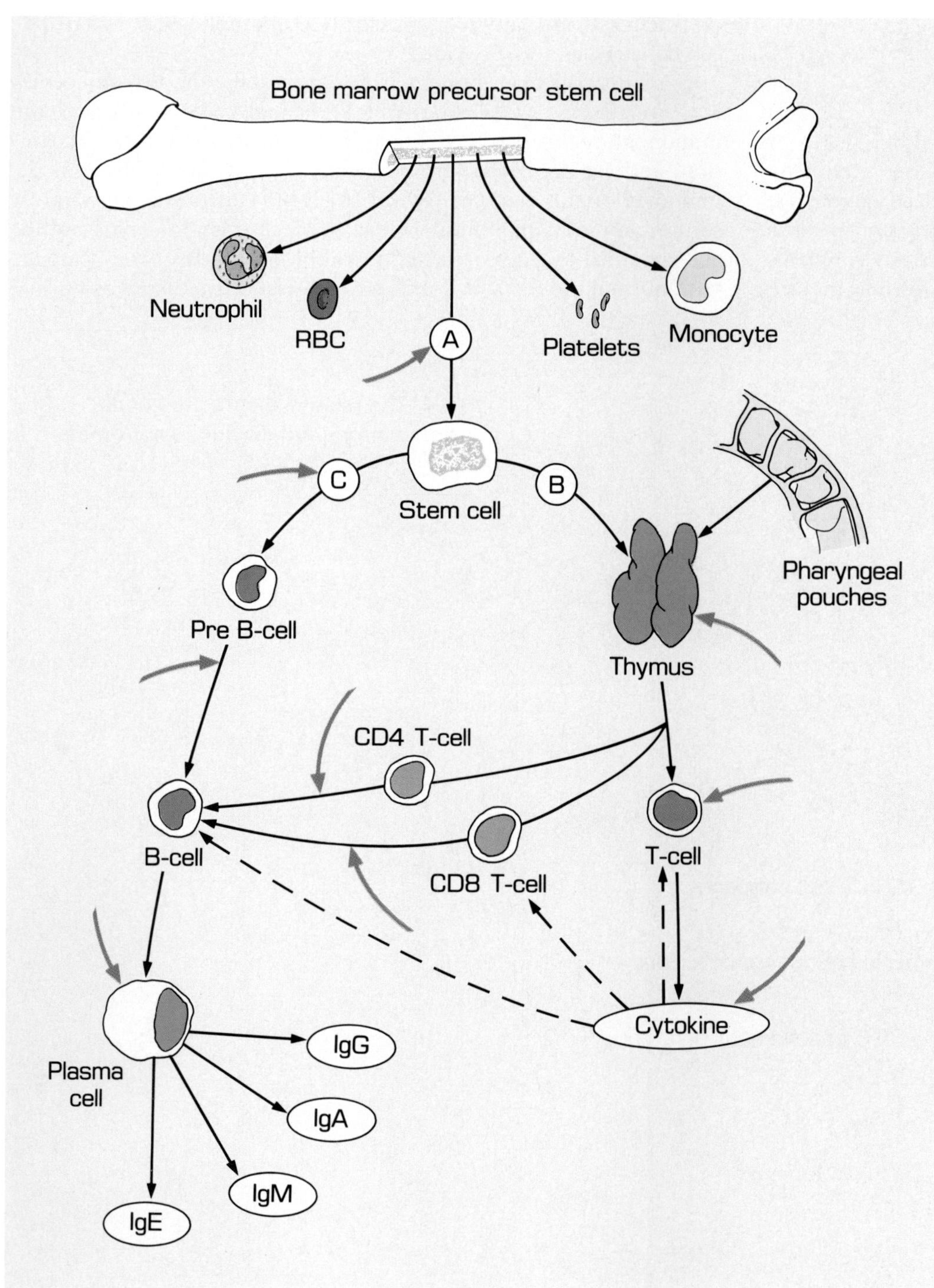

17.5 Diagrammatic representation of T- and B-lymphocyte development from stem cells derived from bone marrow. The arrows indicate the various potential sites of abnormal development. Immune cell defects along pathway A result in combined T- and B-cell immunodeficiencies. Defects at several sites along pathways B or C result in the various T-cell and B-cell deficiencies. (Modified with permission from Waldman *et al.*, 1978.)

thesis by these B-cells, however, does not usually occur during fetal development, but maternal serum IgG does begin to appear in fetal serum by the middle of the second trimester. Through an active placental transport mechanism, maternal IgG continues to increase in fetal serum and at the time of birth achieves a fetal cord serum concentration of 110% that of adults. Maternal serum IgM, IgA, and IgE do not normally cross the placenta. After delivery, the maternal IgG in the infant's serum decreases, being catabolized with a half-life of 3 weeks; it is usually not detectable after 6 months of age. The synthesis of the infant's endogenous serum IgM, IgG, IgA, and

COMBINED T- AND B-LYMPHOCYTE DEFICIENCIES

1. **Severe Combined Immunodeficiency Disease (SCID)**
   SCID with adenosine deaminase deficiency
2. **Ataxia telangiectasia**
3. **Wiskott–Aldrich syndrome**
4. **Hyper-IgE syndrome**

17.6 Combined T- and B-lymphocyte deficiencies.

T-LYMPHOCYTE (CELL-MEDIATED) DEFICIENCIES

1. **DiGeorge syndrome (thymus agenesis)**
2. **Nucleoside phosphorylase deficiency**
3. **Chronic mucocutaneous candidiasis**

17.7 T-lymphocyte (cell-mediated) deficiencies.

B-LYMPHOCYTE (ANTIBODY) DEFICIENCIES

1. **X-linked agammaglobulinemia (Bruton's)**
2. **Common variable immunodeficiency**
3. **IgG subclass deficiency**
4. **IgA deficiency**
5. **Antibody deficiency with normal Ig**
6. **Transient Ig deficiency of infancy**

17.8 B-lymphocyte (antibody) deficiencies.

IgE increases after birth, as indicated in **17.9**. Therefore, for the first several months of age, the infant's serum IgG is a sum of maternal (exogenous) and infant (endogenous) IgG. Lowest IgG levels occur at 3–4 months of age. If the infant's endogenous synthesis of IgG is temporarily delayed, a transient or physiologic hypogammaglobulinemia of infancy can occur, as described below. If there is an intrauterine infection with antigenic stimulation, then IgM may be synthesized, along with lesser amounts of IgA and IgG, by the fetus prior to delivery. This is detectable in cord blood for serologic diagnosis of intrauterine disease.

PATHOGENESIS

The immunodeficiency diseases make up a group of illnesses that are heterogeneous in not only their clinical and immune expression, but also in their basic pathophysiologic mechanisms. The faulty genes in some of the inherited immunodeficiencies have been localized to specific sites on the X-chromosome (**17.10**). These include X-linked hypogammaglobulinemia (Bruton's agammaglobulinemia), X-linked immunodeficiency with hyper-IgM, Wiskott–Aldrich syndrome, X-linked severe combined immunodeficiency (SCID), X-linked lymphoproliferative disease (Duncan's syndrome), properdin deficiency, and chronic granulomatous disease (CGD). The abnormal gene in the DiGeorge syndrome has been localized to chromosome 22, the faulty gene for the adenosine deaminase deficiency with SCID to chromosome 20, the gene for purine nucleoside phosphorylase (PNP) deficiency to chromosome 14, the gene for ataxia telangiectasia to chromosome 11, and that for leukocyte adhesion deficiency to chromosome 21 (**17.10**).

Recent advances in molecular biology have helped identify the primary biologic defect in a small but growing number of these inherited deficiencies, which can be designated as inborn errors of the immune system. In X-linked hypogammaglobulinemia, there is

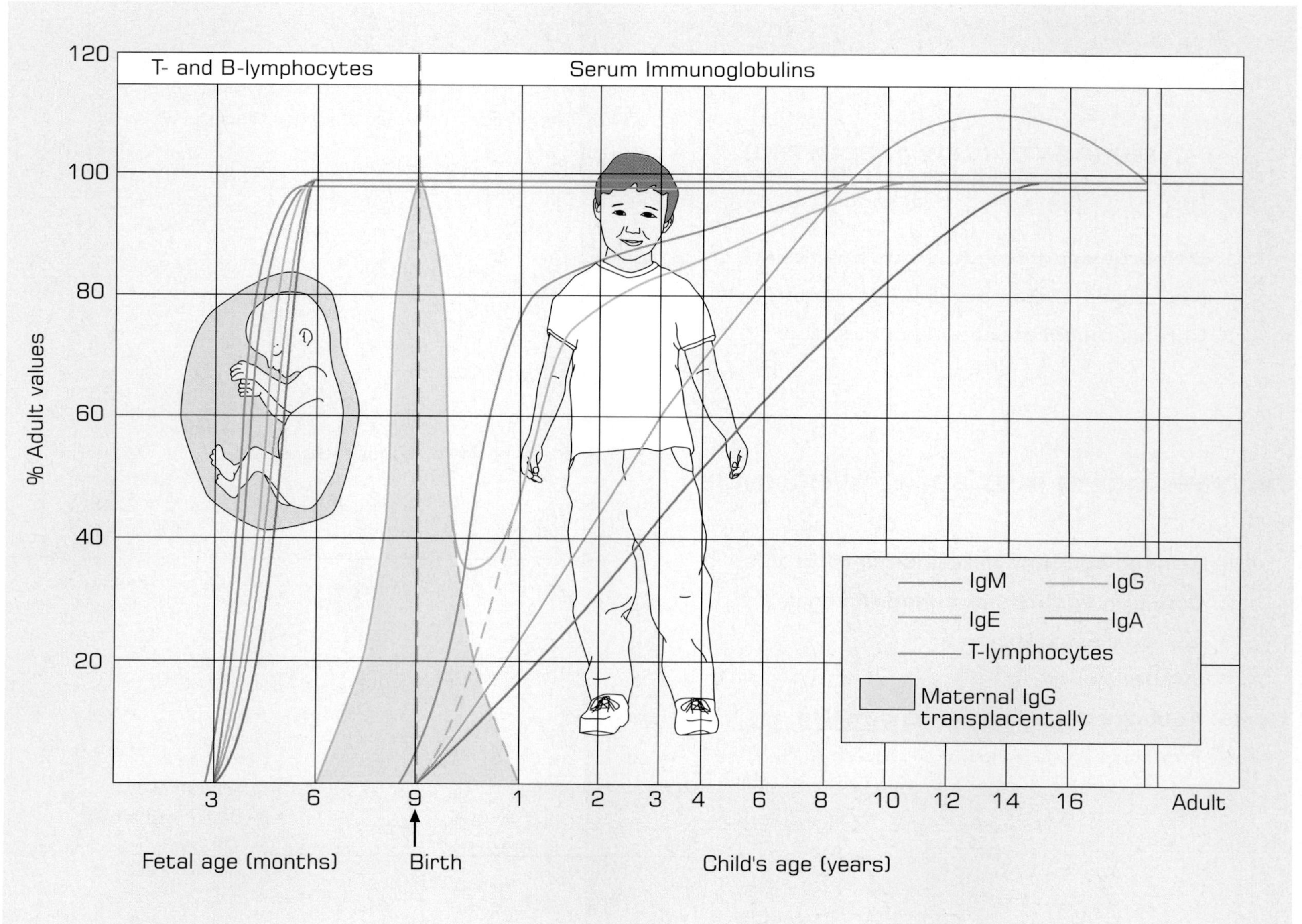

17.9 Both T-lymphocytes and B-lymphocytes appear in fetal tissues as early as at 8–12 weeks' development. B-lymphocytes capable of initiating IgG, IgA, and IgM synthesis are present by 12 weeks of gestation. Serum IgG, IgA, IgM, and IgE as percentages of the normal adult values in the fetus, child, adolescent, and adult.

an intrinsic defect of pre-B to B-cell differentiation due to a defect of B-cell-specific tyrosine kinase (btk). In SCID, a point mutation of the alpha subunit of the IL-2 receptor leads to defective development of T- and B-lymphocytes. Defective synthesis of the CD_{40} ligand required for the immunoglobulin isotype switch from IgM to IgG synthesis has been found in patients with X-linked immunodeficiency with hyper-IgM. In leukocyte adhesion deficiency (LAD), there is an abnormal beta chain subunit of CD_{18}, which results in deficiency of the adhesion protein LFA and several complement receptors (CR_3).

In patients with adenosine deaminase deficiency and SCID, the T- and B-cell deficiencies are due to the toxic metabolites which build up due to the interruption of purine catabolism because of the enzyme deficiency (**17.11**). Adenosine deaminase (ADA) catalyzes the conversions of adenosine into inosine and deoxyadenosine into deoxyinosine; in its absence there is excessive deoxyadenosine which inhibits DNA synthesis. A similar situation exists in patients with PNP deficiency. PNP catalyzes the conversions of inosine into hypoxanthine and of deoxyguanosine into guanine, the step in purine metabolism beyond that catalyzed by ADA (**17.11**). The

CHROMOSOMAL MAP LOCATIONS OF PRIMARY IMMUNODEFICIENCY DISORDERS

Disorder	Chromosome	Locus
X-linked severe combined immunodeficiency	X	q13.1–13.3
X-linked agammaglobulinemia	X	q21.3–22
Immunodeficiency with hyper-IgM	X	q24–27
Wiscott–Aldrich syndrome	X	p11.22–11.3
Adenosine deaminase deficiency	20	q13.11
Purine nucleoside phosphorylase deficiency	14	q13.1
DiGeorge anomaly	22	q11.2 (10p)
Ataxia telangiectasia	11	22–23
Leukocyte adhesion deficiency	21	q22.3

17.10 Chromosomal map locations of primary immunodeficiency disorders.

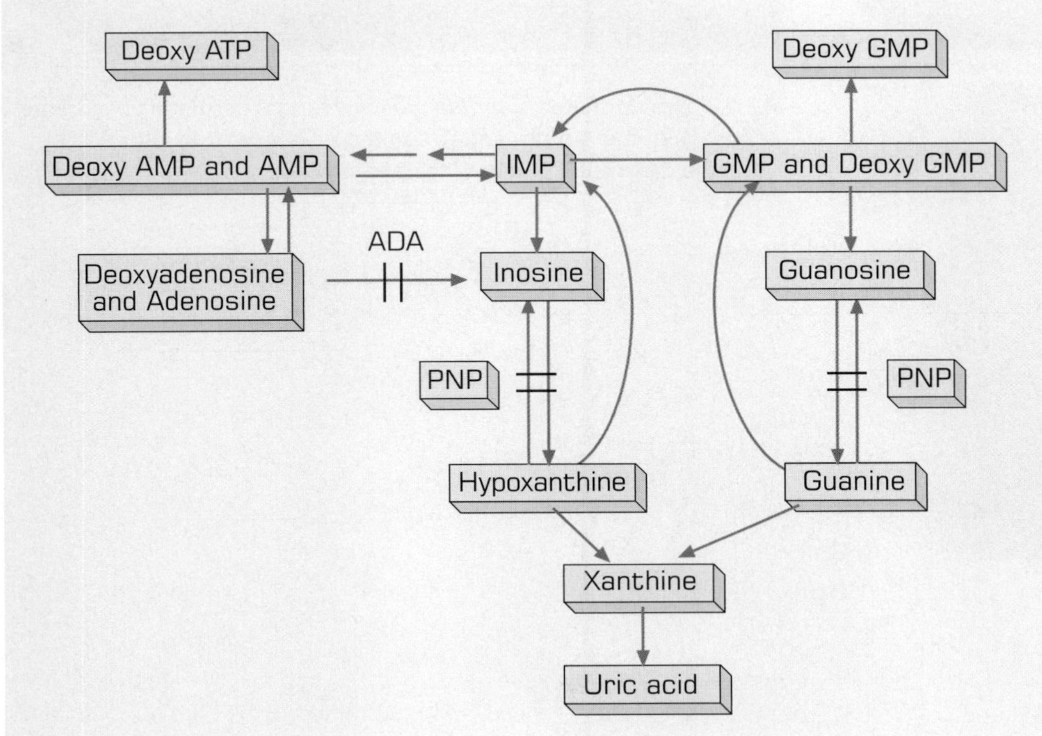

17.11 Steps in the purine catabolic pathway. One form of severe combined immunodeficiency is associated with a defect in adenosine deaminase (ADA), which catalyzes the conversions of adenosine into inosine and deoxyadenosine into deoxyinosine. In purine nucleoside phosphorylase (PNP) deficiency, the enzyme PNP that catalyzes the conversions of inosine into hypoxanthine and guanosine into guanine (and their deoxy derivatives) is absent or abnormal (ATP, adenosine triphosphate; AMP, adenosine monophosphate; IMP, inosine monophosphate; GTP, guanosine triphosphate; GMP, guanosine monophosphate).

excess of deoxyguanosine also inhibits DNA synthesis. It has been postulated that there is greater T- and B-cell immunodeficiency with ADA deficiency than with PNP deficiency because resting T-cells are destroyed by deoxyadenosine, whereas only dividing T-cells are killed by deoxyguanosine. It is anticipated that additional biologic defects in the other immune deficiencies will soon be identified with further refinement of the tools of molecular biology.

CLINICAL PRESENTATIONS

COMBINED T- AND B-LYMPHOCYTE IMMUNODEFICIENCIES

Complete T- and B-cell immunodeficiencies

Severe Combined Immunodeficiency Disease. Severe combined immunodeficiency disease (SCID) is a congenital deficiency of both T- and B-cells that may represent a defect in stem-cell maturation. Sporadic, sex-linked, and autosomal-recessive expressions of SCID have been reported. Inherited deficiency of the enzyme ADA is associated with autosomal-recessive inheritance in 20% of SCID patients, and its pathogenesis involves the accumulation of purine metabolic substrates that are toxic for both T- and B-lymphocytes (see **17.11**).

Infants with deficiencies of both cell-mediated (T-cell) and antibody (B-cell) immunity present with severe, recurrent, bacterial (as well as viral, fungal, and protozoan) infections within the first few months of life. These are often associated with diarrhea. These infants may be suspected as having deficiencies by their poor response to appropriate anti-microbial therapy. Presenting symptoms often include candidiasis (**17.12**). Pneumonia due to *Pneumocystis carinii* or virulent bacteria is common, and the thymus is absent on chest radiography (**17.13**). Hypoplastic tonsils and lymph nodes are also common. Laboratory abnormalities include blood lymphopenia, decreased serum IgG, IgA, and IgM, and defective lymphocyte responses to mitogens, such as phytohemagglutinin. The thymus is histologically dysplastic (**17.14**).

The infant with SCID must be placed in protective isolation and given appropriate supportive therapy, including replacement

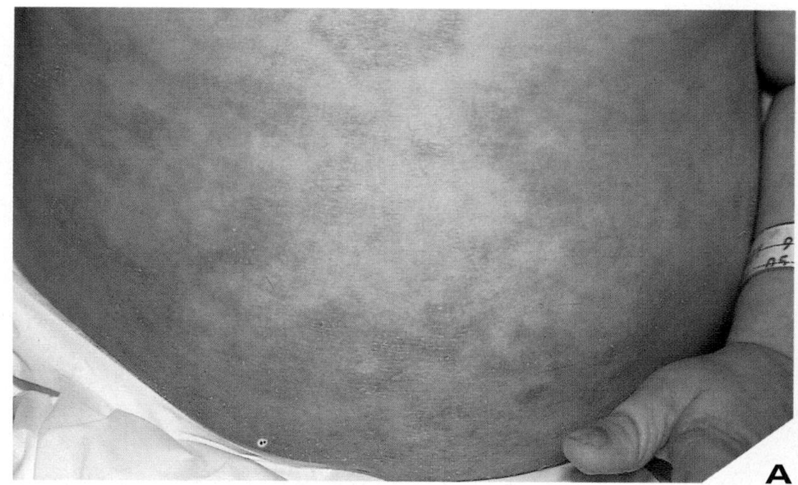

A

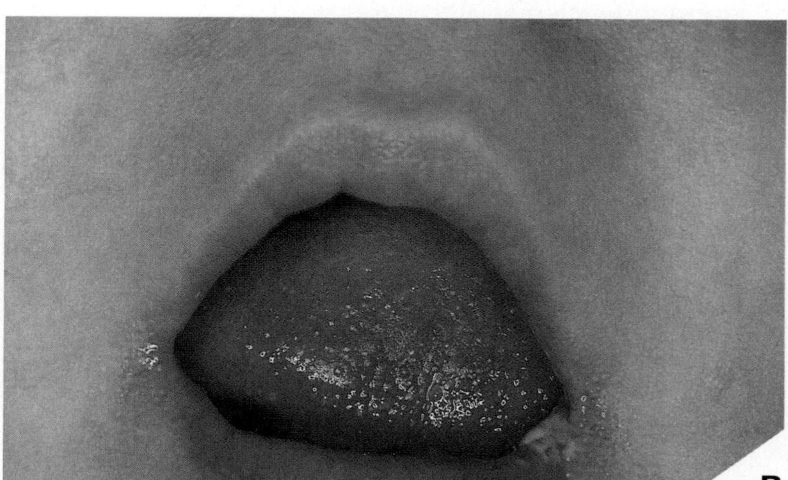

B

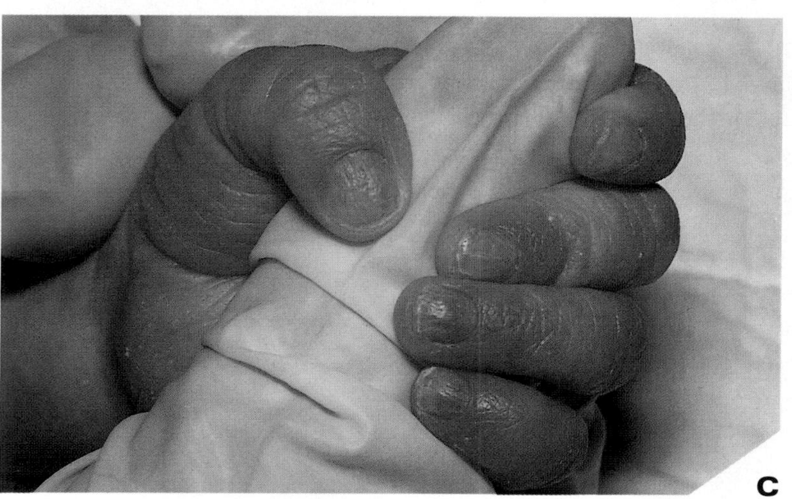

C

17.12 Disseminated *Candida albicans* fungal dermatitis (A) on the trunk, (B) in the mouth, and (C) on the nails of a child with SCID. Note the dystrophic appearance of the nails.

γ-globulin and prophylactic trimethoprim-sulfa anti-microbials. All administered blood products must be irradiated to prevent the potential development of severe graft-versus-host disease. SCID is fatal by 1–2 years of age, unless the patient is immunologically reconstituted by bone marrow transplantation. No live (attenuated) vaccines can be given to these or other immunodeficient patients because of the risk of vaccine infections.

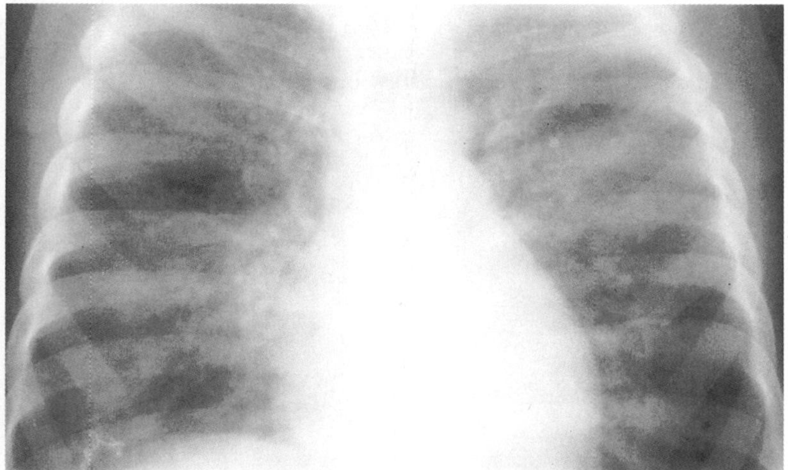

17.13 Chest radiograph of infant with SCID. Note the absent thymic shadow and bilateral pulmonary infiltrates. Sutures indicate the site of lung biopsy which documented the presence of *Pneumocystis carinii.*

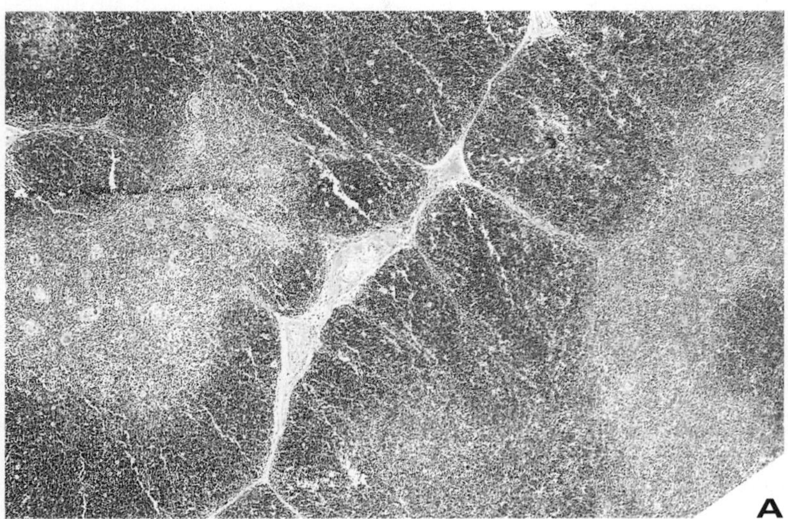

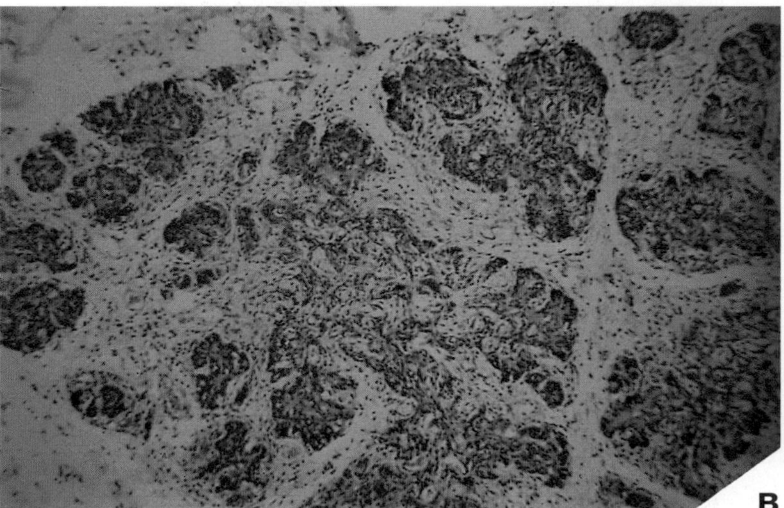

17.14 Histology of (A) the normal thymus as compared to that of (B) the dysplastic thymus found in SCID. Note the lack of normal lobulation and corticomedullary differentation, the decreased numbers of lymphocytes, and the absence of Hassall's corpuscles in the thymus of SCID.

Partial T- and B-cell immunodeficiencies

Wiskott–Aldrich syndrome. Wiskott–Aldrich syndrome is an X-linked recessive disorder characterized by eczema and thrombocytopenia with cutaneous petechiae (**17.15**). The recurrent infections usually begin in infancy. The most commonly reported immunologic defect is the inability to form antibodies to bacterial capsular polysaccharide antigens, but some patients also manifest a partial defect in T-lymphocyte responses.

Ataxia telangiectasia. Ataxia telangiectasia is an autosomal-recessive multi-system syndrome with telangiectasia, progressive ataxia, and variable immunodeficiency. Most patients develop ocular telangiectasia (**17.16**) and cerebellar ataxia during the first 6 years of life. This progressive, variable immunodeficiency consists of selective IgA deficiency and depressed T-cell function. IgG and IgG subclass deficiencies have also been reported. Sinusitis and pulmonary infections are quite frequent. These patients, as well as patients with other immunodeficiencies, have a high incidence of neoplasia.

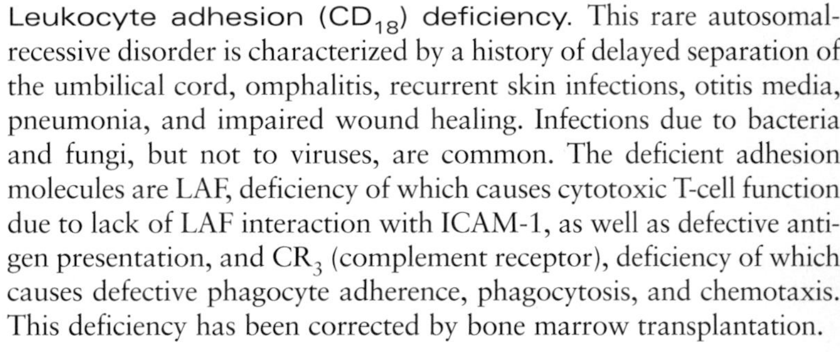

Leukocyte adhesion (CD_{18}) deficiency. This rare autosomal-recessive disorder is characterized by a history of delayed separation of the umbilical cord, omphalitis, recurrent skin infections, otitis media, pneumonia, and impaired wound healing. Infections due to bacteria and fungi, but not to viruses, are common. The deficient adhesion molecules are LAF, deficiency of which causes cytotoxic T-cell function due to lack of LAF interaction with ICAM-1, as well as defective antigen presentation, and CR_3 (complement receptor), deficiency of which causes defective phagocyte adherence, phagocytosis, and chemotaxis. This deficiency has been corrected by bone marrow transplantation.

Hyper-IgE syndrome. Hyper-IgE syndrome is an infrequent autosomal-recessive immunodeficiency characterized by marked increases in serum IgE. Recurrent staphylococcal infections, pruritic eczematoid dermatitis, and coarse facial features are typical (**17.17**). Especially common are recurrent staphylococcal skin infections, including impetigo and furuncles, as well as staphylococcal pneumonia with lung abscesses and pneumatocele formation (**17.18**). Candidiasis is frequent. Immunologic findings include

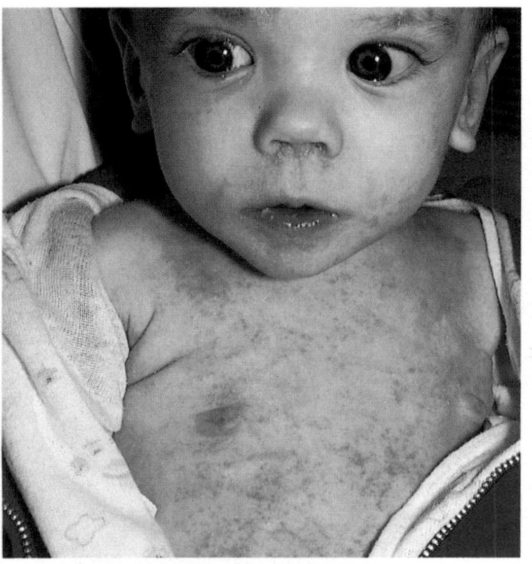

17.15 Child with Wiskott–Aldrich syndrome. The skin eruptions on the trunk and face are eczematoid and pruritic, but not always similar to atopic dermatitis in flexural distribution. Many of these patients have thrombocytopenia, which results in petechiae of varying distribution and intensity.

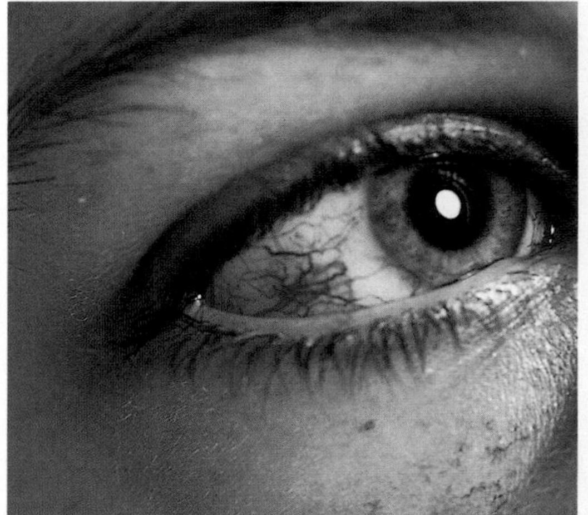

17.16 Scleral telangiectasia typical of ataxia telangiectasia. Other findings characteristic of this disorder include cerebellar ataxia and variable T- and B-cell immunity. (Reproduced with permission from Skoner *et al.*, 1992.)

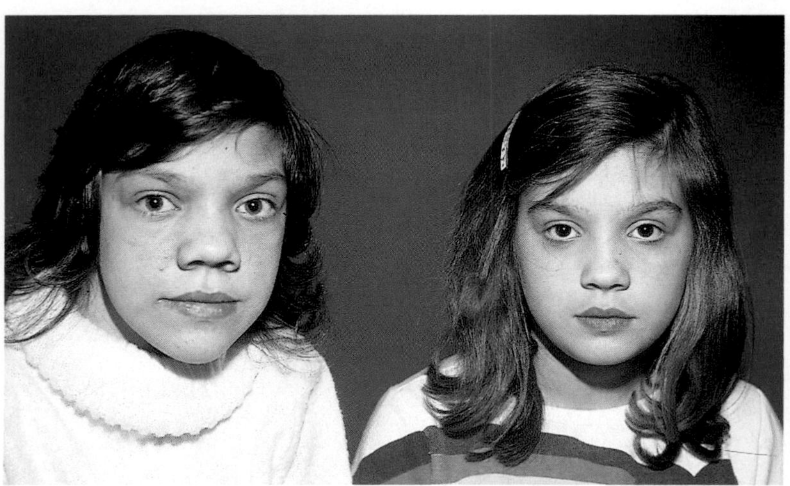

17.17 Coarse facial features of female with hyper-IgE syndrome (left). Her sister (right) has an IgA deficiency. Although distinct syndromes, these illustrate the frequency with which immune deficiencies are observed in family members of IgA deficient patients. (Reproduced with permission from Skoner *et al.*, 1992.)

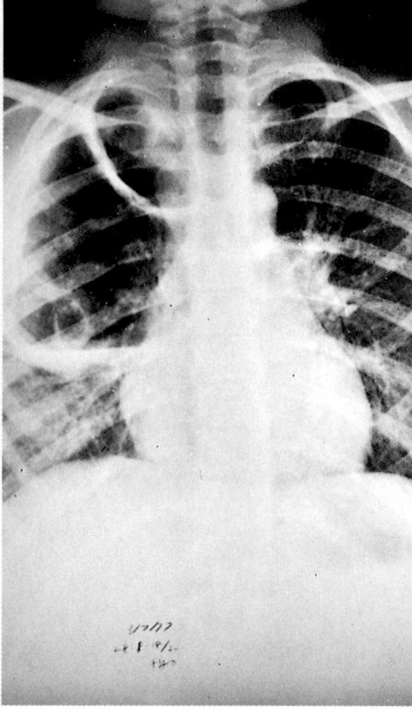

17.18 Clearly defined pneumatocele in the right lung of a patient with hyper-IgE syndrome. This type of lesion is frequently associated with *S. aureus* pneumonia. (Reproduced with permission from Skoner *et al.*, 1992.)

eosinophilia, elevated IgE levels, abnormal cell-mediated immunity, and, in certain patients, abnormal leukocyte chemotaxis.

Acquired immunodeficiency syndrome. Acquired immunodeficiency syndrome (AIDS) is a secondary immunodeficiency disorder caused by the human immunodeficiency virus (HIV). As outlined in **17.19**, those at risk to develop AIDS include homosexuals, intravenous drug abusers, recipients of contaminated blood products (hemophiliacs), Haitians, and infants born to infected mothers. Since its initial description in 1978, many millions of infections and clinical cases, including infants and children, have been reported world-wide; the illness has achieved epidemic proportions. The non-specific complaints of fatigue, malaise, weight loss, fever, and lymphadenopathy may be present for up to one year before infection becomes apparent. Approximately 30% of cases present with skin lesions and tumors consistent with Kaposi's sarcoma (**17.20**). The remaining 70% have undue susceptibility to infection with *Cytomegalovirus, Cryptococcus, Toxoplasma, Herpes, Candida,* or *Mycobaterium* species. The most frequent and devastating infection is due to *P. carinii,* which often leads to pneumonia, disseminated disease, and eventually death. Predisposing these patients to the infectious and malignant complications is a T-cell immune dysfunction. Laboratory tests show lymphopenia, cutaneous delayed hypersensitivity anergy, a marked decrease in CD_4 T-helper cells, and an increase in CD_8 T-suppressor cells. Lymphocyte stimulation with mitogens and antigens is decreased. Serum immunoglobulins are usually increased, but antibody response can be altered.

A screening test to detect antibodies to the HIV organism has been developed, but a positive result only indicates prior exposure to the virus. Since many antibody-positive individuals are totally asymptomatic, the percentage of exposed persons who will ultimately develop AIDS is, as yet, unknown. γ-Globulin supplemental therapy is beneficial in pediatric AIDS patients, but not in adults. Supportive therapy with anti-microbials and agents such as azidothymidine (AZT) is helpful, but definitive therapy is not available. The development of a vaccine to prevent this syndrome and its epidemic spread is needed.

PEOPLE AT RISK OF DEVELOPING AIDS

1. Homosexuals
2. Intravenous drug abusers
3. Recipients of contaminated blood products (e.g., hemophiliacs)
4. Haitians
5. Infants born to infected mothers

17.19 Populations at increased risk of developing AIDS.

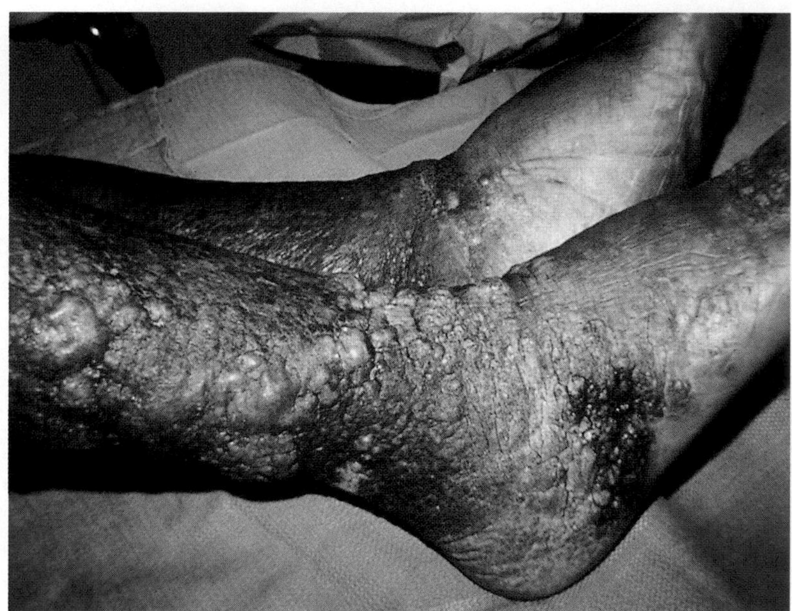

17.20 Cutaneous manifestations of Kaposi's sarcoma. The purplish, hyperpigmented plaques and nodules, with edema of the lower extremities, are characteristic of the condition. (Reproduced with permission from Skoner *et al.*, 1992.)

T-LYMPHOCYTE (CELLULAR) IMMUNODEFICIENCIES

DiGeorge syndrome (anomaly)

DiGeorge syndrome is characterized by deficient T-lymphocytes with normal or near-normal B-lymphocytes, serum IgG, IgA, and IgM. This pure T-cell deficiency results from the abnormal development of the third and fourth branchial pouches during embryogenesis and manifests thymic hypoplasia. Since the parathyroid gland and the cardiovascular system also develop from the same branchial pouches, these patients frequently present with signs of hypocalcemic tetany, seizures, and congenital heart disease within the first few days of life. Associated abnormalities may include esophageal atresia, hypothyroidism, and unusual facies (**17.21**). Because of these multiple anomalies, it has been proposed that this condition be designated DiGeorge anomaly; it may be a polytypic field defect of diverse etiology involving cephalic neural crest cells. The thymus provides the appropriate microenvironment for lymphoid tissue to mature into functioning T-lymphocytes. With a defective thymus, normal T-cell development does not occur and the T-cell immunodeficiency may manifest as overwhelming infection with fungi or viruses. Yet, the T-cell defect may be transient, resolving spontaneously. These infants have been successfully reconstituted with fetal thymus implants.

Purine nucleoside phosphorylase deficiency

Purine nucleoside phosphorylase deficiency is a rare autosomal-recessive disorder. Deficiency of this enzyme of the purine salvage pathways results in the accumulation of toxic deoxyribonucleotides with progressive lymphopenia and poor response of T-cells to mitogens. The humoral (B-cell) immunity remains virtually unimpaired. In addition to recurrent opportunistic infections, these patients are predisposed to lymphoproliferative disorders, such as lymphoma.

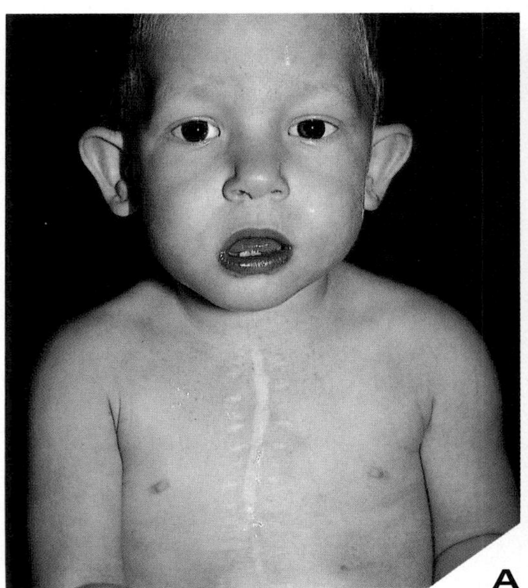

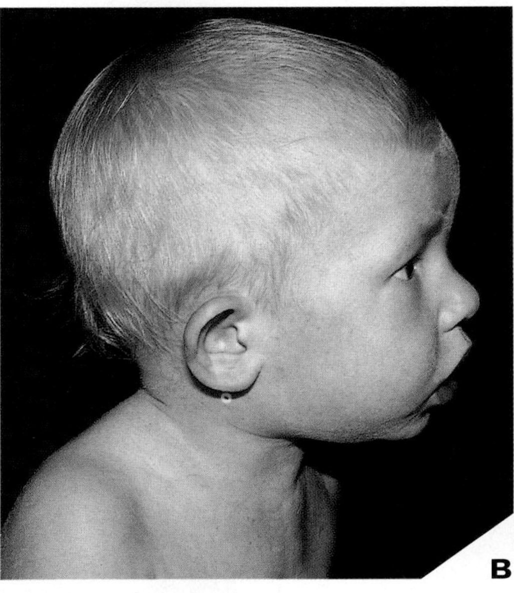

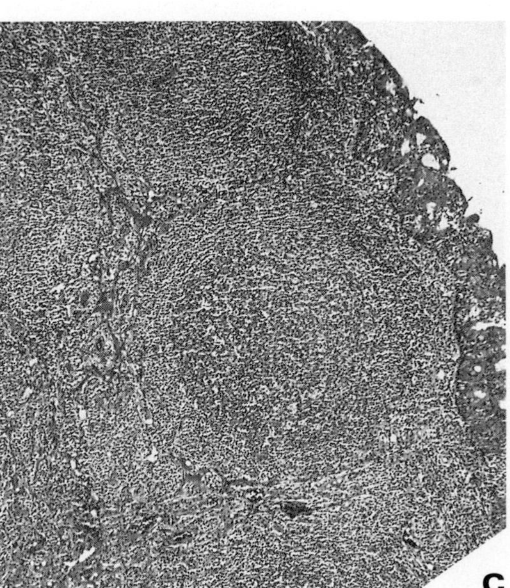

17.21 Facial features of a child with DiGeorge syndrome: (A) frontal and (B) Lateral views. Note the micrognathia, hypertelorism, and malformation of the ears, and midline thoracotomy scar following repair of a congenital heart defect. (C) Photomicrograph of a resected adenoid from a child with an isolated T-cell defect associated with DiGeorge syndrome. The lymphoid follicles are well-formed, having light and dark portions, and a surrounding mantle of small cells. However, the paracortex between the follicles is virtually devoid of lymphoid T-cells. Immunoglobulin-producing plasma cells are present. This lymphoid tissue is a mirror image of that shown in **17.24B**. hematoxylin and eosin × 121. (A and B: Reproduced with permission from Skoner *et al.*, 1992; C: Courtesy of Dr. Ronald Jaffe.)

Chronic mucocutaneous candidiasis

Chronic mucocutaneous candidiasis is characterized by superficial, persistent, and recurrent candidial infections of the mucous membranes, skin, and nails (**17.22**). Endocrinopathy is often associated, and variants of this syndrome may include hypoparathyroidism and polyendocrinopathy. This illness may be sporadic or familial, and the age of onset of symptoms varies. Immunologic abnormalities include absence of delayed cutaneous hypersensitivity to *Candida* and lack of lymphokine production by *Candida*-stimulated lymphocytes. T- and B-cell enumeration, as well as serum immunoglobulins and functional antibodies, appear normal. Long-term antifungal therapy with ketoconazole, administered orally, has resulted in dramatic clinical improvement and decreased morbidity (**17.23**). Treatment with cytokine transfer factor is sometimes helpful.

B-CELL (ANTIBODY) IMMUNODEFICIENCIES

Congenital hypogammaglobulinemia

Congenital hypogammaglobulinemia, also referred to as Bruton-type agammaglobulinemia, may be X-linked or autosomal-recessive. During the first few months of life, affected infants usually appear clinically well due to placentally acquired maternal antibodies. As the maternal antibodies are catabolized, however, these infants develop recurrent or chronic infections with virulent bacterial pathogens, such as *Streptococcus pneumoniae* and *Haemophilius influenzae*. Upper and lower respiratory tract infections, such as sinusitis, otitis media, and pneumonia, are most common.

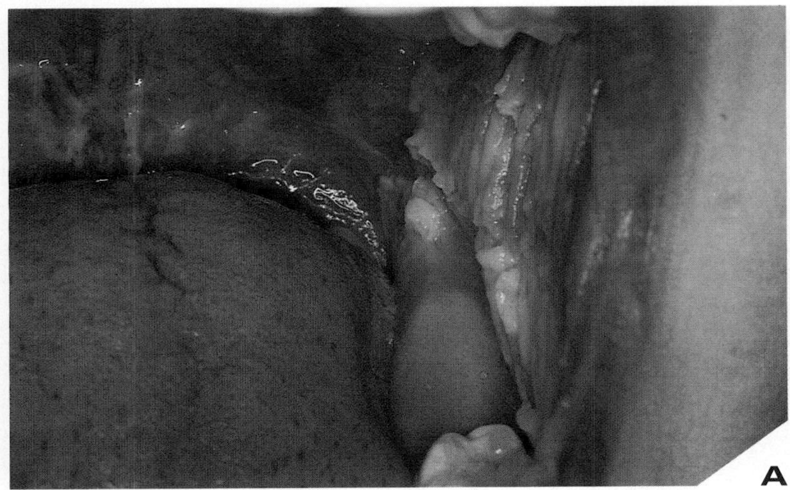

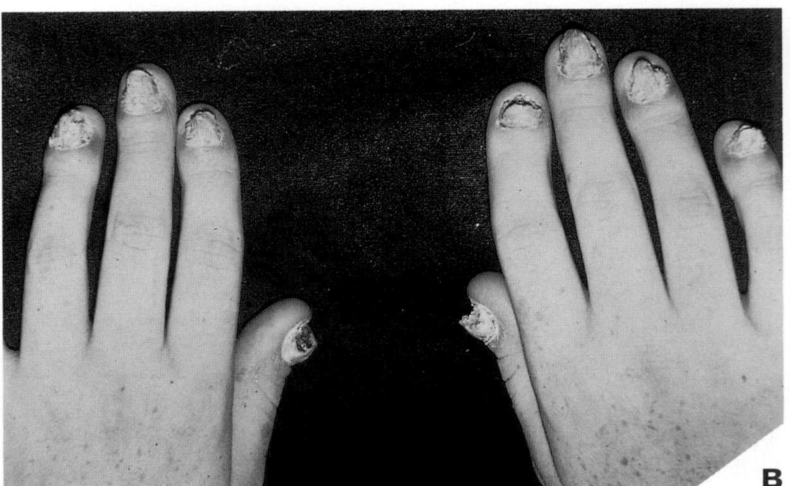

17.22 Diffuse mucocutaneous involvement with *C. albicans* in a patient with chronic mucocutaneous candidiasis. Lesions involving (A) the oral mucosal surfaces and (B) the nail beds are almost always present and recalcitrant to therapy with topical anti-fungal agents.

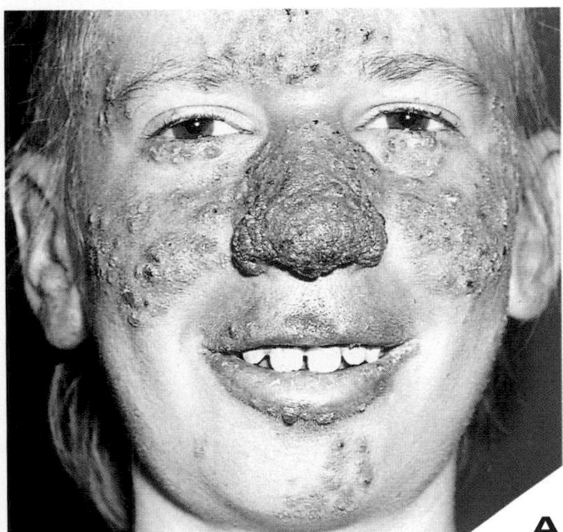

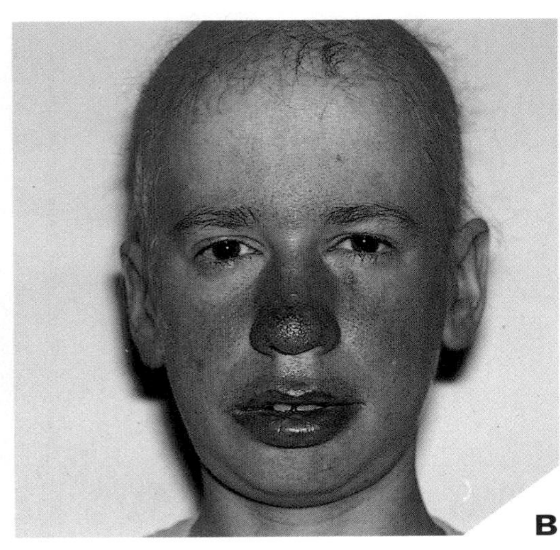

17.23 Patient with chronic mucocutaneous candidiasis (A) before and (B) after treatment with oral ketoconazole. (Reproduced with permission from Skoner *et al.*, 1992.)

Sepsis, meningitis, and skin infections also occur. As a result of these infections, bronchiectasis develops with chronic cough, increased sputum production, and abnormal chest radiographs (**17.24**). These children have little adenoidal, tonsillar, and other lymphoid tissues (**17.25**); what lymphoid tissues they do possess lack plasma cells able to produce immunoglobulin, and lack the ability to form germinal follicles in response to antigen (see **17.24B**). In any child who has recurrent infections with virulent bacterial pathogens, the diagnosis of hypogammaglobulinemia should be considered and confirmed by finding markedly decreased serum IgG, IgA, or IgM. Survival to adulthood is possible with early diagnosis, accompanied by monthly γ-globulin replacement and antibiotic therapy directed against the infectious organisms. Recently, the genetic abnormality has been identified as mutations and/or deletions in the Bruton tyrosine kinase (Btk) encoding gene.

Common variable immunodeficiency

Common variable immunodeficiency patients also present with recurrent infections. There is considerable variability in the clinical course of this syndrome, as well as in the serum IgG, IgA, and IgM levels (which on occasion may even appear normal). Unlike congenital hypogammaglobulinemia, B-cells are usually present in the blood and tissues of common variable immunodeficiency patients, even though tissue plasma cells are deficient. Beside recurrent respiratory tract infections, these patients frequently have gastrointestinal complaints and may manifest gastroenteropathy. They also have an increased number of autoantibodies and may manifest symptoms of collagen-vascular disease. Documentation of functional antibody deficiency is helpful. Defective T-cell immunoregulation has been described in a few patients, but clinical expression of T-cell deficiency is rarely observed.

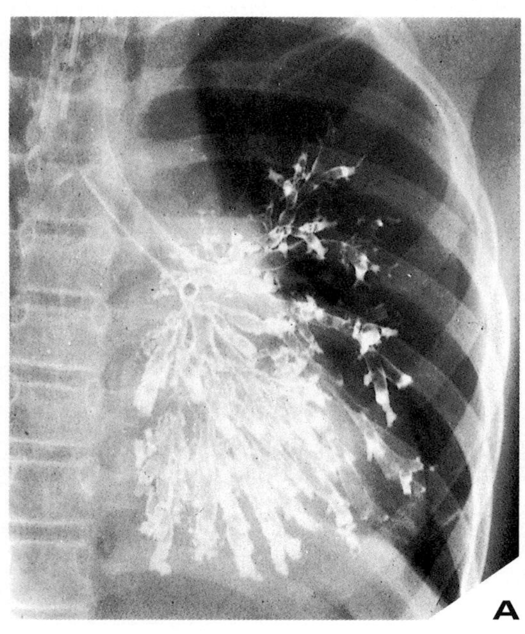

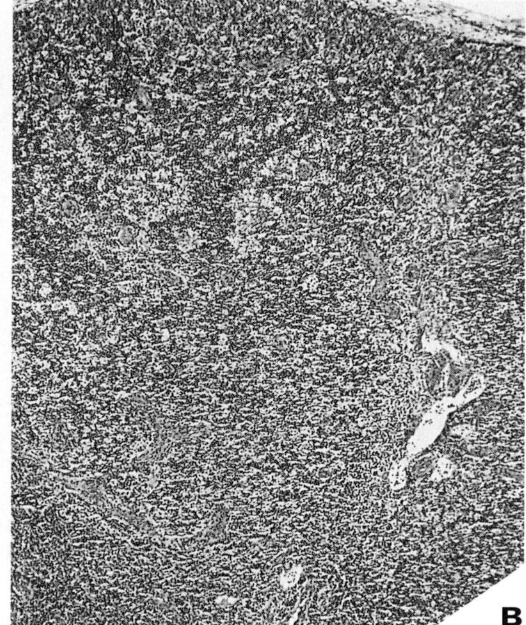

17.24 (A) Bronchogram demonstrating bronchiectasis of the left lower lobe in an older child with hypogammaglobulinemia. Symptoms consisted of chronic cough and sputum production. The child was treated with antibiotics and γ-globulin replacement. (B) Low-power photomicrograph of a lymph node biopsy from a 1-year-old child with hypogammaglobulinemia. No lymphoid follicles are visible, and no germinal centers are detected. Most of the node is paracortex, characterized by the presence of high-walled venules and a 'starry sky' appearance. No immunoglobulin-producing plasma cells were detected in this section. The tissue is a mirror image of that shown in *Figure 17.21C*. (Hematoxylin and eosin stain × 121). (A: Reproduced with permission from Skoner *et al.*, 1992; B: Courtesy of Dr. Ronald Jaffe.)

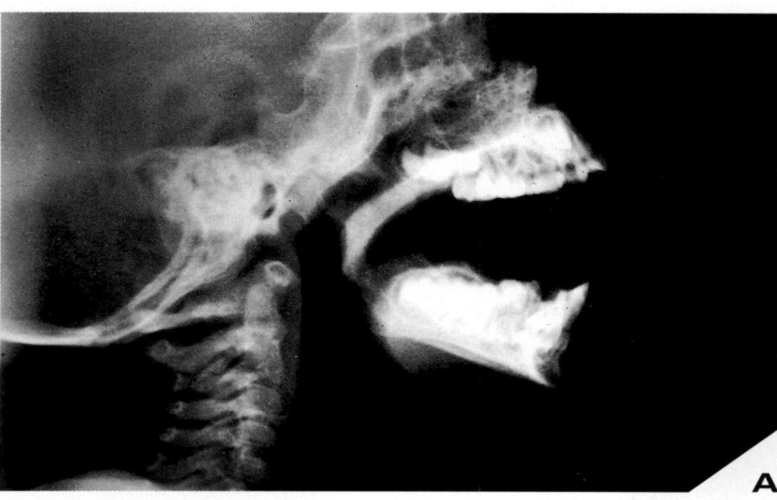

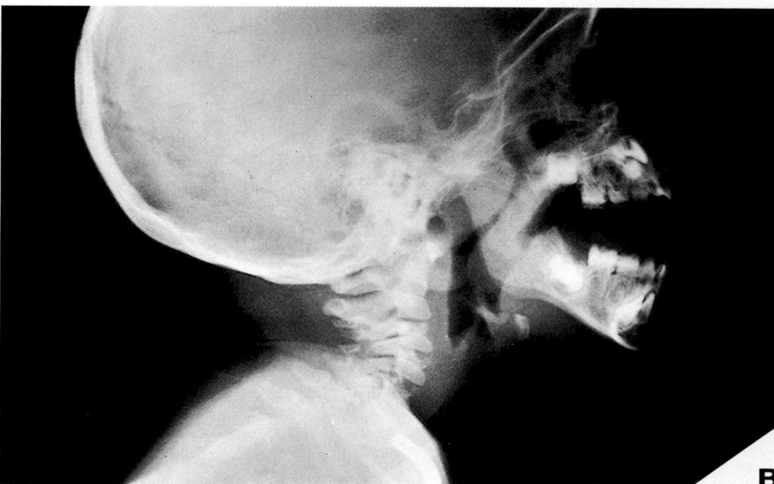

17.25 (A) Lateral neck radiograph showing absent adenoid shadow in a child with congenital hypogammaglobulinemia. (B) Lateral neck radiograph showing normal adenoid shadows in a child with no immunodeficiency. (Reproduced with permission from Skoner *et al.*, 1992.)

IgG subclass deficiency

IgG consists of four subclasses, IgG_1, IgG_2, IgG_3, and IgG_4. The IgG_1 subclass accounts for 60% of total IgG, and shows antibody activity to most microbial protein antigens, such as tetanus and diphtheria. The IgG_2 subclass accounts for 20% of total IgG and contains antibodies to microbial polysaccharide antigens, such as *S. pneumoniae* and *H. influenzae* capsular antigens. IgG_3 antibody activities make up about 15% of the total IgG. A portion of the IgG_4 antibodies may mimic IgE antibody, with its capacity to initiate histamine release from basophils and mast cells.

Some patients with recurrent infections and IgA deficiency or low normal IgG levels have been found to have a deficiency of IgG_1 and/or IgG_2. These patients have recurrent infections of the respiratory tract, but do not usually have a paucity of lymphoid tissue. Laboratory confirmation of these IgG subclass deficiencies also requires documentation of functional antibody deficiency prior to initiation of replacement IgG therapy.

Immunodeficiency with hyper-IgM

This X-linked recessive disease of males is characterized by low IgG and IgA, but normal or elevated polyclonal IgM, with normal numbers of B-lymphocytes. The numbers of T-lymphocytes are also normal, and there is normal T-cell function. These patients have increased and recurrent pyrogenic respiratory tract infections, and may also have neutropenia and manifest autoimmune disorders. They benefit from gammaglobulin therapy. The abnormal gene has been identified as the ligand for CD_{40} on B-cells, and this may provide for future gene therapy.

Selective IgA deficiency

Selective IgA deficiency is the most common humoral antibody deficiency, affecting about one out of every 500 individuals. Only about 50% of these affected individuals manifest symptoms, while the other 50%, despite mucosal, secretory, and serum IgA deficiencies, are clinically well and asymptomatic. These patients may have normal IgG and IgM immunoglobulins. Most cases are sporadic, but siblings may manifest IgA or other immunodeficiencies. Recurrent infections of the sinuses (**17.26**) and middle ear are frequent, but lower respiratory disease is unusual, unless another form of immunodeficiency, such as IgG_2 subclass deficiency, co-exists with the IgA deficiency. IgA-deficient patients have an increased incidence of allergy, chronic diarrhea, neoplasia, collagen vascular disorders, and autoimmune syndromes.

Transient hypogammaglobulinemia of infancy

Transient hypogammaglobulinemia of infancy is a self-limited antibody deficiency that begins at 3–6 months of age and usually lasts 6–18 months. These infants may or may not have increased susceptibility to infection, and physical examination may reveal a paucity of tonsils and lymph nodes. This, however, is not always the case. Thrush is uncommon. These infants show the usual decline in placentally transferred immunoglobulins over the first months of life, but they fail to synthesize IgG until much later than normal. Serum IgM and IgA develop normally and help distinguish transient hypogammaglobulinemia from congenital hypogammaglobulinemia. Circulating B-cells are normal or near-normal in number and distribution, and a thymus is present on chest radiography. These patients have normal antibody responses to diphtheria and tetanus toxoids, usually well before the IgG levels become normal. Premature infants are especially prone to this disorder because of the lower levels of transplacental IgG at birth (*see* **17.9**). While temporary exogenous γ-globulin replacement therapy is occasionally used, spontaneous recovery usually ensues by 9–15 months of age. Levels of immunoglobulins become normal by 2–4 years of age. Following recovery, there is no recurrence or evidence of permanent immune-system abnormality.

PHAGOCYTIC DISORDERS

Polymorphonuclear leukocytes and mononuclear cells play vital roles in the defense against acute infections. Normal neutrophil numbers, intact neutrophil chemotaxis, phagocytosis, and intracellular killing are all necessary for the rapid elimination of microorganisms that invade skin or mucous membranes. Neutropenia may be the result of decreased production, which has been associated with adverse reactions to medications or has an autoimmune basis. Patients with neutropenia are highly vulnerable to bacterial infections, as are other patients with disorders of phagocyte function (**17.27**).

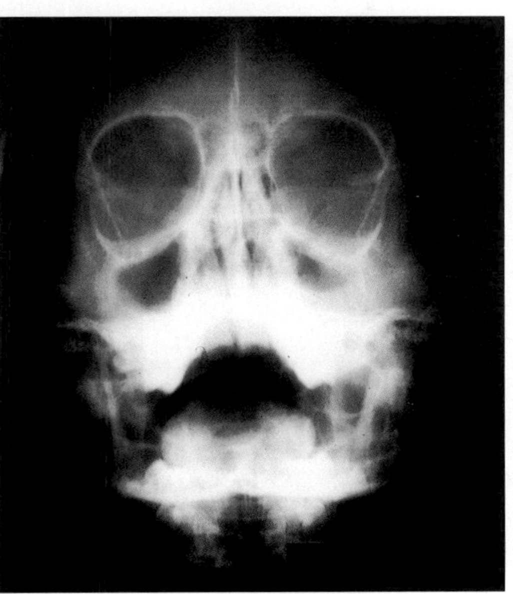

17.26 Maxillary sinusitis in a child with IgA deficiency. (Courtesy of Dr Gilbert Friday.)

PHAGOCYTIC DISORDERS

Defects of microbicidal activity
- Chronic granulomatous disease
- Myeloperoxidase deficiency
- Chediak–Higashi syndrome
- Glucose-6-phosphate dehydrogenase deficiency

Defects of cell locomotion
- Hyper-IgE syndrome
- Actin dysfunction
- Glycoprotein deficiency
- Adhesion molecule deficiency

17.27 Diseases characterized by phagocytic dysfunction or deficiency.

Chronic granulomatous disease

Chronic granulomatous disease is one example of neutrophil dysfunction. Phagocytosis and chemotaxis are intact, but the killing of ingested microorganisms is defective, due to an abnormal leukocyte oxidative metabolism. Intracellular survival of ingested bacteria, even those not typically associated with granuloma formation, can lead to the development of granulomatous lesions. This syndrome usually expresses X-linked recessive inheritance, but females are occasionally affected. These patients become symptomatic early in life, and the presenting complaints include severe, recurrent *Staphyloccocus aureus* infections of the skin and lymph nodes that heal slowly. Suppurative infections often require surgical drainage in addition to antibiotics. Pneumonitis develops into pneumatoceles, and osteomyelitis is common. Hepatosplenomegaly is a constant finding and granulomatous inflammations and involvement of the reticuloendothelial system are typical. Therapy with interferon and antibiotics, especially trimethoprim sulfa, appears beneficial.

COMPLEMENT SYSTEM DISORDERS

The complement system, comprising nine distinct serum proteins designated C_1–C_9, is activated by immune reactions via either the classic or alternative complement pathways. Complement immune functions include:

- Enhancement of phagocytosis (opsonization).
- Viral neutralization.
- Mediation of inflammation via chemotaxis.
- Alteration of vascular permeability.
- Cell lysis.
- Modulation of the immune response.

Although rare, inherited quantitative or functional deficiencies of the complement components have been reported. Their clinical presentations vary, but collagen vascular diseases and recurrent pyrogenic infections predominate.

MUCOSAL AND SKIN BARRIER DISORDERS

Mucosa and skin are crucial barriers in preventing the entrance of microbes and antigens into the body. Host respiratory and gastrointestinal mucosal defense mechanisms are aided by secretory antibodies (predominantly IgA) in the pharynx, bronchi, and intestines. In addition, other factors such as salivary lysozyme, intestinal enzymes, and forceful coughing help in the removal of pathogens.

Dysfunctional cilia syndrome

Initially reported by Kartagener, the dysfunctional cilia syndrome is characterized by defective mucociliary transport and the triad of chronic sinusitis, bronchiectasis, and situs inversus viscerum (**17.28**), although situs inversus is not universal. Some patients are infertile with poorly motile spermatozoa. The ciliary dysfunction impedes mucous clearance and produces the following:

- Early onset of chronic rhinorrhea.
- Chronic otitis media.
- Nasal polyps.
- Chronic sinusitis with opaque sinuses on radiography.
- Chronic productive cough.
- Bronchiectasis.
- Digital clubbing.

Electron microscopic analysis of cilia obtained from biopsy of the nasal or tracheobronchal mucosa (**17.29**) or analysis of spermatozoa documents the abnormality. Therapy with antibiotics is supportive.

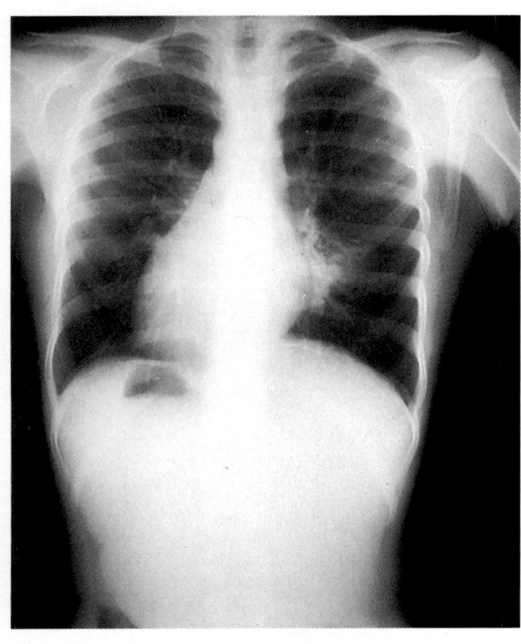

17.28 Dextrocardia and situs invertus of abdominal organs in a patient with Kartagener's syndrome and dysfunctional cilia syndrome. The abnormal ciliary motion is thought to result in malrotation during embryrogenesis. (Reproduced with permission from Skoner *et al.*, 1992.)

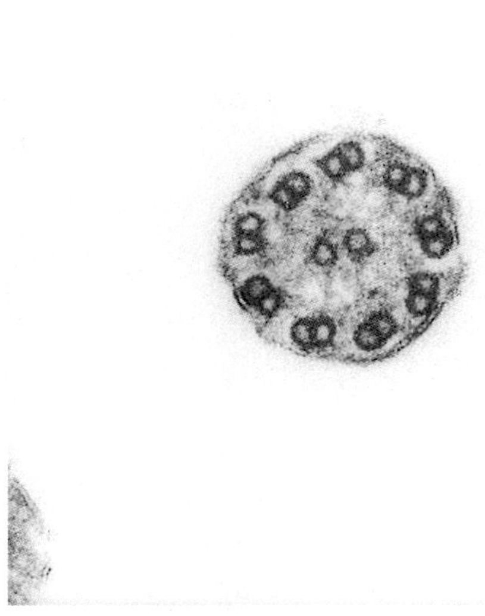

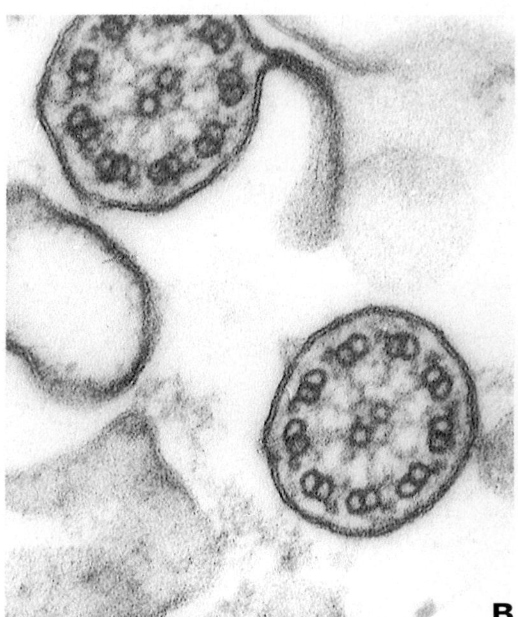

17.29 (A) Electron micrograph of cilia from patient with dysfunctional cilia syndrome. Note the absence of dynein arms from the outer doublets. (B) Normal cilia with dynein arms. (Reproduced with permission from Bluestone and Stool, 1983.)

DIAGNOSIS

In all cases of immunodeficiency, laboratory tests are needed to confirm the diagnosis. If a B- or T-cell immunodeficiency is suspected, the initial laboratory tests (**17.30**) include a complete blood count (CBC), with differential and platelet count, and measurement of IgG, IgM, and IgA serum levels. A CBC establishes anemia, thrombocytopenia, or neutropenia. A lymphopenia (less than 1500 cells/ml^3) suggests T-cell immunodeficiency. Serum immunoglobulin levels must be interpreted carefully, with an eye toward age variations. In older children and adults, an IgG level of less than 300 mg/dl indicates a significant antibody deficiency.

Usually, if the screening tests are all normal, most B-cell immunodeficiency diseases can be excluded. However, if the history is unusually suspicious, further advanced testing must be done. In immunized subjects, antibody titers to tetanus, diphtheria, rubella, poliovirus, *H. influenza*, or *S. pneumoniae* antigens can be used to estimate IgG function. In non-immunized patients, antibody titers should be obtained before and 2 weeks after tetanus or other immunizations. An inadequate response (less than a four-fold rise in titer) is suggestive of antibody deficiency, regardless of the immunoglobulin levels. Immunodeficient patients should never be immunized with live (attenuated) vaccines, because they may be unable to inactivate the attenuated organisms.

All humans, except young infants and individuals with blood type AB, have IgM isoagglutinins (anti-A and/or anti-B antibodies). These antibodies are selectively deficient in certain immunodeficiencies (e.g., Wiskott–Aldrich syndrome). IgG subclass determinations are indicated if IgG levels are normal or near-normal, but antibody function is deficient. These determinations should also be done in symptomatic, selective IgA deficiency, since IgG_2 subclass deficiency is present in some of these cases. If local infections are severe, secretory IgA levels (e.g., in tears or saliva) can be measured. If immunoglobulin levels are low, enumeration of B-cells should be performed. Normally, 5–10% of peripheral blood lymphocytes are surface membrane immunoglobulin-positive. Isolated absences of IgE are rare and of not much clinical significance. IgE levels are high in chemotactic disorders, partial T-cell immunodeficiencies, allergic disorders, and parasitism.

The presence of lymphopenia is suggestive of a T-cell immunodeficiency; however, lymphopenia may not always be present. An absent thymic shadow on a chest roentgenogram in the newborn period is suggestive of T-cell deficiency, particularly before the onset of infection or other stress that may shrink the thymus. Delayed hypersensitivity skin tests with *Candida* are valuable in screening for T-cell deficiencies after 1 year of age.

In advanced evaluation of cellular immunodeficiencies, enumeration of T-lymphocytes is essential (see **17.30**). Most laboratories use various monoclonal mouse antisera that react with T-cell surface receptors, thus allowing enumeration of T-cell subpopulations by fluorescent microscopy or automated fluorescent-activated cell sorting. CD_8 monoclonal antibodies define suppressor/cytotoxic T-cells and CD_4 monoclonal antibodies define helper/inducer T-lymphocytes. The ratio between helper and suppressor T-cells, which is normally about 2:1, may be characteristically reversed in AIDS, thus providing valuable diagnostic information. Monoclonal antibodies are also available to identify activated T-cells, natural killer cells, and other T-cell receptors. Other useful 'advanced' tests measure lymphocyte proliferation when cultured in the presence of mitogens (e.g., phytohemagglutinin, concanavalin A, irradiated allogeneic leukocytes) or antigens (e.g., tetanus, *Candida)* to which the patient has been previously exposed. T-cell immunodeficiencies manifest low proliferative responses. Procedures are also available to assess production of cytokines following mitogenic or antigenic

LABORATORY TESTS IN B-CELL AND T-CELL IMMUNODEFICIENCIES

	Screening tests	Advanced tests
B-cell deficiency	IgG, IgM, IgA serum levels Pre-existing Ab: e.g., polio, rubella, tetanus, diphtheria, isoagglutinins	B-cell enumeration IgG subclass, IgE levels Lateral pharyngeal roentgenogram for adenoid size Ab responses to vaccines such as tetanus, killed polio, pneumococcal polysaccharide, etc.
T-cell deficiency	Lymphocyte count and morphology Thymic size by chest roentgenogram Delayed skin tests – e.g., *Candida*, Trichophyton, tetanus toxoid	T-cell enumeration Proliferative responses to mitogens, antigens, allogenic cells T-cell subsets, including CD_4/CD_8 Cytokine, MIF assays Enzyme assays (ADA, PNP) Adhesion molecules

Abbreviations: Ab, antibody; ADA, adenosine deaminase; MIF, migration inhibition factor; CD_4, T-helper; CD_8, T-suppressor; PNP, purine nucleoside phosphorylase.

17.30 Laboratory tests for diagnosis of B- and T-cell immunodeficiencies.

stimulation (e.g., migration inhibition factor deficiency in chronic mucocutaneous candidiasis). In some forms of T-cell immunodeficiency, enzymes of the purine pathway, ADA or PNP, are deficient and can be assayed. A lymph node biopsy may be indicated in the presence of lymphadenopathy or to exclude malignancy. Finally, biopsies of the skin, liver, or thymus may be of value in certain patients.

Tests for phagocytic and complement deficiencies (**17.31**) are indicated in patients with convincing histories of immunodeficiency, but normal B- and T-cell immunity. In addition to a CBC, initial screening should include determination of IgE levels and a nitroblue tetrazolium (NBT) dye test. The advanced tests include special staining of the granulocytes and quantitative assays for myeloperoxidase, alkaline phosphatase, and esterase. Phagocytosis is also assessed by measuring the uptake of latex particles or bacteria by isolated granulocytes or monocytes. Then, microbial killing by neutrophils is measured. Cell movement can be assessed by a Rebuck skin window, in which the skin is superficially abraded with a scalpel and coverslips placed over this site. An abnormality of chemotaxis can be confirmed by an *in vitro* chemotactic assay in which one measures migration of granulocytes or monocytes toward a chemoattractant using a chemotactic Boyden chamber. Other specialized tests to define phagocytic defects include assays for granulocyte oxidant product (chemoluminescence, superoxide) and granulocyte mobilization.

Screening for complement abnormalities is done by measuring total activity (CH_{50}) and serum C_3 and C_4 levels. Low levels of these may be followed by the measurement of the individual components of complement. Assays of serum opsonic, chemotactic, or bactericidal activities can also be used to assess complement function.

PREVENTION AND TREATMENT

REPLACEMENT THERAPIES

The recognition of immunodeficiency as the basis for a patient's recurrent infections calls for prompt implementation of a treatment program that will not only reverse the clinical course of the current infection, but will also prevent the patient's undue susceptibility to future infection. As outlined in **17.32**, this approach requires the availability of therapeutic procedures or agents that will correct, replace, or modulate the host's immune deficiency. The first such therapeutic agent was γ-globulin, pooled from human sera that showed antibody activity. In 1953, Colonel Bruton documented that intramuscular γ-globulin given monthly reduced the frequency and severity of the bacterial infections associated with X-linked hypogammaglobulinemia. This therapy benefits most patients with B-cell immunodeficiency manifested by serum IgG deficiency, IgG subclass deficiency, and associated functional antibody deficiency. Patients with isolated serum IgA deficiency that is not accompanied by IgG subclass or functional antibody deficiency should not receive gammaglobulin therapy. It is contraindicated in the management of isolated IgA deficiency, since several instances of anaphylaxis following γ-globulin administration were attributed to IgE antibodies reacting with trace amounts of IgA in the pooled γ-globulin. The recent development of γ-globulin for intravenous use has opened another dimension for replacement therapy, since much larger amounts of IgG can now be administered. The clinical considerations for giving γ-globulin intravenously versus intramuscularly are compared in **17.33**. Intravenous γ-globulin is best for most clinical immunodeficiencies.

LABORATORY TESTS IN PHAGOCYTIC AND COMPLEMENT DEFICIENCIES

	Screening tests	Advanced tests
Phagocytic deficiency	NBT test	Phagocytic and bactericidal activity Rebuck skin window
	IgE level	Random mobility and chemotaxis
Complement deficiency	Total (CH_{50}) activity C_3 level C_4 level	Component assays – immunochemical or functional Opsonization Inhibitor assays

Abbreviations: NBT, nitroblue tetrazolium; CH, hemolytic complement; C, complement; Ig, immunoglobulins.

17.31 Laboratory tests for phagocytic and complement deficiencies.

RECONSTITUTION THERAPIES

Transplantation therapies

The development of bone marrow transplantation has provided the opportunity to immunologically reconstitute certain patients with severe T-cell deficiencies. The use of such techniques has been very successful for the reconstitution of SCID patients when an HLA-identical sibling donor is available. Since the SCID patient's T- and B-cell deficiencies markedly suppress their graft-rejection reaction, there is little need for immunosuppression prior to or after the bone marrow transplant. The use of an HLA dissimilar bone marrow results in a fatal graft-versus-host reaction in the SCID recipient, unless mature T-lymphocytes are removed from the donor bone marrow cells by either lecithin-separation or monoclonal antibody techniques. The use of these T-cell-depleted bone marrow preparations has provided clinicians with the option of using one of the

TREATMENT PROGRAMS FOR IMMUNODEFICIENCY

Type of therapy	Immunodeficiency
Reconstitution	
Bone marrow transplant	SCID
Thymus	DiGeorge syndrome
Gene therapy[a]	ADA deficient SCID (experimental)
Replacement	
Intravenous or intramuscular γ-globulin	Hypogammaglobulinemia with deficient IgG, IgG subclass or functional antibody
Enzymes (ADA, PNP)	ADA and PNP deficiencies
Supplemental	
Cytokines	
Interferon	
Transfer factor	Chronic granulomatous disease, Chronic mucocutaneous candidiasis
Interleukins	
Anti-microbial agents	
Anti-viral	AIDS
Anti-fungal	Chronic mucocutaneous candidiasis
Anti-bacterial	Immune deficiency with severe bacterial infections

[a]Gene therapy has been used in four ADA SCID patients and is experimental.

17.32 Programs for the treatment of various immunodeficiencies.

Ig REPLACEMENT THERAPY: COMPARISON OF DELIVERY ROUTES

Intramuscular	Intravenous
Dosage limited	Higher dosages (increased benefit)
Less expensive	More expensive
More convenient	Less convenient
More painful	Less painful

17.33 γ-Globulin replacement therapy: intramuscular versus intravenous routes of delivery.

SCID patient's parents or non-HLA identical siblings as a donor. The use of fetal thymic or liver implants for therapy of SCID is no longer recommended. However, fetal thymic implants successfully reconstitute the immune systems of DiGeorge syndrome patients. The use of enzyme replacement with naturally occurring sources of ADA or PNP for these deficiencies has had limited clinical benefit, but has provided the basis for future attempts using recombinant DNA engineering technology.

Gene therapy

The identification and cloning of specific genes involved in the pathogenesis of immunodeficiency has enabled the initiation of a new area of potential reconstitution, namely by gene therapy. Currently, the leading candidate for gene therapy is SCID with ADA deficiency. The ADA gene has been cloned and inserted via a viral vector into the mature T-cells of two such patients, who are, at the time of writing, undergoing periodic infusions of these reconstituted T-cells, with apparent partial reconstitution. A further seven such patients are currently undergoing gene therapy with the ADA gene inserted into their lymphoid stem cells, which are then infused back into the patient. If successful in these initial experiments, other candidates for gene therapy will include PNP deficiency and LAD deficiency.

SUPPLEMENTAL TREATMENTS

Supplemental therapy with interferon has improved the clinical course of patients with chronic granulomatous disease. Transfer factor, another cytokine, has benefited patients with chronic mucocutaneous candidiasis. As additional cytokines, including the lymphocyte growth factors and interleukins, are better characterized, they should provide a source of more therapeutic agents for immunodeficiency diseases.

The judicious use of appropriate anti-microbial agents continues to play an important role in the management of patients with recurrent infections due to immunodeficiencies. Anti-microbials should be used in maximum dosages to reverse acute or recurrent infectious processes. In addition, prophylactic antibiotics, at times, deserve clinical trials to prevent infections.

REFERENCES

Blaese RM, Culver KW: Gene therapy for primary immunodeficiencies. *Immunodef Rev*, **3**:329–349, 1992.

Bluestone C, Stool S: *Pediatric Otolaryngology,* Vol. 1., W.B. Saunders, Philadelphia, 1983.

Bower DL, Lane HC, Fauci AS: Immunologic abnormalities – acquired immunodeficiency syndrome. *Prog Allergy*, **37**:202, 1986.

Buckley, RH: Immunodeficiency diseases. *JAMA*, **258**:2841, 1987.

de Saint-Basile C, Fisher A: X-linked immunodeficiencies: clues to genes in T- and B-cell differentiation. *Immunol Today*, **12**:456–461, 1991.

Rosen FS, Cooper MD, Wedgewood RJ: The primary immunodeficiencies. *N Engl J Med*, **311**:235, 1984.

Rubinstein A: Acquired immunodeficiency in children. *Pediatr Rev*, **10**:165, 1988.

Skoner DP, Stillwagon PK, Friedman R, Fireman P: Pediatric allergy and immunology, in Ziteleli BJ, Davis HW (eds): *Atlas of Pediatric Diagnosis,* Gower, New York, 1992.

Stiehm ER: Immunodeficiency disorders: general considerations, in Stiehm ER (ed.): *Immunologic Disorders in Infants and Children,* W.B. Saunders, Philadelphia, 1992.

Stiehm ER: New and old immunodeficiencies. *Pediatr Res*, **33**:52–58, 1993.

Waldman TA, Blaese RM, Broder S, Krakauer RS: Disorders of suppressor immunoregulatory cells in the pathogenesis of immunodeficiency and autoimmunity. *Annal Int Med.* 88:226-238, 1978.

WHO, Primary Immunodeficiency Diseases: Report of a World Health Organization Scientific Group. *Clin Immunol Immunopathol*, **40**:166, 1986.

CHAPTER 18

Drug Allergy

Leslie C. Grammer

Immunologically mediated adverse drug reactions or drug allergy and/or hypersensitivity account for 6–10% of all adverse drug effects. There are a number of specific characteristics that are generally helpful in distinguishing drug allergy from other adverse drug reactions. They tend to occur in only a small fraction of patients, are reproducible with minute amounts of the drug, can mimic other allergic reactions, and they do not resemble other known pharmacologic effects. These distinguishing characteristics are listed in **18.1**.

Many drug-hypersensitivity reactions can be classified according to the Gell and Coombs schema. **18.2** is a synopsis of the clinical manifestations and mechanism of each reaction type. Penicillin has been associated with all of them. These mechanisms are schematically depicted in **18.3**. In the Type I or anaphylactic mechanism, allergen is recognized by IgE bound by receptors to mast cells or basophils. The crosslinking of IgE by allergen results in cellular release of mediators, such as histamine, leukotrienes, and prostaglandins. The cytotoxic or Type II mechanism involves antibody recognition of cell-bound antigen; this antibody fixes complement, which causes cell damage. Antigen–antibody lattices or complexes are formed in the Type III or Arthus mechanism; complement is fixed and some components of the complement cascade act as chemoattractants to cells that mediate inflammation. Sensitized T-lymphocytes recognize antigen presented by macrophages in the delayed hypersensitivity or Type IV mechanism. This recognition results in T-cell activation and release of cytokines, that then mediate inflammation, primarily by recruitment of non–sensitized cells. In addition to those drug hypersensitivities that are classifiable

CHARACTERISTICS OF DRUG ALLERGY/HYPERSENSITIVITY

1. Occur in only a small fraction of patients.
2. Can be reproduced by very small dose of drug.
3. Will subside within several days to weeks following discontinuation of drug.
4. Manifestations differ from any known pharmacologic ones.
5. Can mimic other known allergic reactions, including serum sickness and anaphylaxis.
6. Hypersensitivity can manifest as pulmonary infiltrates with eosinophilia, drug fever, and lupus syndrome.
7. Onset is usually after several days, but within several months of administration of a drug.
8. Immunologic mechanism is demonstrable or the putative mechanism.

18.1 Chief characteristics of drug allergy and hypersensitivity.

EXAMPLES OF DRUG ALLERGY DUE TO PENICILLIN CATEGORIZED ACCORDING TO GELL AND COOMBS REACTION TYPE

Clinical manifestations	Gell and Coombs reaction type	Mechanism
Anaphylaxis, bronchospasm, urticaria, angioedema	I. anaphylactic	Antigen crosslinks IgE on cell surface, resulting in mediator release
Hemolytic anemia due to binding of drug to red cells	II. cytotoxic	Cell-bound antigen reacts with antibody thus activating complement, and producing cell injury
Serum sickness	III. Arthus phenomenon	Formation of antigen–antibody complexes that activate complement, resulting in recruitment of macrophages and leukocytes that cause tissue damage
Contact dermatitis with topical application	IV. delayed hypersensitivity	Sensitized T-lymphocytes release cytokines that attract other cells which cause tissue inflammation

18.2 Penicillin has been associated with all four of the Gell and Coombs reaction types. The table lists the clinical manifestations and underlying mechanisms for each of these reactions.

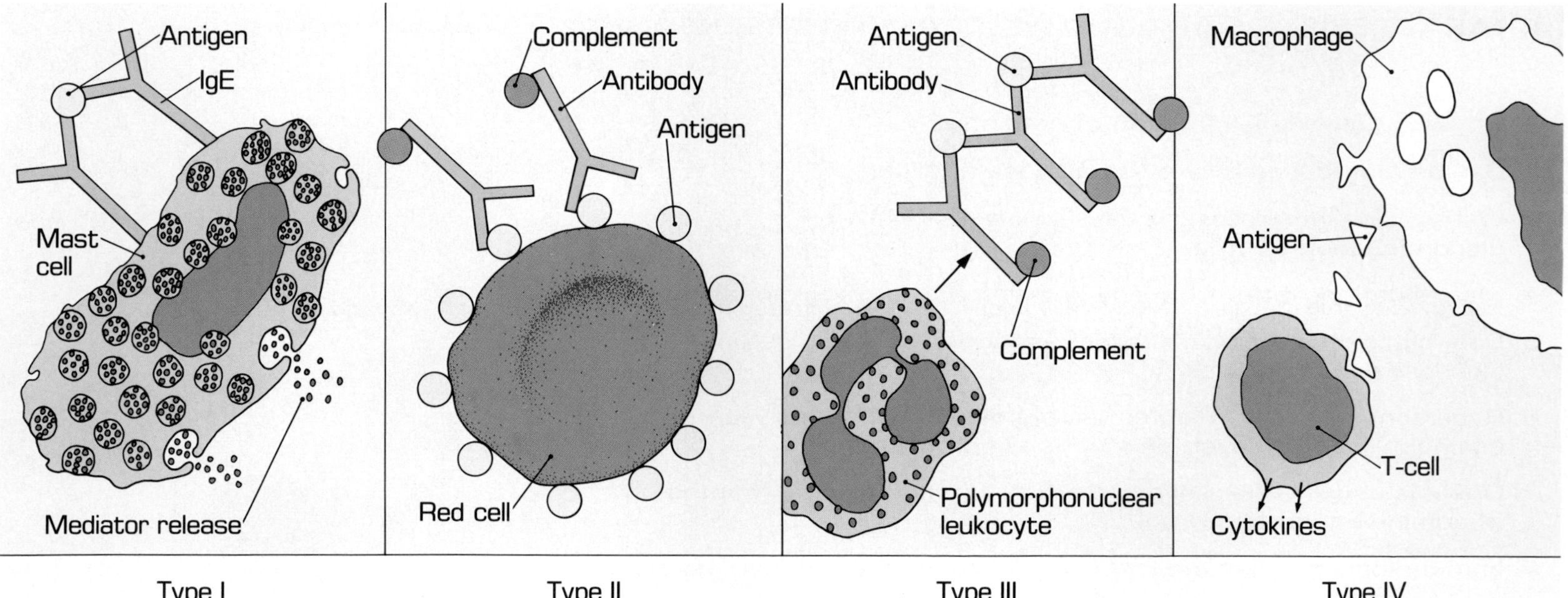

18.3 Schematic representation of the mechanisms underlying the four Gell and Coombs reaction types. The Type I or anaphylactic reaction arises when a drug allergen crosslinks IgE molecules on the surfaces of mast cells, precipitating the release of inflammatory mediators. The Type II or cytotoxic reaction occurs when antibodies bind to cell-bound antigens. The antibodies fix complement which causes cell lysis. The Type III reaction or Arthus phenomenon involves formation of antigen–antibody complexes that fix complement, several components of which are chemoattractants to cells that cause inflammation. The Type IV reaction, delayed hypersensitivity, occurs when sensitized T-cells recognize antigens presented by macrophages. This process activates the T-cells resulting in the release of cytokines.

according to the Gell and Coombs schema, there are other adverse reactions which appear to be immunologically mediated that do not fit into this schema. Examples include pulmonary infiltrates from nitrofurantoin and interstitial nephritis from methicillin. Further, there are also adverse drug reactions that closely mimic the manifestations of immunologically mediated reactions, but no immunologic mechanism can be demonstrated. An example would be the anaphylactoid reactions to opiates that have been described in certain cases.

EPIDEMIOLOGY

The frequency of adverse drug reactions is not precisely known. In cross-sectional studies of hospitalized patients on medical floors, the estimates of prevalence of adverse drug reactions range from 6–15%. The estimated prevalence for other hospital services, such as psychiatry, surgery, pediatrics, and obstetrics–gynecology, is generally lower, ranging from 1–6%. Of all adverse reactions, approximately 6–10% are believed to represent drug hypersensitivity. It has been estimated that the risk of allergic reaction is about 1–3% for most drugs. In practice, penicillins and sulfonamides account for a significant proportion of drug allergy. Although apparently not immunologically mediated, aspirin and other non-steroidal anti-inflammatory drugs are also frequent causes of adverse reactions that mimic drug allergy: urticaria, angioedema, and bronchospasm. A list of drugs that have been implicated frequently in allergic drug reactions is given in **18.4**.

IMMUNOGENICITY OF DRUGS

Molecular weight of 3–5 kdaltons (kDa) and multivalency are generally required for a compound to be immunogenic. Therefore, with the exception of a few protein drugs, such as insulin or streptokinase, very few drugs are complete antigens. The vast majority of drugs are organic chemicals with molecular weights less than 1 kDa, which function as a univalent ligand. Based on the reports of Landsteiner, it is generally acknowledged that low molecular weight drugs (haptens) are not immunogenic unless they are bound to a high molecular weight (>5 kDa) substance, usually a protein (carrier).

Beta–lactam antibiotics are reactive with proteins and can directly haptenize carrier proteins. Most drugs, however, are not chemically reactive with proteins. It is probable that the haptens from most drugs are reactive metabolites of the parent compound that then bind to carrier proteins; certainly, this is the case with metabolites of penicillin. Studies of human IgE to sulfonamides

DRUGS FREQUENTLY IMPLICATED IN ALLERGIC REACTIONS	
Penicillins and cephalosporins	Antihypertensive agents (hydralazine, methyldopa)
Sulfonamides	Antiarrhythmia agents (quinidine, procainamide)
Antituberculous drugs (isoniazid, rifampin)	Antisera and vaccines
Nitrofurans	Organ extracts (ACTH, insulin)
Antimalarials	Heavy metals (gold)
Griseofulvin	Allopurinol
Sedative-hypnotics (barbiturates)	Penicillamine
Anticonvulsants (hydantoin, tegretol)	Enzymes (chymopapain, L-asparaginase, streptokinase)
Phenolphthalein	Antipsychotic tranquilizers (phenothiazines, tricyclics)

18.4 Listing of the drug groups most frequently implicated in allergic drug reactions. (Adapated with permission from De Swarte, 1993.)

have demonstrated the N[4]-sulfonamidoyl determinant to be the major sulfonamide haptenic determinant. For most other allergenic drugs, the formation of reactive metabolites and their conjugation with carrier proteins is somewhat speculative. In the absence of the relevant drug haptens, immunologic assessment is, of course, impossible.

CLINICAL PRESENTATION

The clinical presentations of drug allergy can take many different forms and they are generally not pathognomonic for drug hypersensitivity. That is, similar clinical presentations can be the result of exposure to other allergens or they can be associated with other non-immunologic diseases. Dermatologic manifestations are the most common manifestation of drug allergy. However, many other organ systems can be involved, either alone or in combination, in a patient with drug allergy. It should be appreciated that in many reactions which are believed to be drug allergy, a definitive immunologic mechanism has not been established. A list of the clinical presentations of drug allergy is given in **18.5**.

Anaphylaxis, a potentially life-threatening condition, can include any or all of the following: hypotension, bronchospasm, laryngeal edema, angioedema, or generalized urticaria. If the antigen has been ingested, gastrointestinal symptoms, such as nausea, vomiting, diarrhea, or cramping, may be prominent. Symptoms usually begin within 30 minutes of drug exposure and generally subside within 24 hours. Penicillin is one drug for which frequency of anaphylactic reactions is reported; the estimates range from 0.7–10%. Other drugs that have been implicated frequently in anaphylactic symptoms include radiocontrast material, plasma expanders, and non-steroidal anti-inflammatory drugs, such as aspirin. None of these agents is thought to cause anaphylaxis via an IgE mediated mechanism.

Serum-sickness-like reactions usually occur 1–3 weeks after drug exposure. Because of this latent period, it is imperative to question a patient about any drugs that may have been ingested in the previous month. The symptoms may include fever, urticaria and/or angioedema, arthralgias, joint effusion, lymphadenopathy, and occasionally neuritis (brachial plexus). Renal disease is usually not detected in humans, although it is prominent in animal models. Symptoms may last from several days to several weeks. Other

CLINICAL PRESENTATIONS OF DRUG ALLERGY

Single organ system involvement

Dermatologic manifestations[a]

Respiratory or pulmonary manifestations
- Asthma
- Acute infiltrative reactions (probably allergic)
- Hypersensitivity pneumonia
- Pulmonary infiltrates with eosinophilia
- Nitrofurantoin reactions

Hematologic manifestations
- Eosinophilia
- Drug-induced immune cytopenias:
  - Thrombocytopenia
  - Hemolytic anemia
  - Agranulocytosis

Hepatic manifestations
- Cholestasis
- Hepatocellular damage

Renal manifestations
- Glomerulonephritis
- Nephrotic syndrome
- Acute interstitial nephritis

Multisystem involvement
- Anaphylaxis
- Serum sickness
- Drug fever
- Drug-induced lupus erythematosus
- Vasculitis

[a]See Figure 18.6.

18.5 Listing of the various single organ and multi-system manifestations of drug allergy. (Adapated with permission from De Swarte, 1993.)

multi-systemic clinical presentations of drug allergy include drug fever, drug-induced lupus erythematosus, and vasculitis.

Of all the organ systems affected by drug allergies, the most frequently involved is the skin (**18.6**). While exanthematous eruptions are the most common manifestations, drug allergy can result in almost any type of cutaneous eruption. Other common dermatologic manifestations include urticaria, angioedema, and, from topical medications, contact dermatitis. Less common presentations include fixed drug eruptions, from such medications as phenolphthalein, photosensitivity, from drugs such as doxycycline, and erythema multiforme from penicillins and sulfa drugs. On rare occasions, dermatologic manifestations occur that are severe enough to be potentially life-threatening. These include exfoliative dermatitis and Stevens–Johnson syndrome, a fulminant variant of erythema multiforme with cutaneous and mucous membrane involvement. Uncommon dermatologic presentations of drug allergy include purpura, erythema nodosum, and Lyell's syndrome. Various other dermatologic manifestations are shown in **18.7–18.10**.

Though the skin is most commonly involved, drug allergy can involve other single organ systems. Examples would be the pulmonary reactions induced by nitrofurantoin, thrombocytopenia induced by sulfonamides, hepatitis induced by halothane, and acute interstitial nephritis induced by methicillin.

DIAGNOSIS

The diagnosis of drug allergy may be fairly straightforward sometimes, but this is not usually the case. As indicated in **18.11**, the most important diagnostic tool is the history. First, it is imperative to have a complete and accurate list of all the drugs taken by the patient over the previous month. If a physician does not specifically ask about such non-prescription drugs as aspirin, the patient may not volunteer this information. Second, it is necessary to study the patient's manifestations, to see if they are consistent with known drug allergies. As discussed above, it is important to recognize the protean nature of drug allergy and that it is not confined to 'rashes'. Finally, it is important to consider the temporal relationship between exposure(s) to the drug and onset of clinical manifestations. If a patient is receiving a drug for the first time, allergy generally does not occur until several days have passed. However, it usually occurs within several months. That is, if a patient has been

DERMATOLOGIC PRESENTATIONS OF DRUG ALLERGY

Most common	Less common	Uncommon
Exanthematous eruptions	Fixed drug eruptions	Purpura
Urticaria	Erythema multiforme:	Lyell's syndrome
Angioedema	Steven–Johnson syndrome	Erythema nodosum
Contact dermatitis	Exfoliative dermatitis	
	Photosensitivity	

18.6 Dermatologic manifestations are the most common symptoms of allergic drug reactions. The table lists these presentations in order of frequency. (Adapted with permission from De Swarte, 1993.)

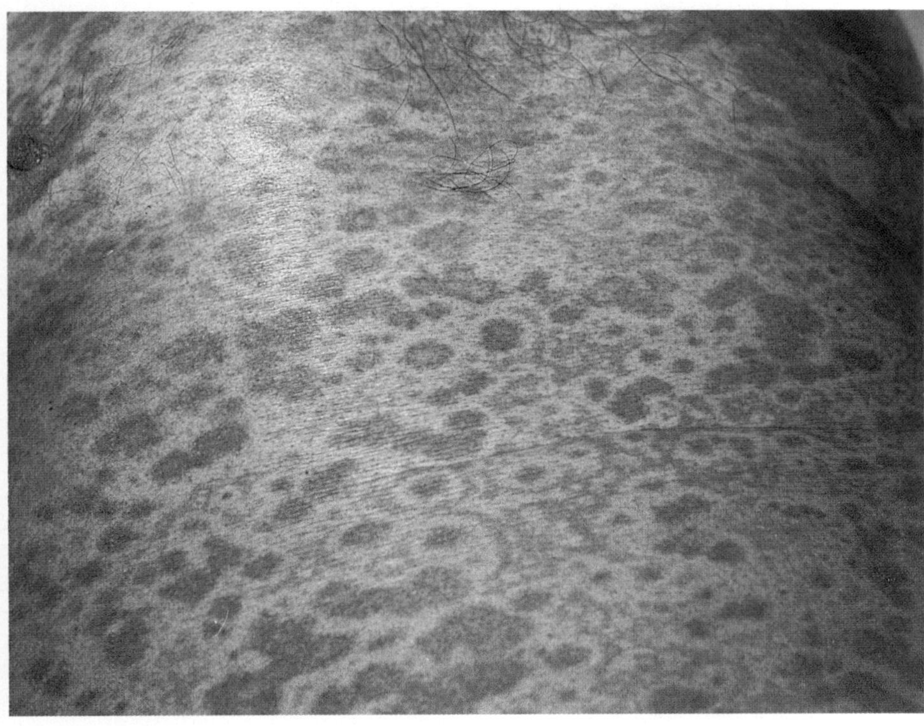

18.7 Drug eruption caused, in this case, by allergy to ampicillin. These lesions are usually pruritic and confluent and tend to show widespread distribution. (Reprinted with permission from duVivier, 1986.)

receiving a drug on a daily basis for over a year, that drug is not likely to be the cause of drug allergy. If a patient has received a drug in the past, sensitization may already have occurred and drug allergy may appear immediately upon re-administration.

There are numerous *in vitro* tests that have been utilized in the investigation of drug allergy. Among these are histamine-release, radioallergosorbent test, immunoassays for specific IgG or IgM, lymphocyte reactivity as measured by lymphokine production or lymphocyte transformation, and agglutination and lysis of blood cells in the presence of the suspected drug and the patient's serum. With the exception of the last, which may be clinically useful in the evaluation of immunologically mediated cytopenias, *in vitro* tests are rarely of clinical value, even though they may be valuable research tools.

In vivo testing for drug allergy, that is, cutaneous testing or provocative test dosing, may be clinically indicated in selected cases. It must be recognized that a serious limitation of cutaneous testing is the dearth of appropriate multivalent test reagents or drug metabolites. This is primarily because the antigenic determinants which result in drug allergy are unknown for most drugs. If a patient has a history compatible with drug allergy, cutaneous tests are negative, and there is a clear indication for a drug reaction, provocative test dosing may be considered. In this method of testing, the initial dose is one that would not cause a serious reaction. Subsequent doses represent incremental increases. An example is given in **18.12**. At each dose increment, it is imperative to ascertain whether or not any symptoms have occurred before proceeding to the subsequent dose.

It is important to appreciate the difference between provocative test dosing and desensitization. The former describes the incremental administration of a drug to which a patient is probably not allergic, even though the history is somewhat suggestive of an allergic reaction. On the other hand, if true IgE-mediated allergy exists, the incremental administration of the drug is termed desensitization, as

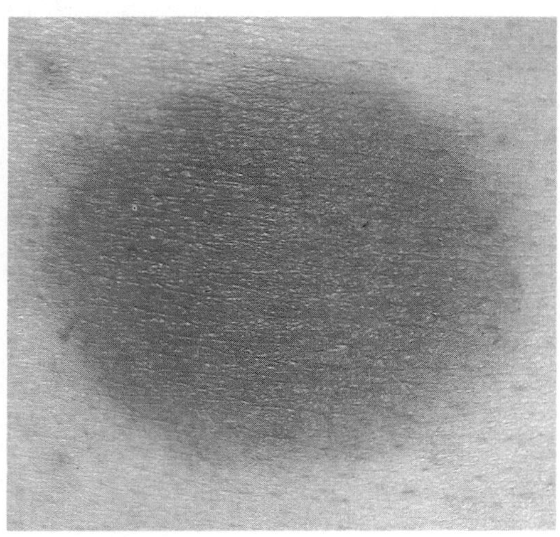

18.8 Single, well-demarcated, red-dish lesion of a fixed drug eruption. The chief feature of such reactions is that they occur in the same site each time the particular allergen is ingested. Lesions develop within hours of ingestion, and subside rapidly, often leaving the skin characteristically hyperpigmented. (Reproduced with permission from duVivier, 1986.)

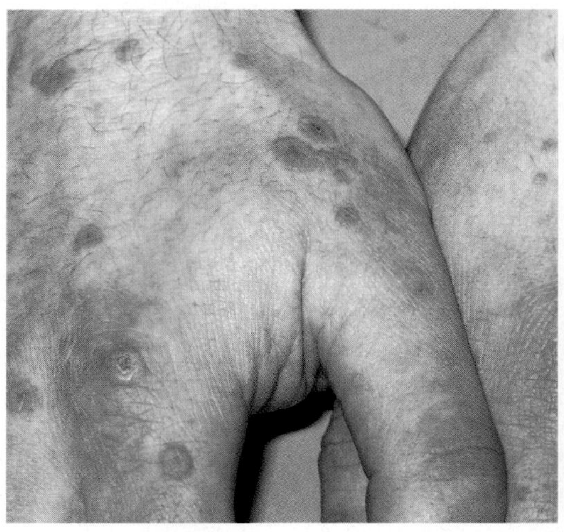

18.9 Iris-type lesions of erythema multiforme. These lesions typically occur on the extremities, particularly the hands, forearms and feet. They can be precipitated by exposure to a number of agents, including sulfonamides, barbiturates and phenylbutazone. (Reproduced with permission from duVivier, 1986.)

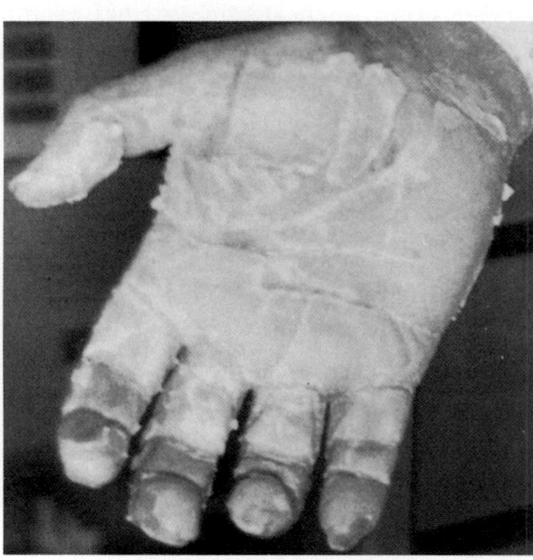

18.10 Exfoliative dermatitis of the hand in a patient with Stevens–Johnson syndrome secondary to administration of allopurinol.

it converts the patient from a state of sensitivity to non-sensitivity to the drug. The mechanism is not entirely clear, but it may be the result of graded antigen-binding of specific IgE or of controlled mediator release. An example of a desensitization schedule for insulin is given in **18.13**. In a sense, desensitization is a treatment for drug allergy; however, since it is so closely associated with cutaneous testing and

DIAGNOSIS OF DRUG ALLERGY

1. **History**
   Careful, complete drug history.
   Clinical manifestations consistent with drug allergy: a temporal relationship between drug exposure and onset of clinical manifestations consistent with drug allergy.
2. ***In vitro* testing**
   Research tool.
   Generally of no clinical value.
3. ***In vivo* testing**
   Clinically indicated in selected cases.
   Cutaneous testing.
   Provocative test dosing.

18.11 Guidelines for the diagnosis of drug allergy.

EXAMPLE OF PROVOCATIVE TEST DOSE SCHEDULE

Route	Dilution
Prick test	1:1000[a]
Intradermal test	1:10,000
Intradermal test	1:1000
Intradermal test[b]	1:100
Intradermal test[b]	1:10
Intradermal test[b]	Full strength

[a]If the previous reaction was severe, a more dilute solution can be used.
[b]As more concentrated solutions can be irritating, the subcutaneous route may be the most appropriate.

18.12 Typical protocol for provocative test dosing. Following each dose increment, it is necessary to assess the patient and determine whether or not any symptoms of allergy have developed. (Adapted with permission from De Swarte, 19893.)

INSULIN DESENSITIZATION SCHEDULE

Day	Time	Insulin (units)	Method
1	8 am	10^{-5}	Intradermal
	12 noon	10^{-4}	Intradermal
	4 pm	10^{-3}	Subcutaneous
2	8 am	10^{-2}	Subcutaneous
	12 noon	10^{-1}	Subcutaneous
	4 pm	1.0	Subcutaneous
3	8 am	2.0	Subcutaneous
	12 noon	4.0	Subcutaneous
	4 pm	8.0	Subcutaneous
4	8 am	12.0	Subcutaneous
	12 noon	16.0	Subcutaneous
5	8 am	20.0	Subcutaneous
6	8 am	25.0	Subcutaneous

18.13 Typical desensitization schedule for insulin-allergic patients. Though the protocols may be similar, it is important to appreciate the difference between provocative test dosing and densitization. The former is a diagnostic technique; the latter, a treatment.

test dosing, it is considered with those topics which are diagnostic. **18.14** indicates agents for which desensitization can be carried out.

Prior to cutaneous testing, test dosing, or desensitization, it is important that there be a clear indication for the drug, that the risks and benefits of drug administration be explained to the patient, and that the medical records document indications, informed consent, and administration schedule.

TREATMENT AND PREVENTION

If drug allergy is suspected, it is important to discontinue the offending drug. Patients often receive multiple drugs and it may be impossible to determine which is the offending agent. It is generally appropriate to discontinue all non-essential drugs and to replace any necessary drugs with non-cross-reacting substitutes. In some very rare circumstances, it may be necessary to continue administering a drug to which the patient is allergic. An example would be continuing sulfa for an AIDS patient with toxoplasmosis brain abscess and sulfa allergy. This would be done only with informed consent and careful consideration of the risks and benefits. Corticosteroids may be required to allow continued administration of an essential, non-replaceable drug to which a patient is allergic.

Treatment of cutaneous eruptions is dependent upon the severity. If the cutaneous manifestations are mild, antihistamines alone generally suffice. However, if the cutaneous eruption is severe or progressive, prednisone, 60 mg daily or b.i.d., is administered until there is improvement; on improvement, prednisone dosage should be tapered rapidly.

Treatment of anaphylaxis due to drug allergy is comparable to that of anaphylaxis from other causes (*see* Chapter 4). The initial treatment for adults consists of subcutaneous or intramuscular 1:1000 epinephrine, 0.3 ml; this may be repeated twice at 15 minute intervals. Depending upon the manifestations of anaphylaxis, additional therapy may be indicated. For example, patients who are hypotensive may require fluids and vasopressors; patients who have bronchospasm may require an aerosolized B_2 agonist and/or intravenous aminophylline 6 mg/kg over 30 minutes. Those who have laryngeal edema may require tracheostomy.

If a patient has a truly essential indication for radiocontrast media (RCM), pretreatment has been useful in reducing the number of repeat anaphylactoid reactions. Low osmolality contrast material also reduces the risk. Pretreatment medications include prednisone 50 mg at 13 hours, 7 hours, and 1 hour before RCM administration; diphenhydramine hydrochloride 50 mg 1 hour before; and albuterol 4 mg at 1 hour before. Albuterol may be contraindicated if the patient has coronary artery disease or an arrhythmia. It is, of course, necessary to document the risks and benefits of the RCM administration and the patient's informed consent.

Prevention of drug allergy is obviously a desirable goal. Several important prevention guidelines are listed in **18.15**. First, there is

AGENTS FOR WHICH DRUG DESENSITIZATION PROTOCOLS ARE PUBLISHED

1. Insulin
2. Penicillin
3. Heterologous antisera
4. Tetanus toxoid
5. Sulfa
6. Furosemide
7. Measles mumps rubella (MMR) vaccine

18.14 Agents for which drug desensitization protocols are published. (Patterson *et al.*, 1994)

PREVENTION OF DRUG ALLERGY

1. Prescribe drugs only if essential.
2. Prior to prescribing drugs, obtain a thorough, careful drug history; drugs to which patients have had reactions, or cross-reacting drugs should not be prescribed.
3. Perform cutaneous tests prior to administration of foreign antisera.
4. If an allergic drug reaction occurs, fully inform the patient Medical records should reflect the incident.
5. Report adverse drug reactions, such as drug allergy, to the FDA; this is especially important for newly introduced drugs.

18.15 Key measures for the prevention of drug allergy.

the obvious principle of prescribing drugs only when clearly indicated. Next, patients should be carefully questioned about previous drug reactions so that they are not given drugs to which they may be allergic. There are some agents, such as foreign antisera, to which many are allergic; cutaneous testing must be performed prior to administration. If a patient experiences an allergic reaction, the patient or responsible person should be informed so that he or she can avoid the drug in the future. The medical record should reflect this information and, in selected patients, Medic-Alert tags may be appropriate.

Finally, adverse reactions such as drug allergies should be reported to the relevant agency, especially in the case of drugs that are relatively new. In the US, physicians are urged to call or write to pharmaceutical manufacturers and the Office of Epidemiology (HFN-700), Center for Drug Evaluation and Research, FDA, Parklawn Building, Rockville, MD 20857, USA. FDA reporting forms (Form 1639a) can be obtained from the FDA, and are also available in *FDA Drug Bulletin*, *AMA Drug Evaluations*, and *Physician's Desk Reference*. In emergent situations, the FDA may be contacted by calling 301/443-4980.

In the UK, doctors are advised to report adverse reactions to any therapeutic agent to the CSM. This may be done by using yellow prepaid cards—bound in the *British National Formulary*—or by dialing 100 and asking for CSM Freephone. All suspected reactions to newer products should be reported, as well as serious suspected reactions and delayed effects.

ACKNOWLEDGEMENT

I am appreciative of the review and comments of Drs Richard DeSwarte and Roy Patterson.

REFERENCES

DeSwarte RD: Drug allergy, in Patterson R, Grammer L, Greenberger P, Zeiss CR (eds): *Allergic Diseases, Diagnosis and Management*, J.B. Lippincott, 1993.

du Vivier A: Drug and toxic eruptions of the skin, *Atlas of Clinical Dermatology*, W.B. Saunders, Chapter 14, 1986.

Patterson R, DeSwarte RD, Greenberger PA, Grammer LC: Drug allergy and protocols for management of drug allergies. *NER Allergy Proc*, **15**:239, 1994.

Index